Handbook of Acquired Communication Disorders in Childhood

Handbook of Acquired Communication Disorders in Childhood

Bruce E. Murdoch, PhD, DSc
Center for Neurogenic Communication Disorders Research
The University of Queensland, Australia

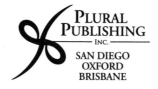

PLURAL
PUBLISHING
INC.
SAN DIEGO
OXFORD
BRISBANE

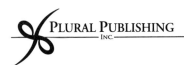

5521 Ruffin Road
San Diego, CA 92123

e-mail: info@pluralpublishing.com
Web site: http://www.pluralpublishing.com

49 Bath Street
Abingdon, Oxfordshire OX14 1EA
United Kingdom

FSC
Mixed Sources
Product group from well-managed
forests and other controlled sources

Cert no. SW-COC-002283
www.fsc.org
© 1996 Forest Stewardship Council

Typeset in 11/13 Palatino Book by Flanagan's Publishing Services, Inc.
Printed in the United States of America by McNaughton and Gunn

Library of Congress Cataloging-in-Publication Data

Murdoch, B. E., 1950-
    Handbook of acquired communication disorders in childhood / Bruce E. Murdoch.
        p. ; cm.
    Includes bibliographical references and index.
    ISBN-13: 978-1-59756-054-2 (alk. paper)
    ISBN-10: 1-59756-054-5 (alk. paper)
    1. Communicative disorders in children. 2. Communicative disorders in children $x
Treatment. I. Title.
    [DNLM: 1. Language Disorders—complications. 2. Child. WL 340.2]

RJ496.C67M87 2010
618.92'855—dc22

                                                                    2010052046

Contents

Preface

Currently, few resources are available to pediatric clinicians to guide their management of children with acquired speech and language disorders. In particular, although a plethora of excellent texts addressing brain-based communication impairments in adults are available, until now no single text has provided a comprehensive coverage of the major neurologic conditions associated with the occurrence of acquired speech and language disorders in children.

In writing this text my aim was to provide a comprehensive coverage of the neuropathologic basis, neurology, clinical symptomatology, prognosis, assessment, and treatment of acquired language and motor speech disorders resulting from a variety of conditions that cause damage to the brain in childhood. To this end, in addition to the more commonly recognized acquired child-hood speech and language disorders, such as those associated with traumatic brain injury, cerebrovascular accidents, and brain tumor, the current book also includes coverage of less well-recognized communicative impairments associated with neurologic disorders caused by cerebral anoxia, inborn errors of metabolism, neural tube defects, infections, radiation induced brain damage, and convulsive disorders.

It is the author's hope that this book not only will provide pediatric clinicians with a valuable resource to aid determination of appropriate treatment strategies, but also will serve as a stimulus for further research by future generations of neuroscientists, speech-language pathologists, and so forth to further our understanding of these disorders and increase our ability to facilitate their rehabilitation.

Bruce E. Murdoch

This book is dedicated to the numerous children and adolescents with a variety of neurologic conditions who have willingly served as participants in the research that forms the basis of this volume. Their smiles freely given and their determination to succeed in the face of adversity have provided the inspiration for the writing of this text.

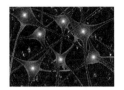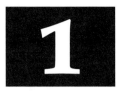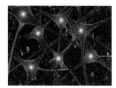

1

Introduction to Acquired Speech and Language Disorders in Childhood

Introduction

Speech and language disorders occurring in childhood can be divided into acquired disorders and developmental disorders. Acquired speech-language disorders are disturbances in speech-language function that result from some form of cerebral insult after language acquisition has already commenced (Hécaen, 1976). The cerebral insult, in turn, can result from a variety of etiologies, including head trauma, brain tumors, cerebrovascular accidents, infections, convulsive disorders (intractable epilepsy), and electroencephalographic abnormalities (Miller, Campbell, Chapman, & Weismer, 1984). Typically, these children have commenced learning language normally and were acquiring developmental milestones at an appropriate rate prior to injury.

Developmental disorders of speech and language, on the other hand, are those that begin prior to the emergence of language (i.e., between birth and one year of age). Consequently children with developmental speech and language disorders have never developed speech and language abilities normally. Although it is usually presumed that primary developmental speech and language disorders are caused by dysfunctioning of the central nervous system, in most cases they have an idiopathic origin (i.e., the cause is unknown). Developmental speech and language disorders, however, can occur secondary to conditions such as peripheral hearing loss, mental retardation, cerebral palsy, child autism, birth trauma, and environmental deprivation.

Of the two types of childhood speech and language disorders, the acquired variety most closely resembles the acquired adult communicative disorders and is the focus of this book. Despite this, the application of adult criteria and classifications to acquired speech and language disorders in children is problematic. It is important to remember that children, depending on age, are either beginning to develop or are still developing speech and language concurrent with damage to the central nervous system. Consequently interactions between the acquired and developmental mechanisms of motor speech and language disorders in children may complicate the use and application of adult classifications in the pediatric population (Murdoch & Hudson-Tennent, 1994). Currently, the impact of a congenital or acquired central nervous system lesion on the developmental continuum of speech and language is unknown.

The difference in potential for the central nervous system to recover from, or compensate for, brain injury exhibited by children and adults is also a significant factor that limits the application of adult criteria to childhood speech and language disorders. Specifically, the potential of the central nervous system to recover from brain trauma sustained at a young age has often been reported as favorable relative to the recovery expected following brain damage in adults. It also is possible that the relationship between site of lesion and type of speech and/or language impairment determined in adults may not be readily applicable to the developing central nervous system.

Although for many decades attempts were made to categorize acquired childhood aphasia using adult aphasia classification systems (e.g., Goodglass & Kaplan, 1972), these attempts largely failed. The mere intention to compare language impairment in children to that exhibited by adults violates the nature of the developing brain and does not take the most essential variables and features that determine the latter into account. The developing brain displays progressive and regressive events dur-

ing which axons, dendrites, synapses, and neurons show exuberant growth and major loss leading to a remodeling of neural circuitry ("wiring"). This time period for remodeling is hypothesized to be a time during which environmental factors can have a major impact on cortical organization. Different neural systems and associated capabilities are affected by environmental input at highly variable time periods, supporting the idea that they develop along distinct time courses (Maurer & Lewis, 1998). Hence, differences in the rate of differentiation and degree of specialization are apparent within language as well. For example, aspects of semantic and grammatical processing differ markedly in the degree to which they depend on language input. Specifically, grammatical processing appears more vulnerable to delays in language experience compared to semantics (Neville & Bavelier, 2000). However, it is not only developmental plasticity that distinguishes an infant's brain but it is also the form of plasticity these brains exhibit in response to brain damage in the course of recovery that is significantly higher in the pediatric population.

In particular, there appear to be two major differences between acquired aphasia in children and aphasia in adults. First, the recovery process is described as being more rapid and complete in children (Lenneberg, 1967). Second, in the majority of cases, acquired childhood aphasia is predominantly nonfluent, its major features being mutism and lack of spontaneity of speech (Alajouanine & Lhermitte, 1965; Fletcher & Taylor, 1984; Hécaen, 1976). Furthermore, with some rare exceptions, the acquired aphasia in children does not appear to fall into clear-cut syndromes evocative of the well-known aphasia subtypes described in adults (Chapter 2).

As in the case of acquired aphasia, the application of adult systems to the classification of acquired childhood dysarthria is problematic. The classification system devised by Darley, Aronson, and Brown (1975) is currently the most commonly used system for the classification of adult dysarthria. Their system, also known as the Mayo Clinic Classification System, identifies six different types of dysarthria (flaccid, spastic, hypokinetic, hyperkinetic, ataxic, mixed dysarthria) that presumably reflect underlying pathophysiology (i.e., spasticity, weakness, etc.) and correlates with the site-of-lesion in the nervous system. Whether or not this same system can be used for the developing central nervous system, however, is still in debate. Some studies have reported an inconclusive relationship between site and features of pediatric dysarthria (Bak, van Dongen, & Arts, 1983). Investigations that have attempted to compare the features of pediatric dysarthria following damage to the cerebellum and brainstem with those of adult dysarthric speakers with damage to the same areas have also been equivocal. Comparisons between the deviant speech characteristics identified for adults and children with acquired dysarthrias have revealed some overlap, but differences also have been evident that require further investigation (Murdoch & Hudson-Tennent, 1994). Unfortunately, at present there is a paucity of literature available that provides a clear description of the nature and course of specific forms of childhood dysarthria, and no neurobehavioral classification system equivalent to the Mayo Clinic classification currently exists for acquired childhood dysarthria. Consequently many clinicians resort to use of the Mayo Classification system to classify their child clients with dysarthria. The problems associated with applying adult classification to acquired childhood dysarthria are discussed more fully in Chapter 11.

Definitions

The three basic neurologic processes involved in the efficient execution of speech production are presented in Table 1–1.

Impairment of each of these three processes results in a distinctive communication disorder. Impairment in the

Table 1–1. Basic Processes Involved in Speech Production

1. A concept of the speech output has to be formed and symbolically formulated for expression as speech—disruption at this level is associated with APHASIA

2. The symbolically formulated concept of speech output has to be externalized as speech through the concurrent motor functions of respiration, phonation, resonance, articulation, and prosody—disruption at this level is associated with DYSARTHRIA

3. Prior to externalization as speech, a program has to be developed which determines the sequence of muscle contractions required to produce individual sounds and words that comprise the intended speech output—disruption at this level leads to APRAXIA OF SPEECH

first process involving the organization of concepts and their symbolic formulation and expression is caused by pathologic processes that damage the cerebral hemisphere that contains the speech-language centers, thereby leading to aphasia. Aphasia has been defined as the loss or impairment of language function caused by brain damage. It is an impairment, due to brain injury, of the capacity to interpret and formulate language symbols. Aphasia is a multimodality disorder (i.e., it manifests in difficulties in speaking, reading, and writing) and involves a reduction in the capacity to decode (interpret) and encode (formulate) meaningful linguistic elements (i.e., words [morphemes] and larger syntactical units such as sentences). The aphasic patient is impaired in the comprehension, formulation, and expression of language although the relative amount of loss in each of these areas varies between one type of aphasia and another (see Chapter 2). All aphasic patients however, do show some loss in all three of these areas.

Impairment in the second process involving the motor production of speech is associated with dysarthria, a group of speech disorders resulting from interference with any of the basic motor processes involved in speech production (a more complete definition of dysarthria is given in Chapter 11). Damage located at a number of different sites in the nervous system including the cerebrum, brainstem, or cerebellum can be associated with dysarthria, in each case a different type of dysarthria resulting (see Chapter 11).

Impairment of the third process involving the programming of motor actions involved in speech production is caused by damage to those circuits located in the cerebrum devoted to the selection and sequencing of sensorimotor programs that determine the sequence of muscle contractions required to produce speech. Such impairment leads to a communication disorder called apraxia of speech (verbal apraxia). Apraxia of speech is, therefore, a "phonetic-motoric disorder of speech production caused by inefficiencies in the translation of well-formed and filled phonological frames into previously learned kinematic information used for carrying out intended movements" (McNeil, Robin, & Schmidt, 2008, p. 264). The condition manifests primarily as errors in the articulation of speech and secondarily by what are thought by many researchers to be compensatory alterations of prosody (e.g., pauses, slow rate, equalization of stress). It is a disorder in which the individual has difficulty speaking because of a cerebral lesion that prevents executing voluntarily and on command the complex sequence of muscle contractions involved in speaking, although the muscles of the speech mechanism are neither paralyzed nor weak. The clinical features and neurologic basis of apraxia of speech are described in detail in Chapter 11.

Whereas aphasia is considered to be a language disorder, dysarthria and apraxia of speech are motor speech disorders involving disruption of the motor control of speech. Although each of these three disorders is distinctive, it should be remembered that they can occur in combination and consequently a neurologically disordered patient may exhibit the characteristics of more than one of these disorders. Many aphasic patients, for instance, may exhibit some apraxic elements and also some type of dysarthria.

Neuropathologic Substrate of Acquired Childhood Speech and Language Disorders

Any type of neuropathology capable of producing structural alterations in an appropriate portion of the brain, whether that be the cerebral cortex, subcortical structures, brainstem, or cerebellum, is capable of producing a communication deficit in the form of either a speech or language disorder or both. Widely diverse disease processes affecting particular brain structures may produce similar abnormalities in brain function. Consequently, it is the neuroanatomic location of the brain damage rather than the causative agent that largely determines the nature of the communicative deficit. The specific causative disease, however, can usually be identified by certain characteristics of the patient's history, the specific pattern of neurologic dysfunction, and by appropriate laboratory and/or clinical examinations.

Although acquired childhood speech and language disorders can be caused by a similar range of disorders of the nervous system as their adult equivalents, the relative importance of each of the different causes to the occurrence of language disturbances in children differs from the situation seen in adults. The major acquired disorders of the nervous system that produce speech and/or language impairments in children include traumatic brain injury (TBI), cerebrovascular disease, brain tumors, infections, and convulsive disorder. The present chapter provides a brief introduction to each of these conditions. Further details together with a comprehensive description of the specific speech and language impairments associated with each of these disorders of the nervous system are provided in subsequent chapters of this book.

Traumatic Brain Injury (TBI)

In the majority of cases of acquired childhood speech and language disorders reported in the literature the cause is TBI resulting from head injury. Head injuries can be divided into two major types: closed-head injuries and open-head injuries. In a closed-head injury the covering of the brain remains intact even though the skull may be fractured. An open-head injury differs from a closed-head injury in that the brain or meninges are exposed. By far the majority of traumatic head injuries in both children and adults in civilian life are closed-head injuries.

Damage to the brain following TBI may be either focal, multifocal, or diffuse in nature. In general, closed-head injuries tend to produce more diffuse pathology whereas open-head injuries are associated with more focal pathology. Brain contusions (bruises), lacerations, and hemorrhages can be caused at the time of head injury from either the direct trauma at the site of impact on the skull, acceleration of the brain against the bony shelves of the skull (e.g., the sphenoidal ridge) or from contracoup trauma that occurs when the brain strikes the skull on the side opposite the point of insult. Brain and Walton (1969) indentified three different destructive forces that are applied to the brain at the moment of impact: compression or impression that forces the brain tissue together, tension that pulls the brain apart, and shearing produced by rotational acceleration and that develops primarily at those points where the brain impinges on bony or ligamentous ridges with the cranial vault. The primary mechanism producing brain injury following closed-head injury is diffuse axonal damage in the white matter occurring at the time of impact and caused by a shearing mechanism arising from rotational acceleration.

It has often been reported that children show a striking rate of recovery following closed-head injury. Some authors have suggested that one of the reasons for the good prognosis for recovery in childhood is that the degree of brain damage following head injury is less in children than in adults, due in part to the different nature of their head injuries as well as to differences in the basic mechanisms of brain damage following head injury. Most childhood head injuries result from falls or low speed accidents. Consequently, many pediatric head injuries are associated with a lesser degree of rotational acceleration and therefore, presumably, with a lesser amount of brain damage (Levin, Benton, & Grossman, 1982). Jamison and Kaye (1974) noted that persistent neurologic deficits were only present in children injured in road traffic accidents which, by their nature, are likely to yield greater diffuse brain injury. Likewise, a study conducted by Moyes (1980) showed road traffic accidents to be the most common cause of long-term morbidity following childhood head injury. In addition, Strich (1969) suggested that the shearing strains produced by rotational acceleration in head trauma are less pronounced in smaller brains.

Although the rate of spontaneous recovery in children following closed-head injury is often described as excellent, persistent long-term language disorders have been reported (Gaidolfi &

Vignolo, 1980; Jordan, Ozanne, & Murdoch, 1988; Satz & Bullard-Bates, 1981) and even when specific linguistic symptoms resolve cognitive and academic difficulties often remain. The speech-language disorders associated with childhood TBI together with the mechanisms of head injury are discussed in detail in Chapters 3 and 12.

Cerebrovascular Accidents

Cerebrovascular accidents or strokes are spontaneous interruptions to the blood supply to the brain, arising from either occlusion of the cerebral blood vessels (ischemic stroke) or in some cases from rupture of one of the cerebral blood vessels (hemorrhagic stroke). Although cerebrovascular accidents are much less common in children than in adults, they occur more frequently than is commonly thought and are a significant cause of morbidity and mortality in the childhood population. Banker (1961) reported that of 555 childhood autopsy cases studied by him, death was due to a cerebrovascular accident in 48 (8.6%).

The three major characteristics of cerebrovascular accidents include: (1) an abrupt onset of focal brain dysfunction; (2) the disability produced (including any speech or language deficit) is worst at onset or within a short period of onset; and (3) if the patient survives, the disability tends to improve, in some cases partially, in others almost totally.

Cerebrovascular accidents can be divided into two major types, ischemic strokes and hemorrhagic strokes. Ischemic strokes occur when the supply of blood to part of the brain suddenly becomes inadequate for the brain cells to function. Hemorrhagic strokes occur when a blood vessel ruptures and blood either rushes through the brain tissue destroying it (intracerebral hemorrhage) or collects outside the brain in one of the spaces between the meninges causing compression of the brain within the skull.

Ischemic Stroke

Ischemic strokes can arise in two ways: first through occlusion of the vessel by thrombus formation (cerebral thrombosis) and second through occlusion of the vessel by an embolus (cerebral embolism). Approximately two-thirds of ischemic strokes are caused by thrombosis whereas one-third are attributed to embolism. Thrombosis is most commonly associated with atherosclerotic changes in the blood vessel wall. However, it also can be associated with inflammatory disorders that affect the blood vessels such as giant-cell arteritis, syphilitic endarteritis, and systemic lupus erythematosus among others.

The potential sources of emboli are remarkably widespread, with most emboli originating from the heart as a result of small pieces of mural thrombosis (from the walls of the heart) becoming dislodged from the cardiac wall by atrial fibrillation or other cardiac arrhythmia. Cardiac surgery and bacterial endocarditis are less common but also real sources of emboli.

Of central importance in both types of ischemic stroke is that they deprive brain tissue of needed oxygen. Both thrombosis and embolism cause acute ischemia in the tissues receiving their vascular supply from the occluded vessel which, in turn, produces an area of cell death (infarct). Embolic infarctions develop much more rapidly than thrombotic infarcts. Both neurons and the myelinated pathways are affected but the white matter is considerably less sensitive to ischemia than gray matter (i.e., the cortex). The center of an infarct will be totally destroyed, but toward the periphery there may be preservation of white matter pathways and there is often a surrounding zone of lesser ischemia in which cells cease to function on a temporary basis, but cell death does not occur. In time, some of these injured neurons recuperate sufficiently to resume function and many white matter pathways survive to carry impulses again. This delayed return of function to certain areas within an infarct provides one explanation (but not the only one, e.g., reduction in degree of associated edema etc. is another) of the spontaneous recovery so often seen in many types of aphasias. The final outcome of an infarct is a cystlike area from which both neurons and white matter have disappeared, surrounded by a scarred, sclerotic zone of glia.

Thrombic stroke usually develops abruptly, often during sleep or shortly after rising. In some cases, however, it may be preceded by transient "warning" signs in which case it has a stepwise onset over several hours or days. Thrombotic strokes are the most common type of cerebrovascular accident. Embolic strokes are almost always abrupt in onset and the patient is only rarely forewarned by transitory symptoms.

Hemorrhage Stroke

Hemorrhage stroke may have a sudden onset with evolution to maximum deficit occurring in a smooth fashion over several hours. Cerebral hemorrhage, when the result of vascular disease (as opposed to trauma, etc.), is most often associated with hypertension but it may occur with a variety of pathologies affecting the cerebral vessels such as aneurysm, angioma, arteriovenous malformation, blood dyscrasia, or arteritis. Anti-coagulant therapy (e.g., warfarin therapy) is acknowledged as a frequent cause of cerebral hemorrhage that can lead to the production of speech and language disorders.

Most hemorrhages occur during activity and without warning. Onset therefore is abrupt and is associated with severe headache, vomiting, and often loss of consciousness. The most common site for intracerebral hemorrhages is the region of the internal capsule in which case the patient suddenly complains of something wrong in the head, followed by headache, dysarthria, and/or aphasia, paralysis down the opposite side of the body, and variable alterations in consciousness. With brainstem hemorrhage there usually is rapid loss of consciousness and often death in a short time. Cerebellar hemorrhages are associated with vertigo, nausea, and ataxia followed by coma and often death. Overall, the prognosis for recovery for hemorrhagic strokes is poorer than for ischemic strokes.

Intracerebral hemorrhages usually involve deeper structures of the brain than the cerebral cortex and produce brain damage both by local destruction and by compression of surrounding brain tissue. The force of blood coming from a ruptured blood vessel directly damages the brain tissue. This extravasated blood forms a clot called a hematoma which increases in size and displaces surrounding brain tissue. The intracranial pressure increases as the clot develops causing compression of the brain tissue. Secondary rupture into the ventricular system or subarachnoid space may also occur. Emergency evacuation of the intracerebral clot is of value in aiding the relief of symptoms in some cases.

In addition to hypertension, rupture of the intracranial aneurysms is another major cause of hemorrhagic strokes. An aneurysm is a thin-walled enlargement of a blood vessel usually found in the circle of Willis or its major branches. Aneurysms tend to occur at junctions or bifurcations and are believed to represent congenital deficiencies in the development of the vessel wall. They tend to increase in size and may produce cranial nerve palsies or focal seizures by compression of adjacent structures prior to rupture. Rupture usually occurs during activity and produces severe headache, collapse and unconsciousness. Generally, bleeding occurs into the subarachnoid space but also may occur into the brain tissue forming an intracerebral hemorrhage. In the latter case prolonged unconsciousness and focal signs such as hemiplegia, hemianesthesia, and aphasia also may occur.

A full discussion of the cerebrovascular disorders most commonly associated with the occurrence of acquired speech and language disorders in children is presented in Chapter 2.

Brain Tumors

Intracranial brain tumors are a recognized cause of acquired speech and language disorders in children. Such tumors may be either benign or malignant. Tumors affecting the central nervous system are said to be primary tumors if they grow from cells within the cranial cavity itself, or secondary (metastases) if they travel to the brain from a primary tumor elsewhere in the body (e.g., lungs).

Brain tumors produce symptoms in three ways. First, because tumors are "space occupying lesions," as they develop they cause the intracranial pressure to rise, leading to compression and distortion of surrounding brain structures. Second, as tumors grow they may disrupt the blood supply to specific regions of the brain or may interrupt the circulation of cerebrospinal fluid, such as by compressing the ventricles or occluding the cerebral aqueduct, thereby leading to increased intracranial pressure. Third, the tumor may directly damage the brain tissue in a localized area. The direct effect produces symptoms and signs (e.g., paralysis down one side of the body, epileptic fits, etc.) that become gradually worse and more extensive as the tumor grows, in complete contrast to the sudden onset of a cerebrovascular accident.

Intracranial tumors can be divided into two major types, namely, intracerebral tumors and extracerebral tumors. Intracerebral tumors are those that directly involve the cerebral tissues while extracerebral tumors arise from tissues outside the brain itself (e.g., the meninges and skull bones). By far the majority of intracerebral neoplasms are gliomas that develop from the supporting tissue of the brain (i.e., the neuroglial cells), tumors of nerve cells being rare. The various types of glioma take their names from the particular neuroglial cells involved and include astrocytomas, oligodendrocytomas, and microgliomas. Some intracerebral tumors called ependymomas develop from the cells lining the ventricles (ependymal cells) whereas others called medulloblastomas develop from primitive cells in the roof of the fourth ventricle. Any variety of intracerebral tumor is capable of producing a speech and/or language disturbance dependent upon its location in the brain. On the other hand, language disorders are rarely caused by extracra-

nial tumors which include among others growing from the meninges (meningiomas), sheaths of peripheral nerves (neurofibromas, e.g., acoustic neuromas), the skull bone (osteomas), and the pituitary gland (e.g., various adenomas). These tumors are mostly benign and do not directly cause destruction of cerebral tissues as in the case of intracerebral tumors but instead may produce abnormal neurologic signs as a result of distortion or displacement of cerebral tissue.

Although intracerebral tumors cause language disorders more often than extracerebral tumors, in neither variety does aphasia usually become a major complaint until late in the course of the disease. The reason why aphasic symptoms usually only appear late in the disorder is that intracerebral neoplasms infiltrate the cerebral tissues widely before producing focal destruction. Furthermore, extracerebral tumors tend to develop slowly, allowing considerable accommodation by the cerebral tissues with only minimal disruption of functions until late in the course of the disorder. If aphasic symptoms do appear early in the development of a tumor, it usually is because the tumor has either disrupted the cerebral blood supply or interfered with the circulation of cerebrospinal fluid. Although the particular neurologic signs, including any speech or language disorder, associated with the presence of a tumor may give some indication as to the location of that tumor in the brain, due to the local effects of the tumor, it must be remembered that distortion and/or compression of cerebral tissue may actually occur at a distance from where the tumor is located. Consequently, the particular speech-language deficit exhibited may have no direct relationship with the location of the tumor itself.

Neoplasms of the posterior cranial fossa (i.e., those involving the cerebellum, pons, fourth ventricle and cisterna magna) occur more frequently in children than supratentorial tumors. Cerebellar astrocytoma is one of the most common types of posterior fossa tumor in childhood, occurring most frequently in children between 5 and 9 years of age (Cuneo & Rand, 1952; Matson, 1969). Fortunately, cerebellar astrocytomas are also highly curable and have an excellent prognosis following surgical removal. Medulloblastoma is also one of the most frequent tumor types involving structures within the posterior cranial fossa in children. Generally, these latter tumors involve children at a younger age than do cerebellar astrocytomas, their maximum incidence being within the age range of 3 to 7 years (Delong & Adams, 1975). Although initially cerebellar astrocytoma and medulloblastoma may present in a similar manner the prognosis of these two tumor types is quite different. Although astrocytoma has a very favorable prognosis medulloblastoma has a poor prognosis for recovery. A third frequently encountered tumor of the posterior cranial fossa is the ependymoma. These neoplasms grow from the floor of the fourth ventricle and affect children of a similar age to the medulloblastomas, and like the latter tumor type, ependymoma has a poor prognosis with a high proportion of tumors recurring after surgical removal. A more complete description of the major types of brain tumors associated with the occurrence of speech and language disorders in children is presented in Chapter 4.

Considering their location in the central nervous system, it would not be expected that posterior fossa tumors would cause language problems. A number of secondary effects, however, are associated with these tumors which can, in some cases, lead to language deficits. Surgical removal of tumors in some cases may be the cause of speech and language deficits due to associated damage to structures such as the cerebellum. Furthermore, many posterior fossa tumors either originate from or invade the fourth ventricle. As a result hydrocephalus may occur following obstruction to the flow of cerebrospinal fluid. Subsequent compression of the cerebral cortex can then lead to malfunctioning of the central speech-language centers. In addition, radiotherapy and chemo-therapy (see Chapter 4) administered after surgical removal of posterior fossa tumors to prevent tumor spread or recurrence has been implicated in the occurrence of speech and language disorders in both adults and children.

The effects of intracranial tumors on speech and language functions in children are discussed in detail in Chapters 13 and 4, respectively.

Infections

Che nervous system and its coverings can be infected by the same microorganisms that affect other organs of the body. Infections of the nervous system are classified according to the major site of involvement and type of infecting organism. Infection of the meninges (usually the leptomeninges) is called meningitis while inflammation of the brain is referred to as encephalitis. In some cases both the meninges and brain may be infected, a condition called meningoencephalitis. Inflammation of the spinal cord is known as myelitis.

Infections of the central nervous system can be caused by viruses, bacteria, protozoa, and fungi. Most varieties of intracranial infection produce rather widespread neurologic symptomatology and any associated language disorder therefore is liable to be lost among other neurobehavioral and cognitive dysfunctions. Occasionally, however, a significant speech and/or language disorder can be traced to a central nervous system infection. Currently, the most common infection reported to give rise to acquired aphasia syndromes is herpes simplex encephalitis.

Acquired speech and language disorders in children also can result from the formation of intracerebral abscesses. A cerebral abscess is a pus-filled cavity in the brain that develops around a localized bacterial infection. Abscesses most commonly develop in the frontal and temporal lobes. Prior to antibiotic drugs, temporal lobe abscesses were a frequent source of aphasia secondary to chronic ear infections. In a manner similar to other types of "space-occupying lesions" such as intracerebral tumors, as it grows an abscess can produce symptoms by compressing and distorting surrounding brain structures and by interrupting the vascular supply or the flow of cerebrospinal fluid.

A detailed description of the major infectious disorders associated with the occurrence of acquired language disorders in children is presented in Chapter 6.

Convulsive Disorder

Acquired aphasia with convulsive disorder was first described by Landau and Kleffner (1957). In this condition the child's language deteriorates in association with the epileptiform discharges seen in their electroencephalogram. In some cases the language deterioration is either preceded, accompanied, or followed by a series of convulsive seizures (van de Sandt-Koenderman, Smit, van Dongen, & van Hest, 1984). Although seizures do occur often, they are not the defining feature of this syndrome.

Onset of the Landau–Kleffner syndrome is usually between 2 and 13 years of age, with the initial loss of language function occurring most frequently between 3 and 7 years of age. Males are affected twice as often as females. Although the cause of Landau-Kleffner syndrome is unknown, several hypotheses on the pathogenesis of this disorder have been proposed. Some authors have postulated that the language regression results from functional ablation of the primary cortical language areas by persistent electrical discharges (Landau & Kleffner, 1957; Sato & Dreifuss, 1973). The characteristics of the language disorder shown by children with Landau-Kleffner syndrome are discussed in Chapter 9.

Other Etiologies

In addition to the etiologies outlined above, acquired childhood speech and language disorders can also occur in association with a range of other conditions the most important of which include: Acute lymphoblastic leukemia (see Chapter 4); inborn errors of metabolism (e.g., galactosemia and phenylketonuria) (see Chapter 5); neural tube disorders (e.g., spina bifida) (see Chapter 8); and conditions associated with acute cerebral anoxia (e.g., accidental suffocation; near-drowning etc.) (see Chapter 7).

Recovery in Acquired Childhood Speech-Language Disorders

A variety of opinions have been expressed in the literature on the prognosis for recovery from acquired childhood aphasia. These opinions range from declarations of complete recovery or near complete recovery (Alajouanine & Lhermitte, 1965) to more guarded predictions of only partial recovery, when the influence of other factors such as site and extent of lesion are taken into account. A number of researchers have reported that brain lesions involving left language areas in children have relatively mild sequelae on language development, in comparison to lesions acquired later in adulthood, both in the case of pre-, peri-, or postnatal (before 6 months of age) focal brain injuries and in the case of lesions occurring after language onset (Bates et al., 1997; Bottari, Cipriani, Chilosi, & Pfanner, 2001; Vargha-Khadem, O'Gorman, & Watters, 1985; Vicari et al., 2000). The excellent recovery of language in children generally has been attributed to an enhanced reorganization potential of the developing brain and interpreted in relation to the concepts of "plasticity" and "equipotentiality" of the immature brain. Plasticity defines a general property of the brain and refers to the compensatory mechanisms underlying lesion-induced neurofunctional reorganization.

Some authors (e.g., Van Hout, Evrard, & Lyon, 1985), however, do not agree with the assertion that children recover more completely and rapidly than adults. Woods and Carey (1979) for instance went as far as to state that any child over the age of 1 year who received an aphasia-producing lesion in the left hemisphere is likely to have their performance on verbal tasks permanently impaired. Hécaen (1983) also recommended caution before concluding that complete recovery is to be expected in cases of acquired childhood aphasia.

One reason for the controversy is that many authors, when describing the recovery of language function in children with acquired aphasia, make reference only to "clinical recovery." Despite apparent "clinical recovery," however, some authors suggest that subtle language deficits may persist in the long-term, even in cases where the injury to the left hemisphere occurred at an early age (Alajouanine & Lhermitte, 1965; Vargha-Khadem et al., 1985).

The literature relating to the prognosis of acquired childhood aphasia was reviewed by Satz and Bullard-Bates (1981). They concluded that, although the majority of children with this condition showed spontaneous recovery, it by no means occurs in all cases. In 25 to 50% of the cases they reviewed in the studies, aphasia remained unremitted 1 year postonset. A recovery period extending up to 5 years in cases of acquired childhood aphasia was suggested by Carrow-Woolfolk and Lynch (1982). Importantly, even in those cases where recovery is reported to occur, serious cognitive and academic difficulties often remain and a majority of children with acquired childhood aphasia, even after apparent recovery, have difficulty following a normal progression through school (Chadwick, 1985; Hécaen, 1976; Martins, 2004; Satz & Bullard-Bates, 1981).

A number of different theories have been proposed to explain the mechanism of recovery in children with acquired aphasia. As indicated earlier, the often reported good recovery shown by children with acquired aphasia is taken by some investigators as indicating the "plasticity" of the immature brain whereby language function is assumed by nondamaged areas of the brain, including the nondamaged portions of the left hemisphere and/or the intact right cerebral hemisphere. Alajouanine and Lhermitte (1965) believed that a child's brain has anatomic–functional plasticity such that the neural networks of the injured hemisphere and more so of the sound hemisphere take part in a new functional organization to compensate for the damaged area. Van Hout et al. (1985) also suggested that the plasticity of the young brain probably accounts for the rapid disappearance in some cases of the positive signs of aphasia. The authors, however, were of the opinion that the process is limited when the lesion is located in the left temporal lobe and some additional right hemisphere damage impedes the right hemisphere taking over the language functions. As evidence against the theory of transfer of language function, Satz and Bullard-Bates (1981) suggested that the speed of recovery sometimes witnessed in children with acquired aphasia is incompatible with a transfer of language to and the learning of language by the right hemisphere.

Another theory proposed to explain the difference in the prognosis of aphasia in children and adults is what Zangwill (1960) called the "equipotentiality hypothesis." According to this theory, at birth each cerebral hemisphere has the same potential to develop language function and that speech and language functions are progressively lateralized and cerebral dominance established as the child matures (Lennenberg, 1967). If the equipotentiality hypothesis is true, it could be expected that aphasia would occur more commonly in children with right cerebral lesions than adults with right cerebral lesions. In recent years, however, support for the equipotentiality hypothesis has declined in that several studies have shown that the frequency of aphasia from right cerebral lesions in right-handed children is similar to that in right-handed adults (Carter, Hohenegger, & Satz, 1982; Satz & Bullard-Bates, 1981).

One explanation for the good recovery shown by some children with acquired aphasia is that favored by some authors and known as the "displacement phenomenon" (Satz & Bullard-Bates, 1981). According to this theory both cerebral hemispheres contain mechanisms for language. Consequently, the right hemisphere (minor hemisphere) has for a time the capacity to subserve speech and language function if the left (dominant) hemisphere is damaged in early life. It is proposed that under normal circumstances the language mechanisms in the right hemisphere are inhibited by those in the left such that only the left hemisphere develops complex language function. When the left hemisphere is damaged, however, the right hemisphere is released from inhibition, allowing it to assume a greater role in language function. The critical period for this release may be only up to 2 to 4 years of age.

A number of different factors have been identified by various authors that may influence the prognosis of acquired childhood aphasia. These factors include: the site of lesion, the size and side of lesion, the cause, the associated neurologic disturbances, the age at onset, the type and severity of the aphasia, and the presence of electroencephalographic abnormalities. Each of these factors is discussed in more detail in Chapter 2.

References

Alajouanine, T., & Lhermitte, F. (1965). Acquired aphasia in children. *Brain, 88,* 653–662.

Bak, E., van Dongen, H. R., & Arts, W. F. M. (1983). The analysis of acquired dysarthria in childhood. *Developmental Medicine and Child Neurology, 25,* 81–94.

Banker, B. Q. (1961). Cerebral vascular disease in infancy and childhood. *Journal of Neuropathology and Experimental Neurology, 20,* 127–140.

Bates, E., Thal, D., Aram, D., Eisele, J., Nass, R., & Trauner, D. (1997). First words to grammar in children with focal brain injury. *Developmental Neuropsychology, 13,* 275–343.

Bottari, P., Cipriani, P., Chilosi, A., & Pfanner, L. (2001). The Italian determiner system in normal acquisition, specific language impairment, and childhood aphasia. *Brain and Language, 77,* 283–293.

Brain, L., & Walton, J. N. (1969). *Brain's diseases of the nervous system* (7th ed.). New York, NY: Oxford University Press.

Carrow-Woolfolk, E., & Lynch, J. (1982). *An integrative approach to language disorders in children.* Orlando, FL: Grune & Stratton.

Carter, R. L., Hohenegger, M. K., & Satz, P. (1982). Aphasia and speech organization in children. *Science, 218,* 797–799.

Chadwick, O. (1985). Psychological sequelae of head injury in children. *Developmental Medicine and Child Neurology, 27,* 72–75.

Cuneo, H. N., & Rand, C. W. (1952). *Brain tumors of childhood.* Springfield, IL: Charles C. Thomas.

Darley, F. L., Aronson, A. E., & Brown, J. R. (1975). *Motor speech disorders.* Philadelphia, PA: W. B. Saunders.

Delong, G. R., & Adams, R. D. (1975). Clinical aspects of tumours of the posterior fossa in childhood. In P. J. Vinken & G. W. Bruyn (Eds.), *Handbook of clinical neurology: Tumours of the brain and skull.* Amsterdam, the Netherlands: North-Holland.

Fletcher, J. M., & Taylor, H. (1984). Neuropsychological approaches to children: Towards a developmental neuropsychology. *Journal of Neuropsychology, 6,* 39–57.

Gaidolfi, E., & Vignolo, L. A. (1980). Closed head injuries of school-age children: Neuropsychological sequelae in early adulthood. *Italian Journal of Neurological Science, 2,* 65–73.

Goodglass, H., & Kaplan, E. (1972). *The assessment of aphasia and related disorders.* Philadelphia, PA: Lea & Febiger.

Hécaen, H. (1976). Acquired aphasia in children and the ontogenesis of hemispheric functional specialization. *Brain and Language, 3,* 114–134.

Hécaen, H. (1983). Acquired aphasia in children: Revisited. *Neuropsychologia, 21,* 581–587.

Jamison, D. L., & Kaye, H. H. (1974). Accidental head injury in children. *Archives of Diseases of Childhood, 49,* 376–381.

Jordan, F. M., Ozanne, A. E., & Murdoch, B. E. (1988). Long-term speech and language disorders subsequent to closed head injury in children. *Brain Injury, 2,* 179–185.

Landau, W. M., & Kleffner, F. R. (1957). Syndrome of acquired aphasia with convulsive disorder in children. *Neurology, 10,* 915–921.

Lenneberg, E. (1967). *Biological foundations of language.* New York, NY: Wiley.

Levin, H. S., Benton, A. L., & Grossman, R. G. (1982). *Neurobehavioral consequences of closed head injury.* New York, NY: Oxford University Press.

Martins, I. P. (2004). Persistent acquired childhood aphasia. In F. Fabbro (Ed.), *Neurogenic language disorders in children* (pp. 231–251). Amsterdam, the Netherlands: Elsevier.

Matson, D. D. (1969). *Neurosurgery of infancy and childhood.* Springfield, IL: Charles C. Thomas.

Maurer, D., & Lewis, T. L. (1998). Overt orienting toward peripheral stimuli: Normal development and underlying mechanisms. In J. E. Richards (Ed.), *Cognitive neuroscience of attention: A developmental perspective* (pp. 51–102). Hillsdale, NJ: Lawrence Erlbaum.

McNeil, M. R., Robin, D. A., & Schmidt, R. A. (2008). Apraxia of speech: Definition and differential diagnosis. In M. R. McNeil (Ed.), *Clinical management of sensorimotor speech disorders* (pp. 249–264). New York, NY: Thieme.

Miller J. F., Campbell, T. F., Chapman, R. S., & Weismer, S. E. (1984). Language behavior in acquired aphasia. In A. Holland (Ed.), *Language disorders in children*. Baltimore, MD: College-Hill Press.

Moyes, C. D. (1980). Epidemiology of serious head injuries in childhood. *Child Care, Health and Development, 6,* 1–9.

Murdoch, B. E., & Hudson-Tennent, L. J. (1994). Differential language outcomes in children treated for posterior fossa tumours. *Aphasiology, 8,* 507–534.

Neville, H. J., & Bavelier, D. (2000). Specificity and plasticity in neurocognitive development in humans. In M. S. Gazzaniga (Ed.), *The new cognitive neurosciences* (pp. 83–98). Cambridge, MA: MIT Press.

Sato, S., & Dreifuss, F. E. (1973). Electroencephalographic findings in a patient with developmental expressive aphasia. *Neurology, 23,* 181–185.

Satz, P., & Bullard-Bates, C. (1981). Acquired aphasia in children. In M. T. Sarno (Ed.), *Acquired aphasia*. New York, NY: Academic Press.

Strich, S. J. (1969). The pathology of brain damage due to blunt injuries. In A. E. Walker, W. F. Caveness, & M. Critchley (Eds.), *The late effects of head injury* (pp. 501–524). Springfield, IL: Charles C. Thomas.

van de Sandt-Koenderman, W. M. E., Smit, I. A. C., van Dongen, H. R., & van Hest, J. B. C. (1984). A case of acquired aphasia and convulsive disorder: Some linguistic aspects of recovery and breakdown. *Brain and Language, 21,* 174–183.

Van Hout, A., Evrard, P., & Lyon, G. (1985). On the positive semiology of acquired aphasia in children. *Developmental Medicine and Child Neurology, 27,* 231–241.

Vargha-Khadem, F., O'Gorman, A. M., & Watters, G. V. (1985). Aphasia and handedness in relation to hemispheric side, age and injury and severity of cerebral lesion during childhood. *Brain, 108,* 677–696.

Vicari, S., Albertoni, A., Chilosi, A., Cipriani, P., Cioni, G., & Bates, E. (2000). Plasticity and reorganization during language development in children with early brain injury. *Cortex, 36,* 31–36.

Woods, B. T., & Carey, S. (1979). Language deficits after apparent clinical recovery from childhood aphasia. *Annuals of Neurology, 6,* 405–409.

Zangwill, O. L. (1960). *Cerebral dominance and its relation to psychological function*. Springfield, IL: Charles C. Thomas.

PART A

Acquired Language Disorders in Childhood

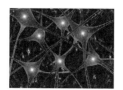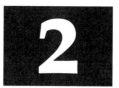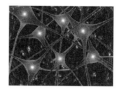

2

Acquired Childhood Aphasia

As outlined in Chapter 1, acquired childhood aphasia is a language disorder resulting from a cerebral lesion sustained in childhood subsequent to onset of language acquisition. Until the late 1970s, our understanding of the clinical features of this condition was dominated by a historic view that had evolved since the first description of acquired childhood aphasia in the mid-19th century (Cotard, 1868). According to the historic view, the symptoms most often reported to be characteristic of acquired childhood aphasia included: initial mutism (suppression of spontaneous speech), followed by a period of reduced speech initiative; a nonfluent motor-type language impairment; simplified syntax (telegraphic expression); no (or rare) accompanying comprehension deficit or other features of a fluent aphasia (e.g., jargon, logorrhea, paraphasia); impairment in naming; a concomitant dysarthria; and disturbances in reading and writing (primarily in the acute stage

postonset). In addition, acquired childhood aphasia was usually regarded as being rare and transitory in nature with most affected individuals exhibiting good recovery. Furthermore, many authors considered that unlike adult aphasia, the clinical presentation of acquired childhood aphasia was not dependent on the localization of the lesion (i.e., acquired childhood aphasia is nonfluent irrespective of lesion site) and that although infrequent in adults, aphasia frequently occurred in association with right cerebral hemisphere lesions in children.

In 1978, the publication of a landmark paper on changing patterns of childhood aphasia by Woods and Teuber (1978) triggered a major re-think of the historic description of acquired childhood aphasia and the implied dissimilarities in the neurology of language in children and adults. Specifically, Woods and Teuber (1978) reported the presence of jargon aphasia in a 5-year-old boy as an "unexpected finding." In support of their finding, further reports in the literature published since the late 1970s have also documented the presence of fluent aphasia with paraphasia in children with acquired aphasia. Collectively, these reports question the validity of the historic description of acquired childhood aphasia and have altered our clinical insights into this condition (Paquier & van Dongen, 1996).

Clinical Features of Acquired Childhood Aphasia

The controversy over the clinical features of acquired childhood aphasia, at least in part, may be due to the presence of methodological limitations in many of the studies in this area that have prevented identification of definitive profiles of the linguistic characteristics of acquired childhood aphasia. These limitations, often resulting from restrictions on the number of subjects available, include factors such as: the inclusion of a diverse range of causes of acquired aphasia; the use of nonspecific methods of lesion localization (e.g., the identification of brain lesions on the basis of the presence of a hemiplegia); the failure to exclude cases with possible bilateral brain damage (e.g., as occurs after traumatic brain injury or infectious disorders); and the inclusion of subjects of different ages before and after the onset of brain damage. Furthermore, prior to the 1980s, most reports of the language characteristics of acquired childhood aphasia were of a descriptive nature with very few standardized language assessments being utilized. Fortunately, in recent studies more objective measures of language performance have been used and more accurate methods of lesion localization (e.g., neuroimaging) employed. Despite this, the prob-

lem of groups of mixed pathology and diverse age ranges persist.

Historic Descriptions of Acquired Childhood Aphasia

Acquired childhood aphasia largely has been regarded as being characterized by aphasia of the nonfluent type ever since the first reports of the condition in the mid-19th century (Bernhardt, 1885; Cotard, 1868; Freud, 1897). Indeed, even until the early 1980s nonfluency was frequently described as the most prevailing clinical feature of acquired aphasia in children (Carrow-Woolfolk & Lynch, 1982; Satz & Bullard-Bates, 1981). In addition, many of the earlier reports noted that children with acquired aphasia exhibit simplified syntax (Alajouanine & Lhermitte, 1965) or telegraphic speech (Guttmann, 1942) without describing the spoken syntax of these children in detail. Although there is general agreement that expressive language problems are common in acquired childhood aphasia, there has been considerable debate over the years concerning the presence of deficits in auditory comprehension and other symptoms of fluent aphasia in this group of children. Most of the early descriptions of acquired childhood aphasia indicated that fluent aphasia and receptive disorders of oral speech such as literal and verbal paraphasic errors, logorrhea and perseverations only rarely are found in children with this condition. The majority of early researchers considered impairments in auditory comprehension to be a rare occurrence in children with acquired aphasia (Bernhardt, 1885; Guttmann, 1942). Approximately one-third of the children with acquired aphasia examined by Alajouanine and Lhermitte (1965) were reported to exhibit auditory comprehension deficits. Furthermore, it has been suggested that when present, disturbances in auditory comprehension occur almost exclusively in the early stages postonset of aphasia and disappear rapidly and almost completely (Hécaen, 1976, 1983). Consequently, the variability relating to the presence of impaired auditory comprehension abilities in children with acquired aphasia reported in the literature may be accounted for by the fact that different authors examined the language abilities of children with acquired aphasia at different stages postonset.

Further confusion as to the presence or absence of symptoms of fluent aphasia, such as auditory comprehension deficits in acquired childhood aphasia arises when patient age is taken into consideration. Some evidence is available to suggest that the primarily nonfluent pattern of aphasia is only prevalent in children who are less than 10 years of age at the onset of aphasia (Alajouanine & Lhermitte, 1965; Guttmann, 1942; Poetzl, 1926). For example, Alajouanine and Lhermitte (1965) reported that the predominant features of the acquired aphasia demonstrated by children at less than 10 years of age included: decreased auditory comprehension; severe writing deficit; and no logorrhea, paraphasias, or perseveration. In contrast, the acquired aphasia noted to be demonstrated by children greater than 10 years of age by these authors was a more fluent form of aphasia, with paraphasia present, less frequent articulatory and phonetic disintegration, and disturbed written language. Contrary to these findings, however, other authors have expressed the opinion that the nonfluent type of aphasia is the pattern present in older children as well as younger ones (Assal

& Campiche, 1973; Basser, 1962; Benson, 1972; Hécaen, 1976). Although unable to confirm a relationship between aphasia type and age, Hécaen (1976) postulated a relationship between lesion site and aphasia type. He reported that children with acquired aphasia resulting from anterior lesions presented with an initial mutism while those with temporal lobe lesions showed comprehension deficits in the acute stages that resolved within one year. On the basis of a review of the literature up to 1978 relating to acquired childhood aphasia, Satz and Bullard-Bates (1981) concluded that the clinical presentation is predominantly nonfluent with rare or absent paraphasias and logorrhea, but disorders of auditory comprehension, naming, and writing may co-exist. They stipulated that at that time it was unclear how those clinical patterns related to age and maturational effects or to lesion, its size, cause, type, site, or the time after the lesion.

Another frequently reported characteristic of the classic description of acquired childhood aphasia is a period of mutism that may last from a few days to months. Indeed, a reduction in all expressive activities, including oral, written and gestural, has been reported to occur in children with acquired aphasia (Alajouanine & Lhermitte, 1965). Mutism has been described as the chief characteristic of acquired childhood aphasia by Branco-Lefèvre (1950) and Alajouanine and Lhermitte (1965). Guttmann (1942) noted an absence of spontaneous speech in 14 of his 16 cases of acquired childhood aphasia, mostly in children younger than 10 years of age. Nine of the 15 right hemiplegic subjects (60%) reported by Hécaen (1976) had a period of mutism lasting from 5 days to 3 months. Hécaen (1983) carried out a retrospective study involving 56 children with acquired aphasia ranging from 3.5 to 15 years of age, with brain lesions resulting from a variety of etiologies, including trauma, tumor, and hematoma. Mutism was reported to be the predominant clinical symptom in the initial stage postonset, occurring in 47% of these children with acquired aphasia. When analyzed according to lesion type, however, Hécaen (1983) noted that only 20% of cases with progressive brain lesions (e.g., tumors) exhibited an initial mutism, whereas 85% of acute head trauma patients demonstrated this symptom in the early stages postonset. Furthermore, Hécaen (1983) observed that mutism appeared mostly in children with frontal rolandic lesions (63%) whereas only 10% of children with temporal lesions showed mutism. Following the period of mutism when speech returns, there is often a period during which the aphasic child is unwilling to speak (Alajouanine & Lhermitte, 1965; Guttmann, 1942). This period has also been described as representing a loss or reduction of "speech initiative" (Hécaen, 1976, 1983). Increased incentives and encouragements are required in this period to get the child to produce even the few words they are capable of producing.

Some authors have suggested a purely psychological basis for the initial mutism shown by children with acquired aphasia (Alajouanine & Lhermitte, 1965; Byers & McLean, 1962). Alajouanine and Lhermitte (1965) proposed that the suppression of spontaneous speech might be the result of a psychological reaction experienced by the children in response to their inability to communicate noting that children tend to isolation, refusal, and silence in response to conflict or difficulties. Furthermore, these authors observed that the unwillingness of aphasic children to speak after speech returns is similar to the behavior of normal children when faced with a difficult problem they cannot solve and wish to put aside.

Another characteristic of acquired childhood aphasia noted to be present in classic descriptions of the disorder, particularly in the acute stages postonset, is a naming deficit or poverty of lexical stock (Alajouanine & Lhermitte, 1965; Bernhardt, 1885; Collignon, Hécaen, & Angerlerques, 1968). Hécaen (1976) noted that naming disorders occurred in 46% of his left-hemisphere lesioned participants, with three of the affected cases exhibiting this deficit long-term. Likewise Hécaen (1983) reported that 44% of his sample of acquired childhood aphasics had naming problems (not of a paraphasic type), which tended to persist. Further Hécaen (1983) observed that naming problems are commonly present when the child returns to school and consequently is often mentioned explicitly in their school reports.

A number of the early researchers noted the presence of hesitations in the speech of children with acquired aphasia (Bernhardt, 1885; Guttmann, 1942) possibly representing the outcome of either the dysarthria reported to be present in these children (Guttmann, 1942; Hécaen, 1976, 1983) or alternatively reflecting the word-finding problems reported to occur in this population. Dysarthria has been listed as a common finding in association with acquired childhood aphasia with Hécaen (1983) reporting that 52% of his 56 subjects exhibited a dysarthric disturbance. Alajouanine and Lhermitte (1965) found dysarthria with paralytic and dystonic features in 22 out of their total of 32 cases. According to Hécaen (1983), the factor having the greatest influence in determining the occurrence of dysarthria is the localization of the underlying lesion. Hécaen (1983) reported that 81% of children with anterior lesions exhibited a dysarthria as part of their aphasic disturbance, whereas only 20% of cases with temporal lesions exhibited a dysarthria.

A further characteristic of acquired childhood aphasia often included in historic descriptions of the condition was a disorder vaguely referred to as a "reading problem." The presence of a "reading problem" was reported to be present in 18 out of the 32 children with acquired aphasia examined by Alajouanine and Lhermitte (1965). Unfortunately, however, in the majority of studies reported in the literature no attempt was made to define the nature of the observed reading disturbance in any further detail other than merely to document its presence. Most authors, for instance, give no indication as to the relative effects of the condition on the children's ability to read aloud versus their ability to read for comprehension. It is possible that the general lack of differentiation in most descriptions of the reading abilities of children with acquired aphasia may be due to the fact that reading disorders, although common in the acute stage postonset, in most cases disappear rapidly and completely (Hécaen, 1976, 1983).

A writing deficit is also a commonly reported feature of acquired childhood aphasia included in historic descriptions of the disorder (Alajouanine & Lhermitte, 1965; Branco-Lefèvre, 1950; Hécaen, 1976, 1983). All 32 of the child subjects with acquired aphasia examined by Alajouanine and Lhermitte (1965) exhibited a disturbance in written language, there being a severe disorder in spontaneous writing, writing to dictation, and copying in over half of their subjects. Furthermore, copied writing only was possible in 25% of their cases. Dysorthographia (the misspellings often being based on phonetic disturbance) was also observed in the spontaneous writing and writing to dictation of a number (5 out of 32) of their child cases with acquired aphasia. The writing disorder observed in his subjects was described by Hécaen (1976) as one of the most frequent, most persistent and most variable of all the symptoms of acquired childhood aphasia.

According to the historic description, acquired childhood aphasia is rare, with affected individuals making rapid recovery. The stated rarity (e.g., Cotard, 1868; Denckla, 1979) was in part contributed to by the observation that children who do exhibit acquired aphasia also show rapid recovery of language skills. Bernhardt (1885) stated that childhood aphasia was not rare but because the aphasia was of a transient nature and rarely permanent it often was not reported. In support of Berhardt (1885), Nadoreczny (1926, cited in Guttmann, 1942) also noted that most cases of acquired childhood aphasia recover within a few weeks. The recovery of language in acquired childhood aphasia, however, varies among children. Some children appear to go through the normal language development process as they regain their language skills whereas others skip developmental stages during the recovery process (Basser, 1962; Byers & McLean, 1962). Satz and Bullard-Bates (1981) carried out a comprehensive review of the literature up to 1978 to investigate several aspects of the historic description of acquired childhood aphasia including its purported rarity and rapid recovery. Overall, the findings of their review demonstrated that, although spontaneous recovery is dramatic in the majority of cases, 25 to 50% of reviewed cases still presented with aphasia more than one year postonset clearly illustrating the need to review traditional descriptions of acquired childhood aphasia. On the basis of their review, Satz and Bullard-Bates (1981) stated that if the lesion is unilateral and encroaches on the speech areas then childhood aphasias are not rare. They noted, however, a lower prevalence of unilateral vascular disease in children as compared with adults. Furthermore, they concluded that if the left hemisphere is damaged the risk of language impairment is approximately the same in right-handed children as in adults. Regardless of age (at least after infancy), the risk of acquired aphasia is substantially greater following left-sided rather than right-sided lesions. Finally, they concluded that crossed aphasias, although rare, do exist in left-handed children regardless of age. Since the early 1980s, therefore, it has been recognized that childhood acquired aphasia is not as rare as previously thought and despite the rapid recovery seen in some cases, a sizeable proportion (25 to 50%) of children with acquired aphasia still exhibit aphasic symptoms one-year postonset.

Contemporary Descriptions of Acquired Childhood Aphasia

Since the landmark publication of Woods and Teuber (1978) documenting the unexpected finding of jargon aphasia in a 5-year-old boy, systematic studies of acquired childhood aphasia have refuted the historic description of this disorder showing that: (a) although the majority of cases exhibit a nonfluent type of aphasia, all types of aphasia may be exhibited by children including fluent aphasia, jargon aphasia, and disturbances of oral comprehension (Klein, Masur, Farber, Shinnar, & Rapin, 1992; Paquier & van Dongen, 1996; van Dongen, Paquier, Creten, Borsel, & Catsman-Berrevoets, 2001; Van Hout & Lyon, 1986); (b) positive aphasic symptoms may occur such as paraphasias, circumlocutions, perseverations, and so forth (Van Hout, Evrard, & Lyon, 1985); (c) the extent of recovery does not clearly correlate with age at onset; (d) crossed aphasia does not occur more frequently in children than in adults, and in normal circumstances language develops in the left hemisphere from the outset (Mariën, Paquier, Engelborghs, & De Deyn, 2001; Martins & Ferro, 1997); (e) anatomoclinical correlations are identical in children to those found in adults (Cranberg, Filley, Hart, & Alexander, 1987; van Dongen, Loonen, & van Dongen, 1985; van Dongen et al., 2001); and (f) acquired childhood aphasia does not always show good recovery, with persistent language problems continuing in some cases (Martins, 2004).

Clinical Presentation of Acquired Childhood Aphasia: Nonfluent Versus Fluent

Although traditional neurological tenets claim that the clinical picture of acquired childhood aphasia is nonfluent irrespective of lesion site, over the past three decades a number of case reports of fluent acquired childhood aphasia have demonstrated that the historic views on the uniformity of the clinical picture of acquired childhood aphasia are obsolete (Mariën, Abutalebi, Engelborghs, & De Deyn, 2005; Martins, Ferro, & Castro-Caldas, 1981; Paquier, van Maldeghem, van Dongen, & Creten, 2004; van Dongen et al., 1985; van Dongen et al., 2001;

Van Hout et al., 1985; Van Hout & Lyon, 1986; Visch-Brink & van de Sandt-Koenderman, 1984; Woods & Teuber, 1978). Indeed, a variety of different aphasia types in addition to traditional nonfluent aphasia, have been reported in cases of acquired childhood aphasia including jargon, Wernicke, transcortical sensory, anomic, and conduction aphasia. For example, Woods and Teuber (1978) reported jargon aphasia in a 5-year-old boy, pointing out that the clinical picture of acquired childhood aphasia was not as homogeneous as previously thought. Martins and Ferro (1991) based on an examination of 33 children with acquired aphasia reported cases of Wernicke, transcortical sensory, conduction, and anomic aphasia. Three cases of Wernicke aphasia in young girls aged 9 to 11 years were reported by van Dongen et al. (1985). In two of these latter cases, the acute language disorder eventually progressed from a Wernicke-like presentation toward that of a conduction aphasia. Several other authors also have described conduction aphasia in children, thereby providing further evidence of the heterogeneous clinical presentation of acquired childhood aphasia (Martins & Ferro, 1987; Van Hout et al., 1985). Further examples of anomic aphasia documented in children with acquired aphasia include those reported by Klein et al., (1992), Van Hout (1993), and Hynd, Leathern, Semrud-Clikeman, Hern, and Wenner (1995).

A fluent aphasia was reported by van Dongen et al. (1985) in 3 of the 27 acquired aphasic children referred to their clinic over a four-year period. Their findings demonstrated that an adult-like fluent aphasia can occur in children less than 10 years of age and consequently they challenged the view that acquired aphasia is always non-fluent and devoid of paraphasias. Although all three subjects with fluent aphasia had posterior lesions, van Dongen et al. (1985) emphasized that posterior lesions do not invariably result in fluent aphasia in children.

A case of Wernicke aphasia in a 10-year-old boy resulting from herpes simplex encephalitis was described by Van Hout and Lyon (1986). The symptoms exhibited by this case were similar to those associated with Wernicke aphasia in adults and included a severe comprehension deficit, jargon output, logorrhea, and anosognosia. The recovery pattern exhibited by this case resembled the pattern described for a sensory aphasia by Buckingham and Kertesz (1974). His rapid recovery of writing skills was atypical of that usually reported for cases of acquired childhood aphasias. Thus, the case as described by Van Hout and Lyon (1986) differs considerably from the usual case of acquired childhood aphasia where logorrhea and anosognosia are rare and writing disorders are one of the more persistent language deficits. Van Hout and Lyon (1986) attributed the Wernicke aphasia observed in their subject to the nature of the lesion itself and not to the age of the subject. In herpes simplex encephalitis, the lesions are profoundly destructive (Barringer, 1978) and consequently this condition causes more severe lesions in the temporal lobes than seen in other varieties of lesions that affect the brain in childhood.

Positive Aphasia Signs: Neologisms, Paraphasias, Perseverations, and so forth

Although the majority of historic descriptions of acquired childhood aphasia, such as those reported by Bernhardt

(1885), Guttmann (1942), Alajouanine and Lhermitte (1965), and Hécaen (1976) stressed the absence or rarity of receptive (termed "positive signs" by Van Hout et al., 1985) speech disorders such as paraphasias, logorrhea, and perseveration, especially in children under 10 years of age, this claim frequently has been contradicted in more recent studies that have documented the occurrence of these features in the spontaneous speech and test responses of children with acquired aphasia (Paquier & van Dongen, 1991; Van Hout et al., 1985; Van Hout & Lyon, 1986;). Consequently, although the rarity of paraphasic errors and logorrhea was once thought to illustrate the unique character of acquired childhood aphasia compared to adult aphasia, the findings of recent studies suggest a need to re-appraise the traditional concept of the clinical features of acquired aphasia in children.

As pointed out by Visch-Brink and van de Sandt-Koenderman (1984), the term "rarity" when used to describe the presence of paraphasias in cases of acquired childhood aphasia appears to be used somewhat loosely in the literature. Alajouanine and Lhermitte (1965), who stressed the "rarity" of paraphasias, actually observed paraphasic errors in the spontaneous speech of 7 out of the 32 children with acquired aphasia in their study. Likewise, Gloning and Hift (1970) observed paraphasias in the spontaneous speech of 4 out of 8 of their acquired aphasic children. Included among Guttmann's (1942) subjects were 4 cases described extensively, 2 cases of whom produced paraphasias (1 child for at least a year postonset).

Visch-Brink and van de Sandt-Koenderman (1984) found that, of the 14 children with acquired aphasia they studied, the spontaneous speech of 8 was marked by the occurrence of paraphasias: 4 of these children were reported in detail, with their aphasia classified according to type (fluent/nonfluent/mixed) and their paraphasic errors categorized as literal, verbal, and neologism. They concluded that paraphasias could not be regarded as rare in their sample of children with acquired aphasia as over half of the children produced paraphasias in their spontaneous speech and a single child could produce many paraphasias. Moreover, paraphasias occurred in all forms of aphasia including fluent, nonfluent, and mixed aphasias.

Van Hout et al. (1985) examined from onset of aphasia or emergence from coma 16 children with acquired aphasia, 11 of whom (ranging in age from 4 to 10.8 years) presented with "nonclassic" symptoms. These authors also found paraphasias in the language output of the children once speech reappeared after a period of initial mutism. Indeed, Van Hout et al. (1985) suggested that paraphasias are the rule rather than the exception in acquired childhood aphasia. Furthermore, in half of the cases they studied, paraphasic errors were not limited only to the acute stage postonset. They divided their subjects into three groups according to the evolution of paraphasias over time. In one group the paraphasic errors resolved within a few days; in the second group paraphasia resolved in a few months; and in the third group paraphasia was still present at greater than one-year postonset.

Although it is not immediately clear why the clinical features of acquired childhood aphasia reported by earlier researchers (e.g., Alajouanine & Lhermitte, 1965) differ from those of more recent workers (e.g., van Dongen et al.,

1985), several explanations have been proposed. One possible reason for the disparity could be the difference in the time postonset that the subjects were examined in the different studies. For instance, Visch-Brink and van de Sandt-Koenderman (1984) suggested that it is possible that the presence or absence of neologisms in the spontaneous speech output of children with acquired aphasia might be related to the time postonset that the subjects were examined. In their study, the subjects were examined within a few days postonset of aphasia and neologisms were recorded. On the other hand Alajouanine and Lhermitte (1965) made their observations a number of months postonset and did not report the presence of neologisms in the spontaneous speech of their acquired aphasic children. It is possible therefore, that by the time that Alajouanine and Lhermitte (1965) examined their subjects, a number of symptoms including the presence of neologism, may have disappeared. Van Hout et al. (1985) also suggested that the time postonset may be a factor underlying the disparity between the earlier and more recent studies in terms of whether so called positive signs such as paraphasias, perseveration, stereotypics, etc. were recorded or not. As they observed that some positive signs persisted long after the acute stage in half of the cases they studied, Van Hout et al. (1985) believed that the time postonset of the language examination does not wholly account for the difference in clinical signs described in the earlier versus more recent studies of acquired childhood aphasia.

Another possible reason for the variation in clinical features of acquired childhood aphasia reported in earlier versus more recent studies lies in the nature of the criteria used to select the aphasic subjects. In many earlier studies, subjects were only included if they had a concomitant hemiparesis or hemiplegia, as this was taken as being indicative of the presence of brain damage and hence served to delineate acquired aphasia from developmental language disorders. As pointed out by Woods and Teuber (1978), however, such a selection criterion could result in a bias toward children with anterior lesions and hence a motor-type of aphasia. It is possible, therefore, that this could explain the lack of paraphasias, logorrhea, etc. reported in many earlier studies of acquired childhood aphasia.

van Dongen et al. (1985) suggested that differences in etiology may provide another reason for the discrepancy between reports. They believed that when the etiology is head trauma, recovery may be observed within a short time, so that the fluent characteristics of the aphasia may be either not recognized or not recorded.

Van Hout et al. (1985) proposed that variations in methodology could best account for the differences between their findings and the descriptions of acquired childhood aphasia in earlier studies. As in the majority of other reports, their subjects were also reluctant to speak. If Van Hout et al. (1985) had limited their study simply to a clinical examination of spontaneous speech, as many of their earlier researchers had done, they believed that positive signs such as paraphasias, logorrhea, and so forth would have been "masked" by the children's lack of spontaneity or mutism. They suggested that it was the testing itself and the encouragement they provided that enabled the acquired aphasic children in their sample to overcome their unwillingness to speak and thereby produce the observed positive signs.

Auditory Comprehension Abilities

As stated earlier, the first reports of acquired childhood aphasia noted the rarity or absence of auditory comprehension deficits. More recent studies, however, have reported the presence of transitory comprehension deficits. For instance, Hécaen (1976, 1983) and Alajouanine and Lhermitte (1965) observed transitory comprehension problems in one-third of the children with acquired aphasia that they examined. In contrast to other early authors Guttmann (1942) was one of the first to report "disturbed auditory comprehension" in two out of his 14 subjects with acquired childhood aphasia. In one of the cases, after a temporoparietal lesion, the comprehension deficit was the major symptom of the aphasia. Guttmann (1942) warned, however, that comprehension difficulties could be "disregarded" unless expressive language deficits were also present.

Of the 32 children studied by Alajouanine and Lhermitte (1965) only 10 were noted to have auditory comprehension deficits. These deficits were "marked" in only four of the 10 cases. In all these cases by 6 months after the lesion, comprehension had returned to "near normal" with difficulties encountered only on the most difficult tasks. One-year postonset no auditory comprehension difficulties were noted in any of the ten subjects. Alajouanine and Lhermitte (1965) had divided their 32 subjects into two age groups. In the youngest age group (5 to 9 years old) nearly all (8 out of 9 cases) had comprehension deficits in the initial stages, whereas in the second age group (10 to 15 years old) only two subjects of the 23 had auditory comprehension deficits. Comprehension deficits from this study, therefore, appear more common in children who acquired a brain lesion before 10 years of age.

Hécaen (1983) reviewed 26 children with acquired aphasia between 3.5 and 15 years of age and found no support for the difference between the number of cases with comprehension difficulties in children above and below 10 years of age noted by Alajouanine and Lhermitte (1965). Although Hécaen observed that there were more cases of auditory comprehension deficits in children with left-sided lesions who were less than 10 years of age (i.e., 6 of 14 cases—42%) than in children older than 10 years of age (6 out of 20 cases—30%) this difference was not statistically significant. Neither was there any significant difference in the number of cases with comprehension impairments in relation to sites of lesion (i.e., frontorolandic or temporal) nor cause of lesion (i.e., hematoma, trauma, or tumor/abscess) in the cases studied by Hécaen, although he noted a trend for more cases of comprehension impairment following an anterior lesion or a rapid onset.

The cause most commonly associated with auditory comprehension disorders in children with acquired aphasia is convulsive disorder (Landau & Kleffner, 1957; Miller, Campbell, Chapman, & Weismer, 1984; Rapin, Mattis, Rowan, & Golden, 1977; Worster-Drought, 1971). The nature of these auditory comprehension deficits is discussed further in Chapter 9.

Early studies reporting the nature of comprehension deficits in children with acquired aphasia usually used subjective and/or descriptive notes on the deficits often without reference to the development level of competence expected in the child. Later studies, while using objective assessment procedures (usually versions of the Token Test), tended to cite unitary scores. Only in the most recent publications are the descriptive and standardized assessment methods combined in an effort to understand the nature of the auditory comprehension disorders. These early descriptions contained in case studies demonstrate the variable nature of auditory comprehension deficits seen in children with acquired aphasia. Oelschlaeger and Scarborough (1976) described a 10-year-old child who was "unable to comprehend auditorily any speech stimuli" (p. 283) following a fall from a horse. After therapy, 1-year postonset she still presented with significantly impaired receptive and expressive language skills but was able to answer questions on current activities appropriately.

Severe comprehension difficulties postonset (e.g., inability to identify parts of the face) were also described by Pohl (1979) in a 6-year-old child after a suspected occlusion of the middle cerebral artery. Four months postonset, comprehension had returned to normal while expressive language was at a one to two word level. Visch-Brink and van de Sandt-Koenderman (1984) described four cases with differing degrees of comprehension impairment immediately postonset. The first case scored 37 of a possible 61 on the Token Test (De Renzi & Vignolo, 1962) soon after a subdural empyema. This score improved to 44 correct, 6 weeks later and to 53 of 61 correct 5 months postonset, at which stage the child's expressive language was characterized by mild syntactic difficulties and resolving paraphasias. The

second case recovered comprehension and expressive skills within 14 days of a head trauma. Before recovery mild comprehension difficulties, telegraphic speech and paraphasias were evident. The other two cases presented with severe comprehension deficits. One of the two cases also had long runs of unintelligible speech and showed very slow recovery in both areas of language whereas the other presented with "empty speech" characterized by strings of disconnected words then periods of adequate speech, paraphasias, and paragrammatisms.

Formal assessment results in individual cases of children with auditory comprehension deficits as part of their aphasia, also emphasizes the variable nature of the deficits and the recovery process reported above in the descriptive studies. Van Hout and Lyon (1986) described a 10-year-old boy with a severe comprehension deficit as part of a Wernicke aphasia following herpes simplex encephalitis. In the early stages the child scored below five standard deviations from his age-matched test mean on the Gaddes and Crockett (1975) norms of the Spreen-Benton Neurosensory Center Comprehensive Examination for Aphasia (NCCEA) (Spreen & Benton, 1969). Eight months later he was scoring a 6-year age level for syntactic comprehension but could only identify an object by name 60% of the time. Another 10-year-old child, described by Dennis (1980), presented on the Identification by Name and Sentence subtests of the NCCEA at below the 6-year age level 2 weeks after a cerebrovascular accident. Three months after the accident, Identification by Name was at an age-appropriate level but Identification by Sentence was still at the original 6-year age level. Descriptive notes stated that 3 months after the cerebrovascular accident the subject understood single words and short commands. Test results indicated that comprehension and expressive skills were developing in parallel.

Two cases with subcortical lesions were reported by Aram, Rose, Rekate, and Whitaker, (1983). Only one of the cases had comprehension deficits. These deficits resolved within 2 months. Initially the subject (7 years old) had exhibited an 18-month delay on the Peabody Picture Vocabulary Test (PPVT) (Dunn, 1965) and a 2½-year delay on the Northwestern Syntax Screening Test (NWSST): Receptive (Lee, 1971). The authors suggested that the language deficit, including the moderate comprehension impairment noted in one subject but not in the other, was related to the site of the subcortical lesion.

van Dongen et al. (1985), however, described differing degrees of comprehension impairment in three girls with similar lesion sites, all of which involved Wernicke's area. All three subjects presented with a fluent aphasia. The cause in two cases was trauma, and both of these showed rapid recovery. One of the head trauma subjects had normal conversational comprehension 13 days postonset. The results of her Token Test, however, revealed auditory comprehension deficits as she scored 28 correct of a possible 61 on the test. By 2½ months postonset, both conversational and test performance comprehension were within normal limits. A faster recovery period was noted in the second head trauma subject. Her Token Test results were 52 of 61 and her conversational comprehension was within normal limits 12 days postonset. Initially, she had presented with marked comprehension impairments both on the test results

(i.e., 13 of 61 correct) and in conversation. She also presented as anomic in spontaneous speech. The third subject described by van Dongen et al. (1985) had a suspected hematoma and 2 months later developed convulsions. Although before the onset of convulsions she scored 6 of 10 correct on the easiest part of the Token Test, once the convulsions had commenced this subject could not be assessed using formal test procedures, even though she could understand simple commands. Her expressive language at this stage was described as being comprised of simple words spoken in a telegraphic style. No improvement was noted over the next 2 years.

Studies, using either descriptive or standardized assessment procedures, have demonstrated a range of auditory comprehension deficits in children with acquired aphasia. These findings are contrary to those of the early reports which either suggested that comprehension disorders did not exist in cases of acquired childhood aphasia or they were of a transitory nature. More recent studies have compared groups of children with acquired aphasia either with a group of nonbrain-injured controls or have compared groups of right and left hemisphere-lesioned subjects. Most of these latter studies have served to emphasize the persistent nature of auditory comprehension deficits found in some children with acquired aphasia.

Van Hout et al. (1985) studied 16 children with acquired aphasia between 2 and 13 years of age. They reported that the three youngest subjects (all 2 years old) presented according to the historic description of childhood aphasia, whereas the two oldest subjects (both 13 years old) presented with Broca's aphasia. The remaining 11 subjects did not fit either pattern. They divided these 11 subjects into three groups based on their recovery from paraphasia. The first two groups whose paraphasias resolved either within days or months presented with moderate comprehension deficits, whereas the third group who had paraphasias lasting more than 1 year postonset, presented with severe comprehension impairments. The authors noted that the most common cause in this last group was infection. Decreased receptive language skills or global aphasia were also described as the initial communication deficits in the four children with infections described by Cooper and Flowers (1987). Initial comprehension deficits, however, were noted in their subjects with anoxia, closed head injury, and tumors.

The assessment of Cooper and Flowers' (1987) 15 brain-lesioned children (between 10 and 18 years of age) was carried out 3 to 12 years postonset. When compared with a control group without brain injury the experimental group performed significantly poorer on all assessments of language comprehension. Despite performing significantly poorer on the assessments than a group of controls, Cooper and Flowers (1987) emphasized the heterogeneity of the group pointing out that one subject showed no impairment on any language test whereas three subjects showed impairment on all expressive as well as receptive tests. For this reason they gave individual assessment profiles for all 15 brain-injured subjects. Nine subjects scored greater than two standard deviations below the age mean on the Peabody Picture Vocabulary Test-Revised (Dunn & Dunn, 1981). Of the nine subjects two subjects scored greater than seven deviations below. On the shortened version of the Token Test (De Renzi & Faglioni, 1978) seven of the 15 subjects scored greater than two standard deviations below the mean; however, Cooper and Flowers (1987) claimed that only one of these could be described as having a moderate comprehension deficit. As a group, the brain-lesioned subjects did not perform significantly different from the controls on Parts 1 to 5 of the test; however, there was a statistically significant difference between the scores of the experimental and control groups on Part 6 of the test. This would indicate that as a group, the brain-lesioned subjects had no more difficulty than the control group with the increase in syntactical information load but had more difficulty with increased linguistic complexity.

The proposed difficulties with syntactical complexity is supported by the individual case profiles published by Cooper and Flowers (1987) which showed that their brain-injured subjects had most difficulty with the items containing the instructions "in addition to, if, between" and the item "touch the blue circle *with* the red square." Only one subject had difficulty with the earlier parts of the test. Six of the 15 subjects reported by Cooper and Flowers (1987) had difficulties with the Processing Spoken Paragraphs subtest of the Clinical Evaluation of Language Function (CELF) (Semel & Wiig, 1980). In all cases the authors noted that the subjects appeared to comprehend the questions asked but were unable to recall the appropriate information. Overall, three subjects presented with deficits in all three areas of comprehension assessed; two had problems in lexical and auditory language comprehension; two had problems in lexical and comprehension of contextual language whereas four subjects had one area only of deficit, two in lexical comprehension and one each in auditory language and comprehension of contextual language. No relationships between these results and the side, site, size or cause of the lesion nor the age at injury or after the lesion could be drawn as the subjects differed too widely on all these variables. The study, however, showed conclusively that after a mean length of time postonset of 8 years, residual comprehension deficits were still shown by all but three of Cooper and Flowers (1987) 15 subjects.

Another series of studies have investigated the influence of the side of lesion on comprehension abilities in children with acquired aphasia. Most of these studies have included children who received their brain lesions perinatally or within a few months of birth. Therefore any deficits found when brain-lesioned children are compared with a control group would support the notion of persisting deficits of auditory comprehension.

Twenty-eight children with left hemisphere lesions and 25 with right hemisphere lesions were assessed using the Token Test 2 years postonset (Vargha-Khadem, Gorman, & Watters, 1985). A significant difference was found between the side of the lesion, with the children who had left hemisphere lesions performing more poorly than those with right-sided lesions. The Token Test scores did not correlate with the WISC-R digit span subtest score, leading the authors to conclude that this was a linguistic not a memory deficit. The scores of the children with right hemisphere lesions did not differ from the control group. Vargha-Khadem et al. (1985) also divided the side of the lesion groups into three subgroups based on age at the time of the lesions, that is, prenatal, early postnatal (2 months to 5 years) and late postnatal (5 to 14 years). There was a

trend that the later the injury occurred the greater was the impairment of auditory comprehension.

Significant differences between the auditory comprehension skills of children with right and left hemisphere lesions were also found by Rankin, Aram, and Horwitz (1981). Lexical comprehension measured using PPVT showed that right hemiplegics performed more poorly than left hemiplegics. This pattern of performance was repeated on the measures of syntactic comprehension using NWSST: Receptive (Lee, 1971) and the Token Test, that is, the right hemiplegics performing less well than the left hemiplegics. A closer examination of the components of the Token Test showed that the left hemiplegics showed a progressive decline in correct scores across the five parts of the test whereas the right hemiplegics showed no errors in Part 1 of the Token Test but their performance deteriorated across Parts 2 to 4 with the increase in information load. The right hemiplegics, however, improved their performance on Part 5 which showed they did not have difficulty with syntactic complexity per se. This is in contrast to the findings of Cooper and Flowers (1987).

Aram, Ekelman, Rose, and Whitaker (1985) compared the comprehension skills of children with right and left unilateral brain lesions. Each group of brain-lesioned children was matched to an appropriate control group. Some children had acquired their brain lesions in the first few months of life while others were 18 months to 6 years of age at the time of the lesion. On the PPVT all left-lesioned children scored within the normal range but five of eight scored lower than their control subjects. Similarly, the right-lesioned subjects performed more poorly than their controls. As a group, the left-lesioned subjects performed higher than the right-lesioned subjects. On the NWSST:Receptive the left-lesioned subjects performed less well than their controls whereas there was no difference between the right-lesioned group and their controls.

In another study using the Revised Token Test (McNeil & Prescott, 1978), Aram and Ekelman (1987) assessed the effect of unilateral brain lesions on auditory comprehension skills. In addition they also assessed the effect of the site of lesion and the age at lesion onset on those skills. Seventeen children with left lesions and 11 children with right-sided unilateral lesions between 6 and 17 years of age were assessed. Significant differences between the right- and left-lesioned groups and their respective controls were found for all 10 subtests of the Revised Token Test. As a whole the left-lesioned group performed similarly to their controls on subtests one to three and subtest nine. In subtest 10 the left-lesion group appeared to use a memory strategy to enable them to remember the instructions. Aram and Ekelman (1987) concluded that the left-lesioned group presented with memory difficulties that affected their performance as the information load increased. The right-lesioned group, however, made more errors than their controls but there was no difference in the number of errors with the increase in information or linguistic loading. The authors suggested that this reflected the more impulsive nature of the right-lesioned group. In relation to site of lesion, there was a trend for more errors on the Token Test in the children with left retrorolandic rather than prerolandic lesions. No difference in performance was noted in the site of the right hemisphere lesions or the presence or absence of subcortical lesions. In general, the

earlier the left hemisphere lesions occurred (i.e., less than 1 year of age) the poorer the performance on the Revised Token Test. The reverse was true, however, for right hemisphere lesions. The results for the left hemisphere lesions were in contrast to the results of Vargha-Khadem et al. (1985) who found greater deficits the older the child was at the time of the lesion.

In conclusion, auditory comprehension deficits do exist in children with acquired aphasia, particularly when the brain-lesioned subjects are compared with a group of matched controls. These deficits, although of a subtle nature, occur even when the lesions are acquired at an early age. The extent of the comprehension impairment is variable, as is its recovery. The differences found between right and left hemisphere-lesioned subjects would suggest that side of lesion may influence the level and type of impairment. Further research into the etiology of acquired aphasia is required to determine the influence of cause, size and site of lesion, and time postonset. Certainly, the evidence to date does not support the historical description of auditory comprehension deficits being rare and only of a transitory nature in children with acquired aphasia.

Production Deficits: Simplified Syntax/Telegraphic Speech

In the traditional description of acquired childhood aphasia, as mentioned previously, the aphasia was described as being of a nonfluent type with simplified syntax (Alajouanine & Lhermitte, 1965) or telegraphic speech (Guttmann, 1942). Alajouanine and Lhermitte (1965) noted that children with acquired aphasia tend to use simplified syntax rather than producing syntactical errors per se.

Consequently, they stated that the syntax used by children with acquired aphasia does not resemble the agrammatism seen in adults. Despite the description of simplified syntax from the earliest reports (Bernhardt, 1885) few studies have given detailed descriptions of the syntax used by children with acquired aphasia.

Cooper and Flowers (1987) examined 15 brain-injured children who had acquired neurologic damage between 2 and 12 years of age and were at least 1-year postonset at the time of the study. As a group these brain-injured children scored significantly poorer than a matched control group on the Producing Formulated Sentences subtest of the CELF (Semel & Wiig, 1980). Cooper and Flowers (1987), however, observed a wide variety of language skills within the brain-injured group. Of the 15 subjects, only one achieved a score greater than two standard deviations below the test mean. By examining the case descriptions supplied by Cooper and Flowers (1987) it appears that most syntactical errors were made on the items which required complex sentence structures (i.e., "because," "if," "herself"). Cooper and Flowers (1987) also provided examples of syntactically correct complex sentences produced by these same subjects. These correct sentences, however, tended to have a more stereotypic quality (e.g., "If I tell you, do you promise to keep it a secret? I'll tell my parents about what has gone on at school. I will tell her I'm hungry"). Some acquired aphasia subjects produced agrammatical sentences (e.g., "Himself and herself is a boy or is a gal") whereas others produced simple or incomplete sentences (e.g., "Because today is rainy and wet") perhaps suggesting a semantic rather than syntactic impairment.

A series of studies by Aram and co-workers are the only ones reported that have systematically looked at productive syntactic skills in children with unilateral brain lesions. It should be noted, however, that most of Aram's subjects acquired brain lesions early in life, before they began talking. It was claimed by Aram and her co-workers that children who suffer left hemisphere lesions shortly after birth are at risk for syntactical impairment. Their reasons for this claim was the observation of significant differences between the syntactical abilities of appropriately matched controls and children with left hemisphere lesions and between children with either left or right hemisphere lesions.

Rankin et al. (1981) found three right-hemiplegic children to be markedly below three left-hemiplegic children on the NWSST. A later study by Aram et al. (1985) comparing eight children with right hemisphere lesions and eight with left hemisphere lesions and two appropriate control groups showed that the children with right hemisphere lesions did not differ from their controls on any syntactic measure except for mean length of utterance. The children with left hemisphere lesions, however, differed from their controls on all measures of syntactical skill including the NWSST and measures based on a spontaneous language sample (e.g., mean length of utterance (MLU) and a Developmental Sentence Score (Lee, 1974)). Examination of individual scores of the children with left hemisphere lesions showed that no subject in this group scored higher than the 18th percentile on the NWSST:Expressive.

An extension of this study by Aram, Ekelman, and Whitaker (1986) undertook more detailed analyses of the spontaneous language samples by the eight left- and eight right-lesioned subjects. These analyses showed that the left hemisphere-lesioned subjects performed more poorly than their controls on most measures of simple and complex sentences while the right-lesioned group was similar to their controls in most measures of syntactical ability. The two lesioned groups differed from each other on measures of MLU, mean number of interrogative reversals and "wh-" questions, the percentage of complex sentences attempted, the percentage of complex sentences correct, the number of embedded sentences attempted and the percentage of embedded sentences correct. The right-lesioned subjects differed from their controls on MLU, percentage of all sentences correct, the percentage of simple sentences correct, the total number of main verbs used, the mean number of negatives used and the grammatical markers in error (GME). The only syntactical measures on which the left-lesioned subjects did not differ from their controls were the total number of negatives used, and the use of pronouns or conjunctions. In addition, it was noted that although the left-lesioned group performed more poorly than their controls on most measures of syntax, they did use more simple sentences reflecting their reduced use of complex sentences. Aram, Ekelman, and Whitaker (1986) suggested that these findings are indicative of a developmental immaturity on the part of the left-lesioned subjects. At the same time, the right-lesion group produced a small percentage of their simple sentences correctly when compared with their controls, even though they attempted the same number of simple sentences. Both of these counts were different

between the left-lesion group and their controls. The obviously poorer performance on the left-lesioned subjects when compared with their controls and when compared with the right-lesioned group and their controls is indicative of a susceptibility for expressive syntactic impairments in children with unilateral left hemisphere lesions.

Production Deficits: Expressive Semantic

Two outstanding aspects of expressive semantics are commonly noted in the historic description of acquired childhood aphasia. The first is the presence and often persistence of naming disorders whereas the second is the absence or rarity of paraphasias, jargon and logorrhea discussed in the section on "Positive Aphasia Signs" above. As Carrow-Woolfolk and Lynch (1982) state, "once speech re-emerges children may have name-finding difficulties but they do not display the paraphasic or misnaming symptoms characteristic of adults" (p. 334). (Receptive semantics has been discussed under auditory comprehension.)

Naming disorders in children with acquired aphasia have been described by Hécaen (1983) as frequent and persistent, and are often noted in school reports. He found 15 of his 34 subjects with acquired aphasia (i.e., 44%), between 3.5 and 15 years of age, to have naming disorders. No significant difference was found in the number of subjects with naming disorders when examined for site or cause of lesion or for the age of the subject. In an earlier study of 15 subjects, Hécaen (1976) found naming disorders in seven cases, three of whom showed persistent problems.

Cooper and Flowers (1987) reported a significant difference between the scores achieved by children with acquired aphasia (between 10 and 18 years of age) and those achieved by a non-brain-damaged group on the Boston Naming Test (Kaplan, Goodglass, & Weintraub, 1983), including latency of response, and the Producing Word Associations subtest of the CELF. As their subjects were assessed between 3 and 12 years postonset their findings support the fact that naming difficulties can be of a persistent nature in children with acquired aphasia.

van Dongen and Visch-Brink (1988) also reported severe naming disorders in their six left hemisphere-lesioned children with acquired aphasia in the initial stages. The recovery from the naming disorder, however, differed between a head-injured group and a nonhead-injured group. In the head-injured group recovery was complete within 6 months while the non-head-injured group could not complete a naming test 1 month postonset and recovery was still not complete 1-year postonset. Meanwhile, six subjects with a right hemisphere lesion had scores on the Boston Naming Test within normal limits immediately postonset. The complete recovery of naming abilities in the head-injured population is in contrast to the findings of Jordan, Ozanne, & Murdoch (1988, 1990) (see Ch. 3).

Differences in naming abilities between subjects with right and left hemisphere lesions and control groups have been investigated by several other authors. Also using the Boston Naming Test, Kiessling, Denckla, and Carlton (1983) found that the mean scores for their right and left brain-lesioned children were lower than those for a sibling control group. This difference, however, was not statistically significant, neither was the difference between the Boston Naming Test scores achieved by children with right compared with left-brain lesions. Two studies using the Oldfield and Wingfield Object Naming Test (Oldfield & Wingfield, 1964) however, did find significant differences between controls and brain-lesioned children. Woods and Carey (1979) reported lower scores for children sustaining a left-sided brain lesion after 1 year of age when compared with a nonlesioned control group. Although a difference between children sustaining a brain lesion before 1 year of age, when compared with controls, was not found by Woods and Carey (1979), such a difference was found by Vargha-Khadem et al. (1985) who also used the Oldfield and Wingfield Naming Test. This difference was evident in Vargha-Khadem et al. (1985) prenatal, early postnatal (i.e., the lesion occurring between 2 months and 5 years of age), and late postnatal (i.e., 5 to 14 years of age), left hemisphere-lesioned groups as well as the early postnatal right hemisphere-lesioned group. The results of their study also indicated that the naming disorders were more marked the later the age at which the lesion occurred.

Rankin et al. (1981) compared the language abilities of three right and three left hemiplegic children between 6 and 8 years of age and found no differences between the two groups on the Naming Fluency subtest of the Boston Diagnostic Aphasia Examination (Goodglass & Kaplan, 1972). Two studies by Aram and co-workers, however, found slightly different results. Using the Expressive One-Word Picture Vocabulary Test (EOWPVT) (Gardner, 1979), Aram et al. (1985) found that both right and left hemisphere-lesioned children between 18 months and 8 years of age performed more poorly than their appropriate controls; however, this difference was only statistically significant for the left-lesioned subjects. Aram et al. (1985) noted the wide variation in individual scores in both the lesioned groups. A greater number of subjects with unilateral brain lesions (*n* = 32) between 6 and 17 years of age were assessed by Aram, Ekelman, and Whitaker (1987) to try to clarify the results of the previous studies. Two measures of lexical retrieval were used: the Word-Finding Test (Wiegel-Crump & Dennis, 1984) and the Rapid Automatized Naming Test (RAN) (Denckla & Rudel, 1976). The results indicated that children with left hemisphere lesions required a longer latency to respond than their controls. The type of lexical access on the Word-Finding Test affected the results. For example, rhyming cues produced more errors and longer latencies than semantic or visual cues; however, this was also the general pattern seen in children developing normally and the control groups used in the study. The left hemisphere-lesioned group was also slower to respond for the RAN, having greater difficulty naming objects and colors than letters and numbers. The right hemisphere-lesioned subjects, on the other hand, produced more errors than their controls but did not require a longer latency. In fact, the right-lesioned group responded faster than their controls on all access conditions of the Word-Finding Test. Aram et al. (1987) suggested that a speed-accuracy trade-off occurred with the right-lesioned group. In addition, the right hemisphere-lesioned subjects had more errors that could be attributed to visual processing difficulties. These results led Aram et al.

(1987) to postulate that left hemisphere-lesioned subjects have lexical retrieval problems while errors seen in the right-lesioned group could be attributed to impulsivity or visual processing difficulties. Aram et al. (1987) also looked at the effects of lesion site and age at time of lesion on naming disorders and concluded that various sites of lesions in the left hemisphere can produce word access problems and that there was no clear relationship between degree of lexical retrieval impairment and age at lesion onset.

Production Deficits: Pragmatics

There is a lack of research relating to the pragmatic skills of children with acquired aphasia. Despite that, the presence of pragmatic problems in this population can be determined from a number of reports in the literature that suggest that soon after the onset of aphasia or in connection with the mute phase, children with acquired aphasia are reluctant to communicate (see, "Historical Perspective" above). For instance, Cooper and Flowers (1987) noted that one of their participants (10 years 3 months old) did not initiate any conversation and only rarely spoke during testing when assessed 6 years postonset of anoxic encephalopathy.

Cooper and Flowers (1987) also described one other child with acquired aphasia who had "unusual or inappropriate usage of language" (p. 259). This subject, a 15-year, 6-months male, often focused on inappropriate topics such as sex, bathrooms, marriage, or death. Irrelevant statements on the above topics often occurred when he was attempting to respond to a task. This was the only subject studied by Cooper and Flowers

(1987) who was intellectually impaired following encephalitis 11 years previously. Therefore, it is unclear in this case whether the observed pragmatic problem resulted from a linguistic deficit or whether it was a problem related to the presence of a broader cognitive impairment.

Dennis (1980) reported an in-depth study of a nine-year-old girl 3 months after she had acquired expressive and receptive aphasia with a right hemiparesis due to an arteriopathy of the left cerebral hemisphere. Her comprehension and expressive language skills were developing in parallel. At the time of testing she was still nonfluent but was able to produce and comprehend short sentences. It was noted that this subject often avoided speech situations. Through the use of puppets, Dennis was able to encourage this subject to tell three fairy tales which were subsequently analyzed using Mandler and Johnson's (1977) story grammar procedure. From this analysis it was noted that the subject used semantically impoverished and simplified propositions and also failed to include the various episodes of the story, just giving an overall view of the plot. Dennis (1980) stated that in story retelling younger children emphasize settings, motivation for and outcomes of actions. All of these components of the story, however, were omitted by Dennis's subject, indicating that she did not follow the normal developmental pattern for the acquisition of narrative abilities.

Production Deficits: Phonology

Again the traditional description of acquired aphasia in children makes reference to the presence of concomitant speech disorders often in the form of a dysarthria or sometimes a dyspraxia (see Chapter 11).

A study by Rankin et al. (1981) comparing three right hemiplegic and three left hemiplegic subjects found no difference between the scores achieved by the two groups of subjects on the Templin Sound Discrimination Test (Templin, 1957) but the right hemiplegic group performed more poorly on the Templin-Darley Screening Test of Articulation (Templin & Darley, 1969). Most of the errors made were later developing sounds, thereby leading the authors to suggest that the speech disorder represented an articulation delay rather than dysarthria. The trend of more articulation disorders occurring in children with left unilateral brain lesions than right unilateral brain lesions was supported by Aram et al. (1985). They assessed eight left-lesioned and eight right-lesioned children and two groups of appropriate controls. Although differences between the two lesioned groups and their appropriate controls were not significant, more children in the left-lesioned group were reported to have articulation scores greater than one standard deviation below the test mean on the Photo Articulation Test (PAT) (Pendergast, Dickey, Selmar, & Soder, 1969). Examination of the individual articulation profiles of all children in the study showed that the children with left hemisphere lesions also presented with the greatest number of individual articulation errors. Although subject numbers used by Aram et al. (1985) were small and no significant differences were apparent their findings do suggest that the left hemisphere-lesioned group have more articulation errors than right-lesioned subjects. These speech errors reported by Rankin et al. (1981) and Aram et al. (1985) must be assumed to be articulation errors rather than speech errors associated with dysarthria or dyspraxia by the omission of such statements to the contrary in the two studies. The occurrence of articulatory/phonological disorders in left-lesioned subjects could be anticipated from the syntactic deficits also found in this group (see earlier in this chapter) and the close association between syntactic and phonological disorders seen in children with developmental language impairment (Rapin & Allen, 1987; Wolfus, Moscovitch, & Kinsbourne, 1980).

Written Language Impairments

Written language problems in children with acquired aphasia were described by Hécaen (1976) as the most frequent but the most variable of all aphasic symptoms seen in children in the acute stages. He also claimed that written language disorders tended to be the most persistent symptom, at times being of a permanent nature. He reported written language disabilities in 13 of his 15 subjects, seven of them having persistent problems. Similarly, Alajouanine and Lhermitte (1965) claimed that written language is always disturbed in the period soon after the brain injury is sustained. They found that written language disorders often were more severe than oral language impairments, and that expressive disorders were more frequent than receptive disorders of written language. Their longitudinal study (more than 12 months postonset) of 32 children between 6 and 15 years of age showed that no subject could follow the normal school progression even though 23 of the 32 subjects currently were attending school. The most difficult subjects for the children with acquired aphasia were those involving language skills (e.g., history, English, and foreign languages rather than mathematics). Despite their oral language skills being within normal limits, Alajouanine and Lhermitte's (1965) subjects were unable to learn new information. Byers and McLean (1962), however, attributed the poor academic performance seen in 6 of their 10 subjects with acquired childhood aphasia to visuomotor and visuospatial impairments as all the children's language skills had spontaneously improved. Recently, Cooper and Flowers (1987) assessed the academic performance of 15 brain-injured subjects between 10 and 18 years of age, 3 to 12 years postonset and found the majority of subjects to be experiencing academic difficulties. Seven of the 15 subjects were in full-time special education programs, three were receiving additional resource instruction, whereas of the remaining five in regular classrooms, only one was at a state school in an age-appropriate grade. The academic assessments used by Cooper and Flowers (1987) were the Wide Range Abilities Test (WRAT) (Jastak & Jastak, 1965) for Reading Recognition, Spelling and Arithmetic and the Peabody Individual Achievement Test (PIAT) (Dunn & Markwardt, 1970) for Reading Comprehension.

In contrast to Alajouanine and Lhermitte (1965), the subjects examined by Cooper and Flowers (1987) had most difficulty with the arithmetic subtest. Thirteen of the 14 subjects given the arithmetic subtest scored more than one standard deviation below the test mean, whereas eight scored below the test mean on spelling, five on reading comprehension and three on reading recognition. Only one subject scored below the test mean of all four academic areas and he was the only subject in the study who had cognitive skills with the intellectual handicapped range. Approximately equal numbers of subjects had impairments in one, two or three of the academic areas assessed. No descriptions of the nature of the arithmetical or reading difficulties experienced by these subjects were given by Cooper and Flowers (1987); however, six subjects with spelling difficulties made phonetic errors whereas one subject (following a left cerebrovascular accident) had difficulties with phoneme-grapheme relationships. Hécaen (1983) had also noted acalculia as a major symptom often associated with language impairments in children with acquired aphasia. Recent reviews (e.g., Zubrick, 1988) have emphasized the relationships between linguistic and mathematical skills, which may provide an explanation for the findings of Cooper and Flowers (1987) and Hécaen (1983).

In Hécaen's (1983) study of 56 children aged between 3.5 and 15 years of age he found writing disorders to be the most frequent language disorder, occurring in 63% of the 34 subjects with left hemisphere lesions. Reading problems, however, were only evident in 40% of the subjects with left hemisphere lesions. Hécaen (1983) further investigated the relationship between the number of subjects presenting with reading or writing disorders and the cause, localization of the brain injury and the age of the subject. No significant differences were found for reading disorders but a higher number of subjects under 10 years of age had writing problems (i.e., 90%) than those over 10 years (45%). Hécaen (1983) noted that reading disorders tend to be very common in the early stages postonset but then tend to disappear rapidly and completely, whereas writing disorders may persist.

Alajouanine and Lhermitte (1965) also noted the difference in written language disorders relating to the age of the subjects. All subjects less than 10 years of age presented with severe writing impairments. Although 10 subjects (of 23) over 10 years-of-age had written language comprehension problems, only three of the 10 had severe impairments. Ten subjects also had writing disorders but only four had jargon orthography. Alajouanine and Lhermitte (1965) went on to describe the nature of the written language disorders and their recovery. Eighteen of their 32 subjects presented with alexia (i.e., being totally unable to read letters, syllables or words), a further five subjects could read but had severe difficulties, whereas a further four subjects could read words but not letters. The authors noted the difference between these reading problems and those seen in adults, with only four subjects (all over 13 years of age) presenting with adult-type symptoms. The writing problems of the subjects examined by Alajouanine and Lhermitte (1965) showed a wide range of impairments, with some subjects displaying quite rapid recovery whereas others continued to have severe writing difficulties. Nineteen subjects presented with severe writing impairments in spontaneous writing, writing to dictation or copying. Eight further subjects were unable to copy, whereas a further five children were capable of dictation and spontaneous writing; however, their attempts showed a dysorthographia. These errors generally were of a phonetic nature. Another five subjects (all between 13 and 15 years of age) had jargon distortions in their written work. Six months later, half the 22 subjects assessed by Alajouanine and Lhermitte (1965) had shown improvement in their alexia whereas the other half still showed severe disorders in, or total lack of, reading. The recovery process seen in the subjects less than 10 years of age showed the reacquisition of written language skills that followed the normal developmental progression. Of the 22 subjects, five children who had initially had severe problems now had writing skills within normal limits whereas 14 still showed dysorthographia, but only seven of these cases were severe. Another three subjects had no written language abilities. In all cases, Alajouanine and Lhermitte (1965) noted that the written language skills were delayed when compared with the child's oral language skills. As noted earlier, none of these 32 subjects coped with normal school progression 12 months after their brain injury.

Similar variations in the nature of the reading and/or writing disturbances and their recovery have been noted by several other authors. Severe written language problems were described by Byers and McLean (1962) in their eight children with acquired aphasia. Immediately postonset, when their medical condition had stabilized, none of the eight children could match names and objects or write simple words to dictation, although they could copy. All were able to write letters in alphabetical sequence or numbers in numerical sequence if the sequence was started. However, they could not write or recognize letters out of context nor could they write numbers such as one hundred and twenty-three (i.e., 123). Soon after onset, some subjects could read and write everything expect difficult words whereas others could only spontaneously read a few familiar words. No explanation was given for the rapid recovery or nonrecovery of particular

subjects. Variability in this recovery process can be seen in individual case studies reported in the literature.

Reading impairments have been described in three of the 11 children (between 2 and 13 years of age) studied by Van Hout et al. (1985). One 9-year-old subject was totally unable to read and his writing consisted only of repetitive letters, whereas another subject had reading retardation as his major aphasic symptom. The third subject was described as paralexic in both reading and writing 1 year postonset. Another two subjects were described as having writing disabilities (together with naming difficulties) 3 months postonset. No further details about the nature of the written language problems were given.

Another 9-year-old subject described by Dennis (1980) presented with written language problems which quickly resolved. Two weeks after a cerebrovascular accident the subject was able to write names to objects, read names and sentences for meaning and write simple sentences to dictation; however, her impaired oral skills severely affected her reading skills, even to the point where the subject confused herself by reading instructions aloud. The poorer oral than written language skills are in contrast to those noted by Alajouanine and Lhermitte (1965). Three months postonset, Dennis's (1980) subject achieved age-appropriate scores on subtests for oral reading of simple sentences, reading names and short sentences for meaning, visual-graphic naming and writing to dictation, and copying. Generally, Dennis felt that the subject's written language skills were relatively well preserved in contrast to her oral skills which were at the level of telegraphic utterances and comprehension of simple commands. This pattern of recovery is in contrast to the persisting problems with written language noted by Hécaen (1976, 1983).

Rapid recovery of written language skills was described as unusual by Van Hout and Lyon (1986) when they reported on a 10-year-old boy presenting with Wernicke aphasia after herpes simplex encephalitis. Six days after the coma the subject was only able to make perseverative attempts at writing. Two days later he was able to read words in isolation with rare literal substitutions; however, matching words to objects was not possible. The subject's ability to read text was adequate for four to six lines only, after which perseveration started to interfere. His speed of reading was high. He was unable to tell anything about what he had read and appeared unaware of his problems. One week later his oral reading/decoding skills were normal but comprehension of the text was poor. He was able to match objects to written words better than to oral words. When the subject encountered difficult passages he would comment on the orthographical features of the words (e.g., the subject said, "There is a /p/, one must say /sap/" when he was reading the word "camp" [field]). His writing skills also showed rapid improvement. On day 6 after the coma he was only able to write simple overlearned words, however, there was perseveration of letters. Six days later he was able to write a few sentences to dictation with a few surface or grammatical errors. The legibility of his writing was good. His written naming was slightly better than his oral. In contrast to his written language skills, his arithmetical abilities through the written mode was never impaired; however, he had problems writing numbers such as three hundred and four. As this was

written 3-100-4, Van Hout and Lyon (1986) concluded that these errors were of a syntactic nature.

Three other children with fluent aphasia described by van Dongen et al. (1985) showed evidence of written language problems. A nine-year-old suffering a hematoma was only able to read four words aloud immediately postonset. No information was available for later stages. A 10-year-old showed rapid improvement in his writing to dictation skills following a craniotomy after a closed head injury. Previously, his writing had contained numerous paraphasias. Two months after craniotomy his only aphasic errors were spelling errors when he wrote to dictation. These errors persisted over 8 months but had resolved by 18 months after the injury. Another subject, an 11-year-old, also had normal school performance 18 months after the closed head injury; immediately after the injury, she only was able to write simple words. Her reading initially was unintelligible because of neologisms.

Case studies reported in the literature also describe written language problems associated with subcortical lesions in children. Ferro, Martins, Pinto, and Castro-Caldas (1982) described literal errors in reading 46 days after a right subcortical infarct in a 6-year-old left-handed child. Writing showed spatial dysgraphia and poor handwriting skills. Another subject who presented with oral language deficits and written language problems following a subcortical cerebrovascular accident was reported by Aram et al. (1983). Six and a half months after the accident the 7-year-old was achieving at a level one grade lower than her age-equivalent in spelling and written language. Her reading comprehension, word attack, and mathematical skills, however, were age-appropriate even though she had missed several months of schooling.

Therefore, like oral language skills, varying degrees of written language impairment are seen in children with acquired aphasia and individual cases show individual patterns of deficit and recovery. As a group, however, it would appear that these deficits are more severe in children under 10 years of age (Alajouanine & Lhermitte, 1965; Hécaen, 1976, 1983) and that school performance is affected by the persistent nature of written language and mathematical difficulties (Alajouanine & Lhermitte, 1965; Byers & McLean, 1962; Cooper & Flowers, 1987; Hécaen, 1976, 1983).

Acquired Childhood Aphasia Subsequent to Right Cerebral Lesions

According to historic descriptions of acquired childhood aphasia, instances of crossed aphasia (i.e., aphasia arising from right hemisphere lesions in a right-handed individual) occurred with greater frequency in children than adults suggesting that, at least in the early years, both cerebral hemispheres had a potential role in language. In 1890 Sachs and Peterson postulated that during the first years of life both hemispheres are equally equipped for the development of language and that during the expansion of language functions, the role of the right hemisphere progressively decreases in favor of the left one. Basser (1962) and Lenneberg (1967) later designated this concept as the hypothesis of "hemispheric equipotentiality and progressive lateralization of language development." This position was also supported by Freud (1897) who noted that, unlike

aphasia in adults, acquired aphasia in children occurs relatively frequently after right hemispheric lesions.

Since the 1940s, however, a growing body of evidence has pointed to the untenability of the hemispheric equipotentiality and progressive lateralization hypotheses. In particular, more recent reports demonstrating that acquired childhood aphasia shows remarkable conformity with aphasia in adults whereby the aphasic symptoms seen in children parallel those observed in adults with similar lesion locations, has forced a rethink of the historic views on the neurobiological mechanisms of language acquisition. Woods and Teuber (1978) noted that the incidence of crossed aphasia in children dropped from 33% in studies reported prior to 1940 to 5% in studies documented after 1940. They attributed the earlier reported high incidence of crossed aphasia in children to undetected bilateral cerebral damage, possibly resulting from diffuse brain involvement due to infectious encephalopathics, the drop in incidence noted after 1940 being possibly related to the introduction of antibiotics and mass immunization programs reducing the common occurrence of neurological complications in infectious diseases.

Based on reviews of the literature on acquired childhood aphasia published since 1940, Satz and Bullard-Bates (1981) and Carter, Hohenegger, and Satz (1982) concluded that: (a) the risk of acquired childhood aphasia is substantially greater following left-sided rather than right-sided cerebral lesions, regardless of age (at least after infancy); and (b) if studies including possible cases of undetected bilateral cerebral damage were excluded, and if a correction for covert left-handedness in children aged 5 years or less was introduced, the estimate of the incidence of crossed aphasia in children aged 5 years or less dropped to 6%. Similarly, Mariën, Engelborghs, Vignolo, and De Deyn (2001) based on a review of the literature from 1975 onward, identified only five children (2.7%) in a corpus of 180 dextrals with aphasia following a right hemisphere lesion.

Satz and Bullard-Bates (1981) did not believe that their findings supported the hypothesis of equipotentiality put forward by Basser (1962) and Lenneberg (1967). These authors did state, however, that their findings were in line with studies which have noted a structural asymmetry of the brain at birth (Chi, Dooling, & Gilles, 1977; Galaburda, Le May, Kemper, & Geschwind, 1978) as well as those which have noted functional asymmetry in non-aphasics (Hiscock & Kinsbourne, 1978; Molfese, Freeman, & Palermo, 1975). Furthermore, even in children who have sustained a brain injury very early in life, deficits in lexical and syntactic comprehension, syntactic production, and naming and lexical retrieval have all been reported to be associated with left but not right hemisphere lesions (Aram & Ekelman, 1987; Aram et al., 1986; Vargha-Khadem, O'Gorman, & Watters, 1985; Woods & Carey, 1979). Overall, the above observations on the lower incidence of crossed acquired childhood aphasia reported in more recent studies and the documented presence of longstanding linguistic deficits after early left hemisphere damage, are in agreement with anatomic, behavioral, and electrophysiologic studies (Chi et al., 1977; Davis & Wada, 1977; Foundas, Leonard, Gilmore, Fennell, & Heilman, 1994; Foundas, Leonard, & Heilman, 1995; Nass, Sadler, & Sidtis, 1992; Steinmetz, Volkmann, Jäncke, & Freund, 1991),

suggesting that the left hemisphere is predisposed to develop language and that lateralization has already begun at birth.

Recovery from Acquired Childhood Aphasia

The consequences of cerebral lesions incurred in childhood are generally regarded as less serious than those incurred in adult life (Basser, 1962; Teuber, 1975). Consequently, it generally is agreed that the prognosis for recovery in acquired childhood aphasia is much better than that expected in adult aphasia (Alajouanine & Lhermitte, 1965; Basser, 1962; Guttmann, 1942; Lenneberg, 1967). The often described complete or near-complete recovery of language function following lesions of the left cerebral hemisphere in childhood is frequently cited as being indicative of the "plasticity" of the immature brain, whereby the nondamaged areas of the brain are capable of assuming language function. Although the mechanisms underlying compensation are not fully understood, the good recovery from acquired childhood aphasia has been attributed to processes that include the transfer of language function to the undamaged portions of the left cerebral hemisphere and/or the intact right cerebral hemisphere. Some authors (e.g., Satz & Bullard-Bates, 1981), however, suggest that the speed of recovery sometimes witnessed in children with acquired aphasia is incompatible with a transfer of language to and a learning of language by the right hemisphere.

Another proposed explanation for the often good recovery exhibited by children with acquired aphasia is that both hemispheres contain mechanisms for language and that language therefore need not be relearned in the minor hemisphere. Under normal circumstances, in the majority of children, the language mechanisms in the right hemisphere are inhibited by those in the left such that only the left hemisphere develops complex language function. According to this proposal, damage to the left hemisphere in children causes a "release from inhibition" in the right hemisphere allowing it to assume a greater role in language function.

Although for some time it generally has been believed that the prognosis of acquired aphasia in children is good, the findings of several studies reported in the literature suggest that the recovery is not as complete as stated. In fact, there are a variety of opinions expressed in the literature concerning the prognosis of acquired aphasia in children ranging from favorable declarations of complete recovery to more guarded predictions of only partial recovery. In describing recovery of language function in acquired childhood aphasia, many authors make reference only to "clinical recovery." A number of researchers, however, have emphasized that despite apparent "clinical recovery," subtle but persistent language deficits may persist, even in those cases where the left hemisphere injury was acquired as early as during intra-uterine life (Alajouanine & Lhermitte, 1965; Rankin et al., 1981; Vargha-Khadem et al., 1985; Woods & Carey, 1979).

Satz and Bullard-Bates (1981) reviewed the literature relating to the prognosis of acquired childhood aphasia and concluded that, although spontaneous recovery occurs in the majority of children with this disorder, it by no means occurs in all cases. Of all the cases included in the studies they reviewed, 25 to 50% remained unremitted by one year postonset. Alajouanine and Lhermitte (1965) reported that 75% of their acquired aphasic subjects attained normal or near-normal language by one year postonset. Of the 8 children who had an unfavorable course in their study, 6 had massive lesions, 1 showed mental deterioration, and 1 died. One-third of the children with acquired aphasia studied by Hécaen (1976) attained complete recovery within a period of 6 weeks to 2 years postonset. Carrow-Woolfolk and Lynch (1982) suggested that the recovery period in cases of acquired childhood aphasia may extend up to 5 years. Martins (2004) described eleven children who remained chronically aphasic for 2 or more years following a nonprogressive brain lesion sustained in childhood. Factors identified as being associated with persistent aphasia included a traumatic or infectious etiology, poor verbal comprehension at onset, epilepsy, and lesions involving the historic language areas of the left hemisphere.

Even in those cases where recovery from aphasia occurs, however, there are often serious cognitive and academic problems that remain (Martins, 2004; Satz & Bullard-Bates, 1981). For the majority of children with acquired aphasia appear to have difficulty following a normal progression through school (Chadwick, 1985; Hécaen, 1976). None of the 32 children with acquired aphasia studied by Alajouanine and Lhermitte (1965) showed normal progress in the long-term. According to these authors, school subjects requiring the use of language (first language study, foreign languages, history, geography, etc.) are more difficult for these children than subjects such as mathematics. Martins

(2004) noted that the children in their cohort who appeared to recover from aphasia had significantly lower scores on short-term and working memory tests and also displayed educational difficulties thereby stressing the need for rehabilitation and educational/professional support in the chronic stages of acquired childhood aphasia.

Factors Influencing Recovery from Acquired Childhood Aphasia

A number of different factors that may influence the recovery of language in acquired childhood aphasia have been identified by various authors. These factors include: the site of lesion; the size and side of lesion; the etiology; the associated neurologic disturbances; the age and onset; the type and severity of the aphasia; and the presence of electroencephalographic abnormalities. As pointed out by van Dongen and Loonen (1977), however, the wide diversity of etiologies, severities of aphasia, length of follow-up reported in the various studies of acquired childhood aphasia, make it difficult to work out which of the factors are the most important in determining the final outcome of the aphasia. According to Satz and Bullard-Bates (1981) our current knowledge is inadequate for determining which factors assist and which factors impede recovery.

Influence of Age at Onset

The prognostic factor that has perhaps received the greatest attention in the literature is the age at onset. Lenneberg (1967) stated that the prognosis of acquired aphasia in children is directly related to the age of onset of aphasia and that any aphasia incurred after the age of puberty does not remit entirely. Various authors agree that there are considerable differences in prognosis with age. Penfield (1965) claimed that in children less than 10 years with acquired aphasia, there is a good chance of reacquisition of lost verbal skills within one year, although such recovery may occur at the expense of other nonverbal skills. In support of this claim, Carrow-Woolfolk and Lynch (1982) suggested that children less than 3 years of age with cerebral lesions follow normal language acquisition after an initial pause of all language development. Vargha-Kadem et al. (1985) found that as the age of aphasia onset increases (at least in children more than 5 years old), the language impairment becomes progressively worse. 10 years of age is considered by many authors to be the upper limit for complete language recovery (Oelschlaeger & Scarborough, 1976), cerebral lesions incurred after this time causing a persistent language deficit. There is an unconfirmed premise that cerebral plasticity is lost by the age of 10 years as a result of development of cerebral dominance or laterized specialization of language function.

Despite the support provided by the above studies that age at onset is an important prognostic determinant in acquired childhood aphasia, not all authors have been able to find a relationship between the age at aphasia onset and recovery. Furthermore, a number of reports in the literature actually contradict the information provided by the more supportive studies outlined above. For instance, Hécaen (1976) described three cases of children with acquired aphasia with onset at 14 years of age, but who showed excellent recovery patterns. Although Alajouanine and Lhermitte (1965) reported a difference in the symptomatology between children with acquired aphasia less than 10 years and aphasic children more than 10 years of age, they found no significant difference in the speed of recovery between these two age groups. Likewise, Van Hout et al. (1985) found no direct relationship between the age at onset and the rate of disappearance of paraphasias in children with acquired aphasia. With such conflicting empirical data, it is obvious that as yet the relationship between age at onset and recovery in acquired childhood aphasia is uncertain.

Influence of Type and Severity of Aphasia

With regard to the type of aphasia, Guttmann (1942) emphasized the good prognosis of a purely motor aphasia, especially in young children. van Dongen and Loonen (1977) also found the type of aphasia exhibited in the acute stage postonset to be of prognostic significance. They reported that 5 out of the 6 children with an initial amnestic aphasia recovered from aphasia, but only 1 of the 7 children with mixed aphasia showed recovery. The findings of van Dongen and Loonen (1977) lend support to an earlier claim by Assal and Campiche (1973) that mixed aphasia has a poor prognosis. van Dongen and Loonen (1977) also found a significant relationship between the severity of the comprehension deficit at the onset of acquired childhood aphasia and a poor recovery from aphasia.

Influence of Etiology

No systematic studies relating etiology to recovery from acquired childhood aphasia have been reported in the literature. Guttmann (1942), however, reported that children with head trauma improve more than those with vascular disease. Likewise, van Dongen and Loonen (1977) also found that most children with traumatic aphasia recovered completely. Infection (e.g., encephalitis) was found to be more frequent in children with the most severe aphasia and persistent paraphasias by Van Hout et al. (1985). A number of authors, including Mantovani and Landau (1980) have suggested that the prognosis for recovery from acquired aphasia associated with convulsive disorder is much worse than for other acquired childhood aphasias.

Influence of Extent and Side of Lesion

The findings of a number of studies have suggested a link between the extent of the cerebral lesion and the persistence of aphasic symptoms in children with acquired aphasia (Alajouanine & Lhermitte, 1965; Hécaen, 1976, 1983). As mentioned previously, 6 of the 8 aphasic children with unfavorable language outcomes in the study conducted by Alajouanine and Lhermitte (1965) had extensive cerebral lesions suggesting that the larger the cerebral lesion the poorer the prognosis for recovery. Hécaen (1983) found bilateral lesions frequently linked with persistent aphasic symptoms. Van Hout et al. (1985) also concluded that bilateral lesions may negatively influence the outcome of the language disturbance in acquired childhood aphasia based on their findings that the aphasic children with the most persistent paraphasias and who exhibited the most severe aphasic disorder in their sample, all had bilateral brain lesions. Other authors, including Collignon et al. (1968) and Gloning and Hift (1970) have also stressed that severe bilateral lesions are indicative of a poor prognosis for recovery in acquired childhood aphasia.

As outline above, based primarily on the findings of studies published prior to the 1940s, for many years it was considered that there was a higher incidence of aphasia following right cerebral lesions in children than in adults. This belief led to the formulation of the "equipotentiality hypothesis" which states that at birth, each cerebral hemisphere has the same potential to develop language function and that the lateralization of language and the development of cerebral dominance occurs as the child matures (Lenneberg, 1967). As indicated previously, however, more recent studies have shown that the frequency of aphasia from right cerebral hemisphere lesions in right-handed children is similar to that in right-handed adults (Carter et al., 1982; Satz & Bullard-Bates, 1981). Satz and Bullard-Bates (1981) stated that, after infancy, the risk of aphasia is significantly greater following left brain damage than right brain injury regardless of the age of the individual.

In addition to the extent and side of lesion, it also has been suggested by several authors that the localization of the cerebral lesion influences recovery from acquired childhood aphasia. Van Hout et al. (1985) suggested that the localization of the lesion is a more important prognostic variable than the extent of lesion. Alajouanine and Lhermitte (1965) also indicated that recovery from acquired aphasia in children is dependent on the site as well as the extent and reversibility of the lesion. It should be noted, however, that although these latter authors suggested a link between lesion localization and recovery, they did not provide any specific examples of how the site of the cerebral damage influences the prognosis for recovery. Although Hécaen (1983) found that all language symptoms, including auditory and written comprehension were more disturbed following anterior than following temporal lesions in children, he did not list the site of lesion as a factor involved in the determination of the outcome of the aphasic disturbance.

Influence of the Presence of Encephalographic Abnormalities

The relationship between changes in the electroencephalographic pattern and recovery in children with acquired aphasia is controversial. Some authors have reported that recovery correlates with a disappearance of abnormalities in the electroencephalographic trace while others have been unable to find any link between these two factors. Shoumaker, Bennett, Bray, and Curless (1974) found that improved language abilities in children with acquired aphasia associated with convulsive disorder corresponded with an improvement in the electrocephalographic pattern. Likewise, van Dongen, and Loonen (1977) found that recovery of language function in a group of children with acquired aphasia resulting from a variety of etiologies (including convulsive disorder) was associated with a reduction in electroencephalographic abnormalities. Other authors, however, including Gascon, Victor, Lombroso, and Goodglass (1973) and McKinney and McGreal (1974) were unable to demonstrate a correlation between improved electroencephalographic patterns and improved language. Of the 24 children with acquired aphasia who were reported to have recovered in the study conducted by Alajouanine and Lhermitte (1965), 16 still suffered severe motor sequelae and electroencephalographic disturbances. Alajouanine and Lhermitte (1965) interpreted this finding as an indication that recovery does not result from the reversibility of the lesion.

Influence of Concomitant Neurologic Disturbances

Concomitant neurologic disturbances represent another variable that has been implicated as a factor which influences recovery from acquired childhood aphasia. As in the case of the prognostic variables discussed above, however, the findings reported in the literature relating to the importance of associated neurologic signs as a prognostic indicator in children with acquired aphasia tend to be contradictory. Lange-Cosack and Tepfner (1973) reported that there is a minimal or no recovery in traumatic aphasic subjects who have suffered coma for more than 7 days. On the other hand, Hécaen (1976) questioned the importance of coma as a prognostic indicator in cases of acquired childhood aphasia, he being unable to demonstrate a clear relationship between the occurrence and duration of coma and the severity and persistence of the language deficit.

In summary, although a number of different factors have been suggested as having prognostic significance in acquired childhood aphasia, currently there is an insufficient amount of information available to determine which of these factors are unequivocally favorable or unfavorable for recovery.

Acquired Childhood Aphasia Following Vascular Disorders

In the past, little attention has been paid to the nature of the specific linguistic impairments shown by children with acquired aphasia resulting from different causes. Consequently the general clinical features of acquired childhood aphasia described previously are largely based on the findings of studies that have included aphasic children with a variety of underlying etiologies including trauma, vascular lesions, tumors, infections, and convulsive disorder. As well as influencing the prognosis for recovery of language function in cases of acquired childhood aphasia, there is some evidence that the etiology also has an important influence on the type of aphasia that is exhibited. It is no longer possible to assume that the effects of slow-onset lesions (e.g., tumors) on language are the same as those of rapid-onset lesions (e.g., cerebrovascular accidents and head trauma). In cases of acquired childhood aphasia following vascular lesions, the prognosis for recovery is poorer and the aphasic symptoms more variable and more persistent than in cases associated with other etiologies (Guttmann, 1942; van Dongen & Loonen, 1977). In addition, although acquired childhood aphasia can be caused by a similar range of disorders of the nervous system as adult aphasia, the relative importance of each of the different causes to the occurrence of language disturbances in children differs from the situation seen in adults. For instance, although in peacetime cerebrovascular accidents are the most common cause of aphasia in adults, the most common cause of acquired childhood aphasia is traumatic brain injury. Therefore, instead of describing the linguistic skills of groups of children with acquired aphasia resulting from different causes, as has occurred in the past, there is a need to examine the clinical features and neuropathology of the acquired childhood aphasia associated with each major etiology separately. The neuropathologic basis and clinical features of acquired childhood aphasia associated with cerebrovascular accidents are described further below whereas those associated with acquired childhood aphasia associated with other etiologies including traumatic brain injury, convulsive disorders, metabolic disorders, cerebral anoxia, brain tumors, infectious diseases, and neural tube disorders are described in subsequent chapters of this book.

Vascular Disorders Associated with Acquired Childhood Aphasia

Cerebrovascular disorders constitute a much smaller proportion of the neurological diseases of childhood than adulthood. However, they occur more frequently than generally thought and are a significant cause of morbidity and mortality in the childhood population. The incidence of cerebrovascular accidents in children has been estimated as 2.6 per 100,000.

Virtually all the diseases of blood vessels which affect adults may at some time also occur in children (Bickerstaff, 1972; Salam-Adams & Adams, 1988). Despite this, the causes of vascular diseases of the brain in children differ from those in adults. For instance, degenerative disorders such as atherosclerosis affect primarily the middle-aged and elderly and are rare in childhood (Moosy, 1959). Some vascular diseases of the brain, such as embolism arising from subacute or acute bacterial endocardial valvular disease, occur at all ages whereas others, such as vascular disorders associated with congenital heart disease, are peculiar to childhood.

Acute hemiplegia of childhood is a term used by many pediatricians and neurologists to describe the sudden onset of hemiplegia in children. A wide variety of vascular diseases of the brain, including both occlusive and hemorrhagic disorders, have been described under this heading.

Idiopathic Childhood Hemiplegia

The most commonly reported and dramatic syndrome resulting from an ischemic stroke in childhood is idiopathic childhood hemiplegia. This syndrome involves the sudden onset of hemiplegia as a result of a unilateral brain infarct of unknown origin and can affect children from a few months of age up to 12 years of age (Bickerstaff, 1972). According to Bickerstaff (1972), females are affected more than males in a ratio of about 3 to 2.

The cause of idiopathic childhood hemiplegia has been argued for many years and a variety of possible causes proposed including: polioencephalitis (Strumpell, 1884), encephalitis (Adams, Cammermeyer, & Denny-Brown, 1949; Bernheim, 1956; Brandt, 1962), venous thrombosis (Bernheim, 1956; Brandt, 1962; Norman, 1962), demyelination (Wyllie, 1948), epilepsy (Norman, 1962), and occlusion of the internal carotid artery (Bickerstaff, 1964; Duffy, Portnoy, Mauro, & Wehrle, 1957; Goldstein & Burgess, 1958). Although there appears to be some agreement that arterial occlusion is the most common cause of idiopathic childhood hemiplegia the reason for the occlusion is less certain. For reasons indicated above, atheroma cannot be implicated in childhood. Studies using carotid angiograms have demonstrated the presence of thrombosis of either the common or internal carotid arteries in some cases of idiopathic childhood hemiplegia (Salam-Adams & Adams, 1988).

Bickerstaff (1964) suggested that roughening of the wall of the internal carotid artery as a result of arteritis secondary to throat, tonsillar or cervical gland infection might be the causal factor in some instances. Furthermore, in some reported cases neither angiography nor post-mortem examination was able to demonstrate the presence of vascular lesions, suggesting that in these cases an embolus may have temporarily blocked a cerebral artery and then later broken up before the angiogram was taken or the postmortem performed (Salam-Adams & Adams, 1988).

Other Vascular Occlusive Disorders in Childhood

A number of other vascular occlusive disorders peculiar to childhood can also cause ischemic strokes in children. These disorders include: vascular disease associated with congenital heart disease, arteritis (inflammation of an artery) of various types, sickle cell disease, vascular occlusion associated with irradiation of the base of the brain, moyamoya, and strokes associated with homocystinuria and Fabry disease.

Ischemic strokes associated with congenital heart disease occur most frequently in the first 2 years of life, corresponding to the stage when congenital heart disease has its greatest frequency (6 per 1,000 live births) (Salam-Adams & Adams, 1988). Banker (1961) reported that of the childhood cerebrovascular accident cases examined by him, 28% were associated with congenital heart disease, making it the single most common cause of cerebrovascular accidents in his study.

Various types of arteritis, including that associated with lupus erythematosus and occurring secondary to infections in the tonsillar fossa and lymph glands in the neck, have also been reported to cause ischemic strokes in children (Bickerstaff, 1964; Davie & Cox, 1967; Salam-Adams & Adams, 1988). Lupus erythematosus is a diffuse inflammatory disease that involves the kidneys, skin, hematologic system, the central nervous system, and occasionally the liver. It is more common in females than males with a ratio of about 10 to 1. Although the average onset is around 30 years of age, symptoms can occur in the first decade of life (Bell & Lastimosa, 1980). Neurologic complications have been reported to occur in up to 75% of patients (Tindall, 1980), with seizures being the most common single neurologic symptom. Hemiplegia secondary to cerebral arteritis, which is either transitory or permanent, occurs in approximately 5% of patients with lupus erythematosus. If permanent neurologic loss occurs it is correlated with obstruction of one of the major extracranial or intracranial blood vessels. A case of lymphadenitis (inflammation of the lymph nodes) in the region of the carotid bifurcation and extending to involve the artery was described by Schnüriger (1966, cited in Bickerstaff, 1972). Bickerstaff (1972) reported damage to the carotid artery near its passage past the tonsillar fossa possibly resulting from arteritis due to a throat infection.

Both arterial and venous occlusions leading to cerebral infarction have been observed in children with sickle cell disease, an inherited blood disorder occurring primarily in Blacks (Salam-Adams & Adams, 1988). Likewise, cerebral infarcts have been reported subsequent to cobalt radiation of the base of the brain for treatment of a variety of neoplastic disorders in children, including craniopharyngiomas and pituitary adenomas.

Another vascular disorder of childhood that may cause vascular occlusion of the internal carotid artery is moyamoya disease. Patients with this condition present with headache, seizures, strokelike episodes, visual symptoms and mental retardation as well as, in some cases, a movement disorder, a gait disturbance, and/or a speech deficit. Typically, the symptoms are bihemispheric. Moyamoya disease is characterized by the presence of a network of fine anastomotic blood vessels at the base of the brain called a rete mirabile. The etiology of moyamoya disease is uncertain. There have been some suggestions that the condition is a congenital disorder involving retention of the embryonal rete mirabile. Alternatively, the network of anastomoses may be the consequence of an acquired disorder involving occlusion of the carotid arteries. It is possible, therefore, that several types of arterial disease in childhood may lead to moyamoya.

Complications of certain hereditary metabolic diseases may also occasionally cause occlusive vascular disease in children. Two such conditions where this may occur include homocystinuria and Fabry's disease. Both conditions result from enzyme deficiencies and both, among other effects, may cause structural damage to the blood vessels leading to thrombosis. Homocystinuria, resulting from a lack of cystathionine-synthetase, manifests as mental retardation. Ischemic strokes arising from either arterial or venous thrombosis may be experienced by persons with this disorder in late childhood, adolescence or adult life. Likewise, Fabry disease, a sex-linked disorder affecting males and resulting from a deficiency in galactosyl hydrolase, may cause structural changes in the blood vessels leading to thrombosis and stroke (Adams & Lyon, 1982).

Brain Hemorrhage in Childhood

Spontaneous intracranial hemorrhage is much less common in children than in adults. Two major types of cerebral hemorrhage occur in childhood: one type occurring secondary to hematological diseases such as leukemia, sickle cell disease, hemophilia, and thrombopenic purpura, the second type occurring secondary to vascular abnormalities such as arteriovenous malformations. It is noteworthy that hemorrhage resulting from rupture of saccular (berry) aneurysms is rare in childhood (Bickerstaff, 1972). In addition, the majority of arteriovenous malformations manifest as brain hemorrhage or in some other way during the third decade of life. Only approximately 10% of arteriovenous malformations cause hemorrhage or other problems in childhood.

Clinical Features of Acquired Childhood Aphasia Following Vascular Disorders

Few studies of acquired aphasia secondary to vascular disorders in children have been reported in the literature. Those studies that have been published, however, suggest that the pattern of language symptoms is similar to that seen in cases of adult aphasia of vascular origin (Aram et al., 1983; Dennis, 1980).

Left Hemisphere Lesions

Aram and her co-workers have found that children with unilateral left hemisphere lesions, when compared with a nonlesioned control group, have longer latency times and more errors on lexical retrieval tasks (Aram et al., 1987), more errors on most measures of syntactical abilities, both receptively and expressively (Aram et al., 1985, 1986), and more errors on the Revised Token Test (Aram et al., 1987), which appeared to be related more to a poor memory for the increasing information load than to the increased linguistic complexity. Aram et al. (1987) also found a quantitative and qualitative difference in the number of dysfluencies produced by children with left hemisphere lesions compared with controls matched for age, sex, and socioeconomic status. In particular, the children with left lesions produced more nonfluencies, which appeared to be due to an increase in the number of stuttering-type nonfluencies. The left hemisphere-lesioned subjects also had a slower rate of speech than their controls, which the authors postulated may be related to the longer latency required by these subjects on word-retrieval tasks.

Overall, despite the above noted significantly poorer performance by their subjects with left unilateral brain lesions, Aram and co-workers have stressed the good performance of these subjects on most linguistic tasks. As predicated from the literature, few of these subjects continued to have clinical signs of aphasia 1 year postonset and performed within normal limits on most of the language tests used in these studies. For example, only one of the left-lesioned subjects reached the level of nonfluencies (i.e., 10%) needed to be classified a stutterer, whereas another two subjects fitted the classification of "ambiguous" (Adams, 1980). All the remaining 17 left-lesioned subjects had less than 2% nonfluencies. This good

prognosis, however, does not appear to hold if there are ongoing seizures or if the brain damage is bilateral.

Trauner and Mannino (1986) also reported a good prognosis for their 10 subjects who had a focal cerebrovascular lesion in the neonatal period. They stated that cerebrovascular accidents in the neonatal period are increasingly diagnosed, especially if the presenting symptom is seizures. Aram (1988) also noted a high frequency of cerebrovascular accidents associated with congenital heart disorders in her prelinguistic subjects. Only one of the 10 subjects studied by Trauner and Mannino (1986) showed a mild motor and intellectual delay. Four subjects continued to have seizures, while two (including the mildly delayed subject) presented with microcephaly and one had a mild spasticity in the right leg. Trauner and Mannino therefore concluded that children who suffer neonatal cerebrovascular accidents have a relatively favorable prognosis for normal development, but warned that it is possible for these subjects to present with subtle learning disabilities and attentional or cognitive deficits in the long-term which may affect their academic success. Such long-term problems have also been identified by Aram and co-workers in their left hemisphere-lesioned subjects.

Half of the 20 subjects with left hemisphere lesions studied by Aram and Ekelman (1988a) showed difficulties at school as measured by delayed entry to school, grade repetition, special class placement or need for special academic tutoring. Subsequent assessments have failed to satisfactorily identify the reason for these educational difficulties. The 20 subjects were assessed using the Woodcock-Johnson Psycho-Educational

Battery: Tests of Cognitive Ability and Achievement (Woodcock & Johnson, 1977). Significantly poorer scores were obtained by the left-lesioned subjects than their controls on all clusters except Verbal on Cognitive Ability, all clusters except Knowledge on Scholastic Aptitude, and the Written Language cluster of the Tests of Academic Achievement. Despite the significantly poorer results obtained by all the left-lesioned subjects in these areas, again their overall performance was better than expected from someone having suffered a brain lesion and from what their educational history might indicate. Although neither age at time of lesion nor site of lesion (i.e., pre- or retrorolandic) appeared to account for differences in linguistic performance, the division between cortical and subcortical involvement in the lesion did account for the differences.

A similar distinction between subjects with left cortical and subcortical lesions could be made based on the results of spelling and reading assessment (Aram, Ekelman & Gillespie, 1989). Generally, no significant difference was found between left-lesioned subjects and their controls on multivariate results for any of the five reading or spelling domains assessed despite the lesioned subjects scoring more than 10 percentiles below the mean of their controls. Univariate results did indicate a significantly poorer performance by the left-lesioned subjects on the total reading comprehension and the inferential reading comprehension scores. Again, group performance indicated a high level of performance by the children with unilateral left lesions. Analysis of individual subject scores, however, identified five subjects who had clinical reading or spelling problems. These included children with left subcortical lesions.

In the five children with reading and spelling difficulties of clinical significance one subject had a strong family history of reading difficulties whereas another had a mild phonological-syntactical language disorder before his cerebrovascular accident at 6 years of age. This latter subject presented with a global language and reading disorder. Since the collection of the data, magnetic resonance imaging (MRI) also has shown this subject to have bilateral brain damage, including a small white matter lesion in the right frontal lobe which had not been detected previously by a computed tomography (CT) scan. It is interesting to note that this subject was also the only child examined by Aram and co-workers who still presented with clinical signs of aphasia 1 year after the lesion, and had a marked verbal-performance IQ discrepancy (i.e., VIQ = 79; PIQ = 118). Other subjects with clinical reading and spelling problems also presented with language and verbal memory problems. The language disorders were a moderate global language deficit with a mild dysarthria, and a word-retrieval difficulty associated with a stuttering disorder. There was a trend that suggested the older the child (i.e., the more reading was established) at the time of the lesion the more specific was the resultant reading disorder.

This still leaves six subjects who had been identified as having academic problems who did not present with clinically significant reading disorders. The assessment of mathematical abilities is presently underway, which may identify some of the other underachieving students.

Memory deficits specific to verbal stimuli and in particular the retrieval of verbal stimuli have been found in this group of left-lesioned subjects which also may account for academic failure (Aram, Ekelman, & Fletcher, 1988). In addition to the 11 of 20 left-lesioned subjects identified by Aram and Ekelman (1988a) as having educational difficulties, there were two subjects who had been honors students before their lesion and were now average in their performance and one other student who, although he was coping adequately at school and performed within normal limits on the assessments used in the study, had marked spelling difficulties. Therefore, although left unilateral brain lesions without ongoing seizures result in good recovery of linguistic skills, there are data to suggest a poor academic prognosis. The presenting academic difficulties may range from not achieving at pre-lesion potential to marked reading and/or spelling disorders of clinical significance. This appears to be more likely if the lesion includes the subcortical region.

The nature of the language disorders presenting in children with left hemisphere lesions of vascular origin have been documented in a number of cases studies. In the acute stages these have included comprehension impairment, neologisms, paraphasias, mutism, nonfluent telegraphic style, difficulties on repetition tasks, reading and writing impairments, naming difficulties, dysarthria, oral dyspraxia, poor metalinguistic judgments of grammatical and agrammatical sentences, and simplified story grammar (Aram et al., 1983; Cranberg et al., 1987 [cases 3 to 8]; Cooper & Flowers, 1987 [cases 6, 8, and 16]; Ferro, Martins, Pinto & Castro-Caldas, 1982; van Dongen & Visch-Brink, 1988 [case 4]; Van Hout et al., 1985 [case 1]).

In most cases the clinical signs of aphasia resolved usually within 10 months of the lesion (Aram et al., 1983; Cranberg et al., 1987; Ferro et al., 1982).

The long-term problems that do remain include word-retrieval problems (Aram et al., 1987; Cranberg et al., 1987; van Dongen and Visch-Brink, 1988), difficulty with comprehension of complex syntactic relationships (Cooper & Flowers, 1987; Cranberg et al., 1987) and difficulty producing complex grammatical constructions (Aram et al., 1986; Cranberg et al., 1987). Most of the subjects examined long-term, however, presented with academic difficulties (Aram & Ekelman, 1988a; Cooper & Flowers, 1987; Cranberg et al., 1987).

The type of aphasia seen in the acute stage after a unilateral left vascular lesion was described by Cranberg et al. (1987) in terms of the aphasic syndromes used for the classification of adult subjects. They concluded that the focal lesions seen in five of the six subjects with vascular lesions produced the aphasia type expected from a similar lesion in an adult. However, one child with a posterior cortical lesion displayed a nonfluent (Broca's) type of aphasia instead of the fluent aphasia usually exhibited by adults with such lesions. Although Cranberg et al. (1987) have demonstrated that in the majority of cases the underlying pathology produced similar clinical pictures to adult aphasics in the acute phase, recent studies by Aram and co-workers have shown that the mechanisms underlying the rapid recovery process seen in children with unilateral lesions may differ from those in adults.

Aram and Ekelman (1986) when studying the cognitive profiles of children with unilateral left hemisphere lesions did not find the typical pattern seen in adults where verbal IQ is lower following a left hemisphere lesion. Nor was the performance of the children with left unilateral lesions similar to either adults with left hemisphere lesions or children with developmental language disorders (Aram & Ekelman, 1988b) on the Tallal Repetition Task: A measurement of auditory temporal processing (Tallal, Stark, & Mellitis, 1985). The performance of the lesioned children was also dissimilar to that seen in adults on a probe-evoked potential procedure (Papanicolaou, Di Scenna, Gillespie, & Aram, 1990). Instead, the left hemisphere showed attenuation for the language tasks and the right hemisphere showed engagement in visuospatial tasks suggesting that the language recovery seen in children with brain lesions and further knowledge development involves intrahemispheric functional reorganization.

In summary, children with unilateral vascular lesions in the left hemisphere usually recover adequate language skills. Long-term problems, however, include difficulties with lexical retrieval, syntax, and comprehension as measured on the Revised Token Test. The last area of deficit may be related to a memory deficit, though further research is required. Although language skills may recover, a large percentage of children with left unilateral brain lesions have difficulty coping with school. The exact reasons for this still requires investigation.

Right Hemisphere Lesions

Similar to the children with left hemisphere lesions, children with unilateral right hemisphere lesions show difficulties with school progress. Aram and Ekelman (1988a) found six of their 11 right hemisphere-lesioned subjects showed poor school progress. Four of the children with academic difficulties had repeated a grade, three then going into a special placement. One other subject was in a

special education placement whereas another received extra tutoring. As a group, the subjects with right hemisphere lesions performed more poorly than their controls on all the Cognitive, Academic, Achievement, and Scholastic Aptitude clusters of the Woodcock-Johnson Psycho-Educational Battery (Woodcock & Johnson, 1977) except for the Verbal (Cognitive) cluster (Aram & Ekelman, 1988a). On measures of reading ability, multivariate analysis showed no difference between the controls and the children with right hemisphere lesions on any of the five spelling or reading domains. Two individual subjects, however, met the criteria specified by Aram et al. (1987) for a clinical reading disorder. One of these subjects had a family history of reading problems that would predispose him to difficulties. The other subject had a subcortical lesion. Five other right-lesioned subjects, however, had subcortical lesions and no reading and/or spelling disorders. Both children with problems had difficulty in the areas of reading comprehension, phonetic analysis, and blending and one had difficulty with spelling.

Although language problems appear to account for some of the difficulties experienced at school by children with left hemisphere lesions (Aram et al., 1989), this does not seem to be so in children with right hemisphere lesions, as they presented with relatively few linguistic deficits when compared with controls. Generally, children with right hemisphere lesions have presented with a short mean length of utterance, a higher number of nonfluencies, and a poorer score for expressive and receptive vocabulary (Aram et al., 1985).

Other language deficits noted in children with right unilateral brain lesions, however, have been attributed to poor attention and impulsivity noted during testing sessions. These language deficits include those observed during their performance on the Revised Token Test, lexical retrieval tasks, and the poorer but not significantly different performance of the Tallal Repetition Task (Aram & Ekelman, 1987, 1988b; Aram et al., 1986, 1987). Even a greater number of syntactic errors on simple sentences has been postulated to be related to impulsivity (Aram et al., 1986).

This hypothesis relating poor performance to poor attention is supported by Voeller (1986). While Voeller did not stipulate the cause of the focal right hemisphere lesions in his experimental group the reported findings do support the hypotheses proposed by Aram and co-workers and indicate areas of pragmatic deficit which should be further investigated in children with right hemisphere lesions. Fourteen of the 15 subjects (93%) examined by Voeller (1986) presented with an attention deficit disorder (ADD) using DSM-III criteria. This compares with 3 to 10% for ADD seen in the normal school-age population. Nine of the subjects had atypical prosody described as high pitched with rapid rate, robotlike, or soft and low pitched. Six of these nine subjects also had a gesturing deficit (no more details were given). Teachers commented on lack of eye contact in most subjects. Thirteen subjects had poor peer relationships, seven of whom were described as insensitive whereas others presented as shy and withdrawn. Voeller (1986) assessed the subject's ability to interpret the affective states of others using two tests devised by Tallman (unpublished thesis; cited in Voeller, 1986). In one test the subjects had to point to pictures of people expressing emotions (e.g., "show me the child who

is angry") whereas the other utilized a 20 word sample of speech which had been filtered so only the intonation patterns remained. Again, the subjects had to identify the emotion, reflected by intonation. As a group, the subjects with right hemisphere lesions performed more poorly than their peers than would have been expected. Caution should be used when interpreting these conclusions relating to emotional responses as 8 of the 15 families reported a family history of emotional problems. The high incidence of ADD, however, together with the obvious pragmatic difficulties experienced by the children with right hemisphere lesions highlight areas requiring further research. In addition, 13 of the 15 subjects in the study conducted by Voeller (1986) were in special education placements or in private schools.

It appears, therefore, that children with unilateral cerebrovascular disorders usually recover their linguistic abilities, although children with left hemisphere vascular lesions do show mild linguistic deficits when compared with appropriately matched controls, and children with right hemisphere vascular lesions often show attentional deficits. Vascular lesions in either hemisphere, however, are associated with a poor school performance.

Case Example: Acquired Childhood Aphasia of Vascular Origin

Ronald was an 11-year, seven-month, right-handed boy when he experienced an intracerebral hemorrhage. He initially presented with a left-sided headache, right facial and limb weakness, and intermittent violent movements of his left limbs. On arrival at hospital his reflexes were normal and pupils equal. Ronald lost consciousness soon after admission. A computed tomographic (CT) scan performed on the day of onset indicated a large hemorrhage in the left temporoparietal subcortical region. There was considerable mass effect causing a midline shift of the brain toward the right (Figure 2–1).

A left frontal craniotomy was also performed on the day of admission to hospital to enable evacuation of the hematoma to relieve pressure on Ronald's brain. The cerebrovascular accident ex-perienced by Ronald left him with a severe expressive and receptive apha-sia, dysarthria and right hemiplegia. Ronald showed a gradual increase in his consciousness, mobility, and speech up to his discharge from hospital at two months postonset. However, his severe language impairment persisted and was still evident when assessed at the Centre for Neurogenic Communication Disorders Research, The University of Queensland at 3 years, 6 months pos-tonset. Although a comprehensive lan-guage assessment conducted at that time showed that Ronald exhibited gen-

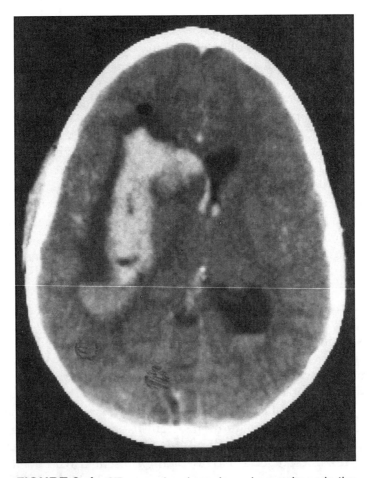

FIGURE 2–1. CT scan showing a large hemorrhage in the left temporoparietal subcortical region.

eral depression in all language areas, his major language problems fell in the areas of confrontation naming, auditory comprehension, repetition, expressive syntax, oral reading, reading comprehension, and spelling. Overall, Ronald's language profile differs in two major ways to historic descriptions of the clinical features of acquired childhood aphasia. First, recovery from acquired childhood aphasia was once thought to be excellent and almost complete. Ronald, however, remained severely language impaired for many years after his stroke. Second, although acquired childhood aphasia is commonly described as being of a nonfluent type, Ronald demonstrated persistent problems in both the expressive and receptive (e.g., auditory comprehension difficulties) aspects of language. It is suggested that the persistent nature of Ronald's language disorder may have been related to the extensive nature of the brain damage caused by his cerebrovascular accident.

References

Adams, M. (1980). The young stutterer: diagnosis, treatment and assessment of progress. *Seminars in Speech, Language and Hearing, 4,* 289–299.

Adams, R. D., Cammermeyer, J., & Denny-Brown, D. (1949). Acute necrotizing hemorrhagic encephalopathy. *Journal of Neuropathology and Experimental Neurology, 8,* 1–29.

Adams, R. D., & Lyon, G. (1982). *Neurology of hereditary metabolic diseases of children.* New York, NY: McGraw-Hill.

Alajouanine, T., & Lhermitte, F. (1965). Acquired aphasia in children. *Brain, 88,* 653–662.

Aram, D. M. (1988). Language sequelae of unilateral brain lesions in children. In F. Plum (Ed.), *Language communication and the brain.* New York, NY: Raven Press.

Aram, D. M., & Ekelman, B. L. (1986). Cognitive profiles of children with early onset of unilateral lesions. *Developmental Neuropsychology, 2,* 155–172.

Aram, D. M., & Ekelman, B. L. (1987). Unilateral brain lesions in childhood: Performance on the Revised Token Test. *Brain and Language, 32,* 137–158.

Aram, D. M., & Ekelman, B. L. (1988a). Scholastic aptitude and achievement among children with unilateral brain lesions. *Neuropsychologia, 26,* 903–916.

Aram, D. M., & Ekelman, B. L. (1988b). Auditory temporal perception of children with left or right brain lesions. *Neuropsychologia, 26,* 931–935.

Aram, D. M., Ekelman, B. L., & Fletcher, J. M. (1988). Verbal and non-verbal memory among children with left and right brain lesions. *Journal of Clinical and Experimental Neuropsychology, 10,* 18.

Aram, D. M., Ekelman, B. L., & Gillespie, L. L. (1989). Reading and lateralized brain lesions in children. In K. von Euler (Ed.), *Developmental dyslexia and dysphasia.* Basingstoke, UK: Macmillan Press.

Aram, D. M., Ekelman, B. L., Rose, D. F., & Whitaker, H. A. (1985). Verbal and cognitive sequelae following unilateral lesions acquired in early childhood. *Journal of Clinical and Experimental Neuropsychology, 7,* 55–78.

Aram, D. M., Ekelman, B. L., & Whitaker, H. A. (1986). Spoken syntax in children with acquired unilateral hemisphere lesions. *Brain and Language, 27,* 75–100.

Aram, D. M., Ekelman, B. L., & Whitaker, H. A. (1987). Lexical retrieval in left and right brain lesioned children. *Brain and Language, 31,* 61–87.

Aram, D. M., Rose, D. F., Rekate, H. L., & Whitaker, H. A. (1983). Acquired capsular/striatal aphasia in childhood. *Archives of Neurology, 40,* 614–617.

Assal, G., & Campiche, R. (1973). Aphasie et troubles du langage chez l'enfant après contusion cérébrale. *Neurochirurgie, 19,* 399–406.

Banker, B. Q. (1961). Cerebral vascular disease in infancy and childhood. *Journal of Neuropathology and Experimental Neurology, 20*, 127–140.

Barringer, J. R. (1978). Herpes simplex infections of the nervous system. In D. Vinken & G. Bruyn (Eds.), *Handbook of clinical neurology* (Vol. 34, pp. 346–368). Amsterdam, the Netherlands: North-Holland/Elsevier.

Basser, L. S. (1962). Hemiplegia of early onset and the faculty of speech with special reference to the effects of hemispherectomy. *Brain, 85*, 427–460.

Bell, R. D., & Lastimosa, A. C. B. (1980). Metabolic encephalopathies. In R. N. Rosenberg (Ed.), *Neurology* (pp. 115–164). New York, NY: Grune & Stratton.

Benson, D. F. (1972). Language disturbances of childhood. *Clinical Proceedings Children's Hospital of Washington, 28*, 93–100.

Bernhardt, M. (1885). Ueber die spastische cerebrale Paralyse im Kindesalter (hemiplegia spastica infantalis), nebst einem Exkurs über: Aphasie bei Kindern. *Archiv für Pathologische Anatomie und Physiologie und für Klinische Medizin, 102*, 26–80.

Bernheim, M. (1956). Thrombophlebitis cerebrales. *Annals of Paediatrics (Basel), 187*, 153–160.

Bickerstaff, E. R. (1964). Aetiology of acute hemiplegia in childhood. *British Medical Journal, 2*, 82–87.

Bickerstaff, E. R. (1972). Cerebrovascular disease in infancy and childhood. In P. J. Vinken & G. W. Bruyn (Eds.), *Handbook of clinical neurology: Vascular diseases of the nervous system part II* (pp. 412–441). Amsterdam, the Netherlands: North-Holland.

Branco-Lefèvre, A. F. (1950). Contribuiçao para o estudo da psicopatologia da afasia em crianças. *Arquivos de Neuro-Psiquiatria (Sao Pãulo), 8*, 345–393.

Brandt, S. (1962). Causes and pathogenic mechanisms of acute hemiplegia in childhood. *Little Club Clinics in Developmental Medicine, 6*, 7–11.

Buckingham, H., & Kertesz, A. (1974). A linguistic analysis of fluent aphasia. *Brain and Language, 1*, 43–61.

Byers, R. K., & McLean, W. T. (1962). Etiology and course of certain hemiplegias with aphasia in childhood. *Pediatrics, 29*, 376–383.

Carrow-Woolfolk, E., & Lynch, J. (1982). *An integrative approach to language disorders in children.* Orlando, FL: Grune & Stratton.

Carter, R. L., & Hohenegger, M. K., & Satz, P. (1982). Aphasia and speech organization in children. *Science, 218*, 797–799.

Chadwick, O. (1985). Psychological sequelae of head injury in children. *Developmental Medicine and Child Neurology, 27*, 72–75.

Chi, J. G., Dooling, E. C., & Gilles, F. H. (1977). Left-right asymmetries of the temporal speech areas of the human fetus. *Archives of Neurology, 34*, 346–348.

Collignon, R., Hécaen, H., & Angerlerques, G. (1968). A propos de 12 cas d'aphasie acquise chez l'enfant. *Acta Neurologica et Psychiatrica Belgica, 68*, 245–277.

Cooper, J. A., & Flowers, C. R. (1987). Children with a history of acquired aphasia: Residual language and academic impairments. *Journal of Speech and Hearing Disorders, 52*, 251–262.

Cotard, J. (1868). *Etude sur l'atrophie cérébrale.* Thesis, Faculté de Médecine, Paris.

Cranberg, L. D., Filley, C. M., Hart, E. J., & Alexander, M. P. (1987). Acquired aphasia in children: Clinical and CT investigations. *Neurology, 37*, 1165–1172.

Davie, J. C., & Cox, W. (1967). Occlusive disease of the carotid artery in children. *Archives of Neurology, 17*, 313–323.

Davis, A. E., & Wada, J. A. (1977). Hemispheric asymmetries in human infants: Spectral analysis of flash and click evoked potentials. *Brain and Language, 4*, 23–31.

Denckla, M. B. (1979). Childhood learning disabilities. In K. Heilman & E. Valenstein (Eds.), *Clinical neuropsychology*. New York, NY: Oxford University Press.

Denckla, M. B., & Rudel, R. G. (1976). Naming of object drawings by dyslexic and other learning disabled children. *Brain and Language, 3*, 1–15.

Dennis, M. (1980). Strokes in childhood 1: Communicative intent, expression and comprehension after left hemisphere arteriopathy in a right-handed nine-year-old. In R. W. Reiber (Ed.), *Language development and aphasia in children* (pp. 79–103). New York, NY: Academic Press.

De Renzi, E., & Faglioni, P. (1978). Normative data and screening power of a shortened version of the Token Test. *Cortex, 14,* 41–49.

De Renzi, E., & Vignolo, L. A. (1962). The Token Test: A sensitive test to detect receptive disturbances in aphasics. *Brain, 85,* 665–678.

Duffy, P. E., Portnoy, B., Mauro, J., & Wehrle, P. F. (1957). Acute infantile hemiplegia secondary to spontaneous carotid thrombosis. *Neurology, 7,* 664–666.

Dunn, L. M. (1965). Peabody picture vocabulary test. Circle Pines, MN: American Guidance Service.

Dunn, L. M., & Dunn, D. M. (1981). Peabody picture vocabulary test-revised. Circle Pines, MN: American Guidance Service.

Dunn, L. M., & Markwardt, F. (1970). Peabody individual achievement test. Circle Pines, MN: American Guidance Service.

Ferro, J. M., Martins, I. P., Pinto, F., & Castro-Caldas, A. (1982). Aphasia following right striato-insular infarction in a left handed child: A clinico-radiological study. *Developmental Medicine and Child Neurology, 24,* 173–182.

Foundas, A. L., Leonard, C. M., Gilmore, R., Fennell, E., & Heilman, K. M. (1994). Planum temporal asymmetry and language dominance. *Neuropsychologia, 32,* 1225–1231.

Foundas, A. L., Leonard, C. M., & Heilman, K. M. (1995). Morphologic cerebral asymmetries and handedness: The pars triangularis and planum temporal. *Archives of Neurology, 52,* 501–508.

Freud, S. (1897). *Infantile cerebral paralysis.* Coral Gables, FL: University of Miami.

Gaddes, W. H., & Crockett, D. J. (1975). The Spreen-Benton Aphasia Tests, normative data as a measure of normal language development. *Brain and Language, 2,* 257–280.

Galaburda, A. M., Le May, M., Kemper, T. L., & Geschwind, N. (1978). Right-left asymmetries in the brain. *Science, 199,* 852–856.

Gardner, M. (1979). Expressive one-word picture vocabulary test. Novato, CA: Academic Therapy Publications.

Gascon, G., Victor, D., Lombroso, C. T., & Goodglass, H. (1973). Language disorder, convulsive disorder and electroencephalographic abnormalities. *Archives of Neurology, 28,* 156–162.

Gloning, K., & Hift, E. (1970). Aphasie im Vorschulalter. *Zeitschrift für Nervenheilkunde, 28,* 20–28.

Goldstein, S. L., & Burgess, J. P. (1958). Spontaneous thrombosis of the internal carotid artery in a seven year old child. *American Journal of Disorders of Childhood, 95,* 538–540.

Goodglass, H., & Kaplan, E. (1972). *The assessment of aphasia and related disorders.* Philadelphia, PA: Lea & Febiger.

Guttmann, E. (1942). Aphasia in children. *Brain, 65,* 205–219.

Hécaen, H. (1976). Acquired aphasia in children and the ontogenesis of hemispheric functional specialization. *Brain and Language, 3,* 114–134.

Hécaen, H. (1983). Acquired aphasia in children: Revisited. *Neuropsychologia, 21,* 581–587.

Hiscock, M., & Kinsbourne, M. (1978). Ontogeny of cerebral dominance: Evidence from time-sharing asymmetry in children. *Developmental Psychology, 14,* 321–329.

Hynd, G. W., Leathern, J., Semrud-Clikeman, M., Hern, K. L., & Wenner, M. (1995). Anomic aphasia in childhood. *Journal of Child Neurology, 10,* 289–293.

Jastak, J. F., & Jastak, S. R. (1965). The wide range achievement test. Wilmington, DE: Guidance Associates.

Jordan, F. M., Ozanne, A. E., & Murdoch, B. E. (1988). Long-term speech and language disorders subsequent to closed head injury in children. *Brain Injury, 2,* 179–185.

Jordan, F. M., Ozanne, A. E., & Murdoch, B. E. (1990). Performance of closed head-injured children on a naming task. *Brain Injury, 4,* 27–32.

Kaplan, E., Goodglass, H., & Weintraub, S. (1983). Boston naming test. Philadelphia, PA: Lippincott Williams & Wilkins.

Kiessling, L. S., Denckla, M. B., & Carlton, M. (1983). Evidence for differential hemispheric function in children with hemiplegic cerebral palsy. *Developmental Medicine and Child Neurology, 25,* 727–734.

Klein, S., Masur, D., Farber, K., Shinnar, S., & Rapin, I. (1992). Fluent aphasia in children: Definition and natural history. *Journal of Child Neurology, 7,* 50–59.

Landau, W. M., & Kleffner, F. R. (1957). Syndrome of acquired aphasia with convulsive disorder in children. *Neurology, 10,* 915–921.

Lange-Cosack, H., & Tepfner, G. (1973). *Das Hirntrauma im Kinder- und Jugendalter.* Berlin, Germany: Springer-Verlag.

Lee, L. (1971). Northwestern syntax screening test. Evanston, IL: Northwestern University Press.

Lee, L. (1974). Developmental sentence analysis. Evanston, IL: Northwestern University Press.

Lenneberg, E. (1967). *Biological foundations of language.* New York, NY: Wiley.

Mandler, J. M., & Johnson, N. S. (1977). Rememberance of things passed: Story structure and recall. *Cognitive Psychology, 9,* 111–151.

Mantovani, J. F., & Landau, W. M. (1980). Acquired aphasia with convulsive disorder: Course and prognosis. *Neurology, 30,* 524–529.

Mariën, P., Abutalebi, J., Engelborghs, S., & De Deyn, P. P. (2005) Pathophysiology of language switching and mixing in an early bilingual child with subcortical aphasia. *Neurocase, 11,* 385–398.

Mariën, P., Engelborghs, S., Vignolo. L. A., & De Deyn, P. P. (2001). The many faces of crossed aphasia in dextral: Report of nine cases and review of the literature. *European Journal of Neurology, 8,* 643–658

Mariën, P., Paquier, P., Engelborghs, S., & De Deyn, P. P. (2001). Acquired crossed aphasia in dextral children revisited. *Brain and Language, 79,* 426–443.

Martins, I. P. (2004). Persistent acquired childhood aphasia. In F. Fabbro (Ed.), *Neurogenic language disorders in children* (pp. 231–251). Amsterdam, the Netherlands: Elsevier.

Martins, I. P., & Ferro, J. M. (1987). Acquired conduction aphasia in a child. *Developmental Medicine and Child Neurology, 29,* 532–536.

Martins, I. P., & Ferro, J. M. (1991). Type of aphasia and lesion localization. In I. P. Martins (Ed.), *Acquired aphasia in children: Acquisition and breakdown of language in the developing brain* (pp. 143–159). Dordrecht, the Netherlands: Kluwer Academic Publishers.

Martins, I. P., & Ferro, J. M. (1997). Recovery of aphasia in children. *Aphasiology, 6,* 431–438.

Martins, I. P., Ferro, J. M., & Castro-Caldas, A. (1981). *Acquired aphasia in children: A longitudinal follow-up study.* Paper presented at the 4th European Conference of the International Neuropsychological Society, Bergen, Norway.

McKinney, W., & McGreal, D. A. (1974). An aphasic syndrome in children. *Canadian Medical Association Journal, 110,* 637–639.

McNeil, M. R., & Prescott, T. E. (1978). *Revised Token Test.* Austin, TX: Pro-Ed.

Miller J. F., Campbell, T. F., Chapman, R. S., & Weismer, S. E. (1984). Language behavior in acquired aphasia. In A. Holland (Ed.) *Language disorders in children.* Baltimore, MD: College-Hill Press.

Molfese, D. L., Freeman, R. B., & Palermo, D. S. (1975). The ontology of brain lateralization for speech and non-speech stimuli. *Brain and Language, 2,* 356–368.

Moosy, J. (1959). Development of cerebral arteriosclerosis in various age groups. *Neurology, 9,* 569–574.

Nass, R., Sadler, A. E., & Sidtis, J. J. (1992). Differential effects of congenital versus acquired unilateral brain injury on dichotic listening performance: Evidence for sparing and asymmetric crowding. *Neurology, 42,* 1960–1965.

Norman, R. M. (1962). Neuropathological findings in acute hemiplegia in childhood.

Little Clubs Clinics in Developmental Medicine, 6, 37–48.

Oelschlaeger, M. L., & Scarborough, J. (1976). Traumatic aphasia in children: A case study. *Journal of Communication Disorders, 9*, 281–288.

Oldfield, R. C. & Wingfield, A. (1964). The time it takes to name an object. *Nature, 202*, 1031–1032.

Papanicolaou, A. C., Di Scenna, A., Gillespie, L. L., & Aram, D. M. (1990). Probe evoked potential findings following unilateral left hemisphere lesions in children. *Archives of Neurology, 47*, 562–566.

Paquier, P., & van Dongen, H. R. (1991). Two contrasting cases of fluent aphasia in children. *Aphasiology, 5*, 235–245.

Paquier, P. F., & van Dongen, H. R. (1996). Review of research on the clinical presentation of acquired childhood aphasia. *Acta Neurologica Scandinavica, 93*, 428–436.

Paquier, P., van Maldeghem, V., van Dongen, H. R., & Creten, W. L. (2004). Recognizable spontaneous language characteristics in a young adult twelve years after she became aphasic as a child. In F. Fabbro (Ed.), *Neurogenic language disorders in children* (pp. 181–197). Amsterdam, the Netherlands: Elsevier.

Pendergast, L., Dickey, S., Selmar, J., & Soder, A. (1969). Photo articulation test. Danville, IL: Interstate Printers and Publishers.

Penfield, W. (1965). Conditioning the uncommitted language cortex for language learning. *Brain, 88*, 787–798.

Poetzl, T. (1926). Ueber sensorische Aphasie im Kindesalter, 2. *Hals N. Ohrenklin, 14*, 109–118.

Pohl, P. (1979). Dichotic listening in a child recovering from acquired aphasia. *Brain and Language, 8*, 372–379.

Rankin, J. M., Aram, D. M., & Horwitz, S. J. (1981). Language ability in right and left hemiplegic children. *Brain and Language, 14*, 292–306.

Rapin, I., & Allen, D. A. (1987). Syndromes in developmental dysphasia and adult aphasia. In F. Plum (Ed.), *Language, communication and the brain*. New York, NY: Raven Press.

Rapin, I., Mattis, S., Rowan, A. J., & Golden, G. S. (1977). Verbal auditory agnosia in children. *Developmental Medicine and Child Neurology, 19*, 192–207.

Sachs, B., & Peterson, F. (1890). A study of cerebral palsies early in life, based upon analysis of one hundred and forty cases. *Journal of Nervous and Mental Disease, 17*, 295–322.

Salam-Adams, M., & Adams, R. D. (1988). Cerebrovascular disease by age group. In P. J. Vinken, G. W. Bruyn, & H. L. Klawans (Eds.), *Handbook of clinical neurology: Vascular diseases part 1*. Amsterdam, the Netherlands: Elsevier.

Satz, P., & Bullard-Bates, C. (1981). Acquired aphasia in children. In M. T. Sarno (Ed.), *Acquired aphasia*. New York, NY: Academic Press.

Semel, E., & Wiig, E. (1980). *Clinical evaluation of language functions*. Columbus, OH: Charles E. Merrill.

Shoumaker, R., Bennett, D., Bray, P., & Curless, R. (1974). Clinical and EEG manifestations of an unusual aphasic syndrome in children. *Neurology, 24*, 10–16.

Spreen, O., & Benton, A. L. (1969). Neurosensory center comprehensive examination for aphasia: Manual of directions. Victoria, B.C.: University of Victoria.

Steinmetz, H., Volkmann, J., Jäncke, L., & Freund, H-J. (1991). Anatomical left-right asymmetry of language-related temporal cortex is different in left- and right-handers. *Annals of Neurology, 29*, 315–319.

Strumpell, A. (1884). Über die acute Encephalitis der Kinder. *Deutsch med. Wschr, 57*, 212–215.

Tallal, P., Stark, R., & Mellitis, D. (1985). Identification of language-impaired children on the basis of rapid perception and production skills. *Brain and Language, 25*, 314–322.

Templin, M. C. (1957). *Certain language skills in children*. Minneapolis, MN: University of Minnesota Press.

Templin, M. C., & Darley, F. L. (1969). Templin-Darley tests of articulation (2nd ed.). Iowa City, IA: University of Iowa.

Teuber, H. L. (1975). Recovery of function after brain injury in man. In R. Porter & D. W. Fitzsimons (Eds.), *Outcome of severe damage of the central nervous system* (CIBA Foundation Symposium No. 34). Amsterdam, the Netherlands: Elsevier/Excerpta Medica.

Tindall, R. S. A. (1980). Cerebrovascular disease. In R. N. Rosenberg (Ed.), *Neurology*. New York, NY: Grune & Stratton.

Torgesen, J. K., & Goldman, T. (1977). Verbal rehearsal and short-term memory in reading disabled children. *Child Development, 48*, 56–60.

Trauner, D. A., & Mannino, F. L. (1986). Neurodevelopmental outcome after neonatal cerebrovascular accident. *Pediatrics, 108*, 459–461.

van Dongen, H. R., & Loonen, M. C. B. (1977). Factors related to prognosis of acquired aphasia in children. *Cortex, 13*, 131–136.

van Dongen, H. R., Loonen, M. C. B., & van Dongen, K. J. (1985). Anatomical basis for acquired fluent aphasia in children. *Annals of Neurology, 17*, 306–309.

van Dongen, H., Paquier, P., Creten, W., Borsel, J., & Catsman-Berrevoets, C. (2001). Clinical evaluation of conversational speech fluency in the acute phase of acquired childhood aphasia: Does a fluency/nonfluency dichotomy exist? *Journal of Child Neurology, 16*, 345–351.

van Dongen, H. R., & Visch-Brink, E. G. (1988). Naming in aphasic children: Analysis of paraphasic errors. *Neuropsychologia, 26*, 629–632.

Van Hout, A. (1993). Acquired aphasia in childhood and developmental dysphasias: Are the errors similar? Analysis of errors made in confrontation naming tasks. *Aphasiology, 7*, 525–531.

Van Hout, A., Evrard, P., & Lyon, G. (1985). On the positive semiology of acquired aphasia in children. *Developmental Medicine and Child Neurology, 27*, 231–241.

Van Hout, A., & Lyon, G. (1986). Wernicke's aphasia in a 10 year-old boy. *Brain and Language, 29*, 268–285.

Vargha-Khadem, F., O'Gorman, A. M., & Watters, G. V. (1985). Aphasia and handedness in relation to hemispheric side, age and injury and severity of cerebral lesion during childhood. *Brain, 108*, 677–696.

Visch-Brink, E. G., & van de Sandt-Koenderman, M. (1984). The occurrence of paraphasias in the spontaneous speech of children with acquired aphasia. *Brain and Language, 23*, 256–271.

Voeller, K. K. S. (1986). Right hemisphere deficit syndrome in children. *American Journal of Psychiatry, 143*, 1004–1009.

Wiegel-Crump, C. A., & Dennis, M. (1984). The word-finding test. Toronto, Canada: The Hospital for Sick Children (unpublished).

Wolfus, B., Moscovitch, M., & Kinsbourne, M. (1980). Subgroups of developmental language impairment. *Brain and Language, 9*, 152–171.

Woodcock, R. W., & Johnson, M. D. (1977). Woodcock-Johnson psycho-educational battery. Hingham, MA: Teaching Resources.

Woods, B. T., & Carey, S. (1979). Language deficits after apparent clinical recovery from childhood aphasia. *Annals of Neurology, 6*, 405–409.

Woods, B. T., & Teuber, H. L. (1978). Changing patterns of childhood aphasia. *Annals of Neurology, 3*, 273–280.

Worster-Drought, C. (1971). An unusual form of acquired aphasia in children. *Developmental Medicine and Child Neurology, 13*, 563–571.

Wyllie, W. G. (1948). Acute infantile hemiplegia. *Proceedings of the Royal Society of Medicine, 41*, 459–466.

Zubrick, A. (1988). *The language of mathematics*. Paper presented at the Annual Conference of the Australian Association of Speech and Hearing, Brisbane, Australia.

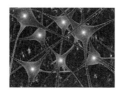 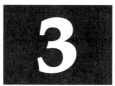 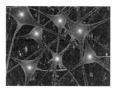

3

Acquired Childhood Aphasia Subsequent to Childhood Traumatic Brain Injury

Introduction

Traumatic brain injury (TBI) has been defined as "an insult to the brain, not of the degenerative or congenital nature, but caused by an external force, that may produce a diminished or altered state of consciousness" (National Head Injury Foundation, 1985). According to this definition, TBI occurs only in cases where the brain damage is caused by an external force and thereby excludes brain insult resulting from other neurologic conditions such as cerebrovascular accidents, tumors, degenerative brain diseases (e.g., Parkinson disease), demyelinating conditions (e.g., multiple sclerosis), and infectious disorders (e.g., encephalitis). TBI, therefore, is the consequence of a head injury in which the severity has been of suffi-

cient magnitude to cause damage to the brain.

Communication impairments are commonly reported sequelae of TBI. Depending on the location of the damage in the nervous system, TBI may be associated with a variety of communication problems including speech disorders, language disorders, or both. When present, communication impairments have important negative implications for the long-term quality of life of child survivors of TBI. Some authors have suggested that communication abilities play the pivotal role in determining the quality of survival after head trauma (Najenson, Sazbon, Fiselzon, Becker, & Schechter, 1978). In children, a communication disorder occurring subsequent to TBI may affect the developmental process of the individual, leading to impairment of further acquisition of speech, language, and social skills.

Epidemiology and Prognosis of Childhood Traumatic Brain Injury

TBI is the leading cause of death and permanent disability in children and adolescents and is the major cause of acquired childhood aphasia. Epidemiologic studies indicate that the incidence of TBI in childhood is approximately 200 per 100,000 per year, with male children having a higher incidence of TBI than female children in a ratio around 1.8:1. Disabilities demonstrated by children who survive TBI range from persistent vegetative state through mental and physical disabilities, language disorders, academic difficulties, and dysarthria.

The prognosis for recovery shown by children who have suffered mild head injuries has been reported to be excellent. Although the prognosis for recovery from severe head injuries is less certain, it is reported to be better than for adults. This difference may be the outcome of two factors. First, it may be due to the different nature of the impacts causing TBI in children versus adults and, second, it may be related to differences in the basic mechanisms of brain damage following TBI in the two groups, which in turn are related to differences in the physical characteristics of children's heads and adult heads. The majority of instances of childhood TBI result from falls (this particularly the case for infants and toddlers) or low-speed (30 to 60 km per hr) pedestrian or bicycle accidents that involve a motor vehicle. Consequently, many pediatric head injuries are associated with a lesser degree of injury resulting from rotational acceleration. Adults, on the other hand, are more likely to sustain TBI as a result of high-speed motor vehicle accidents, which by their nature are more likely to yield greater diffuse brain injury. Despite the fact that motor vehicle accidents may not be the most common cause of head injuries in children, reports are available to suggest that road traffic accidents may be the cause of most of the long-term morbidity and nearly all of the mortality in the pediatric population. In fact, it appears that, in all age groups, the most common cause of head injury associated with acute neurological injury is a motor vehicle accident (Vernon-Levett, 1991).

Evidence is available that indicates that the type of brain injury resulting from severe head trauma depends on the physical properties of the individual's brain and skull. These physical properties are known to differ in a number of ways between children and adults, thereby contributing to different patterns of brain injury following head trauma in each group. First, an infant's brain weight is 15% of body weight progressing through to only 3% of body weight in adults. Second, the existence of unfused sutures and open fontanelles makes the skull of an infant and young child pliable, allowing a greater degree of deformation and possibly a greater ability to absorb the energy of physical impact.

Biomechanics of Traumatic Injury

Brain damage following traumatic head injury may be either focal, multifocal or diffuse in nature and may involve any part of the brain. Consequently, brain damage following head injury can be associated with a variety of communicative deficits depending primarily on the location and extent of the lesion. In general, closed-head injuries tend to produce more diffuse pathology whereas open head injuries usually are associated with more focal pathology.

The communication disorders frequently associated with TBI are the result of complex biomechanical processes associated with a head injury. Therefore, to understand the neuropathophysiologic basis of these deficits, it is necessary to understand the basic mechanical forces involved in causing brain damage subsequent to closed-head trauma. Briefly, the biomechanical forces involved in closed-head injury include compression, acceleration-deceleration, and rotational acceleration, which result in brain tissue being compressed, torn apart by the effects of tension and sheared by rotational forces (Murdoch, 1990).

According to Gennarelli (1993), the application of force to the head results in mechanical loading, which sets off a cascade of physiologic events. Mechanical loading can be initiated by either static or dynamic forces. Static loading results from slow or rapid forces applied to a stationary head so that it is crushed (e.g., compression of the head). The more common type of head injury, however, occurs following dynamic loading. This results from a very brief insult that has either been applied directly to the movable head (impact) or by impacting elsewhere on the body but causing a sudden movement of the head (impulsive) (e.g., whiplash injury sustained in rear-end motor vehicle collisions). Thus, a significant TBI can occur without the victim sustaining a direct blow to the head (Jennett, 1986).

Dynamic loading produces two main mechanical phenomena responsible for pathologic changes in closed-head injury—contact and inertial loading (acceleration) (Gennarelli, 1993; Katz,

1992). Contact loading is a direct result of an impact to the head and leads to local skull distortions or fractures, and contusions or laceration of the brain at the point of contact (i.e., coup contusions). The propagation of shock waves throughout the skull and brain can also occur and may result in small intracerebral hemorrhages in certain vulnerable areas.

Inertial loading or acceleration results from head motion generated by either impact or impulsive forces. This event results in translational or rotational acceleration (Gennarelli, 1993; Pang, 1985). *Translational acceleration* occurs when all parts of the body are similarly accelerated and there is no resultant relative movement taking place among the constituent parts of the brain (Pang, 1985). There is, however, differential movement between the brain and the skull during which the cortex may repeatedly impact against the sharp internal structures of the skull. The predominant injuries resulting from this mechanism are brain contusions, which occur directly opposite the point of impact (i.e., contrecoup contusions).

Rotational acceleration occurs when the head receives a force that does not pass through its center of gravity. This results in the head assuming an angular acceleration and rotating around its own center of gravity. Such acceleration of the head results in a twisting motion between the brain and the skull and causes shear-strain or distortion of the brain tissue (Bigler, 1990; Pang, 1985). Such distortion of the brain tissue results in the permanent stretching or rupturing of neuronal fibers that interconnect different brain regions. The resultant damage is referred to as diffuse axonal injury (DAI) and is widely distributed with most lesions occurring in deep white matter areas of the cerebral hemispheres and in the brainstem (Bigler, 1990).

The biomechanics of closed-head injury are determined largely by the physical and structural properties of the skull and contents (Holbourn, 1943). The brain is a relatively mobile mass of material within a rigid container. Holbourn (1943) considered the most important physical properties of the brain to be its comparatively uniform density, its extreme incompressibility, its small resistance to change in shape, and its high susceptibility to shear-strain damage. During rotational acceleration of the head, the brain does not compress but readily changes shape, or distorts, in an attempt to follow the motion of the skull as it rotates about the brain resulting in shear-strain damage to the brain tissue. Holbourn (1943) described shear-strain distortion as the "type of deformation which occurs in a pack of cards when it is deformed from a neat rectangular pile into an oblique-angled pile" (p. 438). He expounded the view that, following impacts that cause rotational acceleration of the head, shearing distortion takes place in all parts of the brain as it tries to follow the motion of the skull.

At the time of impact, as a result of external forces, the brain moves within the skull, making contact with its rigid walls, with the greatest degree of contact occurring between the soft frontal and temporal lobes and the bony prominences of the skull (e.g., sphenoidal ridge). Consequently, the skull-brain interface also has an important influence on the mechanics of head injury, particularly in relation to sites of lesion (Bigler, 1990). Anatomically, the skull is a spherical vault, with its anterior and middle cranial fossae having rough and irregular bases. The sharp, lesser wing

of the sphenoid bone intervenes between these two fossae. The anterior ventral aspect of both frontal lobes of the brain is separated by a bony protuberance of the ethmoid bone called the crista galli. In adults, the surfaces of the skull in the regions of both the lesser wing of the sphenoid bone and the ethmoid bone are jagged and rough. Many authors view these structures as being directly responsible for "bruising" of surrounding brain tissues following a closed-head injury (Adams, 1975; Bigler, 1990). Holbourn (1943) suggested that the anatomical structures in these areas allow the skull to get a good "grip" on the brain, during rotational acceleration.

Differences in the physical and structural properties of children's heads and adult heads have been implicated as at least part of the explanation for the better prognosis for recovery from TBI reported to occur in children compared to adults (Levin, Ewing-Cobbs, & Benton, 1984). These authors attributed the greater capacity of young children to survive severe closed-head injury, as compared with adults, to anatomic and physical features of head injury that differ between the two populations. Jellinger (1983) also suggested that the morphology of cranial injuries in infancy and childhood is different from that in adults. As indicated earlier, according to Holbourn (1943), the type of brain damage that results from a severe head injury depends on the physical properties of the individual's brain and skull. These physical properties are known to differ in a number of ways between children and adults, thereby contributing to different patterns of brain injury following head trauma in each group (Lindenberg & Freytag, 1969). First, an infant's brain weight at birth is 15% of body weight, progressing through to only 3% of body weight in adults (Friede, 1973). By the end of the second year of life, brain weight is 75% of the adult brain weight and reaches 90% of adult brain weight by the end of the sixth year (Jellinger, 1983). Second, the existence of unfused sutures and open fontanelles makes the skull of an infant and young child more pliable. Some authors have suggested that, because of its elasticity and greater degree of deformation, the skull of an infant absorbs the energy of the physical impact and thereby protects the brain better than the skull of an adult (Menkes & Till, 1995). Other authors, however, believe the greater pliability of the heads of infants makes them more susceptible to external forces than older children and adults. According to Menkes and Till (1995), although deformation of the head absorbs much of the energy of the impact, thereby reducing the effects of acceleration/deceleration, it adds to the risk of tearing blood vessels. A third anatomic difference in the skulls of children versus adults that may aid a better prognosis in the former group is that, unlike adults, the floors of the middle cranial fossa and the orbital roofs in children are relatively smooth and offer little resistance to the shifting brain.

Alternatively, the differences reported in the prognosis for recovery following TBI between children and adults also may be related to the different nature of the impacts causing head injury in these two groups (Hendrick, Harwood-Nash, & Hudson, 1964). As described earlier, most childhood accidents result from child abuse, falls, or low speed (30 to 60 km per hour) pedestrian or bicycle accidents that involve a motor vehicle. Consequently, many pediatric head injuries are associated with a lesser degree of rotational acceleration and, therefore presumably a lesser amount of brain damage (Levin, Benton, & Grossman, 1982). Adults, on the other hand, as well as persons in their late teenage years, are more likely to sustain TBI as a result of high-speed motor vehicle accidents, which by their nature are likely to yield greater diffuse brain injury.

Neuropathophysiology of Traumatic Brain Injury

A knowledge of the neuropathophysiology of closed-head injury provides a framework for predicting and understanding the resultant clinical behaviors and contributes insight into brain-behavior relationships. The principal pathologies associated with closed-head injury have been categorized in various ways. Typically, the divisions involve differentiating focal or diffuse lesions, as well as those that are primary (immediate on impact) injuries and those that are secondary phenomena not attributable to the impact itself. There is evidence, however, that primary and secondary pathologies combine to form marked heterogeneity of injury (Levin et al., 1982; Pang, 1985). The frequent neuropathophysiologic sequelae of closed-head injury are summarized in Table 3–1 and discussed further below.

Primary Neuropathophysiologic Effects of TBI

Primary brain damage occurs at the moment of impact and is the result of the instantaneous events caused by the blow. This damage frequently constitutes the limiting factor for ideal neurologic

Table 3–1. Primary and Secondary Brain Injury After Closed-Head Injury

Lesion	Injury
Primary diffuse	Diffuse axonal injury
Primary focal	Contusions
	Laceration
	Basal ganglia hemorrhage
	Cranial nerve lesions
Secondary diffuse	Cerebral edema
	Raised intracranial pressure
	Ischemia
	Brain shift and herniation
	Cerebral atrophy and ventricular enlargement
Secondary focal	Hematoma:
	• extradural
	• subdural
	• intracranial

recovery (Pang, 1985) and includes DAI, contusions, laceration, basal ganglia hemorrhage, and cranial nerve lesions.

Primary Diffuse Lesions

Diffuse cerebral injury, in the form of widespread damage to the axons in the white matter of the brain, produced at the moment of impact is widely considered to be the primary mechanism of brain damage in individuals with closed-head injury, and a more important factor in determining outcome than the presence of focal lesions (Adams, Mitchell, Graham, & Doyle, 1977; Gennarelli et al., 1982; Strich, 1956, 1961, 1969). This pathologic state, also referred to as diffuse axonal injury (DAI)

was first described by Strich (1956) who determined the presence of diffuse degeneration of the cerebral white matter in the absence of focal pathology in the brains of four survivors of TBI who were quadriplegic and in a profoundly demented or vegetative state. Strich (1956, 1961) concluded that the severe neurologic deficit manifest in these cases was the result of axonal damage produced by mechanical forces shearing the fibers at the moment of impact.

A number of different areas of the brain have been reported to be commonly affected by DAI subsequent to traumatic head injury, including the subcortical white matter of the cerebral hemispheres, the upper brainstem, the superior cerebellar peduncles, and the basal ganglia (Adams, Graham, Murray, & Scott, 1982; Strich, 1969). The interface between the gray and white matter also is commonly involved due to shearing between the different tissue types. Magnetic resonance imaging has identified DAI in the brainstem, hippocampus, corpus callosum, and at interfaces between the brain and dura mater (Guthrie, Mast, Richards, McQuaid, & Pavlakis, 1999).

The concept proposed by Strich (1956, 1961) that DAI is an immediate effect of a closed-head injury has been challenged. Jellinger and Seitelberger (1970), although agreeing that one etiological factor of DAI was mechanical damage to the nerve fibers, suggested that vascular, edematous, and anoxic damage to the cerebral cortex and basal ganglia played a significant role in the pathogenesis of white matter changes. Adams et al. (1982), in a study involving a comparison of fatal head trauma cases with and without DAI, failed to find any significant differences between the two groups with respect to the incidence of cerebral edema or hypoxic brain damage. They concluded that DAI occurs immediately, at the time of impact, and is not secondary to any other form of brain damage. Adams et al. (1982) described DAI in terms of a triad of distinctive features: a focal lesion in the corpus callosum; a focal lesion in the dorsolateral quadrants of the rostral brainstem; and microscopic evidence of diffuse damage to axons, such as axonal retraction balls, microglial stars, and degeneration of specific fiber tracts in the white matter.

The findings of Adams et al. (1982) were supported by those of Gennarelli et al. (1982) who induced DAI in the brains of nonhuman primates by means of imparting angular acceleration. DAI identical to that known to occur in humans subsequent to traumatic head injury was produced and three grades of severity were identified. In the most severe grade, DAI was characterized by a focal lesion in the dorsolateral quadrant of the rostral brainstem in addition to a lesion in the corpus callosum and axonal damage in the cerebral white matter. Gennarelli et al. (1982) concluded that the degree of DAI was directly related to the duration and severity of coma and the clinical outcome. These findings suggest that there is a continuum of axonal injury and were later supported by Blumbergs, Jones, and North (1989) who described similar grades of DAI in humans. According to Adams, Graham, Gennarelli, and Maxwell (1991) even people who have sustained a mild head injury and are rendered unconscious for as little as 5 minutes after injury, have some degree of DAI.

Although DAI is still largely classed as a primary injury, that classification has been further challenged in recent years by Letarte (1999). He argues that, although immediate traumatic axotomy occurs, most of the axonal disruption occurs later. According to Letarte (1999) the majority of axons that eventually will suffer damage remain in continuity immediately after injury, and that it is not until around six hours postinjury that the neurofilaments are destroyed and axotomy occurs (Teasdale & Graham, 1998). The model of axonal injury proposed by Letarte (1999) is different from the immediate, irreversible mechanism described by earlier researchers and implies that the deterioration in patients postinjury may be due to this progressive secondary injury and raises the possibility of developing medical strategies to intervene in this progressive degeneration of axons.

Primary Focal Lesions

A brain contusion (bruise) consists of an area of brain tissue characterized by multifocal capillary hemorrhages, vascular engorgement, and edema. A linear impact on the skull may result in transient distortion and inbending of the bone near to the point of impact causing compression of adjacent brain tissue and bruising of the brain in an area directly below the area of impact. Contusions that occur at the point of impact are termed "coup" contusions. In addition to causing lesions at this site, the impact may cause the brain to strike the skull at a point opposite to the point of trauma, thereby resulting in additional vascular disruption and bruising at this latter site. Contusions of the latter type are termed "contrecoup" contusions. Both coup and contrecoup lesions may cause specific and localizable behavioral alterations that accompany closed-head injury (Lezak, 1983). The symptoms produced by a brain contusion depend on the size and location of the contusion, and may include speech, language, and swallowing disorders. Because intracellular swelling of adjacent structures frequently is associated with contusions, secondary brain damage may develop leading some authors to suggest that the clinical significance of contusions lies more in the risk of the secondary injuries caused by the mass effects than the focal damage itself (Gennarelli, 1993).

Irrespective of the point of impact, brain contusions most often are found in the orbital and lateral surfaces of the frontal and temporal lobes, which occupy the anterior and middle cranial fossae (Auerbach, 1986). The frequent presence of contusions in these sites is due to the brain abrading against the irregular and jagged skull surfaces with which it interfaces (Bigler, 1990). Similarly, the frequent occurrence of contusions on the medial surface of the hemispheres and in the corpus callosum are thought to result from the movement of the brain against the falx cerebri and the tentorium (Gurdjian & Gurdjian, 1976). Previously, contusions were considered to occur only in cortical regions; however, computerized tomographic scans have identified contusions within deep areas of the brain.

When a brain contusion is sufficiently severe to cause a visible breach in the continuity of the brain, it is referred to as a laceration. Lacerations are more typically associated with penetrating head injuries than closed-head injuries and tend to be associated with more severe and prolonged neurologic sequelae than contusions.

Although intracerebral hematoma associated with closed-head injury usually is considered a secondary insult or a primary complication rather than the result of immediate impact injury (Levin et al., 1982), traumatic basal ganglia hematoma has been reported to be indicative of severe primary brain damage (Coloquhoun & Rawlinson, 1989). A distinct and relatively rare traumatic entity, traumatic basal ganglia hematoma, occurs in approximately 3% of severe closed-head injuries. Although it can occur in isolation or in association with other intracerebral hematomas and contusions, most often it is found in patients who have suffered severe diffuse white matter injury (Coloquhoun & Rawlinson, 1989).

A severe closed-head injury can cause dysfunction of a variety of cranial nerves, by either damaging the cranial nerve nuclei in the brainstem or disrupting the nerves themselves in either their intracranial or extracranial course (Murdoch, 1990). Contusions of the brainstem can damage the cranial nerve nuclei leading to flaccid paralysis of the muscles innervated by the affected nerves. In particular, should these affected muscles include the muscles supplied by cranial nerves V, VII, X, or XII, speech disorders may result. The most common cause of damage to the cranial nerves in their intracranial course is fracture of the base of the skull. The facial nerve (VII) is most commonly affected by this condition leading to flaccid paralysis of the muscles of facial expression. Branches of the facial (VII) and trigeminal (V) nerves may be damaged extracranially by trauma to the face. In general, traumatic cranial nerve palsies are permanent, the exceptions being those resulting from contusions of extracranial branches of the nerves (Murdoch, 1990).

Secondary Neuropathophysiologic Effects of TBI

Primary brain injury can generate a variety of secondary insults to the brain, which in turn trigger a pathophysiologic cascade of events. Secondary injury has the potential to be limited with appropriate therapeutic interventions (Gjerris, 1986) and includes cerebral edema, intracranial hemorrhage, ischemic brain damage, pathologic changes associated with increased intracranial pressure (ICP), cerebral atrophy, and ventricular enlargement.

Secondary Diffuse Lesions

According to Bigler (1990), cerebral edema, which involves an increase in brain volume due to an accumulation of excess water in the brain tissue, is "the most common secondary effect of brain injury" (p. 32). Adams, Graham, Scott, Parker, and Doyle (1980) described three types of brain swelling: localized brain swelling, which occurs around a contusion; unilateral brain swelling, which involves diffuse swelling of one cerebral hemisphere; and brain swelling that involves diffuse swelling of both cerebral hemispheres. Edema resulting from TBI is most commonly vasogenic and results from an increase in the permeability of brain capillaries, which allow water and other solutes to exude out into the extracellular spaces within the brain tissue (Levin et al., 1982; Pang, 1985). Various neuropathologic changes may occur as a result of sustained cerebral edema, including stretching and tearing of axonal fibers, compression of brain tissue resulting in cell loss, compression of blood vessels with subsequent infarction of brain tissue, and herniation of the brain (Bigler, 1990).

Elevated ICP occurs when there is an increase in one of the intracranial constituents—blood, brain, cerebrospinal fluid, or extracellular fluid—within the noncompliant skull (Pang, 1985). A sudden increase in ICP is a common finding after closed-head injury, most frequently due to the development of extradural, subdural or intracerebral hematomas, or generalized cerebral swelling. Uncontrolled increases in ICP may cause herniation (a shift of part of the brain to another cranial compartment) and can also impede cerebral blood flow resulting in ischemic brain damage (Levin et al., 1982; Murdoch,

1990; Pang, 1985). Murdoch (1990) described three types of cerebral herniation due to raised ICP following traumatic head injury including: transtentorial herniation, in which the medial portions of the temporal lobes are herniated through the tentorial hiatus, due to an increase in the ICP above the level of the tentorium cerebelli; tonsillar herniation, where the cerebellar tonsils are displaced down though the foramen magnum; and axial herniation, which occurs when there is a downward displacement of the entire brainstem due to increased ICP. Transtentorial herniation causes compression of the brainstem and interferes with the functioning of the reticular formation, thereby leading to a deterioration in the level of consciousness. At the same time, the third cranial nerve is compressed causing pupillary dilation, first on the side of the herniation and later on the other side as well. Eventually, if untreated, compression of the brainstem will lead to death. The level of consciousness and the state of the pupils of the eyes, therefore, are critical factors that require monitoring following closed-head injury. The only structure compressed by tonsillar herniation is the medulla and the first sign of its presence is often respiratory insufficiency or apnea. Although no structures are actually compressed by axial herniation, distortion of the brainstem, caused by its downward displacement, may cause altered levels of consciousness and changes in respiration.

Ischemic brain damage also is widely recognized as a common sequelae of closed-head injury (Adams et al., 1980; Graham, Adams, & Doyle, 1978) and ranges from focal necrosis to wide areas of infarction. Although areas of infarction generally are related to the presence of contusions, hematomas, distortion, and herniation of the brain and raised ICP, Adams (1975) also defined a specific category of ischemic brain damage characterized by different patterns of neuronal necrosis and infarction of the brain, which was not directly associated with these factors. Graham and Adams (1971) analyzed 100 cases of closed-head injury and discovered an unusually high incidence of diffuse neocortical necrosis even after known causes (e.g., cardiac arrest, status epilepticus, contusions, raised ICP, etc.) were eliminated. In a further study of 151 cases, Graham et al. (1978) confirmed a high incidence (91%) of ischemic brain damage following closed-head injury. They also reported that ischemic brain damage following traumatic head injury was more frequently found in the hippocampus (81%) and basal ganglia (79%) than in the cerebral cortex (46%).

The development of cerebral atrophy and ventricular enlargement in the brain following a severe closed-head injury has been frequently documented (Bigler, Kurth, Blatter, & Abildskov, 1993; Cullum & Bigler, 1986). Cullum and Bigler (1986) were able to demonstrate that the average ventricular enlargement in patients with TBI to be twice that of the normal person. They also reported the associated presence of marked cortical atrophy following brain injury, which tended to occur more frequently in the frontal and temporal areas of the brain, as well as in a diffuse pattern throughout the cerebral tissue. Traumatically induced cerebral atrophy and ventricular enlargement have been found to be related to subsequent neuropsychological deficits in complex reasoning and problem solving, memory, language, intellect, and social-emotional functioning (Cullum & Bigler, 1986; Levin et al., 1982).

Secondary Focal Lesions

Intracranial hemorrhages are common complications of a closed-head injury and may involve bleeding into the extradural, subdural, and subarachnoid spaces; into the ventricles; or directly into the brain tissues (Adams, 1975). Although these hemorrhages may occur immediately following impact, their effects usually are not evident until they are of sufficient volume to act as intracranial space-occupying lesions.

Extradural hematomas usually result from laceration of the middle meningeal artery by fractured bone and involve bleeding between the skull bones and the dura mater (Figure 3–1A). Hematomas of this type usually collect and enlarge fairly rapidly and signs of ICP become evident within a short

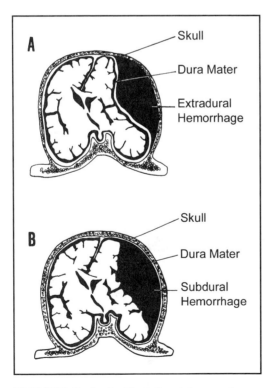

FIGURE 3–1. A. Extradural hemorrhage. **B.** Subdural hemorrhage.

period postinjury. Typically, although the patient may have been knocked unconscious at the time of head injury, consciousness is quickly recovered and then within 1 to 2 hours the patient becomes increasingly drowsy and develops paralysis down one side of the body as a result of compression of the ipsilateral cerebral hemisphere by the expanding hematoma. Eventually, the patient demonstrates pupillary dilation and loses consciousness from compression of the third cranial nerve and brainstem, respectively, as a consequence of herniation of the temporal lobe through the tentorial hiatus. Treatment of an extradural hematoma requires an emergency operation, which involves the drilling of a burr-hole over the bruise site and evacuating the clot. If left untreated, the patient will die as a result of compression of vital centers (e.g., respiratory centers) in the brainstem. Extradural hemorrhage has been reported to occur in approximately 10% of closed-head injured persons (Adams et al., 1980).

Subdural hemorrhage is more common than extradural hemorrhage and is attributed to rupture of small blood vessels within the subdural space leading to bleeding between the dura mater and arachnoid (Figure 3–1B). Adams et al. (1980) recorded an incidence of 45% of subdural hematomas in their series of head injured subjects. Subdural hematomas develop much more slowly than extradural hematomas and consequently, although the neurologic signs and symptoms resulting from associated increased ICP are the same, they appear at a much later time, in some cases days, in others weeks, after the traumatic head injury. If the hematoma develops to the stage of causing transtentorial herniation, as in the case of extradural hematoma, surgical evacuation of the clot is again required to prevent compression of the brainstem.

Subarachnoid hemorrhage occurs following rupture of the blood vessels that cross the subarachnoid space between the arachnoid and pia mater. Such hemorrhages are common occurrences after closed head injury and can be detected by the presence of blood in the cerebrospinal fluid. Although patients with subarachnoid hemorrhages may experience severe headaches and stiffness of the neck for many days, they normally recover spontaneously.

Intracerebral hemorrhages may present in the brain following closed-head injury either singularly or in a multiple format (Adams, 1975). These hematomas usually are directly related to contusions and therefore occur mainly in the subfrontal or temporal regions. Those occurring deep within the brain (e.g., in the basal ganglia) are thought to be due to the effects of shear strains on the small vessels at the moment of impact and are therefore usually regarded as primary injuries. An incidence of 42% of intracerebral hematomas has been reported in a study of closed-head injury subjects by Adams et al. (1980).

Other Complications of Traumatic Brain Injury

In addition to the primary and secondary brain damage outlined above, patients who experience a closed-head injury also may suffer from a number of other medical complications that may impact their quality of life posttrauma. These further complications include: skull fractures, rhinorrhea, and otorrhea, posttraumatic epilepsy, and posttraumatic vertigo.

Skull Fractures

The various different types of skull fracture associated with traumatic head injury are listed in Table 3–2. There is no direct relationship between the severity of any damage to the skull and the extent to which the brain is damaged. Although severe fractures of the skull usually are associated with severe cerebral injury, the brain may be extensively damaged without the skull being fractured. Alternatively, a fracture of the skull may occur without severe damage to the brain. Consequently, the fracture itself is of little importance in relation

Table 3–2. The Different Types of Skull Fracture

Fracture Type	Description
Simple	Cracks or fissures in the skull bone, skin intact
Compound	Cracks in skull bone, scalp also breached
Comminuted	The damage skull bone is broken into several pieces
Depressed	A piece of broken skull bone is driven inward and may cause laceration or compression on the underlying brain tissue

to occurrence of persistent neurologic deficits following traumatic head injury. Rather the presence of neurologic impairments is dependent on the location and extent of damage to the underlying structures, particularly the brain itself. Overall, depressed skull fractures are the most likely to produce severe and permanent neurologic signs due to the possibility of the dislodged piece of bone causing lacerations of the brain tissue.

Rhinorrhea and Otorrhea

These terms refer to the leakage of cerebrospinal fluid from the nose (rhinorrhea) and ear (otorrhea) subsequent to traumatic head injury. Rhinorrhea occurs following fracture of the frontal bone with associated tearing of the dura mater and arachnoid. Otorrhea, on the other hand, is caused by injuries to the base of the skull. As injuries in this latter region often damage the brainstem as well, otorrhea is of more serious prognostic importance than rhinorrhea. Infections and meningitis are potential hazards of both conditions.

Posttraumatic Epilepsy and Posttraumatic Vertigo. Although not incapacitating, these two complications of closed-head injury may have a profound effect on the lifestyle of the head-injured patient. Posttraumatic epilepsy occurs most commonly after penetrating head injuries, the epilepsy being triggered by the formation of scar tissue as a result of brain laceration. The scar may act as an irritating focus to trigger epileptic fits. In some cases, convulsions may occur very shortly after impact (within 24 hours), especially in children. When it occurs in adult head injury cases, however, the epilepsy usually develops within the first 2 years postinjury. Although more common in cases of penetrating head injuries, posttraumatic epilepsy also can occur subsequent to closed-head injuries, and may be triggered by the development of subdural hematomas.

Some degree of vertigo accompanied by vomiting and unsteadiness is common after head injury. Posttraumatic vertigo may last for days or weeks or in some cases may persist for many months.

Medical Management of Traumatic Brain Injury

There are two major components to contemporary treatment of patients with TBI. These include: (1) rapid evacuation of hematomas and control of increasing ICP; and (2) prevention of hypotension and hypoxia and maintenance of cerebral perfusion pressure (CPP) (Letarte, 1999). This current approach, however, has only been implemented since the mid-1980s. It evolved as a consequence of a greater understanding of the mechanisms of cerebral edema and ischemic brain injury brought about by research at the level of cellular physiology.

Until the mid-1980s, the paradigm for treatment of patients with TBI was very much focused on prevention of increasing ICP. There is evidence that, even from the earliest of times, an awareness existed of the special importance of brain swelling on the outcome from head injury. Archeologic findings indicate that in multiple and widespread locations throughout human evolution, trephination was practiced. From the early 1900s to the mid-1950s, rapid evacuation of space occupying lesions, and particularly hematomas, was the principal treatment for head-injured patients, with surgery being the only available treatment method. This treatment, however, was made available only to patients deemed to have space-occupying lesions and, therefore, eligible for surgery. Consequently, many patients who presented as lucid initially went on to deteriorate and often die as the result of untreated space-occupying lesions. Reilly and Adams (1975) reported that many patients with lucid intervals who later died, so-called "talk-and-die" patients, had space-occupying lesions that potentially were treatable. Fortunately, a means of rapidly identifying patients with space-occupying lesions was provided by the introduction of the computerized tomographic (CT) scanner in the mid-1970s. The introduction of this technology also had the effect of intensifying the surgical focus of the treatment of patients with head injury.

Although still focused on the treatment of elevated ICP, nonsurgical therapies for treatment of TBI were introduced in the mid-1950s. The first effective non-operative treatment for elevated ICP became available with the introduction of urea by Javid and Settlage (1956). Urea was followed by mannitol and in rapid sequence by a series of steroids. Parallel and complementary to these developments was the description of a technique by Lundberg (1960) that allowed continuous monitoring of ICP. Consequently, by the early 1960s a means of quantifying cerebral edema as well as methods for treating elevated ICP was available.

The catalyst to changing the paradigm for treatment of patients with head injury from being ICP centered to one that also recognized the need to maintain cerebral perfusion was a publication by Miller and Sweet (1978) that

highlighted ischemia as a significant threat to patients with head injury. This work culminated in Rosner and coworkers (Rosner, 1995; Rosner & Coley, 1986; Rosner & Daughton, 1990) defining a clinical approach to head injury that recognizes ischemia as of equal importance to edema and mass effect in terms of need for treatment.

Letarte (1999) predicted that, in addition to these essential components, a third component in the form of pharmacotherapy will be added to the treatment of patients with TBI early in the new millennium. In particular, pharmacotherapy will aim to combat the neurochemical mediations of secondary injury and will be augmented by new techniques for monitoring brain function such as cerebral blood flow (e.g., xenon CT), brain metabolism (e.g., positron emission tomography [PET]), and global cerebral oxygenation (e.g., jugular bulb monitoring) among others. Using these new techniques, clinicians not only will be able to view the structure of the injured brain but also will be able to map its blood flow and in so doing monitor the adequacy of attempts to maintain CPP. By being able to monitor the metabolism of the brain, clinicians will be able to track markers of neurologic injury and thereby better estimate the severity of the individual's injuries.

Clinical Characteristics of Language Disorder in Childhood Traumatic Brain Injury

Contrary to the traditional view that children make a rapid and full recovery from TBI, over the past two decades a number of studies have documented the existence of persistent language deficits subsequent to severe TBI in children. Gilchrist and Wilkinson (1979) reported that almost two-thirds of young people with severe TBI exhibit aphasic-type disorders. Areas of language function reported to be deficient in children following TBI include: verbal fluency (Chadwick, Rutter, Brown, Shaffer, & Traub, 1981; Chadwick, Rutter, Shaffer, & Shrout, 1981; Jordan, Ozanne, & Murdoch, 1990; Slater & Bassett, 1988); object naming (Jordan, Ozanne, & Murdoch, 1988; Jordan et al., 1990; Levin & Eisenberg, 1979a, 1979b); word and sentence repetition (Levin & Eisenberg, 1979a, 1979b); written output (Ewing-Cobbs, Fletcher, Levin, & Landry, 1985; Ewing-Cobbs, Levin, Eisenberg, & Fletcher, 1987). Unfortunately, the specific methodological approaches employed by different researchers to document the language abilities of children with TBI vary widely from study to study making it difficult to determine the pattern of language impairment in this population. For instance, in some studies, children with TBI have been included in larger groups of children with language difficulties arising from other neurologic conditions (e.g., cerebrovascular accident, brain tumor, etc.) making identification of specific areas of language impairment associated with TBI difficult (e.g., Alajouanine & Lhermitte, 1965; Hécaen, 1976). In addition, whereas some earlier researchers utilized aphasia batteries (e.g., Ewing-Cobbs et al., 1985, 1987; Levin & Eisenberg, 1979a, 1979b) to assess the language abilities of children with TBI, others more recently have used tests more appropriate for use with pediatric subjects (e.g., Jordan et al., 1988). This chapter provides an historical overview of research into the effects of childhood TBI on language abilities in an attempt to establish the status of our

understanding of the nature of language impairments in this population.

Performance on Formal Language Tests

The language abilities of a group of 32 children with acquired aphasia associated with a variety of etiologies, including TBI, cerebrovascular malformation, aneurysm, and occlusion of the middle cerebral artery among others, was evaluated by Alajouanine and Lhermitte (1965). They reported that the most obvious feature of the language disorder exhibited by the children in their group was a reduction in "expressive activities," with each child demonstrating a reduction in oral and written language and a reduction in the use of gestures.

Hécaen (1976) reported the language features of a group of 26 cases of acquired childhood aphasia of mixed etiology, which included 16 cases of head trauma. The associated aphasia was described by Hécaen as being characterized by a period of mutism followed by the recovery of language, marked by decreased initiation of speech, naming disorders, dyscalculia, and dysgraphia. Although less frequent, receptive language disorders were observed in one-third of the children with aphasia examined by Hécaen (1976). Due to the wide range of etiologies included in the subject groups examined by Alajouanine and Lhermitte (1965) and Hécaen (1976), however, any attempts to attribute the language features to any one etiological group such as TBI must of necessity be guarded.

Performance on Standard Aphasia Tests

The early investigations of language in groups composed only of children with

TBI used standardized instruments such as aphasia batteries and tests of specific language behaviors to determine the profile of language impairment. For example, the Neurosensory Center Comprehensive Examination for Aphasia (NCCEA) (Spreen & Benton, 1969) was used by Levin and Eisenberg (1979a) to examine the language abilities of a group of children and adolescents with closed-head injury. Deficits in auditory comprehension were identified in 11% of the group and verbal repetition was impaired in only 4%. Dysnomia for objects presented visually or tactually to the left hand were identified in about 12% of the group studied.

Ewing-Cobbs et al. (1985) also examined the language abilities of a group of children and adolescents with TBI using the NCCEA. Their findings showed that, during the early stages of recovery (less than 6 months posttrauma), a significant proportion of their subjects demonstrated linguistic impairments. In particular, naming disorders, dysgraphia, and reduced verbal productivity were prominent. These authors concluded that the language disorder identified was evidence of a "subclinical aphasia" rather that a frank aphasia disturbance. Ewing-Cobbs et al. (1985) speculated that, from a developmental perspective, the type of speech-language impairment incurred from a TBI is related to the language skills that are in primary ascendancy at the time of the injury. Furthermore, comparison of recovery related to the severity of injury indicated that children with moderate-severe TBI were more likely to demonstrate poorer performance on the naming and graphic subtests when compared to their mildly injured counterparts. In a further study of 23 children and 33 adolescents with TBI, Ewing-Cobbs et al. (1987) iden-

tified "clinically significant language impairment" in a large proportion of their subjects, with expressive and graphic functions most affected.

Performance on Pediatric Language Tests

The most comprehensive series of studies to have documented the language abilities of children with TBI using tests developed for pediatric application is that reported by Jordan and colleagues (Jordan, Cannon, & Murdoch, 1992; Jordan & Murdoch, 1990a, 1993, 1994; Jordan et al., 1988). Jordan et al. (1988) assessed the language abilities of a group of 20 TBI children, between 8 and 16 years of age, at least 12 months postinjury using the Test of Language Development series and the NCCEA. They found the TBI group to be mildly language impaired when compared to the language abilities of a group of age- and sex-matched, nonneurologically impaired controls. In particular, these investigators identified the presence of a specific deficit in naming in the TBI group. The linguistic impairment exhibited by the TBI children studied by Jordan et al. (1988), however, did not conform to any recognized development language disorder. Rather, it was noted by these researchers that the observed language disturbance was similar to that reported to occur following TBI in adults in that their children with TBI also presented with a "subclinical aphasia" characterized by dysnomia. Jordan et al. (1988) concluded that, in contrast to the traditional view that the immature brain makes a rapid and full recovery following traumatic injury, TBI in children can produce long-term and persistent language deficits. In a follow-up study of the same group of children with TBI 12 months later, Jordan and Murdoch (1990a) observed that the naming deficit had persisted while verbal fluency abilities had deteriorated.

The high-level language functioning of a group of 11 children with severe TBI was assessed by Jordan, Cremona-Meteyard, and King (1996). Their findings indicated that the children with severe TBI had a lesser ability to create sentences with reference to social stimuli and a reduced ability to interpret ambiguous or figurative expressions than a group of matched controls. In contrast, Jordan et al. (1996) noted that the children with severe TBI were similar to the control children in their ability to make inferences. Jordan et al. (1992) investigated the linguistic performance of a group of mildly head-injured children in adulthood but failed to identify any persistent linguistic deficits for this group even in the very long term. In contrast, however, Jordan and Murdoch (1994) were able to identify late linguistic sequelae from 10 to 34 years following severe TBI sustained during childhood. Although the overall scores achieved by these subjects fell within the average range on standardized test of adolescent language development, scores were lower for the severely TBI individuals than for controls on measures of lexical recognition and retrieval as well as auditory comprehension of grammatically complex commands. Interestingly, a generalized reduction in linguistic skills across all areas of language competence assessed (syntax, semantics, pragmatics) was noted, suggesting a lack of specificity of linguistic impairment in their sample. It would appear, therefore, that children with mild TBI may be relatively spared in terms of persistent linguistic deficits when com-

pared to their counterparts with severe TBI, although marked variability in linguistic outcomes is evident within the severe TBI group.

As pointed out by Murdoch (1990), although the rate of spontaneous recovery in children following traumatic brain injury is often described as excellent, persistent long-term language disorders do exist. In particular, naming difficulties in children with acquired aphasia are more common than first thought. Written language disorders often are more severe than oral language impairment, and expressive disorders more frequent than the receptive disorders of written language. These findings have recently been confirmed by Lehečková (2004) who documented the long-term language recovery in a Czech-speaking child with aphasia subsequent to severe polytrauma experienced as a result of a motor vehicle accident. Lehečková (2004) reported that the child, an 11-year-old girl, progressed from a global aphasia to a mild amnestic aphasia over a 3½-year period, in the process regaining her ability to use language for communication and reflection. Despite this noted recovery, however, the child failed to re-achieve fluent writing and reading, and exhibited grammatical and lexical problems which, although not apparent in her everyday conversation, continued to restrict her language. In particular, the case reported by Lehečková (2004) was unable to smoothly access the whole lexicon and was insensitive to some complicated grammatical features, especially those with a formal, nonsemantic character. Lehečková (2004) concluded that the aphasic symptoms exhibited by the child with TBI in her study were identical to those of comparable cases of adult aphasia, with the exception that the child continued to develop her linguistic skills beyond the acute stage postonset. Martins (2004) also noted, whereas aphasia recovery in adults is greatest in the first 3 months postonset (Hartman, 1981) with some recovery extending to one year (Basso, 1992), the acquired aphasia exhibited by the children included in her study continued to improve 5 or more years after lesion onset, with consequent changes in the aphasia profile and taxonomic diagnosis. Of relevance to the present chapter is that in 23 of the 50 children examined by Martins (2004), the cause of aphasia was TBI.

In summary, contrary to the long-held view that children make a rapid and full recovery from TBI, a number of studies reported over the past two decades have documented the existence of persistent language deficits subsequent to severe TBI in childhood. In particular, studies of language function after pediatric TBI have shown that expressive oral language skills, including verbal fluency and naming to confrontation, are most consistently compromised, whereas receptive language is less impaired and tends to recovery earlier after injury. The observed language impairment often is characterized initially by reduced verbal output or, in its most severe form, mutism, which is followed in the longer term by subtle high-level language deficits. Subclinical language disturbance, as reflected in impoverished verbal fluency, dysnomia, and decreased word-finding ability, is consistently reported in the literature. Frank aphasia, however, occurs in only a very small proportion of children suffering from TBI, if at all. The pattern of language impairment reported subsequent to childhood TBI is, therefore, similar in many ways to that reported in the literature relating to adult TBI.

Discourse Abilities

As indicated above, traditional studies of the linguistic abilities of children who have suffered a TBI have focused primarily on the use of standard language assessment procedures to document the characteristics of the language impairment exhibited by this population. In particular, many studies have utilized aphasia batteries to describe the linguistic skills of children with TBI. Unfortunately, many authors agree that traditional language measures may not adequately identify the range of language difficulties manifest in persons with TBI (Chapman et al., 1992; Jordan et al., 1992; McDonald, 1992, 1993). In many instances, despite the existence of subtle, high-level linguistic deficits, people with TBI tend to score within normal limits on traditional aphasia tests (Chapman et al., 1992; Jordan et al., 1992; Jordan & Murdoch, 1990a; Levin et al., 1982; McDonald, 1993). Furthermore, despite apparent recovery of language function as identified by structured language measures, both children and adults have been shown to have persistent deficits at the discourse level of language following TBI (Chapman, Levin, Wanek, Weyrauch, & Kufera, 1998; Dennis & Barnes, 1990; McDonald, 1992, 1993; Mentis & Prutting, 1987). Consequently, in an attempt to better define the scope of communicative impairment in children with TBI, many researchers recently have advocated the use of discourse measures to identify those aspects of the language disorder that have proven elusive to traditional language batteries (Dennis & Barnes, 1990; Dennis & Lovett, 1990; Ewing-Cobbs et al., 1985; Jordan et al., 1988).

According to Dennis and Lovett (1990), discourse refers to the use of communicative language in context. Discourse reflects the complex interaction between cognition, linguistic, and information processing abilities (Chapman, Levin, & Lawyer, 1999). Given that children with severe TBI exhibit deficits in a variety of cognitive functions, including attention, memory, visuospatial function, and psychosocial function among others, in addition to linguistic impairments, discourse analysis may provide a better indication of communicative ability following childhood TBI than structured linguistic measures. Although a variety of different discourse types are recognized, including descriptive, conversational, narrative, procedural, and expository discourse, by far the majority of studies that have investigated the discourse abilities of children with TBI have used narrative discourse (Campbell & Dollaghan, 1990; Chapman, 1995; Chapman et al., 1992; Chapman et al., 1998; Dennis, Jacennik, & Barnes, 1994; Jordan, Murdoch, & Buttsworth, 1991).

Performance on Narrative Discourse Tasks

Narrative tasks provide the opportunity to examine "complex language, sequencing of events, children's ability to make information explicit for the listener, and the knowledge of story structure" (Olley, 1989, p. 44). In addition, Liles, Coelho, Duffy, and Zalagens (1989) suggested that story generation tasks are useful in rendering characterizations of language use in high-level TBI subjects. Consequently, the inclusion of narrative tasks in a test battery for children with TBI has been seen by several research groups as having the potential to provide valuable information for documenting further the linguistic characteristics of the TBI population. To that end, Jordan et al. (1991) used a story generation task to examine the story grammar skills and intersentential cohesion abilities of a group of 20 children with TBI aged 8 to 16 years and 1 to 4 years postinjury. Performance of the children with TBI was compared to that of a group of nonneurologically impaired accident victims matched for age, sex, and socioeconomic status. No significant differences were found between the narrative skills of the children with TBI and the matched controls on any of the story grammar measures or use of cohesive devices. Jordan et al. (1991) inferred that the story generation task used in their study may not have yielded optimal narrative performance. In contrast, based on narratives collected during a storytelling task, Chapman et al. (1992) reported deficits in the story grammar skills of 20 children and adolescents with TBI when tested at least 1 year postinjury. In particular, their findings indicated that the discourse of children with severe TBI differed from that of normal controls on both language and information structures, the severe TBI cases producing less language and less information than the normal children in retelling a story. Furthermore, the subjects with severe TBI differed from those with mild/moderate TBI on information structure measures of narratives. The disruption in story structure was reported by Chapman et al. (1992) to be characterized primarily by omission of critical setting and action information.

Chapman et al. (1998) used a storytelling task to investigate the effects of severe TBI on discourse in children who were 6 to 8 years of age at the time of testing. In order to consider the effects of age at injury, these workers compared the narratives of children who sustained a TBI before the age of 5 years to those of children aged greater than 5 years at the time of injury. The results indicated that severe TBI has a deleterious effect on discourse in young children. In particular, Chapman et al. (1998) reported that their TBI cases exhibited marked reductions in the overall amount of information (propositions), in the structural completeness and in the expression of the central semantic meaning (gist) of the story. In contrast, measures of sentential length and complexity did not differ between the severe TBI group and the control subjects. Consistent with the findings of Jordan et al. (1991), the ability of the children with severe TBI to manipulate certain cohesive devices (e.g., use of reference and connectors) was comparable to those of the control subjects. Although no significant differences were found by Chapman et al. (1998) according to age at injury, these researchers suggested that there was a consistent pattern of generally poorer discourse for the early injured group (i.e., less than 5 years of age at the time of injury).

Ewing-Cobbs et al. (1998) examined linguistic structure, cohesion, and thematic recall of the narrative discourse of two groups of children with TBI selected on the basis of the presence or absence of acute language disturbance. A sibling comparison group was also included. Based on a storytelling task, the language-impaired TBI group produced fewer words and utterances than the sibling group, their stories being characterized by fewer complete referential and lexical ties, and more referential errors, which Ewing-Cobbs et al. (1998) suggested were indicative of difficulty conjoining meaning across sentences. In addition, the language-impaired TBI group was reported to recall only one-third of the propositions needed to maintain the story theme and made more errors sequencing the

propositions than the other two groups. The language-impaired TBI group, however, did not differ from the other two groups on measures of rate and fluency of speech production, number or length of mazes, use of conjunctives, or naming errors. Overall, the majority of the findings reported by Ewing-Cobbs et al. (1998) are consistent with those of Chapman et al. (1992) who, as noted earlier, reported a reduction in the number of words, number of sentences and amount of core information retained in the narratives of children and adolescents with severe TBI in conjunction with preservation of syntactic complexity and fluency.

Performance on Conversational Discourse Tasks

To date, only two studies of the conversational discourse abilities of children with TBI have been reported (Campbell & Dollaghan, 1990; Jordan & Murdoch, 1990b). Campbell and Dollaghan (1990) collected a series of spontaneous conversation samples from 9 children and adolescents with TBI over a period of approximately 13 months. At the time of initial assessment 2 to 16 weeks postinjury, significant differences in all measures of expressive language were identified when compared to a normal control group. Significant improvement occurred, however, in the TBI group over the 13 months between the initial and final assessment. Although at the final follow-up the TBI group was reported to produce fewer utterances than controls, their performance on other measures including total number of words, total number of different words, mean length of utterances in morphemes, percentage of complex utterances, and percentage of utterances within mazes was the same as the controls. Campbell and Dollaghan (1990) did note, however, that the patterns of deficit and recovery in the TBI group were heterogeneous with 5 of the 9 TBI cases continuing to exhibit marked deficits. Jordan and Murdoch (1990b) elicited conversations from a group of 20 children with TBI and examined the conversational skills using the Clinical Discourse Analysis (Damico, 1985). No significant differences were found between the performance of the TBI children and a group of matched controls on this measure of conversational competency. Jordan and Murdoch (1990b) cautioned, however, that the children with TBI in their study were all between 1 and 5 years postinjury at the time of testing. They highlighted the need for further research of a prospective nature examining the performance of children with TBI throughout the course of recovery on measures of conversational competency to clarify the relationship between time postinjury and the occurrence of conversational error behaviors.

In summary, evidence is available to suggest that the discourse abilities of children with TBI are impaired in a number of ways compared to normals. As yet, however, the relationship between factors such as age at injury, lesion site and size, severity of injury, and so forth, and the occurrence of deficits in discourse skills is unknown.

Recovery of Language Function Following Childhood Traumatic Brain Injury

The traditionally held viewpoint that the child's brain exhibits a plasticity that enables rapid recovery of function following trauma had its origins in the work of Cotard (1868; cited in Levin et al., 1982). He reported that early or congenital damage to the left cerebral hemisphere did not lead to aphasia. This hypothesis was further supported by studies of a wide variety of brain injury cases, including children suffering congenital vascular disease, hemispherectomy for intractable seizures, as well as traumatic head injury (Lenneberg, 1967; Smith, 1974). In more recent years, however, studies documenting the presence of persistent cognitive, behavioral as well as linguistic impairments subsequent to childhood TBI have cast some doubt on the traditional view of rapid and complete recovery in this population. Despite these doubts, few studies have documented the course of language recovery in children following TBI by way of a series of prospective evaluations.

Prospective Studies of Language Recovery in Childhood TBI

Jordan and Murdoch (1993) followed the course of speech and language recovery of a group of 11 children with TBI over a period of 18 months postinjury. Although their findings confirmed that children with TBI have the potential for significant gains in speech and language skills subsequent to injury, Jordan and Murdoch (1993) noted that few of their subjects recovered to within normal limits on all language measures used, with 2 of the 11 subjects in particular experiencing severe, long-term speech and language deficits. Jordan and Murdoch (1993) commented that, although the patterns of language recovery demonstrated by their subjects were variable and very individual, naming and word-finding abilities as measured on a test of confrontation naming were particularly vulnerable to injury, with the majority of children with TBI experiencing persistent difficulties in this area of linguistic competence. Other authors also have reported dysnomia or word-finding difficulties to be a frequent persistent sequelae to childhood TBI (Ewing-Cobbs et al., 1985; Levin & Eisenberg, 1979a, 1979b; Martins, 2004; Winogran, Knights, & Bawden, 1984).

In a prospective study of 50 children who sustained aphasia as a consequence of a non-progressive brain lesion, Martins (2004) reported that 11 (22%) remained chronically aphasic for 2 or more years postonset. Six of the 11 children with aphasia who did not recover were reported to have had severe head injuries with depressed fractures. Lehečková (2004) reported persistent reading, writing, lexical, and grammatical problems in a Czech child 3½ years subsequent to multiple severe injuries sustained in a motor vehicle accident at 11 years of age.

Factors Affecting Language Recovery in Childhood TBI

A number of factors have been proposed to influence the recovery of language following childhood TBI. These include the severity of the TBI (as measured by the Glasgow Coma Scale [GCS]), the site and size of lesion, and the age at injury. Severity of TBI has frequently been cited as one of the most important variables in determining the recovery of TBI children, with more severe injuries tending to be associated with a poorer long-term prognosis for recovery (Chapman, 1995; Chapman et al., 1998; Jordan & Murdoch, 1993). Discourse measures have been reported to be lower in children who suffered a severe TBI, whereas children with mild TBI perform similarly to

normal controls on discourse tasks (Chapman, 1995, Chapman et al., 1998). Similarly, severity of injury was found to affect the rate of recovery of the TBI children investigated by Jordan and Murdoch (1993). They reported that their children with mild TBI tended to demonstrate most improvements in the language skills evaluated in the first 6 months postinjury. In contrast, the children with severe TBI included in the group investigated by Jordan and Murdoch (1993) demonstrated more gradual improvement in language skills over the 18-month period of their prospective study. Jordan and Murdoch (1993) speculated that the observed differential rate of recovery is related to differences in the initial injury observed in children with severe TBI compared to children with mild TBI. By nature of definition, children with severe TBI are more likely to suffer more extensive diffuse brain injury than their mildly TBI counterparts. Indeed, Bruce, Alavi, Bilaniuk, Colinskas, Obrist, and Uzzell (1981) suggested that the degree of recovery subsequent to TBI is probably dependent on the extent of axonal injury. Jordan and Murdoch (1993) further speculated that, although children with mild TBI suffer less initial trauma in the form of diffuse axonal injury, they still experience the temporary secondary complication typical of TBI, that is, brain swelling. Rapid resolution of such brain swelling may well result in rapid restoration of function, provided there is no persistent local cerebral damage. In contrast, children with severe TBI, as well as experiencing these secondary effects of TBI, also experience more persistent primary axonal damage, leading to their poorer prognosis for recovery.

Despite the support in the literature for the notion that severity of TBI is an important factor influencing the degree of language recovery in children, it is evident that this factor alone does not fully account for degree of recovery in all cases. Examination of recovery patterns on an individual case basis often shows that the recovery patterns exhibited by individual children vary widely. In some cases, children with severe TBI have been reported to show significant recovery of their language abilities while at the same time children with mild to moderate TBI may show poor recovery. For example, 3 of the children included in the prospective study of language recovery carried out by Jordan and Murdoch (1993) had very severe injuries (GCS = 3). Unexpectedly, only 2 of the 3 children experienced severe speech and language deficits in the long term. The third child demonstrated a "significant" recovery of his language skills, although he was reported to demonstrate a marked deficit in naming skills. Chapman, Watkins, Gustafson, Moore, Levin, and Kufera (1997) likewise have noted that severity of TBI does not always correspond to the degree of recovery of discourse abilities in children with TBI.

In addition to severity of injury, the site and size of lesion have been identified as possible factors influencing language recovery following childhood TBI. Although historically it was considered that children did not demonstrate the marked cerebral dominance for language observed in adults, more recent research has challenged this viewpoint, suggesting that significant language impairment is far more likely subsequent to dominant hemisphere damage, rather than nondominant hemisphere damage (Aram, Ekelman, Rose, & Whitaker, 1985; Aram, Ekelman, & Whitaker, 1986, 1987; Carter, Hohenegger, & Satz,

1982; Satz & Bullard-Bates, 1981). Aram et al. (1985, 1986, 1987) reported that the syntactic abilities of children who sustain early left hemisphere vascular lesions are compromised to a greater degree than children with early right hemisphere lesions. As further evidence of lateralization in childhood, Chapman (1997) noted that children with left hemisphere lesions as a consequence of TBI are more likely to show specific language disturbances on traditional language measures than children with an intact left hemisphere. Jordan and Murdoch (1993) suggested that the absence of significant localized damage to the dominant hemisphere may have been an important factor in the good recovery of linguistic competency observed in the majority of children with TBI included in their prospective study.

The size or volume of lesions incurred as a result of TBI also has been reported to be related to language abilities, with larger lesions being associated with greater levels of impairment (Levin, Ewing-Cobbs, & Eisenberg, 1995). In particular, Levin et al. (1995) reported that the volume of left or right frontal lobe lesions in children increased the predictive value of performance on a verbal fluency task as well as on a response modulation task (i.e., respond to one stimulus and withhold response to another stimulus).

The relationship between age at injury and language outcome is somewhat controversial. It has been suggested that brain injury may have its greatest effect on the acquisition of new language skills rather than the recovery of previously established abilities (Hebb, 1942). If true, this hypothesis may explain the noted relatively good recovery of lexical and grammatical aspects of language after brain injury, in that these abilities are often well established in children prior to injury. Consistent with this suggestion are the findings of recent studies that implicate a younger age at injury with a more deleterious impact on long-term language recovery (Chapman et al., 1998; Ewing-Cobbs et al., 1987; Ewing-Cobbs, Miner, Fletcher, & Levin, 1989). Chapman et al. (1998) reported poorer discourse abilities for children who suffered brain injuries prior to 5 years of age than children injured at 5 years of age or older. Likewise, Ewing-Cobbs et al. (1989) identified that children with brain injuries incurred prior to 31 months of age performed more poorly on expressive language tasks than children with brain injuries sustained later than 31 months of age. Also consistent with this pattern, Ewing-Cobbs et al. (1987) noted that written language is more disrupted in children with TBI than adolescents with TBI. Shaffer, Bijur, Chadwick, and Rutter (1980) reported that children who suffer brain injuries prior to 8 years of age have more significant reading problems than children who suffer TBI later in life. Contrary to these findings, Martins (2004) reported that age was not a significant factor for determining prognosis in her group of 50 children who developed aphasia between the ages of 1.5 and 15 years. Rather, Martins (2004) noted that lesion-related variables (size and nature) were the main factors responsible for the outcome.

Latent Behavioral Deficits Following TBI

Retrospective studies of the long-term consequences of TBI have provided evidence that TBI in childhood may lead to the manifestation of behavioral deficits at some later stage in the child's development despite apparent recovery in the short-term postinjury (Bates, Reilly, & Marchman, 1992; Chapman & Levin, 1994). According to Eslinger, Grattan, Damasio, and Damasio (1992), these latent deficits may not be evident until the child with TBI reaches maturity or even, in some cases, enters adult life. Although the mechanism underlying the manifestation of latent behavioral disturbances is not known, Chapman et al. (1999) outlined two possible explanations for their occurrence. First, brain injury may prevent the child from attaining the higher cognitive levels required to support later developmental processes. Second, latent deficits arise from damage to an immature brain region causing a delay of symptoms until that region reaches functional maturity. In fact, the latent deficits may result from an interaction between both of these mechanisms (Chapman et al., 1999).

Differential Recovery of Language Following Childhood TBI

As mentioned earlier in this chapter, the patterns of recovery of linguistic competency exhibited by children following TBI vary greatly from case to case. To illustrate the diversity of these recovery patterns, three cases are presented below. The first case demonstrates what traditionally would be described as a typical recovery pattern and serves to illustrate why children with TBI have, in the past, been renowned for making a rapid and full recovery. The second and third cases, however, show less typical courses of recovery, characterized by persistent significant language impairments.

Case 1: Samantha

Samantha was a 9-year-old right-handed female who was admitted to hospital following a horse riding accident. Although she had not suffered any loss of consciousness immediately following the accident, Samantha was unresponsive to commands. At the time of admission to hospital, she was noted to be irritable and thrashing and her eyes were deviated to the left. Her GCS score was 7 and she demonstrated focal fitting. A computerized tomographic (CT) scan performed shortly after admission revealed no abnormality except for a fracture of the skull in the region of the left occiput.

At 1 day posttrauma Samantha appeared able to recognize her mother but made no attempt to communicate. During the following 24 hours, rapid deterioration of her condition occurred to a state of deep coma. A repeat CT scan at this stage demonstrated the presence of right cerebral edema, with compressed ventricles and some midline shift. The child was electively ventilated and paralyzed for 1 week posttrauma at which time she was weaned off the ventilator and the medication. Focal seizures continued; however, by 9 days postinjury, Samantha was able to open her eyes and shortly after was able to follow simple commands. By 2 weeks postinjury, Samantha was described as bright and enjoyed watching television; however, she still failed to initiate communication and to respond socially. Response to yes/no questions at this time was demonstrated by the use of eye closing. Four weeks after the accident, Samantha showed socially appropriate but simplified language, her speech at this time being described as labored. She was discharged from hospital with regular medical and paramedical follow-up.

Samantha's language abilities were then assessed at regular 6-monthly intervals over an 18-month period postinjury using a battery of standardized language tests which included NCCEA, the Test of Language Development-Intermediate (TOLD-I) (Hammill & Newcomer, 1982), the Boston Naming Test (BNT) (Kaplan, Goodglass, & Weintraub, 1983) and selected subtests of the Clinical Evaluation of Language Functions (CELF) (Semel-Mintz & Wiig, 1982). In addition to these standardized tests, a conversation sample was also collected and analyzed for syntactic adequacy using Prutting and Kirchner's (1987) Pragmatic Protocol.

Samantha's performance on the NCCEA was essentially normal even in the acute stage postinjury and little variability in performance on this test occurred over the 18 month period. At initial assessment 1 month postinjury, Samantha achieved a Spoken Language Quotient of 83 on the TOLD-I, which was just outside the normal range according to the test norms. Based on her performance on the TOLD-I, Samantha made steady gains over the 18-month recovery period and at the final assessment was achieving scores within the normal range for all subtests. A raw score of 38 was achieved at the initial assessment with the BNT, Samantha's performance at this time being marked by numerous semantic errors such as "dice" for "dominoes" and "penguin" for "pelican." Samantha did make continuous quantitative gains in her naming skills over the 18-month test period; however, her performance on the BNT at final contact continued to be marked by semantic errors. At times during the course of the final assessment Samantha requested the first sound of a word to cue her response. The accuracy score achieved by Samantha for the confrontation naming subtest of the CELF was well within normal limits at the initial assessment; however, speed of performance was markedly reduced. By 19 months postinjury, Samantha had little difficulty on the confrontation naming test of the CELF, which requires rapid access of familiar names (for shapes and colors). Performance of the word association subtest of the CELF, which requires the naming of animals and food within a prescribed time period, was within normal limits at each of the test intervals.

Samantha demonstrated well-developed syntactic skills and no deficit areas were identified. Although all communicative acts identified by the Pragmatic Protocol were found to be appropriate, it was noted in the acute stage postinjury, that Samantha's conversational fluency was often interrupted by repetitions and circumlocutory behavior as she appeared to search for the appropriate word. By 18 months postinjury, however, most evidence of word searching behaviors had disappeared, with only the occasional linguistic dysfluency apparent. Based on Samantha's initial conversational sample, it was evident that she had difficulty interpreting jokes in any more than a literal sense and also demonstrated some difficulty understanding complex instructions with frequent repetitions required. At the time of the final assessment, however, Samantha was able to cope with complex verbal instructions; however, she continued to interpret according to literal meaning and demonstrated persistent difficulties with figurative language (e.g., Samantha could only interpret proverbs in a purely literal sense).

In summary, Samantha demonstrated a typical recovery from severe TBI characterized by significant language impairment during the acute stage of recovery, followed by a rapid return of functional communication skills during the first 6 months posttrauma. At the time of initial standardized testing (6 months postinjury) Samantha demonstrated only minimal language impairment, which featured slightly reduced scores on tests of overall language abilities, and evidence of a mild word-finding difficulty. On the basis of the test results and observation and analysis of Samantha's conversational skills over the 18-month period postinjury, it was concluded that Samantha presented with a high-level language deficit affecting both verbal fluency and word retrieval and higher level auditory comprehension abilities.

Case 2: Jane

Jane, a 7-year-old, right-handed female, was admitted to hospital following a motor vehicle-pedestrian accident. On admission to hospital, she presented with a dilated right pupil and left focal fitting involving the entire left arm. Jane was assigned a GCS score of 3 on admission. A CT scan performed shortly after admission demonstrated the presence of a small amount of blood in the right lateral ventricle, in the choroid plexus, and fourth ventricle. A small cerebral contusion also was identified in the right frontal region although no mass lesion was evident. A 5-cm long linear fracture was identified in the outer table of the frontal bone. Jane was intubated and hyperventilated. Intravenous valium was prescribed for fitting.

At 1 day postinjury, Jane presented with decerebrate rigidity with persisting bilateral extensor spasms of both arms and legs. Pupils remained small and only reacted slightly. A repeat CT scan at this time demonstrated scattered hemorrhagic contusions with subarachnoid and intraventricular blood. There was diffuse brain swelling with small cisterns, but no evidence of herniation. Nine days after admission Jane remained in a coma with quadriplegia and decerebrate rigidity. Brainstem function continued to be unstable. An EEG performed 13 days posttrauma indicated a very abnormal pattern with diffuse slow wave activity; however, there were no frank epileptogenic features. At this stage, the child remained unconscious with eyes closed and demonstrated no response to speech. Jane did however, demonstrate suck and swallow reflexes. Two weeks after the accident, Jane developed fitting and there was a slight deterioration in her neurologic state. A CT scan taken 13 days postinjury demonstrated resolving cerebral contusions, normal ventricular size, and generalized cerebral edema. However, no mass lesions were identified.

Three weeks postinjury, Jane spontaneously opened her eyes. It was reported, however, that she demonstrated no comprehension at this time. Jane continued in this state until 8 weeks postinjury at which time medical charts continued to describe her as in a vegetative state. At 9 weeks following the accident, she was discharged from hospital with regular medical and paramedical follow-up.

Evaluation of speech and language skills during the early stages of recovery proved very difficult as the child continued to remain unresponsive to formal evaluation. Recovery of speech and language skills therefore was charted using observational techniques. At 6 weeks postinjury, Jane presented with periods of wakefulness. She was irritable and unresponsive. She demonstrated a severe spastic dysarthria, with extreme oral hypersensitivity and the presence of the primitive oral reflexes (e.g., rooting, bite, suck-swallow, and jaw thrust). Although Jane had begun to take food orally, feeding was a slow and tedious process.

Observation 12 weeks postinjury indicated that Jane had increasing periods of wakefulness and was inconsistently responsive to simple one-part commands (e.g., shut your eyes). Responses, however, were severely limited by her physical condition. Six months after the accident, Jane remained in a severely impaired state. She was alert, could identify body parts and was responsive to simple commands but demonstrated little expressive ability. Vocalizations consisting of /g/ and /n/ plus a vowel were used in a non-communicative manner. At this stage, Jane could produce the reduplicated syllables of /nananana/.

At 10 months postinjury, Jane began to spontaneously utter single words in appropriate contexts. Her first word was reported to be "daddy." The single word stage lasted for only 3 days at which time Jane unexpectedly began to verbalize in well-structured and pragmatically appropriate sentences. Most of Jane's expressions were in response to questions with few spontaneous utterances, and speech was marked by slow and imprecise articulation. Informal assessment at this time indicated the presence of dysarthria, characterized by reduced speech rate, and fatigue with longer utterances. Jane attempted "wh" type questions (what, where, when, why?) and functional questions (e.g., What do you do with a spoon?) with a high degree of accuracy. Tasks involving tactile naming resulted in naming errors characterized by errors within semantic class (e.g., Jane substituted "glass" for "cup" and "pen" for "pencil"). At this time, Jane was diagnosed as having bilateral optic atrophy, with no vision in the left eye and limited vision in the right eye.

Due to Jane's limited concentration span and rapid fatigue, it was not until 12 months postinjury that formal assessment of her language skills could be carried out. During a 4-week period Jane was administered a battery of tests designed to evaluate different aspects of language. As a result of Jane's marked visual impairment, the test battery was somewhat limited but included selected subtests of the NCCEA, the TOLD-I, and selected subtests from CELF. A language analysis was performed using the Language Assessment and Remediation Screening Procedure (LARSP) (Crystal, Fletcher, & Garman, 1976). Jane was reassessed using the same test battery 6 months and 12 months after the initial assessment. At the final assessment (24 months postinjury) the BNT was also included in the test battery.

Subtests of the NCCEA administered at the time of initial testing (12 months postinjury) included: tactile naming (right hand and left hand), sentence repetition, repetition of digits, reversal of digits, word fluency, sentence construction, and articulation. As Jane was able to complete more of the NCCEA subtests at the time of later assessments, additional subtests including visual naming, description of use, identification by name, and identification by sentence were added to the test battery at these later times. Unfortunately Jane's performance on all subtests of the NCCEA was indicative of severe impairment at all assessments. Likewise, Jane's overall language quotient, as determined by the TOLD-I, remained more than 2.5 standard deviations below the mean specified in the test manual for normals for the period of the study and was indicative of a severe persistent language impairment. Subtests for the CELF, which were administered, included: processing relationships and ambiguities; processing spoken paragraphs; and producing word associations. At all occasions of testing, the percentiles achieved by Jane on these subtests fell well below the prescribed range for normals. Jane scored only 6 correct out of a possible 60 on the BNT when administered 24 months postinjury, her performance being marked by the presence of numerous semantic errors.

A syntactic analysis of conversational speech was carried out on a sample of 76 utterances from Jane's initial language assessment (12 months postinjury) using LARSP. Analysis of the therapist-child interaction indicated that much of the sample was dominated by therapist questions, with only limited spontaneous speech on the part of the child (67 responses, 9 spontaneous). Results of the LARSP analysis at this stage placed Jane at Stage III to Stage IV on the LARSP Profile (age equivalence of approximately 2;6 to 3;0). Jane predominantly used utterances involving three clausal elements (subject-verb-object, subject-verb-complement, subject-verb-adverbial) and three phrasal elements (determiner-adjective-noun, preposition-determiner-noun). There was also some evidence of early coordination of sentences using the connective "and." Re-evaluation 6 months later on a sample of 77 utterances indicated that Jane had progressed to Stage V on the LARSP Profile, with some Stage VI structures appearing (age equivalence of approximately 3;0 to 4;6). At this time, Jane used predominantly four and five clausal element structures, with frequent use of coordination, subordination and complex verb phrase structures. There had also been an increase in the number of spontaneous utterances in the sample (58 responses, 19 spontaneous). Twenty-four months postinjury, Jane demonstrated syntactic skills consistent with Stages V and VI of the LARSP Profile. The sample at this time consisted of 94 utterances, with 81 classified as responses and 13 classified as spontaneous.

Overall, Jane exhibited a range of symptoms consistent with those reported in cases of severe TBI (Levin, Madison, Bailey, Meyers, Eisenberg, & Guinto, 1983), including the presence of a persisting period of mutism, followed by a subsequent progression to syntactically intact, although limited, verbalizations. Although Jane could follow simple commands and interact with the environment soon after the return of consciousness, she failed to develop any systematic form of communication for a period of 10 months.

A number of researchers have identified the presence of a period of mutism following severe TBI in children (Hécaen, 1976, 1983; Levin et al., 1983) particularly in the presence of a diffuse increase in brain volume as evidenced in the present case. However, there has been only one reported case of recovery subsequent to such a prolonged period of mutism as documented in the present case (Levin et al., 1983). Other researchers have reported that, of the cases who eventually regained verbal skills subsequent to severe TBI, 98.5% do so within 6 months postinjury (Levin et al., 1982). This would indicate the unlikelihood of the present case regaining verbal skills subsequent to such protracted mutism.

The TBI in the present case was associated with massive cerebral swelling, as evidenced by the early CT scans. Such a generalized increase in brain volume is reported to be common in young patients with 24 hours of severe TBI (Levin et al., 1982; Levin et al. 1983). The resolution of such brain swelling is often thought to be associated with the recovery of function following severe TBI. Consequently, the rapid return of the brain to near-normal proportions in the present case would seem to present a relatively positive prognosis for the rapid return of language function. Based on the CT scan evidence, the brain injury experienced by Jane would seem insufficient to account for the prolonged period of mutism and subsequent language impairment characterized by generalized reduction in communication competency with an accompanying severe word-finding difficulty as documented in her case. Clearly, other factors must be sought to explain the presence of these features.

Snoek, Jennett, Adams, Graham, and Doyle (1979) reported that pathologic findings in the fatal cases of a series of severely TBI children demonstrating generalized cerebral swelling on CT scans identified the presence of diffuse white matter injury, hypoxic cortical damage, cerebral contusion, and signs of increased intracranial pressure. Importantly, the diffuse white matter injury in these cases was discernable only at a microscopic level. Bruce et al. (1981) concluded that the degree of recovery in children following TBI is dependent on the degree of primary axonal injury. It is possible, therefore, that in addition to transient swelling evident on the CT scans, Jane may also have incurred permanent axonal damage at the microscopic level not evident in the CT scans. Although, if present, this permanent damage would serve to explain to some extent the prolonged period of mutism, it fails to explain the abrupt nature of the recovery of functional communication skills.

In summary, Jane's case demonstrates the potential for recovery of at least functional communication skills after the seemingly critical 6-month recovery period following severe TBI in children. It also serves to demonstrate that, contrary to the traditional view that children make a full recovery from TBI, significant linguistic deficits may persist subsequent to severe TBI in some children.

Case 3: Jason

Jason, a 13-year-old, right-handed male, was admitted to hospital subsequent to a cyclist-motor vehicle accident. He had been struck by a motor vehicle and was reportedly unconscious at the scene of the accident. On admission to hospital, he presented with a fixed and dilated pupil and was assigned a GCS score of 3. A CT scan performed shortly after admission demonstrated marked generalized edema, with multiple small contusions. Small high-density areas indicative of hemorrhage were identified in the region of the right anterior lenticulate nucleus and deep in the left temporo-parietal region. There also was a large left fracture in the temporal bone extending across the vertex. Parietal, frontal, and temporal trephine holes were drilled revealing a small acute subdural hematoma, acute traumatic subarachnoid blood, and a tense, swollen brain. The subdural hematoma was evacuated and an intracranial pressure monitor inserted.

Ten days postinjury, Jason began to demonstrate some purposeful movements and was reported to show recognition of some individuals. There was very little lower limb movement and very poor head control. Although cough and gag reflexes were reported to be intact, Jason had poor swallowing skills and was placed on nasogastric feeds. A repeat CT scan 14 days after admission demonstrated scattered intracerebral contusions especially in the left temporal region and widespread edema. A further CT scan performed 21 days postinjury indicated early cerebral atrophy with ventricular dilatation.

Assessment of oral-motor skills at 10 weeks postinjury indicated impaired oral-motor function due to increased tone in the facial muscles, minimal range of jaw movement, presence of primitive reflex patterns (biting, lip retraction), and marked oral and facial hypersensitivity. By 3 months postinjury, Jason showed consistency in response to simple directions (e.g., open your eyes). A CT scan performed 5 months postinjury revealed dilation of both lateral ventricles as well as the third ventricle. There was also an increase in the subarachnoid space in the left temporal region where the left temporal horn of the left lateral ventricle was also more dilated indicative of marked reduction in the volume of the cerebrum on the left.

At 6 months postinjury, Jason demonstrated some consistent yes/no responses and an informal assessment indicated that he could comprehend object names, match pictures, and make requests using an eye-pointing response. By 6 months postinjury, he was able to match words to pictures accurately 80% of the time. At this time, he presented as a spastic quadriplegic.

Formal assessment of language skills using a standardized test battery was not attempted until 12 months postinjury; however, even then due to Jason's severe physical impairments the use of these tests remained limited. Components of the Test of Adolescent Language-2 (TOAL-2) (Hammill, Brown, Larson, & Weiderholt, 1987) and the NCCEA were administered. It must be noted that Jason's communication was entirely dependent on an augmentative communication system, either an adapted computer or a Canon Communicator; hence, in all instances standard procedures for test administration was violated as Jason could not respond in an oral manner. An informal oral-motor assessment was also completed. Testing was carried out at 12 months postinjury and then repeated at 24 months postinjury.

At 12 months postinjury, Jason continued to exhibit severely impaired oral-motor skills. Oral-motor impairment was characterized by a minimal range of jaw movement, the persistence of primitive oral reflexes (jaw extension, bit reflex), extremely limited tongue mobility, reduced tone and mobility of facial muscles, and weakness of the pharyngeal and palatal muscles. Drooling was a constant problem and his vocalizations were limited to three vowels. He could occasionally produce /m/ on command; however, coordination of lip closure and vocalization was extremely poor. The findings were consistent with the presence of a severe mixed spastic/flaccid dysarthria. Reassessment at 24 months postinjury indicated very minimal improvements in Jason's oral-motor skills.

Several subtests of the NCCEA were administered using a "written" response mode or eye pointing in all instances. These subtests included: visual naming; description of use; tactile naming (right and left hand); sentence construction; identification by name; identification by sentence; reading for meaning; writing of names; writing to dictation; and writing (copying). At the time of initial testing, Jason's performance on the visual naming and the description of use subtests were considered to be severely impaired. In contrast, he achieved maximum scores on the subtests of identification by name, reading sentences for meaning and reading words for meaning; hence, his abilities in these areas were deemed to be intact. Performance on the NCCEA, however, was consistent with a marked word-finding difficulty. Jason's written responses were characterized by semantic paraphasic errors (e.g., "comb" became "brush"; "cup" became "bowl") at initial assessment. Marked improvement in scores in all subtests occurred over the 12-month period between initial and follow-up testing.

Due to the severe limitations of Jason's oral communication skills, only the following subtests of the Tests of Adolescents and Adult Language-2 (TOAL-2) were administered: listening/vocabulary; listening/grammar; reading/vocabulary; reading/grammar; writing/vocabulary; and writing/grammar. At both the initial and follow-up assessments, all scores achieved by Jason on these subtests fell below the range of average performance, with only very minimal improvement being evidenced over the 12-month period between tests. In particular, the skill areas most affected by Jason's injury appeared to be those involving a reading component (e.g., reading/grammar, writing/vocabulary, and writing/grammar all required Jason to read the stimulus material).

Overall, Jason demonstrated marked speech and language deficits subsequent to severe TBI. During the early stages of recovery, he remained semicomatose and any form of communication was severely limited for the first

6 months postinjury. Recovery of comprehension skills then proceeded rapidly and Jason was able to demonstrate at least functional comprehension by 12 months postinjury. Severe oral-motor impairment persisted throughout the recovery stage limiting any restoration of verbal communication. Jason continued to be reliant on an augmentative communication system for expressive function.

Performance on tests of overall language function demonstrated the presence of marked impairment in expressive and receptive syntax and expressive and receptive semantics with a particular deficit in word-finding skills. The presence of a deficit in word-finding skills is consistent with much of the research on language recovery subsequent to pediatric TBI, which indicates the persistence of word-finding difficulties (Ewing-Cobbs et al., 1985; Levin & Eisenberg, 1979a). Jason's basic reading skills were preserved as indicated by his performance on the NCCEA subtest of reading for meaning; however, more advanced reading abilities accessed by the reading/vocabulary and reading/grammar subtests of the TOAL-2 were found to be impaired. Although Jason demonstrated a number of language characteristics considered representative of typical recovery subsequent to pediatric TBI, the persistence of his language disorder is not consistent with the traditional view of recovery in this population.

Summary

The three cases of severe TBI presented above have served to highlight the heterogeneity that exists with regard to language recovery in the pediatric TBI population. Despite similar levels of severity (as demonstrated by the GCS scores), each case experienced a remarkably different pattern of recovery of linguistic skills in the long term. It is interesting to note, however, that a number of features were consistent despite the marked variability observed. It would appear that receptive language skills were least affected in each case and, although these were varying degrees of recovery, all three children progressed to a stage of at least functional communication skills. A special feature consistent across the three cases was the presence of a word-finding problem. Word-finding problems have been reported frequently in the literature as the most outstanding feature of the language disorder subsequent to childhood TBI (Levin & Eisenberg, 1979b; Jordan et al., 1988; Winogran et al., 1984).

Based on the observations made with these three cases, it is obvious that children suffering TBI do not present as a homogeneous group with regard to language abilities and consequently cannot be treated using a prescriptive approach. Rehabilitation programs for the child with TBI, therefore, must cater to the specific needs of the child in question. Communication management may require the use of an augmentative communication system in either the acute stage or in the longer term as demonstrated in Case 3, or may require the use of facilitative techniques that enable the child to manage his or her persistent communication deficits more effectively. The fact that all three cases presented demonstrated some degree of word-finding deficit indicates that speech-language pathologists should provide the child with TBI with strategies to overcome word-finding deficits from very early stages in recovery in an attempt to prevent later breakdown of communication in response to this deficit.

References

Adams, J. H. (1975). The neuropathology of head injuries. In P. J. Vinken & G. W. Bruyn (Eds.), *Handbook of clinical neurology: Vol. 23 Injuries of the brain and skull: Part 1* (pp. 35–65). Amsterdam, the Netherlands: North-Holland.

Adams, J. H., Graham, D. I., Gennarelli, T. A., & Maxwell, W. L. (1991). Diffuse axonal injury in non-missile head injury. *Journal of Neurology, Neurosurgery and Psychiatry, 54,* 481–483.

Adams, J. H., Graham, D. I., Murray, L. S., & Scott, G. (1982). Diffuse axonal injury due to non-missile head injury in humans: An analysis of 45 cases. *Annals of Neurology, 12,* 557–563.

Adams, J. H., Graham, D. I., Scott, G., Parker, L. S., & Doyle, D. (1980). Brain damage in fatal non-missile head injury. *Journal of Clinical Pathology, 33,* 1132–1145.

Adams, J. H., Mitchell, D. E., Graham, O. T., & Doyle, D. (1977). Diffuse brain damage of immediate impact type. *Brain, 100,* 489–502.

Alajouanine, T., & Lhermitte, F. (1965). Acquired aphasia in children. *Brain, 88,* 653–662.

Aram, D. M., Ekelman, B. L., Rose, D. F., & Whitaker, H. A. (1985). Verbal and cognitive sequelae following unilateral lesions acquired early in childhood. *Journal of Clinical and Experimental Neuropsychology, 7,* 55–78.

Aram, D. M., Ekelman, B. L., & Whitaker, H. A. (1986). Spoken syntax in children with acquired unilateral hemisphere lesions. *Brain and Language, 27,* 75–100.

Aram, D. M., Ekelman, B. L., & Whitaker, H. A. (1987). Lexical retrieval in left and right brain lesioned children. *Brain and Language, 31,* 61–87.

Auerbach, S. H. (1986). Neuroanatomical correlates of attention and memory disorders in traumatic brain injury: An application of neurobehavioral subtypes. *Journal of Head Trauma Rehabilitation, 3,* 1–12.

Basso, A. (1992). Prognostic factors in aphasia. *Aphasiology, 6,* 337–348.

Bates, E., Reilly, J., & Marchman, E. (1992, October). *Discourse and grammar after early focal brain injury.* Abstract from Presentation at the 30th annual meeting of the Academy of Aphasia Meeting, Toronto, Canada.

Bigler, E. D. (1990). Neuropathology of traumatic brain injury. In E. Bigler (Ed.), *Traumatic brain injury* (pp. 13–49). Austin, TX: Pro-Ed.

Bigler, E. D., Kurth, S., Blatter, D., & Abildskov, T. (1993). Day-of-injury CT as an index to pre-injury brain morphology: Degree of post-injury degenerative changes identified by CT and MR neuroimaging. *Brain Injury, 7,* 125–134.

Blumbergs, P. C., Jones, N. R., & North, J. B. (1989). Diffuse axonal injury in head trauma. *Journal of Neurology, Neurosurgery and Psychiatry, 52,* 838–841.

Bruce, D. A., Alavi, A., Bilaniuk, K., Colinskas, C., Obrist, W., & Uzzell, B. (1981). Diffuse cerebral swelling following head injuries in children: The syndrome of malignant brain edema. *Journal of Neurosurgery, 54,* 170–178.

Campbell, T. F., & Dollaghan, C. A. (1990). Expressive language recovery in severely brain-injured children and adolescents. *Journal of Speech and Hearing Disorders, 55,* 567–581.

Carter, R. L., Hohenegger, M. K., & Satz, P. (1982). Aphasia and speech organization in children. *Science, 218,* 797–799.

Chadwick, O., Rutter, M., Brown, G., Shaffer, D., & Traub, M. (1981). A prospective study of children with head injuries: II Cognitive sequelae. *Psychological Medicine, 11*, 49–61.

Chadwick, O., Rutter, M., Shaffer, D., & Shrout, P. E. (1981). A prospective study of children with head injuries: IV. Specific cognitive deficits. *Journal of Clinical Neuropsychology, 8*, 101–120.

Chapman, S. B. (1995). Discourse as an outcome measure in pediatric head-injured populations. In S. H. Broman & M. E. Michel (Eds.), *Traumatic brain injury in children* (pp. 95–116). New York, NY: Oxford University Press.

Chapman, S. B. (1997). Cognitive-communication abilities in children with closed head injury. *American Journal of Speech-Language Pathology, 6*, 50–58.

Chapman, S. B., Culhane, K. A., Levin, H. S., Harwood, H., Mendelsohn, D., . . . Bruce, D. (1992). Narrative discourse after closed head injury in children and adolescents. *Brain and Language, 43,* 42–65.

Chapman, S. B., & Levin, H. S. (1994, November). *Discourse abilities and executive function in head-injured children.* Paper presented at the American Speech-Language and Hearing Association Convention. New Orleans, LA, USA.

Chapman, S. B., Levin, H. S., & Lawyer, S. L. (1999). Communication problems resulting from brain injury in children: Special issues of assessment and management. In S. McDonald, L. Togher, & C. Code (Eds.), *Communication disorders following traumatic brain injury* (pp. 235–269). Hove, Sussex, UK: Psychology Press.

Chapman, S. B., Levin, H. S., Wanek, A., Weyrauch, J., & Kufera, J. (1998). Discourse after closed head injury in young children: Relation of age to outcome. *Brain and Language, 61,* 420–449.

Chapman, S. B., Watkins, R., Gustafson, C., Moore, S., Levin, H. S., & Kufera, J. A. (1977). Narrative discourse in children with closed head injury, children with language impairment and typically developing children. *American Journal of Speech-Language Pathology, 6,* 66–75.

Coloquhoun, I. R., & Rawlinson, J. (1989). The significance of haematomas of the basal ganglia in closed head injury. *Clinical Radiology, 40,* 619–621.

Crystal, D., Fletcher, P., & Garman, M. (1976). *The grammatical analysis of language disability.* London, UK: Edward Arnold.

Cullum, C. M., & Bigler, E. D. (1986). Ventricle size, cortical atrophy, and the relationship with neuropsychological status in closed head injury: A quantitative analysis. *Journal of Clinical Experimental Neuropsychology, 8,* 437–452.

Damico, J. (1985). Clinical discourse analysis: A functional approach to language assessment. In C. S. Simon (Ed.), *Communication skills and classroom success* (pp. 165–203). London, UK: Taylor & Francis.

Dennis, M., & Barnes, M. A. (1990). Knowing the meaning, getting the point, bridging the gap, and carrying the message: Aspects of discourse following closed head injury in childhood and adolescence. *Brain and Language, 39,* 428–446.

Dennis, M., Jacennik, B., & Barnes, M. A. (1994). The content of narrative discourse in children and adolescents after early-onset hydrocephalus and in normally developing age peers. *Brain and Language, 46,* 129–165.

Dennis, M., & Lovett, M. W. (1990). Discourse ability in children after brain-damage. In Y. Joanette, & H. H. Brownell (Eds.), *Discourse ability and brain damage: Theoretical and empirical perspectives* (pp. 199–223). New York, NY: Springer-Verlag.

Eslinger, P., Grattan, L. M., Damasio, H., & Damasio, A. R. (1992). Developmental consequences of childhood frontal lobe damage. *Archives of Neurology, 49,* 764–769.

Ewing-Cobbs, L., Brookshire, B., Scott, M. A., & Fletcher, J. M. (1998). Children's narratives following traumatic brain injury: Linguistic structure, cohesion and thematic recall. *Brain and Language, 61,* 395–419.

Ewing-Cobbs, L., Fletcher, J. M., Levin, H. S., & Landry, S. H. (1985). Language disorders after pediatric head injury. In J. K. Darby (Ed.), *Speech and language evaluation in neurology: Childhood disorders* (pp. 97–112). Orlando, FL: Grune & Stratton.

Ewing-Cobbs, L., Levin, H. S., Eisenberg, H. M., & Fletcher, J. M. (1987). Language functions following closed head injury in children and adolescents. *Journal of Clinical and Experimental Neuropsychology, 9*, 575–592.

Ewing-Cobbs, L., Miner, M. E., Fletcher, J. M., & Levin, H. S. (1989). Intellectual motor and language sequelae following closed head injury in children and adolescents. *Journal of Pediatric Psychology, 9*, 575–592.

Friede, R. L. (1973). *Developmental neuropathology*. New York, NY: Springer.

Gennarelli, T. A. (1993). Mechanisms of brain injury. *Journal of Emergency Medicine, 11*, 5–11.

Gennarelli, T. A., Thibault, L. E., Adams, H. J., Graham, D. I., Thompson, C. J., & Marcincin, R. P. (1982). Diffuse axonal injury. *Annals of Neurology, 12*, 212–223.

Gilchrist, E., & Wilkinson, M. (1979). Some factors determining prognosis in young people with severe head injuries. *Archives of Neurology, 36*, 355–359.

Gjerris, F. (1986). Head injuries in children: Special features. *Acta Neurochirurgica, Supplement 36*, 155–158.

Graham, D. J., & Adams, J. H. (1971). Ischaemic brain damage in fatal head injuries. *Lancet, 1*, 265–266.

Graham, D. J., Adams, J. H., & Doyle, D. (1978). Ischaemic brain damage in fatal non-missile head injuries. *Journal of Neurological Science, 39*, 213–234.

Gurdjian, E. S., & Gurdjian, E. (1976). Cerebral contusions: Re-evaluation of the mechanism of their development. *Journal of Trauma, 16*, 35–51.

Guthrie, E., Mast, J., Richards, P., McQuaid, M., & Pavlakis, S. (1999). Traumatic brain injury in children and adolescents. *Child and Adolescent Psychiatric Clinics of North America, 8*, 807–826.

Hammill, D. D., Brown, V. L., Larson, S. C., & Weiderholt, J. L. (1987). Test of adolescent language-2. Austin, TX: Pro-Ed.

Hammill, D. D., & Newcomer, P. L. (1982). Test of language development-intermediate. Austin, TX: Pro-Ed.

Hebb, D. O. (1942). The effect of early and late brain injury upon test scores and the nature of abnormal adult intelligence. *Proceeding of the American Philosophical Society, 1*, 265–292.

Hécaen, H. (1976). Acquired aphasia in children and the ontogenesis of hemispheric functional specialization. *Brain and Language, 3*, 114–134.

Hécaen, H. (1983). Acquired aphasia in children: Revisited. *Neuropsychologia, 21*, 581–587.

Hendrick, E. B., Harwood-Nash, D., & Hudson, A. R. (1964). Head injuries in children: A survey of 4465 consecutive cases at the hospital of sick children, Toronto, Canada. *Clinical Neurosurgery, 11*, 45–65.

Holbourn, A. H. S. (1943). Mechanics of head injuries. *Lancet, 2*, 438–441.

Javid, M., & Settlage, P. (1956). Effect of urea on cerebrospinal fluid pressure in human subjects: Preliminary report. *Journal of the American Medical Association, 160*, 943–949.

Jellinger, K. (1983). The neuropathology of pediatric head injuries. In K. Shapiro (Ed.), *Pediatric head trauma* (pp. 143–194). Mount Kisco, NY: Futura.

Jennett, B. (1986). Head trauma. In A. K. Asbury, G. M. McKann, & W. I. McDonald (Eds.), *Diseases of the nervous system* (pp. 1282–1297). Philadelphia, PA: W. B. Saunders.

Jordan, F. M., & Cannon, A., & Murdoch, B. E. (1992). Language abilities of mildly closed head injured children 10 years post-injury. *Brain Injury, 6*, 39–44.

Jordan, F. M., Cremona-Meteyard, S., & King, A. (1996). High-level linguistic disturbances subsequent to childhood closed head injury. *Brain Injury, 10*, 729–738.

Jordan, F. M., & Murdoch, B. E. (1990a). Linguistic status following closed head injury: A follow-up study. *Brain Injury, 4*, 147–154.

Jordan, F. M., & Murdoch, B. E. (1990b). A comparison of the conversational skills of closed head injured children and normal children. *Australian Journal of Human Communication Disorders, 18,* 69–82.

Jordan, F. M., & Murdoch, B. E. (1993). A prospective study of the linguistic skills of children with closed head injuries. *Aphasiology, 7,* 503–512.

Jordan, F. M., & Murdoch, B. E. (1994). Severe closed head injury in childhood: Linguistic outcomes into adulthood. *Brain Injury, 8,* 501–508.

Jordan, F. M., Murdoch, B. E., & Buttsworth, D. L. (1991). Closed head injured children's performance on narrative tasks. *Journal of Speech and Hearing Research, 34,* 572–582.

Jordan, F. M., Ozanne, A. E., & Murdoch, B. E. (1988). Long-term speech and language disorders subsequent to closed head injury in children. *Brain Injury, 2,* 179–185.

Jordan, F. M., & Ozanne, A. E., & Murdoch, B. E. (1990). Performance of closed head injured children on a naming task. *Brain Injury, 4,* 27–32.

Kaplan, E., Goodglass, H., & Weintraub, S. (1983). Boston naming test. Philadelphia, PA: Lea & Febiger.

Katz, M. D. (1992). Neuropathology and neurobehavioral recovery from closed head injury. *Journal of Head Trauma Rehabilitation, 7,* 1–15.

Lehečková, H. (2004). Recovery from aphasia after polytrauma in a Czech child: What is lost and what is left. In F. Fabbro (Ed.), *Neurogenic language disorders in children* (pp. 199–229). Amsterdam, the Netherlands: Elsevier.

Lenneberg, E. (1967). *Biological foundations of language.* New York, NY: John Wiley.

Letarte, P. B. (1999). Neurotrauma care in the new millennium. *Surgical Clinics of North America, 79,* 1449–1470.

Levin, H. S., Benton, A. L., & Grossman, R. G. (1982). *Neurobehavioural consequences of closed head injury.* New York, NY: Oxford University Press.

Levin, H. S., & Eisenberg, G. M. (1979a). Neuropsychological impairment after closed head injury in children and adolescents. *Journal of Pediatric Psychology, 4,* 389–402.

Levin, H. S., & Eisenberg, G. M. (1979b). Neuropsychological outcome of closed head injury in children and adolescents. *Child's Brain, 5,* 281–292.

Levin, H. S., Ewing-Cobbs, L., & Benton, A. L. (1984). Age and recovery from brain damage: A review of clinical studies. In S. W. Scheff (Ed.), *Aging and recovery of function in the central nervous system* (pp. 169–205). New York, NY: Plenum.

Levin, H. S., Ewing-Cobbs, L., & Eisenberg, H. M. (1995). Neurobehavioral outcome of pediatric closed head injury. In S. H. Broman & M. E. Michel (Eds.), *Traumatic head injury in children* (pp. 70–94). New York, NY: Oxford University Press.

Levin, H. S., Madison, C. F., Bailey, C. B., Meyers, C. A., Eisenberg, H. M., & Guinto, F. C. (1983). Mutism after closed head injury. *Archives of Neurology, 40,* 601–607.

Lezak, M. (1983). *Neuropsychological assessment* (2nd ed.). New York, NY: Oxford University Press.

Liles, B. Z., Coelho, C. A., Duffy, R. J., & Zalagens, M. R. (1989). Effects of elicitation procedures on the narratives of normal and closed head injured adults. *Journal of Speech and Hearing Disorders, 54,* 356–366.

Lindenberg, R., & Freytag, E. (1969). Morphology of brain lesions from blunt trauma in early infancy. *Archives of Pathology (Chicago), 87,* 298–305.

Lundberg, N. (1960). Continuous recording and control of ventricular fluid pressure in neurosurgical practice. *Acta Psychiatrica Scandinavica, Supplement 36,* 1–193.

Martins, I. P. (2004). Persistent acquired childhood aphasia. In F. Fabbro (Ed.), *Neurogenic language disorders in children* (pp. 231–251). Amsterdam, the Netherlands: Elsevier.

McDonald, S. (1992). Communication disorders following closed head injury: New approaches to assessment and rehabilitation. *Brain Injury, 6,* 283–292.

McDonald, S. (1993). Pragmatic language skills after closed head injury: Ability to meet the informational needs of the listener. *Brain and Language, 44,* 28–46.

Menkes, J. H., & Till, K. (1995). Postnatal trauma and injuries by physical agents. In J. H. Menkes (Ed.), *Textbook of child neurology* (pp. 557–597). Baltimore, MD: Williams & Wilkins.

Mentis, M., & Prutting, C. A. (1987). Cohesion in the discourse of normal and head injured adults. *Journal of Speech and Hearing Research, 30,* 88–98.

Miller, J. D., & Sweet, R. C. (1978). Early insults to the injured brain. *Journal of the American Medical Association, 240,* 439–442.

Murdoch, B. E. (1990). *Acquired speech and language disorders: A neuroanatomical and functional neurological approach.* London, UK: Chapman & Hall.

Najenson, T., Sazbon, L., Fiselzon, J., Becker, E., & Schechter, I. (1978). Recovery of communicative functions after prolonged traumatic coma. *Scandinavian Journal of Rehabilitation Medicine, 10,* 15–21.

National Head Injury Foundation. (1985). *An educator's manual: What educators need to know about students with traumatic brain injury.* Framington, MA: National Task Force on Special Education for Students and Youths With Traumatic Brain Injury.

Olley, L. (1989). Oral narrative performance of normal and language impaired school aged children. *Australian Journal of Human Communication Disorders, 17,* 43–65.

Pang, D. (1985). Pathophysiologic correlates of neurobehavioural syndromes following closed head injury. In M. Ylvisaker (Ed.), *Head injury rehabilitation: Children and adolescents* (pp. 3–70). Austin, TX: Pro-Ed.

Prutting, C. A., & Kirchner, D. M. (1987). A clinical appraisal of the pragmatic aspects of language. *Journal of Speech and Hearing Disorders, 52,* 105–119.

Reilly, P. L., & Adams, J. H. (1975). Patients with head injury who talk and die. *Lancet, 2,* 375–377.

Rosner, M. J. (1995). Introduction to cerebral perfusion pressure management. *Neurosurgical Clinics of North America, 6,* 761–773.

Rosner, M. J., & Coley, I. B. (1986). Cerebral perfusion pressure, intracranial pressure and elevation. *Journal of Neurosurgery, 65,* 636–641.

Rosner, M. J., & Daughton, S. (1990). Cerebral perfusion management in head trauma. *Journal of Trauma, 30,* 933–940.

Satz, P., & Bullard-Bates, C. (1981). Acquired aphasia in children. In M. T. Sarno (Ed.), *Acquired aphasia* (pp. 75–93). New York, NY: Academic Press.

Semel-Mintz, E., & Wiig, E. H. (1982). *Clinical evaluation of language functions.* Columbus, OH: Charles E. Merrill.

Shaffer, D., Bijur, P., Chadwick, D. F., & Rutter, M. L. (1980). Head injury and later reading disability. *Journal of the American Academy of Child Psychiatry, 19,* 592–610.

Slater, E. J., & Bassett, S. S. (1988). Adolescents with closed head injuries. *American Journal of Diseases of Children, 142,* 1048–1051.

Smith, E. (1974). Influence of site of impact upon cognitive performance persisting long after closed head injury. *Journal of Neurology, Neurosurgery and Psychiatry, 37,* 719–726.

Snoek, J., Jennett, B., Adams, J. H., Graham, D. I., & Doyle, D. (1979). Computerised tomography after recent severe head injury in patients without acute intracranial haematoma. *Journal of Neurology, Neurosurgery and Psychiatry, 42,* 215–225.

Spreen, O., & Benton, A. L. (1969). *Neurosensory Center Comprehensive Examination for Aphasia: Manual of directions.* Victoria, BC, Canada: University of Victoria.

Strich, S. J. (1956). Diffuse degeneration of cerebral white matter in severe dementia following head injury. *Journal of Neurology, Neurosurgery and Psychiatry, 19,* 163–185.

Strich, S. J. (1961). Shearing of nerve fibres as a cause of brain damage due to head injury. *Lancet, 2,* 443–448.

Strich, S. J. (1969). The pathology of brain damage due to blunt injuries. In A. E. Walker, W. F. Caveness, & M. Critchley

(Eds.), *The late effects of head injury* (pp. 501–524). Springfield, IL: Charles C. Thomas.

Teasdale, G. M., & Graham, D. I. (1998). Craniocerebral trauma: Protection and retrieval of the neuronal population after injury. *Neurosurgery, 43,* 723–738.

Vernon-Levett, P. (1991). Head injuries in children. *Critical Care Nursing Clinics of North America, 3,* 411–421.

Winogran, H. W., Knights, R. M., & Bawden, H. N. (1984). Neuropsychological deficits following head injury in children. *Journal of Clinical Neuropsychology, 6,* 269–286.

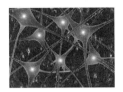 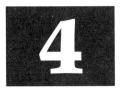 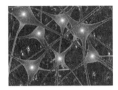

4

Language Disorders Subsequent to Treatment for Childhood Cancer

Introduction

New developments in the treatment of pediatric cancer have resulted in marked improvements in the 5-year survival rates of children treated for neoplastic conditions over recent decades. Although almost always rapidly fatal five decades ago (Southam, Craver, Dargeon, & Burchenal, 1951; Tivey, 1952), the 5-year survival rate of children treated for pediatric leukemia in the 1990s had risen to 72.8% (Boring, Squires, & Tong, 1991), with some survival rates reported to be as high as 80% (Cousens, Ungerer, Crawford, & Stevens, 1990). Currently, the survival rate beyond 5 years for acute lymphoblastic leukemia is approximately 90% (Brière, Scott, McNall-Knapp, & Adams, 2008). Similarly, the survival rates for children diagnosed with brain and central nervous system (CNS) tumors have also shown dramatic improvement from 35% during the period 1960 to 1963 to 59% survival

during the period 1981 to 1986 (Boring et al., 1991). More recently, survival beyond a 5-year survival period for children treated for CNS tumors has been reported to vary between 25 to 85% depending on the type of tumor (Stiller & Bleyer, 2004).

Although indisputably saving the lives of children with neoplastic conditions, the treatments applied to these disorders, including focal or craniospinal radiotherapy and/or chemotherapy, may have some long-term adverse effects on brain structure and function leading to the development of a number of undesirable negative sequelae. These negative sequelae include significant behavioral and neurocognitive deficits (Anclair, Hovén, Lannering, & Boman, 2009; Palmer & Leigh, 2009; Schatz, Kramer, Albin, & Matthay, 2000) as well as speech and language deficits (Buttsworth, Murdoch, & Ozanne, 1993; Hudson & Murdoch, 1992a, 1992b; Jackel, Murdoch, Ozanne, & Buttsworth, 1990; Murdoch & Hudson-Tennent, 1994).

Consequently, the improvement in survival rates of children diagnosed with cancer has lead to allied health professionals, including speech-language pathologists being required to provide rehabilitation and support services to an increasing number of pediatric cancer cases, with attention now being focused on improving the quality of life of survivors of childhood leukemia and brain tumor. It is now recognized that achieving a cure necessitates a fine balance between effective intervention and acceptable neurocognitive morbidity (Askins & Moore, 2008). To reduce morbidity associated with the management of pediatric neoplastic conditions while still maintaining high rates of survival, changes to treatment protocols over the past decade have seen treatments now tailored to risk status (Palmer & Leigh, 2009). Children at a lower risk of relapse are offered risk-adapted treatments with the expectation that they will experience fewer treatment effects and have a better quality of long-term survival (Bhatia & Meadows, 2006). The various treatments applied to pediatric cancer are described in more detail later in this chapter.

Acute leukemias represent the most common type of pediatric malignancy (Parkin, Stiller, Draper, & Bieber, 1988) with brain and spinal tumors being the second most common childhood cancer in the developed countries of North America, Europe, Australasia, and Japan (Heideman, Packer, Albright, Freeman, & Rorke, 1993; Tait, Bailey, & Cameron, 1992). In particular, brain tumors located in the posterior cranial fossa (i.e., infratentorial tumors involving the cerebellum, fourth ventricle and/or brainstem) occur more commonly in childhood than supratentorial neoplasms, accounting for approximately 60% of all intracranial

tumors in the first decade of life (Cohen, Duffner, & Tebbi, 1982). The present chapter reviews the major types of pediatric cancer with regard to their epidemiology, diagnosis, etiology, subtypes, symptomatology, medical course, and prognosis, with emphasis given to posterior fossa tumors and acute lymphoblastic leukemia. The medical treatments applied to the latter conditions are also described as are the clinical features of any associated language disorders.

Major Forms of Childhood Cancer

It has been estimated that 1 in 600 children will develop cancer, and 1 in every 1,000 young adults will be a survivor of childhood cancer. Although posterior fossa tumors account for greater than 50% of brain tumors in children, the most common form of leukemia in childhood is acute lymphoblastic leukemia, with incidence rates at approximately 80% of all leukemia types (McWhirter & Petroeschevsky, 1990).

Pediatric Brain Tumors

Pediatric brain tumors are often clincopathologically, histopathologically, and genetically different from those of adults with significant contrasts having been reported between the incidence, location, and natural history of brain tumors in children compared to their adult counterparts (Becker & Jay, 1990). Although both infratentorial (posterior fossa) and supratentorial brain tumors may occur in children, it has been reported that the percentage of male patients, and the proportion of tumors located in the midline, or in the posterior fossa are significantly higher in children than adults (Nomura, Nishizaki, Tamashita, & Ito, 1998).

Posterior Fossa Tumors

The posterior cranial fossa is that part of the cranial cavity that lies below the level of the tentorium cerebelli. Components of the brain located within the posterior fossa include the cerebellum, fourth ventricle, and brainstem. Due to the prevalence of posterior fossa tumors in childhood, a large proportion of the literature on pediatric intracranial neoplasms has centered on tumors involving brain structures within this region.

Types of Posterior Fossa Tumors. The most common posterior fossa tumors are medulloblastomas, astrocytomas, and ependymomas. Based on a sample of 151 children with posterior fossa tumor, Menkes and Till (1995) reported that 34.4% had medulloblastomas, 21.9% had astrocytomas, and 10.6% ependymomas. Brainstem neoplasms were present in 26.5% of the 151 cases. Similar figures for the occurrence of various posterior fossa tumors were reported by Matson (1956). The major characteristics of medulloblastomas, astrocytomas, and ependymomas are summarized in Table 4–1.

Medulloblastoma. Medulloblastomas account for approximately 40%

Table 4–1. Characteristics of Medulloblastomas, Astrocytomas, and Ependymomas

Feature	Medulloblastoma	Astrocytoma	Ependymoma
Malignancy*	Highly malignant	Grades I to IV	Grades I to IV
Age at onset	4 mo to 16 yr	0 to 16 yr	0 to 7 yr
Male/female ratio	1.3:1	1:1	Reports vary
Incidence (%)**	34.4	21.9	10.6
Origin	Cerebellar vermis	Cerebellar hemisphere	Fourth ventricle
Symptom duration***	1 to 80 mo	2 yr; 4 mo	Unreported
Medical prognosis	Variable	Favorable	Variable
Tumor recurrence	10 to 100% of cases reported	Rare	Common
Symptoms	Headache, nausea, vomiting, gait disturbance, apathy, irritability, neck stiffness/pain, dizziness, papilledema, squint, nystagmus, change in muscle tone, tendon reflex changes, dorsiflexor plantar response, head tilting, visual impairment, limb paresis, facial weakness		

*Based on the Kernohan classification with Grade I being benign and Grade IV highly malignant.
**Proportion of pediatric posterior fossa tumor cases diagnosed by Menkes and Till (1995).
***Average symptom duration reported in 43 cases by Davis and Joglekar (1981).
y = years; m = months.

of all posterior fossa tumors and are highly malignant, rapidly growing brain tumors derived from embryonal cell nests in the posterior medullary velum of the cerebellum. Although usually situated in the midline (i.e., vermis) of the cerebellum (Becker & Hinton, 1986; Dhall, 2009; Heideman et al., 1993; Mabbott, Penkman, Witol, & Strother, 2008; Yachnis, 1997), medulloblastomas subsequently invade the subarachnoid spaces, fourth ventricle, and cerebrospinal pathways and may extend into the cerebellar hemispheres. On neuroradiologic scans, a medulloblastoma characteristically appears as a well-defined, noncalcified, noncystic, slightly dense inferior vermian mass that invades the back of the fourth ventricle (Figure 4–1).

Due to a common presentation in the midline and compression of the fourth ventricle, hydrocephalus is often the earliest and most frequent symptom to accompany medulloblastoma (Heideman et al., 1993). Truncal ataxia and unsteady gait are also characteristic of this type of tumor, in addition to papilledema, headache, emesis, and lethargy (Heideman et al., 1993).

Children have been diagnosed with medulloblastomas between 4 months and 16 years of age with the incidence documented to peak at 5 years of age, although some authors describe a bimodal plateau at 3 to 4 years and again at 8 to 9 years rather than a single peak (Cohen & Duffner, 1984). The incidence of medulloblastoma is slightly higher in males than females (1.3:1). As a consequence of their rapid growth, the time period between onset of symptoms and treatment generally is shorter for medulloblastomas than other pediatric brain tumors. The potential for medulloblastomas to invade adjacent areas of the brain, as well as a common tendency

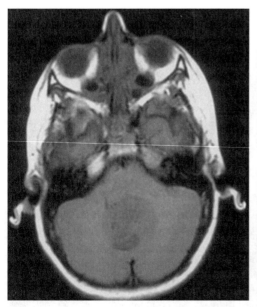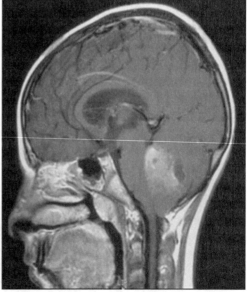

FIGURE 4–1. Axial (*left*) and midsagittal (*right*) magnetic resonance imaging scans demonstrating a 3.2 × 3.3 cm intra-axial medulloblastoma involving the cerebellum in the midline.

to metastasize in the subarachnoid space and disseminate via the cerebrospinal fluid to both neuroaxis sites as well as outside the CNS (at a rate between 5 to 35%) is well documented (Heideman et al., 1993; Plowman, 1992; Yachnis, 1997). Consequently, the primary concern for children with medulloblastomas is the risk of tumor recurrence posttreatment in the posterior cranial fossa and/or the development of supratentorial, spinal cord, or systemic metastases. Where they occur, recurrences usually arise in the first two to three years following treatment with an average survival time for children with recurrence of only 19 months. The prognosis for patients with recurrent medulloblastoma, therefore, is poor. Poor prognostic indicators also include brainstem invasion, incomplete resection, evidence of dissemination, and young age at diagnosis (Plowman, 1992). Currently, the overall 5-year disease-free survival rate for medulloblastoma is approximately 50% and 40% at 10 years for children treated with surgery and craniospinal irradiation, respectively (Menkes & Till, 1995; Tait, Bailey, & Cameron, 1992). Aggressive radiotherapy including the whole craniospinal axis is recommended in cases of medulloblastoma. Medulloblastoma has also been demonstrated to be sensitive to chemotherapy due to its rapid growth and embryonal pathology (Heideman et al., 1993; Neidhardt, Bamberg, & Riehm, 1986). Currently, most treatment protocols in relation to medulloblastoma include chemotherapy for high-risk patients.

Cerebellar Astrocytoma. Cerebellar astrocytomas are derived from and composed of astrocytic neuroglial cells and account for between one-third and 40 to 50% of pediatric posterior fossa tumors (Heideman et al., 1993; van Eys, 1991). These tumors can arise from either the vermis or lateral lobes of the cerebellum and tend to be well circumscribed and often cystic, containing one or more sacs of clear yellow or brown fluid (Tait et al., 1992; Yachnis, 1997). Cerebellar astrocytomas are slow growing and most commonly remain confined to the cerebellum, although extension through the cerebellar peduncles and involvement of the brainstem may occur in rare cases (Figure 4–2). Consequently, these tumors usually are amenable to complete surgical excision.

Astrocytomas are usually assigned a grade from 1 to 4 according to their level of malignancy, with grade 1 being benign and grade 4 highly malignant [Note: Grade 3 and 4 astrocytomas are referred to as glioblastomas]. Fortunately, most cerebellar astrocytomas are low grade (Becker & Jay, 1990; Plowman, 1992; Tait et al., 1992; Yachnis, 1997), with a cystic presentation. Approximately 80 to 85% of cerebellar astrocytomas in children are of the more benign juvenile, pilocytic variety, with the more malignant diffuse form of astrocytoma responsible for 15% (Heideman et al., 1993; Plowman, 1992; Yachnis, 1997). Juvenile astrocytomas, as their name suggests, tend to appear during the first decade of life whereas diffuse astrocytomas usually arise in adolescence. Although juvenile pilocytic astrocytomas are compact, clearly demarcated tumors, diffuse astrocytomas may display diffusely infiltrative edges that infiltrate surrounding brain tissue such as the brainstem and are more prone to malignant transformation (anaplasia) than the juvenile type.

Prognostically, the cerebellar astrocytoma has been described as the most favorable and benign of all childhood

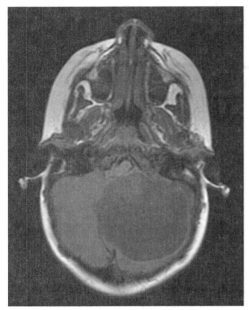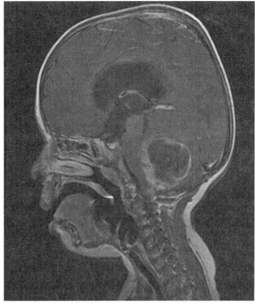

FIGURE 4–2. Axial (*left*) and midsagittal (*right*) postgadolinium magnetic resonance imaging scans demonstrating a 6 × 5 × 4 cm anaplastic pilocytic astrocytoma involving the left cerebellar hemisphere with extension into the vermis and the left side of the pons.

brain tumors (Cohen & Duffner, 1984; Cohen, Duffner, & Tebbi, 1982; Gumbinas, 1983). Survival rates as high as 94% for children with juvenile pilocytic astrocytoma and 38% for children with the diffuse variety have been reported (Becker & Jay, 1990; Becker & Yates, 1986; Heideman et al., 1993). Excellent long-term results following surgical removal are reported for pilocytic variety, with total removal considered the best treatment option (Gumbinas, 1983; Tait et al., 1992; van Eys, 1991). Due to such excellent response rates to surgical intervention, radiotherapy is often not indicated in cases of cerebellar astrocytoma (van Eys, 1991). Postoperative radiotherapy, however, is often employed in patients with diffuse varieties, as total resection is less often achieved (Gumbinas, 1983; Tait et al., 1992).

Because of a slower rate of growth, symptoms associated with cerebellar astrocytoma have been noted to occur for a more extended duration prior to diagnosis (Cohen & Duffner, 1984; Cohen et al., 1982; Gumbinas, 1983; McWhirter & Masel, 1987; van Eys, 1991). As with the medulloblastoma, early indicators are often commonly related to intracranial pressure and present in more than 90% of patients (Heideman et al., 1993). Such symptoms, including headache and vomiting, are often intermittent and likely responsible for length of duration prior to diagnosis (Cohen & Duffner, 1984; Cohen et al., 1982). Midline cerebellar signs have also been suggested to occur in as many as 70% of patients, due to pressure on these structures (Heideman et al., 1993; Plowman, 1992). Other findings associated with cerebellar astrocytoma included papilledema, incoordination, vertigo, head tilt, neck stiffness, irritability, lethargy, and weight loss (Cohen & Duffner, 1984; Cohen et al.,

1982; Delong & Adams, 1975; van Eys, 1991; Wilson, 1975). Specific symptoms often largely depend on the specific location of the tumor within the posterior fossa (Delong & Adams, 1975).

Cerebellar astrocytomas occur most commonly in the first decade of life, with peaks in incidence being reported at 5 to 9 years of age as well as early in the second decade (Becker & Yates, 1986; Cohen & Duffner, 1984; Heidman et al., 1993; Yachnis, 1997). Geissinger and Bucy (1971) reported the average age at diagnosis of cerebellar astrocytoma to be 8 years and 9 months. However, children presenting with this type of tumor at clinics for treatment of associated communication impairment could be expected to vary in age from infancy through adolescence. Males and females appear to be affected equally.

Ependymomas. Ependymomas constitute the third most common posterior fossa tumor in children and are slow growing, predominantly benign neoplasms derived from the ependymal cells lining the ventricles of the brain. Sixty-five to 70% of ependymomas are located in the posterior fossa, with 25 to 30% occurring in the supratentorial region of the brain (Becker & Jay, 1990; Cohen et al., 1982; Heideman et al., 1993; Plowman, 1992). Although they can arise from any part of the ventricular system, in children the most common origins for ependymomas are the roof and the floor of the fourth ventricle (Yachnis, 1997). Subsequent growth of the tumor may lead to occlusion of the cavity of the fourth ventricle, protrusion into the cisterna magna and possible extension through the foramen magnum to overlap the cervical segments of the spinal cord (Figure 4–3). The initial symptoms of ependymoma therefore are those associated with increased intracranial pressure and obstructive hydrocephalus rather than cerebellar signs. Symptoms such as cerebellar dysfunction, nystagmus, dysmetria, and neck pain and stiffness develop later.

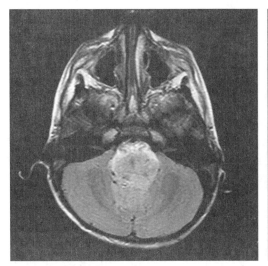 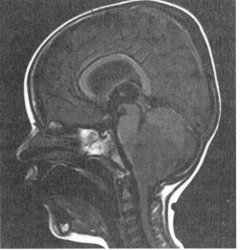

FIGURE 4–3. Axial (*left*) and midsagittal (*right*) magnetic resonance imaging scans demonstrating a 2.9 × 2.6 × 3.2 cm midline ependymoma with associated mass effects and hydrocephaly.

As a consequence of their origin in the roof or floor of the fourth ventricle, complete surgical resection of childhood ependymomas usually is not possible so that recurrence of the tumors in the primary site is common. Development of metastases in other sites, however, is unusual. Because of the high incidence of recurrence, childhood ependymomas have a poor prognosis. Reported rates for tumor recurrence vary with recurrence rates as high as 90% having been reported by some authors (Menkes & Till, 1995) while others estimate the rate to be approximately 30% (Delong & Adams, 1975; Ross & Rubenstein, 1989). If tumor recurrence does occur, it is usually identified within 4 years of the initial diagnosis (Salazar, Castro-Vita, VanHoutte, Rubin, & Aygun, 1983).

A 5-year survival rate of 39% was reported by Naidich and Zimmerman (1984); however, far more favorable survival rates were determined by Salazar et al. (1983), and Ross and Rubenstein (1989). Fifty-one adults and children treated with surgery and radiotherapy for either infratentorial (31 patients) or supratentorial (20 patients) ependymoma (17 patients had grade 1 and 2 ependymomas, whereas 34 had grade 3 and 4 tumors) were reviewed by Salazar et al. (1983). The 10-year survival rates calculated were 75% for low grade and 67% for high-grade ependymomas. Similarly, Ross and Rubenstein (1989) described 15 patients with malignant ependymomas (10 were situated in the posterior fossa) and found 10 patients (67%) to be alive from 15 months to 14 years after surgery.

Salazar et al. (1983) also considered prognostic factors which may influence the survival of patients with ependymoma. A significant difference in median survival times was found for children less than 12 years of age (37 months) at the time of diagnosis and patients older than 12 years at diagnosis (18 months). In contrast, West, Bruce, and Duffner (1985) found that adults had a longer median survival time (52 months) than children 15 years of age or less (28.5 months). Neither tumor position above or below the tentorium, nor the extent of surgical excision, significantly influenced survival in the patients studied by Salazar et al. (1983). The extent of radiation treatment was also correlated with survival. Patients treated with whole-brain irradiation for low-grade tumors and craniospinal irradiation for high-grade tumors had significantly longer survival times than those treated with partial brain irradiation.

The peak incidence of childhood ependymoma has been reported to occur between either 3 and 7 years of age (Delong & Adams, 1975), or 1 and 5 years of age (Naidich & Zimmerman, 1984).

Brainstem Tumors. In addition to the more common posterior fossa tumors outlined above, children can also experience a variety of brainstem tumors. The tumors themselves may vary from benign astrocytomas through to highly malignant glioblastomas.

Brainstem tumors comprise 10 to 20% of all childhood CNS tumors, and most commonly arise from the pons and infiltrate the midbrain, medulla, cerebellum, and/or fourth ventricle (Ater, 1989; Becker & Jay, 1990; Becker & Yates, 1986; Cohen & Duffner, 1984; Cohen et al., 1982; Heideman et al., 1993; McWhirter & Masel, 1987; Plowman, 1992; Tait et al., 1992; van Eys, 1991; Yachnis, 1997). The most common tumor pathology occurring in the brainstem region is the astrocytoma, representing 80% of all brainstem tumors (Becker & Yates, 1986;

Plowman, 1992; Tait et al., 1992; Yachnis, 1997). Due to the large number of nerve pathways and cranial nerve nuclei, tumors occurring in the brainstem region have been reported to have significant impact manifesting in a wide variety of signs and symptoms, such as cranial nerve involvement or palsies, long tract signs, and cerebellar and pyramidal involvement. Seventh nerve palsy (facial weakness) is a common finding, with involvement of the pons and upper medulla producing sixth nerve palsy (squint and head tilt), hearing loss (eighth nerve), and/or dysarthria and dysphagia (IXth and Xth), as well as gait disturbances and ataxia (van Eys, 1991). Signs of intracranial pressure and hydrocephalus are rarely reported unless the tumor is located higher in the mesencephalon (Becker & Jay, 1990). Prognosis is generally considered to be poor (Tait et al., 1992), although survival has been correlated with malignancy of tumor and duration of symptoms prior to diagnosis (Cohen et al., 1982; Heideman et al., 1993).

Treatment for brainstem tumors in childhood often employs the use of radiotherapy, which has been reported to be effective in prolonging survival rates in cases with responses as high as 70% (Plowman, 1992; Tait et al., 1992; van Eys, 1991). Symptomatic improvements have been reported by Heideman and colleagues (1993) in as many as 75% of patients with at least 50 Gy delivered to the tumor. In contrast, surgical removal has largely been considered hazardous and is most often either not performed or resection is extremely limited due to the precarious nature of the location (Becker & Yates, 1986). However, in cases of cervicomedullary tumors, cystic, and more focal lesions, as well as exophytic tumors, partial resection is more often achieved with improved diagnosis (Becker & Jay, 1990; Plowman, 1992). The use of chemotherapy for managing pediatric brainstem tumor has been found to have poor response rates (van Eys, 1991).

Clinical Symptoms of Posterior Fossa Tumors. The presenting signs and symptoms of any posterior fossa tumor type are largely due to increased intracranial pressure that results from the mass effect of the tumor itself, associated edema and obstruction to the flow of cerebrospinal fluid. Destruction or compression of brain tissue may also underlie many of the signs and symptoms observed (Tew, Feibel, & Sawaya, 1984). Symptoms associated with the presence of a brain tumor may be nonspecific or localizing. Nonspecific symptoms (e.g., headache, nausea) could be caused by many other childhood illnesses and do not necessarily suggest neurologic damage, whereas localizing symptoms (e.g., ataxia, nystagmus) imply nervous system involvement.

Symptoms associated with posterior fossa tumors include bifrontal headache, nausea and vomiting, gait disturbance, depressed cerebral function (manifested as apathy and irritability), neck stiffness or neck pain, dizziness, papilledema (edema of the optic disks due to impairment of the venous drainage from the optic nerve and retina subsequent to increased intracranial pressure), squint and nystagmus, alteration of muscle tone, tendon reflex changes, dorsiflexor plantar response, tilting the head away from the side of the tumor, visual impairment, and paresis of limbs (Delong & Adams, 1975; Gol, 1963; Kadota, Allen, Hartman, & Spruce, 1989; Tew et al., 1984). Facial weakness and deafness are rare but have been reported (Delong & Adams, 1975). Although seizures may be the presenting symptom in childhood supratentorial neoplasms (Hirsch Rose, Pierre-Khan, Pfister, Hoppe-Hirsh, 1989), seizures have not been reported in association with tumors of the posterior fossa.

In that they share a cerebellar site, the clinical symptoms of medulloblastomas and astrocytomas essentially are the same. However, the duration between the onset of symptoms and initiation of treatment tends to be much shorter in the case of medulloblastomas (Delong & Adams, 1975), possibly due to the rapid growth of these tumors and the midline position of medulloblastomas. Both of these features result in the early obstruction of the fourth ventricle and interruption of the cerebrospinal fluid flow. The time between onset of symptoms and initiation of treatment in the case of medulloblastomas has been reported to average 5.2 months (range 1 to 80 months), whereas the same period for astrocytoma patients is 2 years 4 months (Davis & Joglekar, 1981). In general, the symptoms associated with ependymomas cannot be distinguished from medulloblastomas and astrocytomas (Delong & Adams, 1975; Naidich & Zimmerman, 1984). However, as ependymomas block the flow of cerebrospinal fluid prior to invading the cerebellum the initial symptoms are those associated with increased intracranial pressure rather than cerebellar deficits.

Medical Treatment of Posterior Fossa Tumors. Treatment of posterior fossa tumors involves surgical removal of the tumor, supplemented in some cases by craniospinal irradiation and, in the case of highly malignant tumors, by chemotherapy. Whether craniospinal irradia-tion and chemotherapy are required is determined by the degree of surgical excision (i.e., whether the tumor has been totally or only partially removed) and the level of malignancy of the tumor.

Access to the posterior cranial fossa is gained by way of a craniotomy through the occipital region of the cranium. Macroscopically, tumor removal is judged as total, subtotal (at least 80% of the tumor is excised), or partial. If the tumor is inaccessible only a biopsy is taken to allow determination of the tumor type. The extent of tumor excision depends on the neurologic deficits that are likely to result from aggressive surgical resection.

The tumor tissue removed at surgery is analyzed and a histologic diagnosis made. Subsequent treatment depends largely on the pathologist's report and the extent of the tumor resection. Most children receive whole brain and/or spinal irradiation with an extra boost to the tumor site. Children with low-grade astrocytomas are often spared craniospinal irradiation, a factor which may lead to a lower incidence of neuropsychological sequelae, including speech and language disorders, in the long term. A course of radiotherapy takes approximately 6 weeks to complete. Completing a course of radiotherapy is a grueling experience for both the child and the family. The child often feels tired, irritable, and nauseated, whereas the family is required to spend many hours each week accompanying the child to the radiotherapy clinic.

Children with highly malignant tumors may also receive chemotherapy. Although postoperative chemotherapy is not administered as routinely as radiotherapy, it has been suggested that when added to a regimen of surgical excision and CNS irradiation, or when implemented in cases of recurrent tumor, chemotherapy will prolong survival time (Horowitz et al., 1988; van Eys, Baram, Cangir, Bruner, & Martinez-Prieto, 1988). Chemotherapy protocols can vary widely in drug selection, dosages, and timing. Both chemotherapy and radiotherapy courses, and the complications which may be associated with such treatments, are discussed in further detail below.

As discussed previously, many patients experience tumor recurrence despite aggressive tumor management at initial diagnosis. Depending on the site and growth characteristics of the recurrent tumor, these patients undergo further surgery, radiotherapy, and/or chemotherapy. In some cases, the additional treatment is described as palliative rather than curative, with the ultimate aim being the alleviation of symptoms and an extension of the expected survival time.

The majority of children with posterior fossa tumors experience hydrocephalus due to ventricular and cerebrospinal fluid pathway obstruction. This symptom is alleviated by the surgical insertion of a shunting system. The most common shunt utilized is a ventriculoperitoneal (VP) shunt, which drains fluid from the lateral ventricles into the peritoneal cavity. The shunting procedure is usually performed prior to surgical excision of the tumor; however, in some cases shunting may not be required until after the tumor has been resected.

Language Disorders Associated with Posterior Fossa Tumors. Although the neuroanatomical location of the majority of childhood brain tumors in the posterior cranial fossa does not lead to the immediate prediction of associated language deficits, there are a number of features of these tumors that could

cause the presence of language impairments in affected individuals. First, treatments such as surgery, radiotherapy, and chemotherapy applied to posterior fossa tumors may lead to impairments in brain structure and function (see below). Second, there now is growing evidence that the cerebellum itself may be involved in language and cognitive function (Murdoch, 2010) such that tumors either originating from or invading the cerebellum may compromise normal language function. Furthermore, the invasion and compression of cerebral tissue as the tumor grows may also result in vascular changes which could be related to dysfunction in the central cortical speech and language centers. Third, indirect effects of tumor growth such as hydrocephalus and increased intracranial pressure caused by obstruction of the flow of cerebrospinal fluid may result in compression of the cerebral cortex leading to impaired language abilities. Prior to examining each of these potential causes of language disorders, however, it is important to first document evidence to support the presence of language impairments in children treated for posterior fossa tumors and to describe the nature of those impairments.

Language Disorders: Evidence from Mixed Etiology Studies. Prior to the 1990s evidence pointing to the presence of language impairments in children treated for posterior fossa tumors was largely confined to studies of acquired childhood aphasia of mixed etiologies that included some children with posterior fossa tumors (Alajouanine & Lhermitte, 1965; Carrow-Woolfolk & Lynch, 1982; Cooper & Flowers, 1987, Hécaen, 1976; Miller, Campbell, Chapman, & Weismer, 1984; van Dongen, Loonen, & van Dongen, 1985). Unfortunately, the majority of these studies did not differentiate between various causes of acquired language disorders, nor did they describe tumor sites or treatments applied.

Alajouanine and Lhermitte (1965) studied 32 children with cerebral lesions between 6 and 15 years of age. Two of these children had undergone surgery for astrocytoma removal; however, the sites of the tumors were not provided. Although a posterior fossa location is more common in children, astrocytomas can also originate in the cerebral hemispheres. Alajouanine and Lhermitte (1965) reported that the reduction of expressive activities (oral, written, and gesture) was the most prominent feature of the acquired language disorders exhibited by the subject group. This reduction of expression was noted in all 32 children and was not related to the presence of dysarthria. No or limited oral expression was also reported in two of the other tumor studies previously discussed (Rekate, Grubb, Aram, Hahn, & Ratcheson, 1985; Volcan, Cole, & Johnston, 1986). However, in the latter studies the reduction in expression could have been caused by the presence of mutism and/or dysarthria and consequently a language disturbance may or may not have existed. Alajouanine and Lhermitte (1965) noted simplified rather than erroneous syntax, and severe reading and writing disturbances. The aphasic characteristics seen in adults such as logorrhea, phonemic or semantic paraphasias, verbal stereotypes, and perseverations were not detected in the cases of acquired aphasia studied. The general pattern of simplified syntax, severe reading and writing disturbances and reduced oral expression is commonly reported in the literature with the addition of comprehension and word-finding difficulties in some cases (Carrow-Woolfolk & Lynch, 1982; Satz & Bullard-Bates, 1981; van Dongen et al., 1985).

Although several authors have attempted to specify a common set of characteristics of acquired childhood aphasia (see Chapter 2) Cooper and Flowers (1987), in a study of children with aphasia resulting from different causes, were unable to identify one particular language deficit or a cluster of deficits as common to their group of brain-injured children. Fifteen children with histories of closed-head injury, stroke, encephalitis, or brain tumor (one patient showed a posterior fossa mass on computed tomography [CT]) were assessed between 1 and 10 years post-onset using a battery of language and academic tests. The subjects performed significantly below a group of non-brain-injured controls in the areas of word, sentence, and paragraph comprehension; naming; oral production of complex syntactic constructions; and word fluency. Within the subject group, language deficits ranged from no or only mild impairment to significant language deficits. Two of the 15 subjects were receiving academic assistance of some kind. In particular, the child who had been treated for posterior fossa tumor when 10, had, when 6 years old, demonstrated aphasia, reduced receptive skills, and monosyllabic verbalizations at diagnosis. Twelve months later, the child was enrolled in full-time special education and was receiving speech therapy, occupational therapy, and physiotherapy. On assessment, particular difficulties were noted on sentence formulation and naming tasks. Unfortunately, details of the medical management of this case were not provided. In his sample of 26 children with cortical lesions Hécaen (1976) also included two cases of tumor. It was found that in one of these cases, the presence of a tumor in the left cerebral hemisphere resulted in muteness lasting 2 months, and articulation, reading, and writing disorders from which there was no change.

Language Disorders: Evidence from Children Treated for Posterior Fossa Tumor. The most comprehensive series of studies of acquired language disorders associated with posterior fossa brain tumor reported to date were conducted by Hudson, Murdoch, and colleagues (Hudson & Murdoch, 1992a, 1992b, 1992c; Hudson, Murdoch, & Ozanne, 1989; Murdoch & Hudson-Tennent, 1994), who described the language abilities of children treated for posterior fossa tumors (Murdoch & Hudson, 1999). A preliminary study reported by Hudson et al. (1989) investigated six children on a case-by-case basis who had undergone surgery for removal of a posterior fossa tumor. Hudson et al. (1989) used a battery of specific language assessments to determine the presence or absence of long-term language deficits in this population and to document the specific characteristics of any identified communication disorder. Findings indicated that language deficits occurred in four of the six cases. In particular, deficits were found to exist in the areas of expressive vocabulary and word-finding, receptive syntax, expressive syntax, and reading. It was noted that the two cases with no identified language deficits were the only children to not receive radiation therapy to the CNS as treatment for their condition, compared to the remaining four cases with identified language disorders. Sev-

eral factors were considered to have influenced the language profiles reported in the researchers' six cases, including age at onset, tumor type, extent of surgical excision, insertion of VP shunts, and the effects of the treatment modalities, radiotherapy, and/or chemo-therapy (Hudson et al., 1989).

In a further study, Hudson and Murdoch (1992a) investigated the presence, nature, and severity of language deficits exhibited by a group of 20 children treated for posterior fossa tumor. Results indicated that the language abilities of the group were significantly reduced compared to those of their peers on both receptive and expressive language tasks in the chronic stage subsequent to treatment. Additionally, deficiencies in the understanding and manipulation of complex and abstract language structures were also noted, indicating overall reduced performance on higher level language tasks particularly in areas involving making inferences from given information, complex sentence generation appropriate to context, and interpreting metaphoric expressions (Hudson & Murdoch, 1992a).

In a prospective study of three children treated for posterior fossa medulloblastoma, Hudson and Murdoch (1992b) reported a considerable degree of variation in language abilities over a 28 month posttreatment follow-up period. Although severe semantic-lexical deficits were found to be present immediately post-treatment in all cases examined, dramatic improvements in semantic abilities were reported in the first 6 months posttreatment via surgery and CNS radiotherapy. Residual word-finding difficulties were also identified at final assessment. In addition to reduced ability on semantic, word-finding, and listening tasks, Hudson and Murdoch (1992b) also reported the presence of some mildly reduced receptive language skills.

The narrative abilities of 16 children treated for posterior fossa tumors were investigated by Hudson and Murdoch (1992c). Their findings indicated that the spontaneously generated narratives of their group of children treated for posterior fossa tumor were similar to their peers, with cohesive adequacy the only discourse feature considered to be reduced.

An examination by Murdoch and Hudson-Tennent (1994) of the individual language abilities of 20 children who had been treated for posterior fossa tumor highlighted the variability of the nature and severity of language deficits exhibited by these children, which ranged from above average language abilities to marked global language deficits. Three of the 20 subjects demonstrated a global language deficit across all receptive and expressive skill areas, whereas 5 of the 20 were shown to have an adequate level of language ability. According to Murdoch and Hudson-Tennent (1994), the remaining 12 subjects evidenced strengths and weaknesses across the various language abilities that were assessed. Six of the 12 participants with variable strengths and weaknesses were documented to experience particular difficulty with expressive semantic and/or syntactic language, with five experiencing deficits predominantly in the area of receptive language. The remaining participant of the 12 demonstrated only word-finding deficits and difficulty on higher level advanced language tasks (Murdoch & Hudson-Tennent, 1994). Seven of the participants examined individually by Murdoch and Hudson-Tennent (1994) were reported

to experience difficulty on tasks requiring naming ability.

More recently, Docking, Murdoch, and Suppiah (2007) examined the language abilities of four children treated with surgery and/or radiotherapy for cerebellar tumor 6 months to 3 years posttreatment. Their findings revealed intact abilities across all four cases on measures of general language ability, including receptive language, expressive language, receptive vocabulary, and naming. Although 2 of 4 cases also demonstrated intact high-level language skills across all measures, the remaining two cases showed specific deficits in linguistic problem solving at 6 months posttreatment. Follow-up assessment of one case demonstrated further decline in this area 12 months later.

In contrast to the impaired language abilities of children treated for posterior fossa tumors involving the cerebellum, relatively intact language skills have been reported in cases where the tumor is restricted to the brainstem alone (Docking, Ward, & Murdoch, 2005; Murdoch & Hudson-Tennent, 1994). Murdoch and Hudson-Tennent (1994) conducted a detailed examination of a child treated for brainstem tumor as part of a study of a larger cohort of 20 children with posterior fossa tumor. Treatment at the age of 2 years, 1 month included surgical removal followed by a combination of both radiotherapy and chemotherapy. Language findings for this child revealed performance within the average range on measures of general language skills, despite some weakness on a sentence-combining task. Four out of five components of an assessment of auditory comprehension were also considered intact. Overall, Murdoch and Hudson-Tennent (1994) concluded that the case treated for posterior fossa tumor with brainstem involvement demonstrated relatively intact language abilities. Similar findings were reported by Docking et al. (2005). These latter researchers examined the general and high-level language abilities of 6 children treated for brainstem tumor, in addition to phonological skills. Group analysis revealed that these children treated for brainstem tumor demonstrated intact language and phonological awareness skills compared to a control group. Individual analysis revealed only 1 of the 6 children treated for brainstem tumor showed evidence of language disturbance, with an additional child demonstrating an isolated mildly reduced score on one phonological awareness task.

Language Disorders: Clinical Implications. The findings of case studies as well as group studies reported in the literature to date indicate that, although not inevitable, language disorders do occur in children in the chronic stage subsequent to treatment for posterior fossa tumors. Furthermore, it is clear that all aspects of language may be compromised in this population and hence, there is a need to monitor both the receptive and expressive language abilities of children treated for posterior fossa tumors throughout their school years.

As yet, no characteristic language pattern has been elucidated to provide clinicians with a starting point for patient management, or to alert them to specific areas of language deficit that may require more in-depth evaluation in tumor cases. Rather, the data available to date indicate the presence of variable language abilities within the tumor population thereby necessitating the need for development and imple-

mentation of individualized therapy programs. Although sharing a common etiology (i.e., posterior fossa tumor), because they represent a variety of tumor types requiring different treatment approaches, children treated for posterior fossa tumors do not represent a homogeneous group. For instance, it is apparent that several complicating factors, such as CNS irradiation, chemotherapy, hydrocephalus, and so forth, may also influence the long-term language abilities of posterior fossa tumor patients, although as yet the precise contribution of these factors to the manifestation of language disorders is unknown. Consequently, therapy for this population can never be prescriptive as it is essential that clinicians evaluate each child's abilities in the context of the tumor treatment being given (e.g., surgery, radiotherapy, chemotherapy), the presence of other complicating factors (such as hydrocephalus and VP shunts), the presence of any intellectual deterioration, the educational status of the child, the involvement of other medical and educational services, and the emotional state of the child and their family.

It is noteworthy that neurologic deterioration can occur from months to years after the completion of treatment of brain tumors (Kun, Mulhern, & Crisco, 1983; Mulhern & Kun, 1985). Consequently, clinicians need to be aware of the need to obtain initial baseline measurements of language abilities from these children and to review them at 6- or 12-monthly intervals for several years whether or not speech pathology was recommended subsequent to the initial assessment. Speech-language pathologists, therefore, need to take an active role in the management of children treated for brain tumors, even if initially intervention does not appear warranted. In particular, the high-level language skills that may influence academic performance should be monitored and, if necessary, the appropriate intervention provided.

Language Disorders: Neuropathologic/Neurophysiologic Basis—Treatment Effects. As outlined above, the treatment of posterior fossa tumors in children usually involves the use of techniques such as surgery, radiotherapy, and chemotherapy. Unfortunately, over recent decades it has become recognized that, despite being essential for survival these techniques may cause structural and functional changes in the brain leading to a number of long-term negative sequelae that may significantly decrease the quality of survival, including possible language and other deficits.

Effects of Surgical Treatment. Recent years have seen significant improvements in the surgical care of children with posterior fossa tumors. Contemporary neuroimaging techniques such as CT and magnetic resonance imaging (MRI) have enabled earlier detection and more accurate localization of tumors. Furthermore, surgical techniques utilizing the operating microscope, microsurgical instrumentation, ultrasound aspirators and lasers combined with a better understanding of homeostasis and three-dimensional neuroanatomy currently enable the modern neurosurgeon to undertake more difficult and aggressive neurosurgical operations than in the past. The goal of most operations is both to biopsy the tumor and to remove as much of it as can be removed without causing or increasing neurologic deficit. Overall, several factors determine the decision to operate: The value of making histologic diagnosis; the need to remove mass effect (e.g., obstruction of the flow of cerebrospinal fluid); and the effect of tumor removal on survival. Unfortunately, many tumors are unable to be surgically excised without risks of surgically mortality or negative neurologic sequelae. Postoperative complications are dependent on several factors including: The experience of the operating surgeon; the preoperative condition of the child; the tumor location; and the extent and care of tumor removal. The presence of severe neurologic deficits in the immediate postoperative period has been reported to be suggestive of a poorer prognosis in terms of a full recovery of neurologic function (Tait et al., 1992).

Effects of Radiotherapy. The effects of irradiation on brain structure and function can be divided into acute reactions, early-delayed reactions and late-delayed reactions. Early or acute reactions are symptoms that occur during treatment and up to 6 weeks posttreatment (Heideman et al., 1993). Considered rarely to be life threatening, acute side effects usually resolve within weeks of treatment completion (Deutsch, 1990b). Although reported to be uncommon, these acute CNS effects may be a consequence of increased pressure of localized or generalized edema, which occurs as a result of radiation to the brain (Ater, 1989; Kun & Moulder, 1993; van Eys, 1991).

Early-delayed effects of radiotherapy treatment are considered to be symptoms that occur approximately 2 to 4 months following treatment completion (and up to 6 months) (Cohen et al., 1982; Heideman et al., 1993). Transient symptoms attributed to temporary demyelination have been seen six to eight weeks after completion of radiotherapy to the brain and spinal cord (Heideman et al., 1993). Reported to be frequent, electroencephalographic changes of slow-wave activity consistent with diffuse cerebral disturbance have also been documented in the early-delayed stages following radiotherapy treatment (Heideman et al., 1993; van Eys, 1991).

Treatment effects that are defined as delayed or late occurring, include symptoms that manifest 6 months to many years following radiotherapy (Cohen et al., 1982; Heideman et al., 1993). As these effects tend to be progressive and more permanent in nature, it is these latter reactions that are more likely to underlie the development of language disorders. Until recently, the survival of children with brain tumors was limited, so that concerns over long-term effects of therapy were considered unnecessary. Radiotherapy was often considered palliative with late effects often not investigated (van Eys, 1991). As children with various types of brain tumors currently have improved prognoses, these long-term effects have important implications (Duffner, Cohen, & Thomas, 1983). The clinical manifestation of long-term effects resulting from radiotherapy is one of insidious progressive deterioration, focal neurologic signs, encephalopathy, dementia, seizures, and many other adverse long-term sequelae that have been implicated as the primary result of radiation therapy (Cohen et al., 1982; Heideman et al., 1993). This damage may lead to neuropathologic changes, second malignancies, motor and sensory changes, and endocrine and cognitive dysfunction (Heideman et al., 1993). Late CNS effects often restrict the dose, volume, and

intensity of treatment (Kun & Moulder, 1993). In fact, modern radiation oncologists now often describe tolerance in terms of doses that would cause particular incidence of brain necrosis or severe damage (Deutsch, 1990b). However, much lower doses can also be associated with late sequelae affecting quality of survival (Deutsch, 1990b).

The primary site of late or delayed radiation-induced damage to the CNS is the glial cells, particularly oligodendroglia, and damage to the vasculature (capillary endothelial cells) (Arya, Gilbert, & Wiedrich, 1986; Heideman et al., 1993; Hoppe-Hirsch, 1993). A spectrum of clinical syndromes may occur, radionecrosis, necrotizing leukoencephalopathy (white matter hypodensity), mineralizing microangiopathy with dystrophic calcification (intracerebral calcifications), cerebral sclerosis, cerebral atrophy, ventricular and subarachnoid space dilatation, and spinal cord dysfunction (Arya et al., 1986; Hoppe-Hirsch, 1993; Plowman, 1992).

The most commonly documented and most severe complication of radiotherapy directed to the CNS is radionecrosis, which commonly develops from 6 months following treatment up to a reported 20 years later (Altman & Schwartz, 1983; Arya et al., 1986; Ater, 1989; Barrett & Donaldson, 1992; Cohen et al., 1982; Di Chiro et al., 1988; Heideman et al., 1993; Kun & Moulder, 1993; Marks, Baglan, Prassad, & Blank, 1981). Radiation necrosis is commonly associated with higher than conventional doses (i.e., greater than 50 Gy over 5 weeks or longer), larger than conventional daily fraction sizes, or the use of combination approaches (Barrett & Donaldson, 1992; Heideman et al., 1993), with an incidence of 5 to 10% of children (between 54 and 60 Gy), and increasing to more than 25 to 50% of cases when doses exceed 65 Gy (van Eys, 1991). Clinically, radionecrosis manifests as seizures and focal neurologic dysfunction, such as headache, personality changes, seizures, hemiparesis, ataxia, and signs of increased intracranial pressure, together with focal neurologic deficits (Heideman et al., 1993).

Another well-documented structural postradiotherapy syndrome associated with CNS damage in childhood brain tumors is necrotizing leukoencephalopathy (Cohen et al., 1982; Duffner et al., 1983; Heideman et al., 1993; Kun & Moulder, 1993). Necrotizing leukoencephalopathy is a subacute syndrome clinically manifesting as lethargy, seizures, perceptual changes, cerebellar dysfunction (spasticity and ataxia), dementia, and pseudobulbar paresis, with characteristic white matter changes observed on both CT and MRI scans (Kun & Moulder, 1993). It is reported to occur almost exclusively when high-dose intravenous methotrexate is involved, usually following normally tolerated doses of radiation (Kun & Moulder, 1993).

Mineralizing microangiopathy with dystrophic calcification, another form of postradiotherapy CNS damage in childhood brain tumors, may occur at total doses greater than 20 Gy, and again can possibly be exacerbated by intrathecal methotrexate or intrathecal cytosine arabinoside (Heideman et al., 1993; Kun & Moulder, 1993). Incidence is reported at greater than 25 to 30% of treated children, although onset is variable (from 9 months following radiotherapy) (Heideman et al., 1993). Clinically, mineralizing microangiopathy may manifest with headaches and seizures (Heideman et al., 1993).

As a consequence of radiotherapy, some neurologic deficits may result due to its detrimental effects on cerebral blood vessels (Hoppe-Hirsch, 1993). Symptomatic cerebrovascular disease may develop, according to Altman and Schwartz (1983), following radiation treatment for CNS tumors. Both Deutsch (1990a) and Cohen et al. (1982) also reported that symptomatic intracranial large-vessel vasculopathy may occur. Cerebrovascular occlusive disease may follow radiation to levels at 50 to 54 Gy, but is most common under 2 years even at lower doses (Wharam, 1983). Endarteritis, a known effect of irradiation, has also been reported as a late consequence of vascular changes (Bamford et al., 1976).

Basal ganglia calcification frequently has been cited as a consequence of childhood cranial irradiation. Lee and Suh (1977) reported two cases of gray matter calcification 10 and 14 years subsequent to radiotherapy in children with an optic glioma and medulloblastoma, respectively. These authors described the cause as related to radiation vasculitis of the small vessels of the brain with hyalinization and calcification noted to result. Hodges and Smithells (1983) documented a case where intracranial calcification developed subsequent to cranial irradiation and partial resection of a cerebellar astrocytoma. Although an initial CT did not reveal evidence of calcification, a follow-up CT five years later revealed a right occipital lobe calcification. It also was reported that a gradual deterioration in intellectual function had been evident since completion of treatment, resulting in the child requiring special education. Murdoch and Hudson (1999) also reported the presence of intracranial calcification in a child who underwent radiotherapy as part of the treatment for a medulloblastoma. A CT scan taken 22 months postradiotherapy revealed the presence of widespread calcification in the temporal fossa, posterior temporal regions and frontal lobes consistent with the effects of radiotherapy (Figure 4–4).

Brain atrophy has also been reported to result following childhood radiotherapy (Davis, Hoffman, Pearl, & Braun, 1986). A retrospective evaluation of 49 children who had received cranial radiotherapy for a primary CNS or skull-based tumor conducted by Davis and colleagues (1986), revealed that the most commonly observed abnormality was generalized atrophy, at an incidence of 51%. This incidence was noted to vary little with age or with use of chemotherapy.

In addition to atrophy, white matter abnormalities also were reported by Davis and colleagues (1986) in 26% of

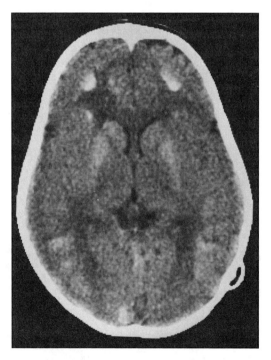

FIGURE 4–4. CT scan of a child performed 22 months postradiotherapy showing widespread intracranial calcification consistent with the effects of radiotherapy.

children studied. Both focal and generalized areas were noted, together with focal calcifications in 9 out of 13 cases. According to Davis et al. (1986), these white-matter abnormalities tended to occur in younger children under 3 years of age, with or without chemotherapy. Calcification was observed in 28% of children, with the most frequent site subcortical at the gray-white junction. Davis et al. (1986) reported that such subcortical calcification was progressive over one or two years and resulted from radiation induced mineralizing microangiopathy and dystrophic calcification with demyelination. Thus, 73% of children in this study had abnormalities unrelated to the tumor itself. In fact, according to Davis et al. (1986), radiotherapy was the primary mode of treatment associated with white matter abnormalities and calcification, which were documented to be more frequent and more severe in children treated prior to 3 years of age.

Therefore, it is clear that potential exists for neuropathologic changes to occur following radiotherapy treatment for childhood brain tumor. The potential for these structural changes to affect various functions of the brain is apparent, including cognition and language function.

Effects of Chemotherapy. Chemotherapy has become an increasingly important part of multimodality treatment planning for children with primary brain and spinal cord tumors, with chemotherapy documented to be of benefit for some forms of childhood primary CNS tumors (Allen, 1991, 1992; Cohen et al., 1982; Packer, Nicholson, & Ryan, 1993).

The most commonly reported agents in the management of childhood brain tumors are alkylating agents such as nitrogen mustard (mechlorethamine), procarbazine, cyclophosphamide, and ifosfamide; the platinum compounds, cisplatin and carboplatin; the nitrosoureas, lomustine and carmustine; plant alkaloids such as vincristine and etoposide; and antimetabolites such as methotrexate. Most of the toxicities are dose dependent, with the amount of drug a patient may tolerate dependent not only on differences in that individuals drug metabolism and organ sensitivity, but also on age and prior therapy (Allen, 1991, 1992).

Although chemotherapy is not considered appropriate for all types of brain tumor, high-grade tumors such as medulloblastoma, primary neuroepithelial tumor, ependymoma, and glioblastoma are intrinsically chemosensitive (Tait et al., 1992). However, randomized clinical trials have so far been able to define only a limited role for chemotherapy (Tait et al., 1992). The main factors considered responsible for reduced effectiveness include limited drug access due to the blood-brain barrier, and tumor cell heterogeneity (Tait et al., 1992). An additional obstacle can be attributed to irradiation of the craniospinal axis temporarily inactivating up to 70% of the total marrow capacity of the patient and thereby decreasing tolerance to chemotherapy (van Eys, 1991).

Although most complications of chemotherapy in children with brain tumor are considered to be acute and short-lived, exceptions do exist (Allen, 1991, 1992). However, long-term effects from chemotherapy have not been considered as severe as morbidity resulting from radiotherapy (Cohen et al., 1982). To a large extent, the CNS is considered protected from the effects of drugs by the blood-brain barrier. However, it is well documented that some chemotherapeutic agents such as methotrexate, may have an adverse effect on the CNS, as well as being implicated in the development of severe irreversible CNS toxicity (Altman & Schwartz, 1983; Arya et al., 1986; Hoppe-Hirsch, 1993).

Neurologic changes have been described in children receiving intrathecal, intraventricular, or high doses of parenteral methotrexate in the absence of radiation (Altman & Schwartz, 1983). However, the toxicity associated with methotrexate supposedly is enhanced in the presence of radiotherapy (Vietti, 1991). Although leukoencephalopathy is well documented as being associated with radiotherapy, it is also well recognized to be exacerbated by methotrexate (Cohen et al., 1982; Heideman et al., 1993). It is considered that this is due to the radiation-induced disruption of the blood-brain barrier increasing the concentration of the methotrexate in the nervous tissue and hence its toxicity (Hoppe-Hirsch, 1993). Other chemotherapeutic agents either cross the blood-brain barrier (enabling them to reach the isolated tumoral cells spreading in the normal nervous tissue) or do not cross the blood-brain barrier (reaching the tumor where the barrier is disrupted) (Hoppe-Hirsch, 1993). The latter variety, however, is considered less toxic (Hoppe-Hirsch, 1993).

Dennis, Spiegler, Hetherington, and Greenberg (1996) have reported that adjuvant chemotherapy for childhood brain tumor evokes a risk of cognitive morbidity, which presently is becoming more evident as children are followed up over longer periods. A study conducted by Sands, van Gorp, and Finlay (1998) documented neuropsychological findings in 10 children who had received conventional induction chemotherapy (vincristine, cisplatin, cyclophosphamide, and etoposide) repeated every three weeks for five cycles, followed by mye-loblative consolidation chemotherapy with autologous bone marrow reconstitution, subsequent to maximal surgical resection. As a group, subjects performed in the low average range of overall intelligence, verbal IQ/verbal reasoning and performance IQ/abstract visual reasoning. Performance was, however, in the average range in areas of reading, spelling and numerics, verbal learning and memory, visual memory, and visuospatial, social-emotional, and behavioral functioning (Sands et al., 1998).

In addition to suggestions of cognitive impairments resulting from neurotoxicities to the brain induced by chemotherapy administered to children with brain tumors, several reports in the literature also implicate chemotherapy as an underlying cause of language problems in children treated for cancer. To date, the majority of these studies have involved examination of children treated with chemotherapy for acute lymphoblastic leukemia (see below). The only study reported to date that has investigated the language and cognitive abilities of children treated with chemotherapy alone for brain tumor was that reported by Sands et al. (1998). Based on an examination of 10 cases these latter researchers reported the presence of significant deficits on language tasks investigating expressive naming and receptive vocabulary.

Summary of Treatment Effects. Although advances in modern medical technology and improvements in treatment regimens have led to increased survival rates for children treated for posterior fossa tumors, evidence is available indicating that the various treatment techniques inclusive of surgery, radiotherapy, and chemotherapy are associated with a number of negative sequelae that have the potential to cause language impairments. Importantly, many of these negative sequelae, including structural and functional changes in the brain may only manifest in the long-term (in some instances many years posttreatment). Consequently, it is important for clinicians to recognize that children treated for posterior fossa tumors may require monitoring for potential language disorders over an extended period of time with intervention applied as required.

Language Disorders: Neuropathologic/Neurophysiologic Basis—Cerebellar Involvement. As outlined above, most posterior fossa tumors either originate from or invade the cerebellum. Although originally confined to the domain of motor control, a series of recent reviews have highlighted a role for the cerebellum not only in movement control but also in language and cognitive function in the adult population (Mariën, Engelborghs, Fabbro, & De Deyn, 2001; Murdoch, 2010). An increasing body of support is also highlighting similar findings in children with acquired lesions (Levisohn, Cronin-Golomb, & Schmahmann, 2000; Riva, 2000). Consequently, direct damage to the cerebellum itself at least partly may contribute to the language impairments observed in children treated for posterior fossa tumors.

Deficits observed in frontal functions following cerebellar lesions in pediatric populations confirm the existence of connections with frontal lobes via the thalamus. Studies of children with acquired cerebellar lesions also appear to support findings in adult studies, whereas furthermore appearing to present a more concordant pattern of specific neuropsychological profiles depending on lesion site. In particular, involvement of the cerebellar hemispheres has been noted in the processing of cognitive functions and has been associated with patterns of site-specific cognitive dysfunctions, whereas lesions of the vermis have been related to behavioral and verbal production disturbances, including anarthric and agrammatic language disturbances (Riva, 2000).

Riva and Giorgi (2000a, 2000b) analyzed the specific functions of both the cerebellar hemispheres and the vermis in examining the cognitive, language, and executive functions of children who had undergone surgical removal of either a cerebellar hemispheric tumor or a vermal tumor. Groups with either left or right involvement were observed to show varying degrees of reduced ability in thinking flexibility and problem solving. Results from the group of hemispheric patients also reportedly confirmed the dissociation of the circuits connecting the cerebellum to the supratentorial associative areas through the thalamus. Specific high-level language deficits, global impairment, and expressive language and syntax were also acknowledged among others to be related to direct impact of cerebellar damage (Murdoch & Hudson-Tennent, 1994).

The right cerebellar hemisphere has been recently considered to maintain substantial responsibility for language processing. Particularly, clinical manifestations resulting from damage to this specific region in children include disturbances in auditory sequential memory, alterations in verbal intelligence, decreased competence in complex language processing, significantly reduced syntactic comprehension, reduced abil-

ities in verbal sequencing and categorical memory, and an interruption of literacy skills. Conversely, damage to the left cerebellar hemisphere has been associated with visual and spatial memory, nonverbal information processing, nonverbal intelligence, and impairments in prosody.

The vermal region has also been specifically implicated in the occurrence of transient mutism following surgical intervention and behavioral disturbances, including a dysregulation of affect. Other areas of disturbance in children have been noted to include verbal fluency, telegraphic speech, reductions in complex language structures, impaired procedural learning and some reports of naming difficulties. The congenital cerebellar condition, global hypoplasia of the vermis or selective hypoplasia of some vermian lobules is frequently observed in children with neurologic diseases. These anatomic alterations are often associated with neuropsychological or developmental disorders resembling mental insufficiency of varying severity with behavioral changes that may even mirror autism. Riva and Giorgi (2000a, 2000b) reported two presentations: namely, postsurgical mutism and behavioral disturbances. These reports of post-surgical mutism evolved either into a historic speech disorder or a language disorder characteristic of agrammatism with intact comprehension. Behavioral disturbances presented as affective and social behavioral alterations ranging in severity from irritability to a more autistic manifestation.

Evidence from childhood studies serves to indicate that the presence of a cerebellar contribution to language and cognition in children reflects observations in adult patients. It also highlights the presence of functional cerebrocerebellar connections early in childhood. Additionally, it has been suggested that the earlier cerebellar damage occurs during development, the greater the subsequent impact on language and cognitive function. Studies examining the role of the cerebellum in children have indicated that damage to specific areas of the cerebellum exerts impact on a distinct range of functions, indicating that functional specialization is also present at a very early age. Consequently, it is possible that direct involvement of the cerebellum may, at least in part, explain aspects of the language disorder reported to occur subsequent to treatment of posterior fossa tumors in children.

Language Disorders: Neuropathologic/Neurophysiologic Basis—Indirect Effects. Intracranial tumors, including posterior fossa tumors, may indirectly cause neurologic compromise through associated increased intracranial pressure. Indeed, increased intracranial pressure is responsible for some of the earliest and most common clinical manifestations of CNS tumors. Symptoms of increased intracranial pressure are commonly considered subacute nonspecific or nonlocalizing (Heideman et al., 1993). Signs and symptoms vary with location, growth rate of the tumor, and age of the patient (according to the extent of cranial bone fusion and degree of CNS maturity) (Heideman et al., 1993; van Eys, 1991). Usually, these symptoms result from a gradual increase in pressure, which causes varying degrees of headache, vomiting, impaired vision, cranial enlargement, convulsions, intellectual disturbances, and possibly language impairments.

Increased intracranial pressure can be caused by the tumor mass or by blockage of the flow of cerebrospinal fluid. The increase in intracranial volume associated with the presence of a space-occupying tumor within a fixed space such as the cranial vault, results in an increase in pressure. This so-called mass effect may be further exacerbated by edema resulting from the growing tumor. Cerebral edema may have greater implications than the tumor itself, with rapid onset, and can cause sudden clinical deterioration. Obstruction of the flow of cerebrospinal fluid leading to hydrocephalus due to the location of the tumor is also a common cause of increased intracranial pressure in children with posterior fossa tumors. For example, as outline above, due to compression of the fourth ventricle by the tumor, hydrocephalus is often the earliest and most common symptom to accompany medulloblastoma. Overall, many of the neurologic, neuropsychological, or intellectual impairments found in children who have survived pediatric brain tumors are considered by several authors to occur as a result of increased intracranial pressure (McWhirter & Masel, 1987; Silverman & Thomas, 1990).

Supratentorial Brain Tumors

The supratentorial region of the brain encompasses the intracranial structures above the level of the tentorium cerebelli. According to Becker and Jay (1990) supratentorial tumors comprise 40% of pediatric brain tumors. These tumors are distributed throughout the cerebral hemispheres (35%), parasellar regions (40%), thalamus and basal ganglia (10%), pineal region (10%), and intraventricular location (3%). Children with supratentorial tumors may exhibit a variety of signs and symptoms that are dependent on the size and location of the tumor (Heideman et al., 1993).

Types of Supratentorial Tumors. Approximately 65% of tumors in the supratentorial region are astrocytomas, with a further 15% noted to be primary neuroepithelial tumors, 15% ependymomas, and 5% distributed among other varieties. Given that the majority of the supratentorial tumors likely to be associated with the occurrence of language impairments are astrocytomas the present chapter will focus on this tumor group.

Supratentorial Astrocytomas. Supratentorial astrocytomas constitute 35% of all childhood CNS tumors, invading either the cerebral hemispheres or the deep midline structures and the basal ganglia (Heideman et al., 1993; Plowman, 1992). The major clinical signs often relate to increased intracranial pressure although seizures are common in up to 25% of patients (Becker & Yates, 1986; Gumbinas, 1983; Heideman et al., 1993). Other signs relate to location and local effects such as focal motor weakness and hemiplegia occurring in up to 40% of children with supratentorial astrocytomas (Becker & Yates, 1986; Heideman et al., 1993; Yachnis, 1997). Prognosis of high-grade supratentorial astrocytomas generally is regarded to be poor, with 5-year survival rates less than 5% (Tait et al., 1992). Treatment for childhood supratentorial astrocytoma involves surgical removal followed by radiotherapy (Tait et al., 1992).

Clinical Symptoms of Supratentorial Tumors. Children with supratentorial tumors may evidence a variety of signs and symptoms which are dependent on the size and exact location of the tumor.

Such signs are commonly nonspecific and nonlocalizing with the potential to precede signs of increased intracranial pressure (Heideman et al., 1993; van Eys, 1991). Following headache, the next most common symptom of a supratentorial tumor is seizures (Heideman et al., 1993; Tait et al., 1992). Approximately 25% of children with supratentorial tumors have seizures as an initial presenting symptom. However, the likelihood of a child presenting with a seizure is dependent on histology, rate of growth, and location of the tumor (Heideman et al., 1993). Slow-growing and superficial tumors have been reported as most likely to result in a convulsion (Heideman et al., 1993). Seizures are frequently grand mal in nature, although complex partial seizures (less dramatic episodes with incomplete loss of consciousness) and partial seizures (transient focal events without loss of consciousness) also have been noted (Heideman et al., 1993). In fact, children who have had supratentorial lesions may continue to experience seizures and require anti-epileptic treatment for many years (Tait et al., 1992).

Peritumoral edema has been documented to be present in many pediatric brain tumors, particularly supratentorial, and can be reduced by corticosteroids. Although able to be reduced prior to craniotomy, intracranial pressure is particularly elevated by tumor mass effect in cases of supratentorial hemispheric tumors (Albright, 1990). Other signs that may occur as a direct effect of a supratentorial tumor include upper motor neuron signs such as hemiparesis, hyperreflexia, and clonus (Heideman et al., 1993; van Eys, 1991). Associated sensory losses also may occur (Heideman et al., 1993; van Eys, 1991). Endocrine changes may develop from hypothalamic or pituitary involvement (Albright, 1990; van Eys, 1991).

Language Disorders Associated with Supratentorial Tumors. To date few reported studies have specifically investigated the language abilities of children treated for supratentorial tumors. Van Lieshout, Renier, Eling, de Bot, and Slis (1990) documented the case of a child who presented with language and memory disturbances as a result of radiotherapy treatment for a thalamic tumor. In particular, the case described by these researchers evidenced a significant impairment of auditory short-term memory, auditory word comprehension, nonword repetition, and syntactic abilities, with mild disturbances of word fluency and naming. However, the most prominent feature was considered to be an auditory-verbal short-term memory deficit, with all verbal deficits appearing related to or impacted by this area. More recently, Docking, Murdoch, and Ward (2003a) examined the general language abilities of six children managed for supratentorial tumor using a comprehensive standardized general language assessment battery, including receptive and expressive components, receptive vocabulary and naming. At a group level, the children treated for supratentorial tumor performed below a matched control group in both general expressive language skills and the total overall language score. Deficits at an individual case level were evident in two cases, with disturbances to expressive language and syntax observed in the general language performance of a child who had undergone surgical treatment for a left parietal astrocytoma and reduced semantic abilities in a child who had been treated for an optic nerve glioma. The remaining four cases with

largely similar profiles in treatment and various tumor locations that included similar sites to those with language deficits, demonstrated intact general language abilities. Docking et al. (2003a) considered a series of factors as influencing the performance of the six cases, such as the long-term presence of the tumor prior to diagnosis, the young age at diagnosis and treatment, and the varied duration posttreatment of the language assessment.

In a follow-up study, Docking et al. (2003b) examined the higher language and phonological awareness abilities of five of the children reported in their previous study. Assessments included measures of receptive and expressive semantic abilities, inferencing, figurative language, and problem solving, as well as comprehensive preliteracy test. As a group, reductions were evident in problem solving, and in the ability to receive and decode content of high-level language when compared to a group of age and gender matched peers. At an individual level, only two of the five children managed for supratentorial tumor demonstrated language deficits. These two cases were noted to be the same children previously identified as having general language deficits. More widespread findings were noted in phonological awareness, with four of the five children treated for supratentorial tumor demonstrating weakness in one or more areas.

Overall, the presence of general and high-level language deficits together with impairments in phonological awareness skills highlights the importance of monitoring these skills in children treated for supratentorial tumor. As in the case of posterior fossa tumors outlined above speech-language pathologists should take an active role in the long-term management of children treated for supratentorial tumors, even if intervention is not initially warranted or has been discontinued.

Acute Lymphoblastic Leukemia

Leukemia is a progressive, malignant disease of the blood-forming organs, marked by distorted proliferation and development of leucocytes and their precursors in the blood and bone marrow. Acute lymphoblastic leukemia (ALL), is the most common cancer presentation in childhood (Butler & Haser, 2006; Pieters & Carroll, 2008). ALL is characterized by an overproduction of immature white blood cells called lymphoblasts. These cells crowd the bone marrow, preventing it from making normal blood cells. They also can spill out into the blood stream and circulate around the body. Due to their immaturity they are unable to function properly to prevent or fight infection. Inadequate numbers of red cells and platelets being produced by the bone marrow leads to anemia and bleeding and/or bruising. Although ALL is a disease of children and adults, it predominantly affects children with an initial peak incidence of the disease occurring between 3 and 5 years of age. The incidence of ALL decreases after 5 years of age, and drops sharply between the ages of 10 and 14 years (Madan-Swain & Brown, 1991). The incidence of ALL is higher in males than in females. One survey in the United States found that, for children under 15 years of age, the annual incidence of ALL among males was 22.3 per million, whereas for females it was 15.7 per million (Young & Miller, 1975).

In past decades, ALL together with most other forms of pediatric cancer was virtually always rapidly fatal (Southam et al., 1951; Tivey, 1952). In more recent years, however, improved therapeutic procedures have greatly improved the survival rate of children with ALL. Currently, the survival rate beyond 5 years for ALL is approximately 90% (Briére et al., 2008). Subsequently, with such advances in treatment, ALL is no longer viewed as an almost invariably fatal disease, but as a life-threatening illness, with long-term disease free survival frequently achieved, and cure as a realistic goal. Although ALL does not directly affect the brain, as outlined earlier in the current chapter, procedures such as radiotherapy and chemotherapy used in the treatment of this disease are known to have negative effects on brain structure and function, which have the potential to cause language and other cognitive impairments (Buttsworth, Murdoch, & Ozanne, 1993; Jackel et al., 1990; Murdoch, Boon, & Ozanne, 1994). Consequently, as a result of the improvements in treatment, a group of children have emerged who, having survived the brain insults sustained from the necessary radio- and chemotherapy, go on to develop undesirable neurological and neuropsychological sequelae, including language impairments (Buttsworth et al., 1993; Lewis, Murdoch, Barwood, Docking, & Gellatly, 2010; Lewis, Murdoch, & Docking, in press; Murdoch et al., 1994). These language impairments are discussed in detail below.

Medical Treatment of Acute Lymphoblastic Leukemia

The likelihood of children surviving ALL has increased in recent decades, due mainly to advances in treatment options including the implementation of CNS prophylaxis (Pieters & Carroll, 2008) for consolidation therapy (see below). Two decades ago, CNS-targeted cranial radiation therapy (CRT) was routinely administered to provide prophylactic CNS therapy in the treatment of ALL. Unfortunately, treatment protocols involving CNS CRT and/or chemotherapy have been implicated in deleterious neurocognitive outcomes for children (Langer et al., 2002; von der Weid, 2001; Waber et al., 2007). Recognition of these potential deleterious effects in recent years has led to a change in treatment protocols used for CNS prophylaxis. In particular, recent years have witnessed a trend to the use of intensive intrathecal chemotherapy with a phasing out of CNS CRT for the purpose of CNS prophylaxis in an attempt to improve both the short-term and long-term outcomes of the treatment for ALL. Consequently, speech-language pathologists when dealing with language disorders subsequent to the treatment for ALL will encounter two differing populations, one where the individual will have been treated with combined chemotherapy and/or CRT and the other with CNS-targeted chemotherapy alone. Details of the language impairments reported to be encountered in each of these populations are provided below. It is worth noting, however, that the different treatment protocols are also reflected in studies that have investigated the language abilities of children treated for ALL. Nineteen of the 22 children investigated by Buttsworth et al. (1993) and all 9 participants in Jackel et al.'s (1990) study, for example, were treated with CRT. In contrast, the two cases reported by Lewis et al. (2010) and the 13 cases examined by Lewis et al. (in press) receive CNS-targeted chemotherapy alone.

Treatment of leukemia is aimed at inducing, consolidating and maintaining remission and involves the use of multiple cytotoxic drugs in complex protocols.

Induction Therapy. According to Miller (1982), there are three aims to the induction of remission in acute lymphoblastic leukemia. These are: (1) to destroy as many leukemic cells as rapidly as possible, (2) to preserve normal hematopoietic cells, and (3) to restore hematopoiesis (production of red blood cells) as quickly as possible. Remission has been reported to occur in 85% of children with ALL when treated with two cytotoxic drugs (usually vincristine and prednisone) in combination (Poplack & Reaman, 1988). An even better remission rate of 95% has been reported when a third agent (e.g., L-asparaginase) is added to the treatment protocol (Miller, 1982). Treatment protocols containing four or more active agents, however, are used only in the treatment of cases with a poor prognosis because they are associated with a higher incidence of complications and toxicity during induction.

Consolidation Therapy. Children with ALL are at risk of developing CNS leukemia, involving leukemic infiltration of the meninges, brain, and cranial or spinal nerves. CNS prophylaxis is aimed at preventing the development of this condition in children with ALL (Littman et al., 1987). The blood-brain barrier, although protecting the CNS by monitoring the chemicals allowed to enter the CNS, does not offer adequate protection from infiltration of leukemic cells. Moreover, systemic chemotherapy has no effect on leukemic cells present in the CNS since the therapeutic agents cannot cross the blood-brain barrier to gain access to the invading leukemic cells. Consequently, the CNS acts as a sanctuary site for leukemic cells that are then able to proliferate and eventually to metastasize to the bone marrow and other peripheral sites and thereby cause a systemic relapse. Without prophylaxis to prevent overt leukemic infiltration of the CNS, many children who survive ALL develop CNS leukemia, which is difficult to eradicate, causes considerable discomfort and is associated with a risk of further neurologic complications (Chessells, 1985a; Ochs et al., 1985).

The incidence of CNS leukemia in children with ALL has been found to be considerably reduced by adequate pre-symptomatic prophylaxis with cranial irradiation in conjunction with intrathecal methotrexate (Hustu & Aur, 1978; Kim, Nesbit, D'Angio, & Levitt, 1972). In fact the risk of developing CNS leukemia can be reduced from as high as 50 to 60% in children receiving minimal or no prophylactic CNS treatment (Green et al., 1980; Littman et al., 1987; Ludwig, Calvo, Kober, & Brandeis, 1987; Moe, 1984) to 3-10% by administering prophylactic cranial irradiation and intrathecal methotrexate during early phases of therapy when no signs of CNS leukemia are present (Chessells, 1985b; Ch'ien et al., 1981; Kaleita & Al-Mateen, 1985; Littman et al., 1987; Moe, 1984; Pinkel, 1979).

Although the need for CNS prophylaxis is unquestionable, evidence is accumulating that suggests that this therapy, especially when it involves the combined use of CRT and chemotherapy, may be associated with adverse long-term sequelae (Langer et al., 2002; Moss, Nannis, & Poplack, 1981; Waber et al., 2007). The increase in the number of survivors of ALL has led to the recognition of some important late sequelae of the disease and its treatment. With improvement in survival, especially for children with the most favorable outlook, there has been a shift to the use of

intensive intrathecal methotrexate to provide CNS-targeted chemotherapy (Butler & Haser, 2006) which is now administered in up to 80% of ALL cases (Ziegler, Dalla Pozza, Waters, & Marshall, 2005). This change in treatment protocol also reflects a shift in emphasis, with almost as much concern now shown for the late effects of treatment as for the improvement of present therapy itself. The potential for language difficulties to emerge following CNS-targeted chemotherapy, however, exists, due to the neurotoxicity of intrathecal methotrexate (Moleski, 2000). Irreversible changes to the white matter tracts of the brain (Carey et al., 2008; Khong et al., 2003) following CNS-directed methotrexate have been identified and include necrotizing leukoencephalopathy, subacute myeloencephalopathy, mineralizing aniopathy, and demyelinization of cerebral white matter (Moleski, 2000). Growth and expansion of white matter begins in infancy, but it is not complete until early adulthood (Anderson, 2007). In order to protect white matter tracts from neurotoxic damage in children, leucovorin (folinic acid) is given as a rescue agent after high-dose methotrexate in current treatment regimens (Prabu & Bakhshi, 2009).

Maintenance Therapy. Maintenance chemotherapy is also an essential part of the treatment of children with ALL. Without some form of maintenance therapy remission in most patients lasts only 1 to 2 months. As in the case of remission induction, most maintenance therapy programs employ a multiple-drug regimen. The choice of drugs varies according to different risk groups. As an example, a multiple-agent regimen may involve reinforcement chemotherapy with periodic (i.e., monthly or quarterly) chemotherapy pulses. The two most frequently administered drugs in reinforcement therapy are methotrexate (administered weekly or twice weekly) and 6-mercaptopurine (daily). In addition, remission appears to be prolonged by intermittent pulses of vincristine and prednisone, with or without L-asparaginase. It must be noted, however, that pulsed chemotherapy may not be required for all patients. As in remission induction it has been found that although multiple-drug regimens are superior to single drug treatments for the purpose of maintenance therapy, adding too many chemotherapeutic agents to the protocol merely serves to increase the toxicity and morbidity associated with the treatment without having any significant effect on remission duration or survival in most patients except perhaps for those with a very poor prognosis.

Adverse Effects of Treatment for Acute Lymphoblastic Leukemia. Negative sequelae of treatment for ALL include structural changes in the brain, neurological dysfunction, and neuropsychological impairments.

Structural Changes in the Brain. Studies using CT scans have identified a number of structural brain abnormalities in leukemic patients who have received CNS prophylaxis. These abnormalities include: focal areas of white matter hypodensity, ventricular dilation, and cerebral calcifications (Ochs et al., 1980, 1986; Peylan-Ramu, Poplack, Pizzo, Adornato, & Di Chiro, 1978; Pizzo, Poplack, & Bleyer, 1979). Microangiopathies (calcification of cerebral blood vessels) have also been identified in patients treated with cranial radiation and intrathecal and intravenous methotrexate (Chi'en et al, 1981; Price & Birdwell, 1978). The findings of several postmortem investigations have also suggested that chemotherapy for the treatment of leu-

kemia might be responsible for inducing structural changes in the brain. Smith (1975) performed autopsies on 20 patients with acute lymphoblastic leukemia, acute myeloid leukemia, hairy cell leukemia, or non-Hodgkin's lymphoma. Ten had received intrathecal methotrexate whereas 10 patients were not given intrathecal therapy. Patients were between 6 months and 67 years of age at the time of diagnosis. Damage to the brain in patients given intrathecal methotrexate included the destruction of oligodendroglial cells, white matter swelling, moderate to severe astrocytosis, petechial hemorrhages, edema, and coagulative necrosis. The damage was confined to the white matter of both the cerebrum and cerebellum.

Although nine of the 10 patients given intrathecal methotrexate also received up to 2400 rads of radiotherapy, Smith (1975) attributed the damage to the course of chemotherapy. She claimed that damage occurring to the brain following radiotherapy usually appears many years after the conclusion of treatment. However, Smith (1975) failed to indicate the delay between the conclusion of chemotherapy and the detection of CNS damage in the 20 patients studied. In addition, it was claimed that the lesion types observed following the irradiation of intracranial tumors differed from those experienced by patients treated with chemotherapy for leukemia. Smith (1975) described irradiation-related damage as being more severe and involving the cerebrovascular system. Although Smith recognized that the relatively low doses of irradiation used to treat patients with leukemia might exacerbate the damage, it was concluded that methotrexate itself directly affects the oligodendrocytes.

Another case of intracranial damage following a course of intrathecal methotrexate was reported by Skul-lerud and Halvorsen (1978). A 2-year-old boy with acute leukemia was given methotrexate intrathecally (6.5 mg per week for 3 weeks followed by monthly injections of 6.5 mg). Radiotherapy was not administered in this case. Twenty-four hours after completing the fifth intrathecal methotrexate treatment, the child developed progressive flaccid pare-sis. Mental deterioration was observed and he died 18 days after the onset of the symptoms. Autopsy revealed areas of incomplete necrosis with astrocytosis on the base of the brain and along the insula, around the foramina of Luschka, and over the superior and inferior colli-culi. Similar lesions were also found over the surface of the cerebellum, par-ticularly over the vermis. In contrast to the findings to Smith (1975), there were no lesions in the central white matter of the brain or spinal cord, or along the ependyma of the ventricles. It was con-cluded that methotrexate alone caused the lesions observed because metho-trexate was the only drug the patient received intrathecally, and as tests showed no evidence of leukemia within the CNS, the cancer could not have caused the damage. Skullerud and Hal-vorsen (1978) also noted that the most extensive tissue destruction occurred in areas which are in direct contact with the cerebrospinal fluid and therefore with the methotrexate.

Neurologic Changes. Progressive dementia was observed by Pizzo, Bleyer, Poplack, and Leventhal, (1976) in a 6-year-old girl undergoing a course of intrathecal methotrexate without radio-therapy for relapse of meningeal leuke-mia. The patient was disoriented to time and place, demonstrated a gait distur-bance and experienced a significant deterioration of reading and arithmeti-cal abilities. Intrathecal methotrexate was discontinued and during the next 6 months the symptoms disappeared completely. The authors surmised that in this case the lack of radiotherapy eliminated the possibility that alteration of the blood-brain barrier enhanced the toxicity of intrathecal methotrexate.

Meadows and Evans (1976) also attributed the neurologic symptoms observed in patients treated for leuke-mia to methotrexate administered to the CNS. Four of the 23 children assessed by them demonstrated severe impair-ments including spastic quadriplegia or paraplegia and limited responsiveness. It must be noted, however, that three of the four severely impaired children also received up to 3400 rads of irradiation. Five of the children assessed by Mead-ows and Evans (1976) demonstrated mild neurologic dysfunction. Two had abnormal psychological test results and three required special education. Of the five patients showing minimal neuro-logic deficits, three were given radio-therapy. However, it was claimed that in two cases the administration of radi-ation followed the signs of minimal cerebral dysfunction. Five of the 23 chil-dren examined by these workers had electroencephalogram abnormalities but were clinically asymptomatic. Nine pa-tients had no signs of neurologic abnor-malities. These nine patients did not receive cranial irradiation, suggesting that methothrexate should not be cited as the sole cause of CNS damage in this study.

Meadows and Evans (1976) observed that the only clinical feature common to the 14 patients with some degree of neurologic impairment was the adminis-tration of methotrexate in high doses (5 to 10 mg per kg per month) over prolonged periods (2 to 7 years). Although it was postulated that radiation may cause changes in the blood-brain barrier allowing methotrexate to diffuse more easily into the white matter, the authors concluded that methotrexate alone does have a direct effect on the nervous system as not all of their patients had received radiotherapy. However, in order to isolate the elements which may contribute to any long-term deficits, it was recommended that patients receive detailed neurologic and psychological examinations before, and at regular intervals after, CNS prophylaxis.

Despite the claims that methotrexate has negative effects on the structure and function of the nervous system, two studies involving relatively large patient groups have failed to detect any long-term damage to the CNS. Ochs et al. (1980) examined 43 children with acute lymphoblastic leukemia. Ten patients were given intrathecal methotrexate while 33 received intrathecal methotrexate in combination with intravenous methotrexate. All patients received weekly oral methotrexate. Patients were assessed using CT between 10 and 59 months (median = 29) after the completion of treatment. It was concluded that none of the 43 patients had evidence of intracerebral calcification or areas of decreased attenuation coefficient (i.e., hypodense areas) on CT scans. Although mild ventricular dilation and visualization of the cortical sulci was detected in four patients, such features were also observed in control subjects.

Neuropsychological Sequelae. In addition to causing structural and neurological abnormalities, a number of recent reports in the literature have indicated that CNS prophylaxis also may have detrimental effects on various neuropsychological functions. Several researchers have reported the presence of intellectual impairment in children treated for acute lymphoblastic leukemia with cranial irradiation and chemotherapy (Duffner, Cohen, Thomas, & Lansky, 1985; Eiser, 1978; Meadows et al., 1981; Said, Waters, Cousens, & Stevens, 1987; Taylor, Also, Phebus, Sachs, & Bierl, 1987). A subtle but significant lowering of intelligence quotients (IQs) was noted in long-term survivors of acute lymphoblastic leukemia by Duffner et al. (1983) and Taylor et al. (1987). It has been suggested that CNS prophylaxis, in the form of cranial irradiation or the combination of radiotherapy and intrathecal methotrexate, is a primary factor in the development of the reported mild neuropsychological deficits (Eiser, 1978; Tamaroff et al., 1982; Tebbi, 1982).

The possibility that a combination of methotrexate and cranial irradiation (2400 rads) could be responsible for intelligence deficits was also noted by Twaddle, Britton, Craft, Nobel, and Kernahan (1983). These investigators estimated pretreatment IQs of leukemic patients and solid tumor patients from corrected measures of sibling IQ. A significant difference between the estimates and posttreatment IQs was found in the acute lymphoblastic leukemia group, but not in the solid tumor group. Twaddle et al. (1983) noted that higher functions of intelligence were particularly affected in the leukemic group, such as verbal associate reasoning and reasoning with abstract material.

In addition to intellectual impairment, other neuropsychological deficits following CNS prophylaxis for acute lymphoblastic leukemia have also been reported in the literature. Memory deficits are frequently noted (e.g., Chessells,

1985a; Copeland et al., 1985; Eiser, 1978; Mulhern et al., 1987). Difficulty in concentration and attention problems also exist (Chessells, 1985a; Said et al., 1987). Reading deficits have been found both in children with acute lymphoblastic leukemia in complete continuous remission (Eiser, 1978) and in leukemic children who have suffered a relapse (Mulhern et al., 1987). In addition, Mulhern et al. (1987) reported spelling and mathematical difficulty in children with acute lymphoblastic leukemia who had suffered a relapse.

Despite the evidence that a combination of chemotherapy and radiotherapy in the form of CNS prophylaxis may have long-term effects on various neuropsychological abilities, the effect of chemotherapy alone on these functions is less certain. Tamaroff et al. (1982) failed to detect neuropsychological deficits following the administration of intrathecal methotrexate. Forty-one children with acute lymphoblastic leukemia were assessed within 1 year of completing a 36-month course of intrathecal methotrexate. Methotrexate was administered at regular intervals in a dose of 6.25 mg per m^2 and was the sole agent of CNS prophylaxis. A control group of 33 children with embryonal rhabdomyosarcoma who had no central nervous disease or treatment also were studied. There was no significant difference in IQ between the two groups for children less than 8 years of age. When children older than 8 years of age were considered, the children with acute lymphoblastic leukemia achieved IQ scores significantly greater than the children suffering from embryonal rhabdomyosarcoma. In addition, 12 of the 21 younger children were reassessed at an average of 57.4 months after the initial examination. No long-term intellectual changes were detected. The authors concluded that intrathecal

methotrexate alone does not have either short-term or long-term effects on general intellectual functioning. Tamaroff et al. (1982) suggested that the 2400 rads of cranial radiation given to patients in other studies may be responsible for any reported deficits or perhaps radiation and methotrexate in combination produce the neurologic deficits.

To examine the effects of contemporary treatment protocols, neurocognitive studies have focused on outcomes following CNS-targeted chemotherapy-only treatments for ALL (see e.g., Buizer, de Sonneville, van den Heuvel-Eibrink, Njiokiktjien & Veerman, 2005; Buizer, de Sonneville, van den Heuvel-Eibrink, & Veerman, 2006; Kingma et al., 2001; Montour-Proulx et al., 2005; Moore et al., 2008; von der Weid et al., 2003). The findings to date have been inconclusive. Substantial negative outcomes in the skill areas of intelligence and memory were identified by Montour-Proulx et al. (2005). In contrast, Buizer et al. (2006) described only subtle behavioral and educational difficulties in children following chemotherapy treatment, whereas Kingma et al.'s (2001) findings suggested children treated with chemotherapy attained normal academic achievements and only slight cognitive impairments. von der Weid and colleagues (2003) contend that although the phasing out of CNS-targeted CRT has led to a reduction in neurocognitive decline associated with treatment, the implementation of CNS-targeted chemotherapy has not averted all negative-related effects.

Language Disorders in Acute Lymphoblastic Leukemia

To date, the most extensive investigations of the language abilities of children treated for ALL are those carried out by

Buttsworth et al. (1993) and Murdoch et al. (1994). Specifically, Buttsworth et al. (1993) compared the performance of a group of 22 children treated for leukemia on a battery of language tests with that of a group of age- and sex-matched nonneurologically impaired control subjects. Murdoch et al. (1994) documented the individual variability in language outcomes demonstrated by children treated for ALL through a detailed case-by-case examination of 23 such children.

Language Disorders in Acute Lymphoblastic Leukemia: Evidence from Group Studies. As a follow-up to the preliminary study reported by Jackel et al. (1990), Buttsworth et al. (1993) examined the language abilities of a larger group (*n* = 22) of children treated for ALL. The subjects included ranged in age from 5;0 to 17;9, with a mean age of 11;2 (SD = 43.1 months). Those experimental subjects included had been treated for ALL at least two months previously. A group of 22 nonneurologically impaired children matched for age and sex served as control subjects. None of the experimental or control subjects had a history of birth trauma, head injury, intellectual impairment, neurologic disorder, or hearing impairment. Children with genetic diseases were excluded from the study as were experimental subjects with a history of speech and/or language disorders prior to diagnosis of ALL. English was the primary language of all subjects included.

A series of language assessments were used to assess a range of linguistic abilities. The principal language test administered was an age-appropriate measure from the Test of Language Development (TOLD) series (Hammill, Brown, Larsen, & Wiederholt, 1987; Hammill & Newcomer, 1982; Newcomer & Hammill, 1982). This series was chosen as

all of the tests contain subtests which assess receptive and expressive linguistic abilities in the areas of syntax and semantics. The TOLD-P (primary) was administered to children between the ages of 4;0 and 8;11. The TOLD-I (intermediate) was administered to children between the ages of 9;0 and 11;11. The second edition of the Test of Adolescent Language (TOAL-2) was used for subjects between the ages of 12;0 and 18;5. The TOLD-I may be used for children as young as 8;6. However, the TOLD-P was chosen for assessment of Case 7 (aged 8;6) because it offers a variety of both auditory and visual stimulus cues, whereas the TOLD-I is purely auditory-based test. Similarly, although the TOLD-I may be used for children up to the age of 12;11, the TOAL-2 was chosen for the assessment of 12-year-olds, because of its greater ability to detect subtle linguistic deficits. The TOAL-2 is composed of subtests assessing grammar and vocabulary skills across reading, writing, listening, and speaking modalities. Tables are provided in the TOLD series manuals to convert raw scores for the subtests into standard scores (mean = 10 ± 3). Quotients (mean = 100 ± 15) are composite scores derived from subtest standard scores to specific areas of language impairment, for example, grammar versus vocabulary deficits, or listening versus speaking impairment. All three tests provide an overall language quotient (Spoken Language Quotient in TOLD-P and TOLD-I; Adolescent Language Quotient in TOAL-2), as well as quotients for listening and speaking. In addition to these quotients, both the TOLD-P and TOLD-I have semantic and syntactic quotients, whereas the TOAL-2 has reading, writing, vocabulary, and grammar quotients.

In conjunction with one of the TOLD series tests, the children all were assessed with three other tests. The Token Test (De Renzi & Faglioni, 1978) was administered to children aged 12 years and older, whereas children younger than 12 years of age were assessed with the Token Test for Children (DiSimoni, 1978). These tests were selected to detect high-level comprehension deficits. The Boston Naming Test (BNT) (Kaplan, Goodglass, & Weintraub, 1983), and the timed subtests (i.e., Subtest 7: Word Series, Subtest 8: Confrontation Naming, and Subtest 9: Word Association) of the Clinical Evaluation of Language Function (CELF) (Semel & Wiig, 1982) were also administered. These assessments of semantic ability were included because semantic skills, particularly word-retrieval abilities, have been known to be affected by diffuse brain lesions in groups such as children with closed-head injury (Jordan et al., 1988) and children after irradiation (Hudson et al., 1989).

With regard to the CELF subtests, there were varying numbers of children used in the comparison groups for each parameter. The Confrontation Naming Subtest yields two scores: the number of items correct, and the minus time (the time taken to complete the task, subtracted from 120 seconds). However, only children in Grade 3 and above are expected to obtain a minus time score. Therefore, mean minus time scores for the Confrontation Naming Subtest of the CELF are calculated for 18 subjects and their controls, Cases 1 to 4 inclusive having been omitted. Mean number correct scores were obtainable for 21 subjects, as Case 1 did not have adequate color knowledge to complete the task.

The findings of the study carried out by Buttsworth et al. (1993) based on performance on the TOLD series of language tests confirmed the preliminary results reported by Jackel et al. (1990)

that children treated for leukemia have impaired language abilities compared to control subjects. In the group of nine children whose ages were greater than 12 years (assessed with the TOAL-2), Buttsworth et al. (1993) observed particularly large discrepancies between the means recorded for the leukemic and control group for Expressive Language, Grammar and Writing Quotients, the children treated for leukemia scoring significantly lower quotients than the control subjects. These authors also observed moderate differences between the mean scores achieved by all 22 leukemic subjects compared to controls for the Overall Language Quotient and Speaking Quotient, and all other measures of the TOAL-2. Although the differences between the mean scores on the remaining subtests of the TOLD-P and TOLD-I were not as large, Buttsworth et al. (1993) reported that the scores obtained by the leukemic children on all subtests of all TOLD series assessments were significantly lower than those obtained by their control subjects.

Buttsworth et al. (1993) reported that the ability of the older children treated for leukemia included in their study to follow spoken commands (as measured by the Token Test) was also significantly lower than their controls, a result which concurs with the findings of Taylor et al. (1987). A similar result, however, was not found for the younger children treated for ALL who were assessed on the Token Test for Children.

Naming ability was assessed by Buttsworth et al. (1993) using the BNT. They found that the ALL group had a significantly lower mean BNT score than their control subjects. Taylor et al. (1987) who used the Expressive One-Word Picture Vocabulary Test (like the BNT a picture-naming test), however, failed to find a significant difference in the ability to name between ALL subjects and their healthy siblings. Unlike Jackel et al. (1990) and Taylor et al. (1987) no problem was observed by Buttsworth et al. (1993) to be present in their leukemic group with regard to confrontation naming and word fluency as measured by the timed subtests of the CELF. The disparity between the findings of Buttsworth et al. (1993) and the results of Taylor et al. (1987) may lie in the different assessment tools. Taylor et al. (1987) used the Stroop Color Test and Word Fluency Test from the Spreen-Benton Aphasia Test (Gaddes & Crockett, 1975) to assess confrontation naming and word fluency, respectively. Alternatively, the use of different control groups (age- and sex-matched by Buttsworth et al. [1993]; sibling control subjects in the study by Taylor et al. [1987]) may be reflected in the difference in naming skills.

The disparity between the results obtained by Buttsworth et al. (1993) for the BNT compared with the subtests of the CELF could be due to the nature of the naming tasks involved. The BNT is a confrontation naming task that draws on the subject's existing vocabulary, and on their ability to search for, find, and generate the target word if it is present in their vocabulary. The Confrontation Naming Subtest of the CELF, although it is also a convergent task, does not explore vocabulary since there are only seven target words (red, blue, black, yellow, circle, square, triangle), but required rapid recognition of the stimulus, selection of, and production of the appropriate label for the stimulus item. The Word Association Subtest of the CELF, unlike the previous two naming tasks is a divergent task and needs different semantic-lexical abilities for its successful completion (e.g., generation of many items within a semantic category, determining the category boundaries, rejecting items outside the category).

Expression and Reading Comprehension was found by Taylor et al. (1987) to be deficient in ALL subjects compared with their siblings; similarly, Waber et al. (1990) found Reading and Spelling (assessed by the Wide Range Achievement Test) in both male and female ALL subjects to be lower than normative test data expectations. This agrees with the low scores on Reading, Writing, and Written Language Quotients reported by Buttsworth et al. (1993).

Although the findings of the study carried out by Buttsworth et al. (1993) are suggestive of a link between the treatment process and the occurrence of language disorders in children treated for ALL, it is not possible to attribute the language impairment to a single cause such as the radiotherapy and\or the chemotherapy used in the treatment of this condition. As pointed out earlier in this chapter, radiotherapy has been identified as a possible cause of linguistic deficits in children treated for brain tumors (Hudson et al. 1989). Radiation dosage following surgery for brain tumors, however, is much greater (5000–6000 rads) (Curnes et al., 1986; Marks et al., 1981) than the doses used for childhood ALL (1800 or 2400 rads). The findings of Buttsworth et al. (1993), however, do suggest that even low levels of radiation may contribute to language deficits in some children.

Other than CNS prophylaxis involving cranial irradiation, with or without intrathecal therapy, the other risk factor most often implicated in neuropsychological problems in children treated for ALL is the patient's age at the time of CNS prophylaxias (Ochs & Mulhern, 1988). Buttsworth et al. (1993), however, were unable to demonstrate a correlation between age at diagnosis or radiation dosage and language quotients achieved on the TOLD series by their cohort of children treated for ALL. They cautioned, however, that their sample size was small and that the treatment protocols used on their 22 leukemic subjects were heterogeneous. The children assessed in their study ranged from patients treated in the 1970s to those whose treatment finished in the early 1990s, leading to differences in the treatment protocols used. In addition, as pointed out by Bleyer (1990), by the early 1990s advances in the diagnosis and treatment of ALL had made it possible to tailor therapy to the individual needs of subgroups of patients, rather than using the same treatment on every patient with ALL. A number of other researchers have considered the effect of age at diagnosis and dosage of cranial irradiation on neuropsychological abilities. Several investigators have reported that younger children (below 5 years of age) treated for ALL have more severe neuropsychological aftereffects than older children (Jannoun, 1983; Moore, Kramer, & Albin, 1986; Said et al., 1987). Moore et al. (1986) attributed this to enhanced vulnerability of the brain to biological insults during the period of rapid development (Dobbing, 1968). Others, however, did not find this effect (Jackel et al., 1990; Whitt, Wells, Lauria, Wilhelm, & McMillan, 1984). Tamaroff et al. (1982) found no difference in the cognitive effects of cranial irradiation with doses of 2400 and 1800 rads. According to Said et al. (1987), neuropsychological outcome is better following the reduced dose of 1800 rads of cranial irradiation, if distinct treatment protocols are compared and large numbers of cases are considered. The effects of age at treatment, sex of the subject, and dosage of cranial irradiation on language outcome in leukemic children, as well as the relationship between their cognitive and language abilities, requires ongoing investigation utilizing a large pool of subjects treated with similar protocols.

In addition to language difficulties, some of the children treated for ALL examined by Buttsworth et al. (1993) also had academic difficulties. Of the 12 younger children in their group who were attending primary school, two were experiencing difficulty and had repeated grades. Five of the nine older children had academic problems, especially in mathematics and English. Difficulties reportedly became more noticeable in high school. Academic performance has received consideration in the ALL literature. The Wide Range Achievement Test (WRAT) (Jastak & Jastak, 1978), which considers reading, spelling, and arithmetic, frequently has been used to measure academic performance of ALL subjects and controls. Significantly poorer WRAT outcomes have been reported for leukemic patients than their siblings (Taylor et al., 1987) and solid tumor control subjects (Copeland et al., 1985; Moore et al., 1986; Waber et al., 1990). Studies that have compared the WRAT results of leukemic subjects who had received cranial irradiation with those of subjects who had received prophylaxis consisting of drug therapy only, have not identified significant differences between these two treatment groups (Whitt et al., 1984; Copeland et al., 1985; Ochs, Parvey, & Mulhern, 1986).

In summary, the findings of group studies reported to date indicate that language deficits may occur in children subsequent to treatment for ALL. Clinicians need to be aware of the possibility of language impairment as part of the late effects of treatment, so that such children can receive early remediation in areas of deficit, and thus maintain the highest quality of life possible. Routine language assessment of each individual may not be possible (or even necessary) in a busy clinic, but early detection and intervention should be a realistic goal.

Language Disorders in Acute Lymphoblastic Leukemia: Evidence from Case Studies. Although the findings of Buttsworth et al. (1993) indicated that, as a group, children treated for leukemia have significant language deficits compared to control subjects, when examined individually it is apparent that the language abilities of the children treated for ALL included in their study varied considerably from individual to individual. Some of the leukemic subjects demonstrated normal (or in one case above average) language abilities whereas others had significant language problems. In addition, the performance of the leukemic subjects on specific language tasks varied widely. Although some of the children treated for ALL demonstrated one or two particularly weak (or strong) areas of language ability that functioned to depress (or elevate) their overall language score, other subjects showed a relatively consistent performance across all language areas. Consequently, it was felt by Buttsworth et al. (1993) that by presenting their data on a group basis only, that important information concerning the variety of language outcome following treatment for ALL may have been lost. As a follow-up to their earlier study, therefore, Murdoch et al. (1994) examined the language abilities of the same children treated for ALL (with the addition of one further child) on an individual

basis to enable any observed language problem to be described and discussed with reference to individual variables relating to personal details, medical history, treatment factors, etc.

Language Disorders in Acute Lymphoblastic Leukemia: Evidence from Children Treated with CNS-Targeted Chemotherapy Alone. To date, only two studies have investigated the language abilities of children treated with CNS-targeted chemotherapy alone. In the largest study, Lewis et al. (in press) investigated the general and high-level language abilities of 13 children treated with a CNS-targeted chemotherapeutic regimen for ALL. The results identified the presence of impaired expressive language skills and reduced proficiency with figurative language in the children treated for ALL compared to a matched control group suggesting that impaired language skills may follow contemporary treatments for ALL. Lewis et al. (in press) concluded that their findings should alert clinicians to the potential for language difficulties following the sole use of CNS-targeted chemotherapy in the treatment of ALL and the need for long-term monitoring of such children. Declining receptive and high-level language skills over a 2-year period were reported in a pilot study of 2 children treated with CNS-targeted chemotherapy for ALL by Lewis et al. (2010).

Language Disorders in Acute Lymphoblastic Leukemia: Clinical Implications. Based on the findings of group studies and case studies reported in the literature to date, it is apparent that although not mandatory, language disorders may occur in children subsequent to treatment for leukemia. A large variation in the language abilities of children who have undergone such treatment has been observed, ranging from above normal to severely impaired language function. Although routine assessment of this population by speech-language pathologists does not appear warranted, health professionals, parents, caregivers, and teachers of leukemic children need to be aware of the possibility of children treated for ALL developing language disorders, particularly as part of the long-term effects of treatment. Certainly, there is a need for hospital-based speech-language pathologists to take an educative role with medical and other professionals working in oncology units to alert them to the possible negative linguistic outcomes in children treated for ALL. Furthermore, considering the negative effect of linguistic impairment on later learning and academic achievement, speech-language pathologists working in community and educational settings need to actively educate parents, caregivers, and teachers of children treated for leukemia as to the possible long-term effects of that treatment with a view to encouraging such persons to refer these children for early consultation with relevant professionals.

Case Examples

The cases described below have been selected to represent the range of language outcomes reported for children treated for posterior fossa tumors and ALL. In each case the language battery administered comprised the age-appropriate tests selected from the Test of Language Development (TOLD) series, the Token Test for Children (DiSimoni, 1978), Subtests 7, 8, and 9 of the Clinical Evalua-

tion of Language Functions (CELF) (Semel & Wiig, 1982), the Boston Naming Test (BNT) (Kaplan et al., 1983), and the Test of Language Competence (TLC) (Wiig & Secord, 1985). According to each subject's age, the test administered from the TOLD series was either:

■ Test of Language Development-Primary (TOLD-P) (Newcomer & Hammill, 1982) (age range 4;0 to 8;11);
■ Test of Language Development-Intermediate (TOLD-I) (Hammill & Newcomer, 1982) (age range 8;6 to 12;11);
■ Test of Adolescent Language 2 (TOAL-2) (Hammill et al., 1987) (age range 12;0 to 18;5);

Posterior Fossa Tumor: Examples

Case 1: Cerebellar Astrocytoma

At the age of 5;1, Jacinta underwent investigations for a 1-month history of vomiting, headaches, and transient incidences of slurred speech. A CT scan revealed the presence of a 5-cm mass in the right cerebellar hemisphere extending across the midline and involving the vermis (Figure 4–5). The fourth ventricle was displaced to the left and anteriorly and high-grade obstructive hydrocephalus was observed. Jacinta underwent the total excision of a large cerebellar astrocytoma and subsequently experienced a rapid, uneventful recovery. No further treatments, including radiotherapy, were required.

Language assessments were performed 1 year, 2 months postsurgery. At this time Jacinta was aged 6;3 and was

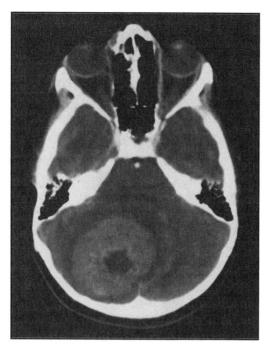

FIGURE 4–5. Case 1: Cerebellar astrocytoma. Preoperative CT scan showing a 5-cm mass in the right cerebellar hemisphere extending across the midline.

succeeding in Grade 1 as well as at extra-curricular activities such as piano and ballet classes.

TOLD-P. Jacinta obtained above average quotients on all of the language areas assessed by the TOLD-P.

Token Test for Children. An Overall Age Scaled Score of 506 was achieved on the Token Test for Children. This is slightly above the test's average range of 495 to 505.

CELF. Jacinta performed above criterion on Subtests 7, 8, and 9 of the CELF.

BNT. Jacinta achieved a score of 47 out of a possible 60 items on the BNT. This

is above the range of 20–34 (mean = 29) obtained by the Grade 1 children assessed by Kaplan et al. (1983).

Summary of Language Abilities. Jacinta achieved above average language scores on the tests administered.

Case 2: Juvenile Pilocytic Astrocytoma

Pamela was admitted to hospital at the age of 3;2 for the investigation of a 3-week history of papilledema and an unsteady, wide-based gait. A CT scan indicated the presence of a partly cystic, soft tissue mass just to the left of the midline in the posterior fossa. The tumor measured 4.5 cm in diameter and was displacing the fourth ventricle laterally to the right. Resultant obstructive hydrocephalus was observed with dilation of the third and lateral ventricles. A right VP shunt was inserted to relieve the hydrocephalus and 4 days later a posterior fossa craniotomy was performed. A juvenile pilocytic astrocytoma was subtotally removed. Pamela was discharged from hospital 2 weeks after tumor resection and continued to make a steady, uneventful recovery. No further treatments, including radiotherapy, were required.

Pamela's language abilities were assessed at four years two months post-surgery when she was aged 7;4. At this time, she was a Grade 2 student in a multiage Grade 1 and 2 combined class and was receiving eight hours individual tutoring each week. She had just been accepted into a small remedial class. Pamela presented as an enthusiastic, talkative child who enjoyed the assessment tasks presented to her over three testing sessions.

TOLD-P. Pamela scored an Overall Language Quotient of 74, which was below the average score of 85 to 115 provided by the TOLD-P. Closer examination of Pamela's TOLD-P results indicated that her expressive language skills were in advance of her receptive language abilities. Her Listening Quotient of 64 was greater than 2 SD below the test's mean of 100. This score resulted from poor performances on the Picture Vocabulary and Grammatic Understanding subtests of the TOLD-P. Pamela demonstrated difficulty comprehending the verb tenses and negative structures included in the Grammatic Understanding Subtest. Only Pamela's Speaking Quotient (i.e., expressive semantics and syntax) fell within the test's normal range. The Semantics and Syntax Quotients obtained by Pamela were below average due to her below average receptive subtest scores and borderline expressive results. It was noted during testing that Pamela did not have difficulty remembering the test instructions or sentences, and could often repeat them or correct her response two test items later. This finding suggested the presence of a slowed language processing ability.

Token Test for Children. Pamela experienced no difficulty completing Parts I to IV of the Token Test for Children, however, her performance deteriorated during Part V when concepts and dependent clauses were introduced. Pamela frequently used repetition of the instruction as a strategy, but still manipulated the tokens incorrectly.

As observed during administration of the TOLD-P, Pamela was able to remember the instructions, irrespective of their length, but failed to process complex structures and concepts.

CELF. Pamela performed within normal limits on Subtests 7, 8, and 9 of the CELF.

BNT. Pamela achieved a low score of 16 on the BNT, a score markedly below the normal range of 34 to 45 specified by the test norms.

Summary of Language Abilities. Pamela exhibited a generalized language impairment with particular difficulties being evident on receptive language tasks. Expressive skills were shown to be at a borderline level. It is noteworthy that language impairments were evident despite an absence of CNS prophylaxis in Pamela's medical history.

Case 3: Medulloblastoma

Following a 1-month history of unsteady gait and intermittent headaches, vomiting, and blurring of vision, Marcus collapsed and hit his head. A CT scan identified a calcified tumor of the fourth ventricle and associated hydrocephalus (Figure 4–6). Marcus underwent surgery for the insertion of a right external ventricular drain and subtotal removal of a medulloblastoma. The tumor was found to fill the fourth ventricle, obstruct the aqueduct and was adherent to the right wall of the fourth ventricle. Marcus made a rapid recovery and was discharged from hospital 7 days postsurgery. A CT scan performed at the conclusion of craniospinal irradiation showed no evidence of residual ventricular tumor. Eight months posttreatment, a CT scan revealed mild cerebral atrophy due to whole brain irradiation but no signs of recurrent or residual tumor.

Language assessment was carried out at 1 year, 11 months postsurgery, at which time Marcus, aged 14;11, was

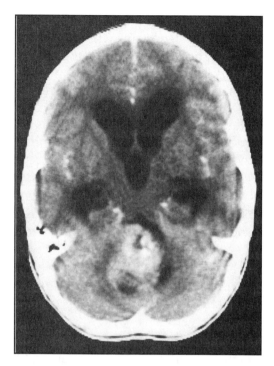

FIGURE 4–6. Case 3: Medulloblastoma. Preoperative CT scan showing a calcified medulloblastoma of the fourth ventricle and associated hydrocephalus.

experiencing moderate academic difficulties in a normal Grade 9 class.

TOAL-2. All but one of the language quotients obtained by Marcus fell greater than 2 SD below the test mean. His expressive semantic and syntactic skills were marginally above the other language measures as reflected by the Speaking Quotient. Examination of the specific TOAL-2 subtests indicated that most difficulty was experienced comprehending spoken and written syntactic structures, as well as writing grammatically correct sentences.

Token Test for Children. Although Marcus was aged 14;11 at the time of testing, the Token Test for Children was admin-

istered to supplement the information provided by the TOAL-2. His auditory comprehension abilities were shown to be below average relative to the data provided for children aged 12;6. Marcus made errors in token selection and in the concepts presented in Part V.

CELF. All three timed subtests of the CELF were scored above criteria.

BNT. Marcus performed within normal limits, correctly naming 41 of the 60 items on the BNT.

TLC. Overall, Marcus performed poorly on tasks involving high-level language competencies. A standard score within the normal range was obtained for Subtest 3 (Recreating Sentences), which corresponds to his best performance on the TOAL-2-Subtest IV (Speaking/ Grammar).

Summary of Language Abilities. The global reduction in language functioning, as indicated by the TOAL-2, the Token Test for Children and the TLC, could have been anticipated in the presence of the generalized cerebral atrophy revealed by CT. Receptive language skills were slightly more impaired than expressive abilities.

Case 4: Ependymoma

Ben presented for neurologic examination at the age of 13;3 following a 2-month history of headaches, slurred speech, and mild ataxia. A CT scan showed an infiltrating, low density, mass lesion in the cerebellum (Figure 4–7). Marked hydrocephalus was also present. A VP shunt was inserted to alleviate the hydrocephalus, and 1 week later

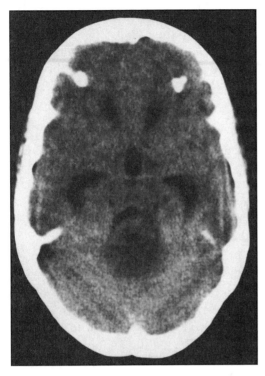

FIGURE 4–7. Case 4: Ependymoma. Preoperative CT scan showing a posterior fossa ependymoma in the midline and slightly to the left of the midline.

an ependymoma was partially removed. Immediately following surgery, truncal ataxia was observed but speech was described as clear. Recovery was rapid and Ben was discharged 6 days after tumor excision. A course of craniospinal irradiation followed, involving a total radiation dose of 5000 rads. A CT scan performed at the conclusion of treatment indicated the presence of residual ependymoma in the superior vermian cistern and mild ventromegaly. No further treatment was provided.

At the time of his language assessment two years four months postsurgery, Ben was in Grade 10. Parental and school reports indicated that although Ben had been a very high achiever premorbidly, he was now failing all subjects.

TOAL-2. Most of the language quotients obtained by Ben were within the test's normal range. Listening/Grammar was the only subtest for which a below average standard score was obtained and as a result, a below average auditory comprehension (Listening) Quotient was recorded as well as low-average Receptive Language (auditory and reading comprehension) and Grammar Quotients.

CELF. All three tests of rapid language retrieval and production were scored above criteria.

BNT. Ben correctly named 56 of the 60 BNT items.

TLC. Ben demonstrated an average level of language competency as determined by TLC.

Summary of Language Abilities. Ben made a rapid recovery following partial resection of an ependymoma. Overall, he exhibited intact language skills.

Case 5: Juvenile Cerebellar Astrocytoma

Peter experienced a 6-month history of vomiting, headaches, and coughing, followed by the development of ataxia, prior to the diagnosis of a cerebellar juvenile astrocytoma at age 12;1. Following surgery to insert a right VP shunt, Peter was drowsy and exhibited a left facial paresis and left upper limb paresis. No improvement occurred before the posterior fossa craniotomy was performed 13 days later. An astrocytoma, 5 cm in diameter, was completely resected from the midline and left side of the cerebellum. Peter was mute postsurgery and exhibited a poor recovery. Three days after tumor removal, he became cyanosed due to a collapsed left lung and had to be re-intubated for 2 days. One week after this incident, Peter was still drowsy and exhibited a left hemiparesis but was able to move all limbs on request. A CT scan revealed a right-sided extradural hemorrhage that was immediately evacuated with resultant improved consciousness. One month after tumor removal, a follow-up CT scan revealed the presence of a densely calcified membrane associated with a right-sided epidural collection. The collection did not appear to have as much mass effect as the previous extradural hemorrhage. The collection and calcified membrane were removed at a fourth operation. Peter exhibited a more rapid recovery than was previously experienced. His hemiparesis resolved, however, he remained ataxic. At this time, he was able to obey simple commands and identify some body parts. Two shunt revisions were required during the 4 years following tumor removal. Three years after the initial surgery, recurrent astrocytoma was detected adjacent to the left cerebellar peduncle. This was subtotally resected, after which a rapid, uneventful recovery was made. Neither radiotherapy nor chemotherapy was included in Peter's treatment regimen.

At the time of language assessment, four years nine months after tumor diagnosis, Peter exhibited a small residual tumor in the posterior fossa, which was being regularly monitored. He was ataxic and used a wheelchair most of the time. His coordination and hearing were deteriorating as the need for further surgery approached. Peter had withdrawn from school at the age of 15. According to his parents, Peter had been an excellent scholar prior to tumor diagnosis.

TOAL-2. Due to poor vision and a marked fine motor deficit, Peter was unable to complete the five subtests of the TOAL-2 which involved reading, writing, and picture stimuli. Subtests II (Listening/Grammar), III (Speaking/Vocabulary), and IV (Speaking/Grammar) were completed, resulting in a Speaking Quotient of 82. No other language quotients could be calculated. Peter's comprehension of syntax (Subtest III) was shown to be in advance of his expressive syntactic abilities (Subtest IV).

CELF. Although Subtest 7 was scored above criterion, Subtests 8 and 9 were scored below criterion on the CELF. The presence of a severe dysarthria inhibited the rapid production of language during these tasks.

BNT. Impaired vision prevented Peter's completion of the BNT.

TLC. Fatigue and an inability to see the written and picture stimuli included in the TLC prevented the administration of this test.

Summary of Language Abilities. Peter presented with severe communication and physical disabilities. The TOAL-2 indicated the presence of an expressive language deficit, which may have been exacerbated by Peter's attempts to overcome poor intelligibility. Factors that may have contributed to Peter's poor functional status include the additional surgical procedures experienced, the episode of cyanosis, the mass effect of the extradural hemorrhage and the epidural collection, the recurrent tumor, and the prolonged premorbid symptoms that most likely were signs of hydrocephalus.

It is noteworthy that Peter exhibited severe language problems despite the presence of several factors in his history that would normally imply a good prognosis. These factors include, his relatively older age at diagnosis, tumor type, and lack of chemotherapy and radiotherapy in his treatment regimen.

Acute Lymphoblastic Leukemia: Examples

Case 1: Joanne

Joanne was diagnosed with acute lymphoblastic leukemia at the age of 2;4. Intrathecal methotrexate (together with other, non-intrathecal drugs) was administered as induction therapy. CNS prophylaxis consisted of intrathecal methotrexate, vincristine, and 6-mercaptopurine. No radiotherapy was administered. Methotrexate was administered both intrathecally and systemically (together with other cytotoxic drugs) for maintenance therapy. Treatment ceased after 26 months, when the subject was aged 4;6. At the time of language assessment, 6 months after completion of treatment, Joanne presented as a lively, outgoing 5-year-old girl who was attending and enjoying preschool.

Joanne achieved below average scores on the TOLD-P in the subtests of receptive semantics (Picture Vocabulary), and syntactic comprehension (Grammatic Understanding). Scores for the other subtests of the TOLD-P were within the average expected for her age, although the scores for expressive syntax (Sentence Imitation) and auditory discrimination (Word Discrimination) were at the lower end of the normal range. Joanne obtained a below average Overall Language Quotient, and below average quotients for Listening and Semantics. The other language quotients were in the average range. Her Overall Score of 489 on the Token Test for Children was more than 2 SD below the age mean of 500 and reinforced the indication of poor syntactic comprehension. The fact that Joanne had difficulty distinguishing between the labels "yellow" and "green," however, no doubt contributed to the low score. The errors she made, though, were not solely a result of this lack of color knowledge, as they also included shape errors (i.e., circle versus square) and prepositions as well.

Of the three CELF subtests selected it was not possible to administer Confrontation Naming, since this subtest requires the child to be capable of generating the color and shape of 36 items, and Joanne could not consistently name colors. She knew five of the days of the week required in the Producing Word Series, and thus performed above criterion in comparison to normative data provided in the test manual. The score achieved in Producing Word Associations was also above criterion.

Joanne performed poorly on the BNT correctly naming only 15 out of the 60 items. This score was considerably lower than the mean of 29.6 achieved by the group of five-year-old children tested by Kaplan et al. (1983). Overall, the language tests indicated that Joanne had a mild language impairment, with particular difficulties being experienced in the areas of expressive and receptive semantics and syntactic comprehension. As Joanne had only recently commenced preschool, there was an insufficient history on which to judge the presence of any academic difficulties. Consequently, it is difficult to gauge whether the depressed language scores represent a language delay that eventually may "catch up" to normal development, or an impairment that will remain as Joanne matures. As the treatment for ALL began at an age when Joanne would be expected to be acquiring language, it may be that the intensive chemotherapy has slightly delayed the acquisition of normal language skills, rather than actively impairing her existent language abilities.

Case 2: Greta

Greta was a girl aged 5;11. Diagnosis of ALL was made at the age of 1;9 and treatment commenced immediately. Intrathecal methotrexate was administered as part of the induction of remission. CNS prophylaxis consisted of a total dose of 1800 rads of radiation, as well as intrathecal methotrexate, vincristine, cyclophosphamide, and ara-C. Maintenance treatment ran for 20 months, and included systematic (but also intrathecal) administration of methotrexate. Greta was aged 3;8 when maintenance therapy ceased. At the time of language assessment 27 months later, Greta presented as a cooperative, although timid girl, who was enjoying Grade 1 at school.

All subtests and quotients of the TOLD-P were within the normal range. Greta's Overall Score on the Token Test for Children was normal for her age with all subtests, except one, being within 1 SD of the mean. The exception was Part 4, where Greta seemed to experience a lapse of concentration, which she regained for the fifth subtest after encouragement from the examiner.

The Producing Word Series and Confrontation Naming Subtests of the CELF were above criterion. The Producing Word Associations Subtest fell below criterion. As all items generated were good examples of the given category, the limited number of category members

generated could have been the result of shyness, rather than word retrieval problems or vocabulary restrictions.

Greta scored 23 (out of a possible 60) on the BNT. According to the "norms" provided in the test manual, the age-expected score is 29.6. Twenty-nine of the 60 items were simply unknown to Greta, which is not unexpected in a 5-year-old child. Of the items that Greta attempted to name, the errors were mainly semantic (e.g., boat, sailboat for "canoe") or perceptual (e.g., pencil for "dart"). Naturally, in a 5-year-old, these errors are more indicative of intelligent guessing than of a word-finding problem, as they would be in an adult.

At a time more than two years after cessation of treatment for ALL, Greta's language was found to be developing normally. Academic performance was difficult to gauge, as she had only been attending her first year of school for 3 months.

Greta was less than two years old at the time of diagnosis (and therefore CNS prophylaxis). Children under five years of age are thought to be most vulnerable to the effects of CNS prophylaxis (Eiser & Lansdown, 1977). As cognitive deficits associated with prophylactic CNS chemotherapy may not manifest until several years after diagnosis (e.g., Brown et al., 1992; Pfefferbaum-Levine et al., 1984; Rubenstein, Varni, & Katz, 1990), it would be necessary to monitor Greta on a long-term basis in order to be satisfied that CNS prophylaxis has left no legacy of language impairment.

Case 3: Nicola

Nicola was diagnosed with ALL at the age of 2;11. Following induction, she received a radiation dosage of 1800 rads (given in 12 fractions) and intrathecal methotrexate as part of CNS prophylaxis. There was a slight problem establishing an appropriate dosage in the maintenance stage of treatment owing to drug toxicity. Nicola received approximately 75% of the recommended dosage. Treatment was completed at the age of 4;8, 21 months after ALL was diagnosed. Nicola's language was assessed when she was aged 6;4, 20 months after completion of treatment. She presented as an outgoing child with a cheerful interest in the world, who was enjoying Grade 1 at school.

Nicola obtained scores within the normal range on all subtests and quotients of the TOLD-P. Both the Overall and the individual subtest scores of the Token Test for Children were at or above the age-expected mean; indeed, Nicola obtained a score of 507 for Part 4, which was greater than 1 SD above the mean for normal subjects. The three CELF subtests were above criterion. The score of 30 achieved on the BNT was in accord with the published mean of 29 expected for her age. In addition, it compared favorably with the score of 31 achieved by an age- and sex-matched control. In summary, Nicola's language ability was found to be competent and well within the normal limits for her age.

Case 4: Mark

Mark was admitted to hospital with a diagnosis of ALL at the age of 3;8. CNS prophylaxis included a radiation of 1800 rads. Treatment was completed 24 months later when he was aged 5;8. At the time of language assessment, Mark was aged 7;1, and had been in complete continuous remission for 17 months. He was in Grade 2 at the local primary school, and appeared to be coping satisfactorily. His mother was of the opinion

that he was lacking in concentration; this problem had not been reported by his teacher. In addition, his mother felt that Mark was "not as bright" as he had been prior to the treatment for ALL. Mark presented as a friendly boy who cooperated cheerfully for all tasks.

Mark obtained below average scores on the TOLD-P in the subtests of receptive semantics (Picture Vocabulary) and phonology (Word Articulation). Receptive syntax (Grammatic Understanding) was at the lower end of the average range, whilst the other subtests were in the average range, some at the higher end of the average range, which resulted in a wide variety of quotients. Mark obtained average Overall, Speaking, Semantic and Syntax Quotients, and a below average Listening Quotient.

Despite the below average listening skills demonstrated in the TOLD-P, Mark's scores on the Token Test for Children were all within the normal range for both age and grade. All three subtests of the CELF were above criterion. Mark achieved a score of 36 on the BNT, which was close to the published "mean" of 37 expected for children in Grade 2.

With one exception, Mark's language skills were average for his age. The exception was the below average Listening Quotient he obtained on the TOLD-P. This quotient was determined at by combining the results of the receptive semantics and receptive syntax subtests, both of which were low. Since his ability to follow multi-step spoken instructions was average, an explanation was sought to reconcile the apparent disparity between different listening tasks and scores. Both TOLD-P tasks were picture-pointing tasks, where the examiner names a stimulus word (for semantics) or sentence (for syntax), and the subject selects one out of a choice of four (or for syntax, three) pictures. Thus, the child must process the visual information (from the pictures) in order to correctly select the match for the auditory information supplied by the examiner. It may be that Mark was too anxious to point to a picture, and was not allowing sufficient time to process both the visual and auditory information in order to make the correct response for these tasks.

Case 5: Luke

Luke was diagnosed with ALL at the age of 4;7. The CNS prophylactic stage of therapy included a radiation dosage of 1800 rads. Maintenance therapy was completed 24 months after ALL was diagnosed, when Luke was aged 6;7.

The language test battery was administered when Luke was aged 7;8, 13 months after treatment for ALL had been discontinued. He was in complete continuous remission, and was attending a local church school where he was repeating Grade 1. He was on a waiting list to be seen by a speech-language pathologist, and his mother was anxious for him to receive some form of specialist assistance. Luke presented as a quiet child, who cooperated for all tasks. His ability to concentrate on the tasks seemed limited, but could be regained by an encouragement to keep attending.

Luke achieved below average scores on the TOLD-P in the subtests of expressive syntax (Sentence Imitation and Grammatic Completion), auditory discrimination (Word Discrimination), and phonology (Word Articulation). The other three subtests were within the normal range, although receptive syntax (Grammatic Understanding) was at the

lower end of the normal range. Consequently, Luke obtained a below average Overall Language Quotient and below average quotients for Speaking and Syntax. Other language quotients were within normal limits.

Luke performed poorly on the Token Test for Children, with only one subtest (Part 1) falling within the normal range expected for his age. The other four subtests and the Overall Score were 2 or more SDs below the age-expected mean. Parts 3 and 5 were 2 SDs below the mean, Part 4 was 3 SDs below the mean, the Overall Score was 4 SDs below the mean, and Part 2 was greater than 4 SDs below the mean. These low scores would appear to reflect the findings of poor auditory memory reported in the neuropsychological tests. It was interesting to note that Luke did not utilize any strategies, such as verbal repetition of examiner's instruction, to assist him in carrying out the instruction.

Luke achieved a score of 36 on the BNT, which was comparable with the published age-expected mean of 27. The BNT score, taken in conjunction with the two vocabulary subtests of the TOLD-P (where Luke's scores were average) would suggest that his vocabulary and naming ability are normal for his age. However, the Confrontation Naming Subtest of the CELF was below criterion indicating that speed of naming may be slower than average. The other two subtests of the CELF were above criterion.

Luke's language skills were below the normal expectation for his age, with the exception of semantic ability, which was average. The disparity between his average Listening Quotient on the TOLD-P (made up of the Picture Vocabulary and Grammatic Understanding Subtests) and his low scores on the Token

Test for Children may lie in the differences in the tasks involved. The two TOLD-P subtests involve picture-pointing, with a one in three or one in four chance of the correct answer, whereas the Token Test for Children requires a correct action to be made in response to instructions of increasing length and complexity.

Luke's pattern of language deficits seems to be similar to the pattern of language deficits reported by Taylor et al. (1987), who compared leukemic subjects with their healthy siblings, and found that the leukemic subjects performed less well than their siblings on tasks requiring speed and accuracy (such as word fluency and contingency naming) and on tasks requiring the ability to follow multiple element directions (Token Test for Children). Although Luke's word fluency (Producing Word Associations Subtest of the CELF) was above criterion, the other findings agree with his language deficits.

References

Alajouanine, T., & Lhermitte, F. (1965). Acquired aphasia in children. *Brain, 88,* 653–662.

Albright, A. L. (1990). Surgery in the management of childhood brain tumours. In M. Deutsch (Ed.), *Management of childhood brain tumors* (pp. 175–186). Boston, MA: Kluwer Academic.

Allen, J. C. (1991, 1992). Complications of chemotherapy in patients with brain and spinal cord tumors. *Pediatric Neurosurgery, 17,* 218–224.

Altman, A. J., & Schwartz, A. D. (1983). The late effects of cancer treatment. In A. J. Altman, & A. D. Schwartz (Eds.), *Malignant diseases of infancy, childhood and adolescence* (2nd ed., pp. 560–576). Philadelphia, PA: W. B. Saunders.

Anclair, M., Hovén, E., Lannering, B., & Boman, K. K. (2009). Parental fears following their child's brain tumor diagnosis and treatment. *Journal of Pediatric Oncology Nursing, 26,* 68–74.

Anderson, V. (2007). Childhood white matter injuries: What are the issues? *Developmental Neuropsychology, 32,* 619–623.

Arya, S., Gilbert, E. F., & Wiedrich, T. A. (1986). Complications of treatment of neoplasia in childhood, including second malignancies. In M. Finegold (Ed.), *Pathology of neoplasia in children and adolescents* (Vol. 18, pp. 433–464). Philadelphia, PA: W. B. Saunders.

Askins, M. A., & Moore B. D. (2008). Preventing neurocognitive late effects in childhood cancer survivors. *Journal of Child Neurology, 23,* 1160–1171.

Ater, J. L. (1989). Brain tumors. In R. A. Gottlieb & D. Pinkel (Eds.), *Handbook of pediatric oncology.* Boston, MA: Little, Brown.

Bamford, F. N., Morris Jones, P., Pearson, D., Ribeiro, G. G., Shalet, S. M., & Beardwell, C. G. (1976). Residual disabilities in children treated for intracranial space-occupying lesions. *Cancer, 37,* 1149–1151.

Barrett, A., & Donaldson, S. S. (1992). Radiation therapy. In P. A. Voute, A. Barrett, & J. Lemerle (Eds.), *Cancer in children: Clinical management* (3rd revised ed., pp. 42–50). Berlin, Germany: Springer-Verlag.

Becker, L. E., & Hinton, D. (1986). Primitive neuroepithelial tumors of the central nervous system. In M. Finegold (Ed.), *Pathology of neoplasia in children and adolescents* (Vol. 18, pp. 397–418). Philadelphia, PA: W. B. Saunders.

Becker, L. E., & Jay, V. (1990). Tumors of the central nervous system in children. In M. Deutsch (Ed.), *Management of childhood brain tumors* (pp. 5–51). Boston, MA: Kluwer Academic.

Becker, L. E., & Yates, A. J. (1986). Astrocytic tumors in children. In M. Finegold (Ed.), *Pathology of neoplasia in children and adolescents* (Vol. 18, pp. 373–396). Philadelphia, PA: W. B. Saunders.

Bhatia, S., & Meadows, A. T. (2006). Long-term follow-up of childhood cancer survivors: Future directions for clinical care and research. *Pediatric Blood and Cancer, 46,* 143–148.

Bleyer, W. A. (1990). Acute lymphoblastic leukemia in children: Advances and prospectus. *Cancer, 65,* 689–695.

Boring, C. C., Squires, T. S., & Tong,T. (1991). Cancer statistics 1991. *CA: Cancer Journal for Clinicians, 41,* 19–36.

Brière, M. E., Scott, J. G., McNall-Knapp, R. Y., & Adams, R.L. (2008). Cognitive outcome in pediatric brain tumor survivors: Delayed attention deficit at long-term follow-up. *Pediatric Blood and Cancer, 50,* 337–340.

Brown, R. T., Madan-Swain, A., Pais, R., Lambert, R. G., Baldwin, K., Casey, R., . . . Kamphaus, R. W. (1992). Cognitive status of children treated with central nervous system prophylactic chemotherapy for acute lymphocytic leukemia. *Archives of Clinical Neuropsychology, 7,* 481–497.

Buizer, A. I., de Sonneville, L. M. J., van den Heuvel-Eibrink, M. M., Njiokiktjien, C., & Veerman, A. J. P. (2005). Visuomotor control in survivors of childhood acute lymphoblastic leukemia treated with chemotherapy only. *Journal of the International Neuropsychological Society, 11,* 554–565.

Buizer, A. I., de Sonneville, L. M. J., van den Heuvel-Eibrink, M. M., & Veerman, A. J. P. (2006). Behavioral and educational limitations following chemotherapy for childhood acute lymphoblastic leukemia or a Wilms' tumor. *Cancer, 106,* 2067–2075.

Butler, R. W., & Haser, J. K. (2006). Neurocognitive effects of treatment for childhood cancer. *Mental Retardation and Developmental Disabilities Research Reviews, 12,* 184–191.

Buttsworth, D. L., Murdoch, B. E., & Ozanne, A. E. (1993). Acute lymphoblastic leukaemia: Language deficits in children posttreatment. *Disability and Rehabilitation, 15,* 67–75.

Carey, M. E., Haut, M. W., Reminger, S. L., Hutter, J. J., Theilmann, R., & Kaemingk, K. L. (2008). Reduced frontal white matter volume in long-term childhood leukemia survivors: A voxel-based morphometry study. *American Journal of Neuroradiology, 29,* 792–797.

Carrow-Woolfolk, E., & Lynch, J. I. (1982). *An integrated approach to language disorders in children.* Orlando, FL: Grune & Stratton.

Chessells, J. M. (1985a). Cranial irradiation in childhood lymphoblastic leukaemia: Time for reappraisal? *British Medical Journal, 291,* 686–687.

Chessells, J. M. (1985b). Risks and benefits of intensive treatment of acute leukaemia. *Archives of Disease in Childhood, 60,* 193–195.

Ch'ien, L. T., Rhomes, J. A., Verzosa, M. S., Coburn, T. P. Goff, J. R., Hustu, H. O., . . . Simone, J. (1981). Progression of methotrexate-induced leukoencephalopathy in children with leukaemia. *Medical and Pediatric Oncology, 9,* 133–141.

Cohen, M. E., & Duffner, P. K. (1984). *Brain tumors in children: Principles of diagnosis and treatment.* New York, NY: Raven Press.

Cohen, M. E., Duffner, P. K., & Tebbi, C. K. (1982). Brain tumors in children: Diagnosis and management. In C. K. Tebbi (Ed.), *Major topics in pediatric and adolescent oncology* (pp. 240–289). Boston, MA: G. K. Hall Medical Publishers.

Cooper, J. A., & Flowers, C. R. (1987). Children with a history of acquired aphasia: Residual language and academic impairments. *Journal of Speech and Hearing Disorders, 52,* 251–262.

Copeland, D. R., Fletcher, J. M., Pfefferbaum-Levine, B., Jaffe, N., Reid, H., & Maor, M. (1985). Neuropsychological sequelae of childhood cancer in long-term survivors. *Pediatrics, 75,* 745–753.

Cousens, P., Ungerer, J. A., Crawford, J. A., & Stevens, M. M. (1990). The nature and possible causes of deficit after childhood leukemia. Brain impairment: Advances in applied research. *Proceedings of the Fifteenth Annual Conference of the Australian Society for the Study of Brain Impairment,* pp. 173–181.

Curnes, J. T., Laster, D. W., Ball, M. R., Moody, D. M., & Witcofski, R. L. (1986). MRI of radiation injury to the brain. *American Journal of Roentgenology, 147,* 119–124.

Davis, C. H., & Joglekar, V. M. (1981). Cerebellar astrocytomas in children and young adults. *Journal of Neurology, Neurosurgery and Psychiatry, 44,* 820–828.

Davis, P. C., Hoffman, J. C. Jr., Pearl, G. S., & Braun, I. F. (1986). CT evaluation of effects of cranial radiation therapy in children. *American Journal of Roentgenology, 147,* 587–592.

Delong, G. R., & Adams, R. D. (1975). Clinical aspects of tumours of the posterior fossa in childhood. In P. J. Vinken & G. W. Bruyn (Eds.), *Handbook of clinical neurology: Tumours of the brain and skull* (Vol. 18, Part III, pp. 387–411). Amsterdam, the Netherlands: North-Holland.

Dennis, M., Spiegler, B. J., Hetherington, C. R., & Greenberg, M. L. (1996). Neuropsychological sequelae of the treatment of children with medulloblastoma. *Journal of Neuro-Oncology, 29,* 91–101.

De Renzi, E., & Faglioni, P. (1978). Normative data and screening power of a shortened version of the token test. *Cortex, 14,* 41–49.

Deutsch, M. (1990a). Late sequelae in survivors of childhood brain tumors. In M. Deutsch (Ed.), *Management of childhood brain tumors* (pp. 481–492). Boston, MA: Kluwer Academic.

Deutsch, M. (1990b). Radiotherapy. In M. Deutsch (Ed.), *Management of childhood brain tumors* (pp. 187–232). Boston, MA: Kluwer Academic.

Dhall, G. (2009). Medulloblastoma. *Journal of Child Neurology, 24,* 1418–1430.

Di Chiro, G., Oldfield, E., Wright, D. C., De Michele, D., Katz, D. A., Patronas, N. J., . . . Kufta, C. (1988). Cerebral necrosis after radiotherapy and/or intraarterial chemotherapy for brain tumors: PET and neuropathologic studies. *American Journal of Roentgenology, 150,* 189–197.

DiSimoni, F. (1978). *The Token Test for Children.* Hingham, MA: Teaching Resources.

Dobbing, J. (1968). Vulnerable periods in the developing brain. In A. N. Davison & J. Dobbing (Eds.), *Applied neurochemistry* (pp. 287–316). Oxford, UK: Blackwell Scientific.

Docking, K., Murdoch, B. E., & Suppiah, R. (2007). The impact of a cerebellar tumour on language function in childhood. *Folia Phoniatrica et Logopaedica, 59,* 190–200.

Docking, K., Murdoch, B. E., & Ward, E. C. (2003a). General language abilities following management of childhood supratentorial tumour: Part 1. *Acta Neuropsychologica, 1,* 260–283.

Docking, K., Murdoch, B. E., & Ward, E. C. (2003b). High-level and phonological awareness abilities of children following management for supratentorial tumour: Part II. *Acta Neuropsychologica, 1,* 367–381.

Docking, K., Ward, E. C., & Murdoch, B. E. (2005). Language outcomes subsequent to treatment of brainstem tumour in childhood. *NeuroRehabilitation, 20,* 107–124.

Duffner, P. K., Cohen, M. E., & Thomas, P. (1983). Late effects of treatment on the intelligence of children with posterior fossa tumors. *Cancer, 51,* 233–237.

Duffner, P. K., Cohen, M. E., Thomas, P. R. M., & Lansky, S. B. (1985). The long-term effects of cranial irradiation on the central nervous system. *Cancer, 56,* 1841–1846.

Eiser, C. (1978). Intellectual abilities among survivors of childhood leukaemia as a function of CNS irradiation. *Archives of Disease in Childhood, 53,* 391–395.

Eiser, C., & Lansdown, R. (1977). Retrospective study of intellectual development in children treated for acute lymphoblastic leukaemia. *Archives of Disease in Childhood, 52,* 525–529.

Gaddes, W. H., & Crockett, D. J. (1975). The Spreen-Benton Aphasia Tests: Normative data as a measure of normal language development. *Brain and Language, 2,* 257–280.

Geissinger, J. D., & Bucy, P. C. (1971). Astrocytomas of the cerebellum in children: Long term study. *Archives of Neurology, 24,* 125–135.

Gol, A. (1963). Cerebellar astrocytomas in children. *American Journal of Diseases of Children, 106,* 21–24.

Green, D. M., Freeman, A. I., Sather, H. N., Sallan, S. E., Nesbit, M. E., Cassady, J. R., . . . Frei, E. III. (1980). Comparison of three methods of central nervous system prophylaxis in childhood acute lymphoblastic leukaemia. *Lancet, 315,* 1398–1402.

Gumbinas, M. (1983). Tumors of the central and peripheral nervous system. In A. J. Altman, & A. D. Schwartz (Eds.), *Malignant diseases of infancy, childhood and adolescence* (2nd ed., pp. 347–367). Philadelphia, PA: W. B. Saunders.

Hammill, D. D., Brown, V. L., Larsen, S. C., & Wiederholt, J. L. (1987). Test of adolescent language 2: A multidimensional approach to assessment. Austin, TX: Pro-Ed.

Hammill, D. D., & Newcomer, P. L. (1982). Test of language development-intermediate. Austin, TX: Pro-Ed.

Hécaen, H. (1976). Acquired aphasia in children and ontogenesis of hemispheric functional specialization. *Brain and Language, 3,* 114–134.

Heideman, R. L., Packer, R. J., Albright, L. A., Freeman, C. R., & Rorke, L. B. (1993). Tumors of the central nervous system. In P. A. Pizzo & D. G. Poplack (Eds.), *Principles and practice of pediatric oncology* (2nd ed., pp. 633–681). Philadephia, PA: J. B. Lippincott.

Hirsch, J. F., Rose, C. S., Pierre-Kahn, A., Pfister, A., & Hoppe-Hirsch, E. (1989). Benign astrocytic and oligodendrocytic tumors of the cerebral hemispheres in children. *Journal of Neurosurgery, 70,* 568–572.

Hodges, S., & Smithells, R. W. (1983). Intracranial calcification and childhood medulloblastoma. *Archives of Disease in Childhood, 58,* 663–664.

Hoppe-Hirsch, E. (1993). Intellectual and psychosocial complications of posterior fossa tumor surgery and supplemental (radiation therapy/chemotherapy) treatment. In A. J. Raimondi, M. Choux, & C. Di Rocco (Eds.), *Posterior fossa tumors* (pp. 194–200). New York, NY: Springer-Verlag.

Horowitz, M. E., Mulhern, R. K., Kun, L. E., Kovnar, E., Sanford, R. A., Simmons, J., . . . Jenkins, J. III. (1988). Brain tumors in the very young child: Postoperative chemotherapy in combined-modality treatment. *Cancer, 61,* 428–434.

Hudson, L. J., & Murdoch, B. E. (1992a). Chronic language deficits in children treated for posterior fossa tumour. *Aphasiology, 6,* 135–150.

Hudson, L. J., & Murdoch, B. E. (1992b). Language recovery following surgery and CNS prophylaxis for the treatment of childhood medulloblastoma: A prospective study of three cases. *Aphasiology, 6,* 17–28.

Hudson, L. J., & Murdoch, B. E. (1992c). Spontaneously generated narratives of children treated for posterior fossa tumour. *Aphasiology, 6,* 549–566.

Hudson, L. J., Murdoch, B. E., & Ozanne, A. E. (1989). Posterior fossa tumours in childhood: Associated speech and language disorders post-surgery. *Aphasiology, 3,* 1–18.

Hustu, H. O., & Aur, R. J. A. (1978). Extramedullary leukemia. *Clinical Hematology, 7,* 313–337.

Jackel, C. A., Murdoch, B. E., Ozanne, A. E., & Buttsworth, D. L. (1990). Language abilities of children treated for acute lymphoblastic leukaemia: Preliminary findings. *Aphasiology, 4,* 45–53.

Jannoun, L. (1983). Are cognitive and educational development affected by age at which prophylactic therapy is given in acute lymphoblastic leukaemia? *Archives of Disease in Childhood, 58,* 953–958.

Jastak, J. F., & Jastak, S. R. (1978). *The Wide Range Achievement Test: Manual of instructions* (rev. ed.). Wilmington, DE: Jastak Associates.

Jordan, F. M., Ozanne, A. E., & Murdoch, B. E. (1988). Long-term speech and language disorders subsequent to closed head injury in children. *Brain Injury, 2,* 179–185.

Kadota, R. P., Allen, J. B., Hartman, G. A., & Spruce, W. E. (1989). Brain tumors in children. *Journal of Pediatrics, 114,* 511–519.

Kaleita, T. A., & Al-Mateen, M. (1985). Subacute necrotizing leukoencephalopathy in after treatment for acute lymphocytic leukemia (Letter to the Editor). *New England Journal of Medicine, 312,* 317.

Kaplan, E., Goodglass, H., & Weintraub, S. (1983). *Boston Naming Test.* Philadelphia, PA: Lea & Febiger.

Khong, P-L., Kwong, D. L. W., Chan, G. C. F., Sham, J. S. T., Chen, F-L., & Ooi, G-C. (2003).

Diffusion-tensor imaging for the detection and quantification of treatment-induced white matter injury in children with medulloblastoma: A pilot study. *American Journal of Neuroradiology, 24,* 734–740.

Kim, R., Nesbit, M. E., D'Angio, G. D., & Levitt, S. H. (1972). The role of central nervous system irradiation in children with acute lymphoblastic leukemia. *Radiology, 104,* 635–641.

Kingma, A., van Dommelen, R. I., Mooyaart, E. L., Wilmink, J. T., Deelman, B. G., & Kamps, W. A. (2001). Slight cognitive impairment and magnetic resonance imaging abnormalities but normal school levels in children treated for acute lymphoblastic leukemia with chemotherapy only. *Journal of Pediatrics, 139,* 413–420.

Kun, L. E., & Moulder, J. E. (1993). General principles of radiation therapy. In P. A. Pizzo & D. G. Poplack (Eds.), *Principles and practice of pediatric oncology* (2nd ed., pp. 273–302). Philadelphia, PA: J. B. Lippincott.

Kun, L. E., Mulhern, R. K., & Crisco, J. J. (1983). Quality of life in children treated for brain tumours. *Journal of Neurosurgery, 58,* 1–6.

Langer, T., Martus, P., Ottenmeier, H., Hertzberg, H., Beck, J. D., & Meier, W. (2002). CNS late effects after ALL therapy in childhood. Part III: Neuropsychological performance in long-term survivors of childhood ALL: Impairments of concentration, attention, and memory. *Medical and Pediatric Oncology, 38,* 320–328.

Lee, K. F., & Suh, J. H. (1977). CT evidence of grey matter calcification secondary to radiation therapy. *Computerized Tomography, 1,* 103–110.

Levisohn, L., Cronin-Golomb, A., & Schmahmann, J. D. (2000). Neuropsychological consequences of cerebellar tumour resection in children: Cerebellar cognitive affective syndrome in a paediatric population. *Brain, 123,* 1041–1050.

Lewis, F. M., Murdoch, B. E., Barwood, C., Docking, K. M., & Gellatly, A. (2010). Language outcomes following treatment for acute lymphoblastic leukaemia with CNS chemotherapy: A two-year follow-up study. *Asia Pacific Journal of Speech, Language, and Hearing, 13,* 51–60.

Lewis, F. M., Murdoch, B. E., & Docking, K. M. (in press). An investigation of general and high level language skills in children treated with CNS-targeted chemotherapy for acute lymphoblastic leukemia. *Journal of Medical Speech-Language Pathology.*

Littman, P., Coccia, P., Bleyer, W. A., Lukens, J., Siegel, S., Miller, D., . . . Hammond, D. (1987). Central nervous system prophylaxis in children with low risk acute lymphoblastic leukaemia (ALL). *International Journal of Radiation Oncology, Biology, and Physics, 13,* 1443–1449.

Ludwig, R., Calvo, W., Kober, B., & Brandeis, W. E. (1987). Effects of local irradiation and I.V. methotrexate on brain morphology in rabbits: Early changes. *Journal of Cancer Research and Clinical Oncology, 113,* 235–240.

Mabbott, D. J., Penkman, L., Witol, A., & Strother, D. (2008). Core neurocognitive functions in children treated for posterior fossa tumors. *Neuropsychology, 22,* 159–168.

Madan-Swain, A., & Brown, R. T. (1991). Cognitive and psychological sequelae for children with acute lymphocytic leukemia and their families. *Clinical Psychology Review, 11,* 267–294.

Mariën, P., Engelborghs, S., Fabbro, F., & De Deyn P. P. (2001). The lateralized linguistic cerebellum: A review and a new hypothesis. *Brain and Language, 79,* 580–600.

Marks, J. E., Baglan, R. J., Prassad, S. C., & Blank, W. F. (1981). Cerebral radionecrosis: Incidence and risk in relation to dose, time, fractionation and volume. *International Journal of Radiation Oncology, Biology, and Physics, 7,* 243–252.

Matson, D. D. (1956). Cerebellar astrocytoma in childhood. *Pediatrics, 18,* 150–158.

McWhirter, W. R., & Masel, J. P. (1987). *Paediatric oncology: An illustrated introduction.* Sydney, Australia: Williams & Wilkins.

McWhirter, W. R., & Petroeschevsky, A. L. (1990). Childhood cancer incidence in

Queensland, 1979–1988. *International Journal of Cancer, 45,* 1002–1005.

Meadows, A. T., & Evans, A. E. (1976). Effects of chemotherapy on the central nervous system. *Cancer, 37,* 1079–1085.

Meadows, A. T., Massari, D. J., Ferguson, J., Gordon J., Littman, P., & Moss, K. (1981). Declines in IQ scores and cognitive dysfunctions in children with acute lymphocytic leukaemia treated with cranial irradiation. *Lancet, ii,* 1015–1018.

Menkes, J. H., & Till, K. (1995). Postnatal trauma and injuries by physical agents. In J. H. Menkes (Ed.), *Textbook of child neurology* (pp. 557–597). Baltimore, MD: Williams & Wilkins.

Miller, D. R. (1982). Acute lymphoblastic leukemia. In C. K. Tebbi (Ed.), *Major topics in pediatric and adolescent oncology* (pp. 2–43). Boston, MA: Hall Medical.

Miller, J. F., Campbell, T. F., Chapman, R. S., & Weismer, S. E. (1984). Language behaviour in acquired childhood aphasia. In A. Holland (Ed.), *Language disorders in children.* Baltimore, MD: College-Hill Press.

Moe, P. (1984). Recent advances in the management of acute lymphoblastic leukaemia. *European Paediatric Haematology and Oncology, 1,* 19–28.

Moleski, M. (2000). Neuropsychological, neuroanatomical and neurophysiological consequences of CNS chemotherapy for acute lymphoblastic leukemia. *Archives of Clinical Neuropsychology, 15,* 603–630.

Montour-Proulx, I., Kuehn, S. M., Keene, D. L., Barrowman, N. J., Hsu, E., Matzinger, M-A., . . . Halton, J. (2005). Cognitive changes in children treated for acute lymphoblastic leukemia with chemotherapy only according to the Pediatric Oncology Group 9605 Protocol. *Journal of Child Neurology, 20,* 129–133.

Moore, I. M., Kramer, J., & Ablin, A. (1986). Late effects of central nervous system prophylactic leukemia treatment on cognitive functioning. *Oncology Nursing Forum, 13,* 45–51.

Moore, I. M., Miketova, P., Hockenberry, M. Krull, K., Pasvogel, A., Carey, M. E., . . . Kaemingk, K (2008). Methotrexate-induced alterations in beta-oxidation correlate with cognitive abilities in children with acute lymphoblastic leukemia. *Biological Research for Nursing, 9,* 311–319.

Moss, H. A., Nannis, E. D., & Poplack, D. G. (1981). The effects of prophylactic treatment of the central nervous system on the intellectual functioning of children with acute lymphoblastic leukemia. *American Journal of Medicine, 71,* 47–52.

Mulhern, R. K., & Kun, L. E. (1985). Neuropsychologic function in children with brain tumours: III. Interval changes in the six months following treatment. *Medical and Pediatric Oncology, 13,* 318–324.

Mulhern, R. K., Ochs, J., Fairclough, D., Wasserman, A. L., Davis, K. S., & Williams, J. M. (1987). Intellectual and academic achievement status after CNS relapse: A retrospective analysis of 40 children treated for acute lymphoblastic leukemia. *Journal of Clinical Oncology, 15,* 933–940.

Murdoch, B. E. (2010). The cerebellum and language: Historical perspective and review. *Cortex, 46,* 858–868.

Murdoch, B. E., Boon, D. L., & Ozanne, A. E. (1994). Variability of language outcomes in children treated for acute lymphoblastic leukaemia: An examination of twenty-three cases. *Journal of Medical Speech-Language Pathology, 2,* 113–123.

Murdoch, B. E., & Hudson-Tennent, L. J. (1994). Differential language outcomes in children following treatment for posterior fossa tumours. *Aphasiology, 8,* 507–534.

Murdoch, B. E., & Hudson, L. J. (1999). Language disorders in children treated for brain tumours. In B. E. Murdoch (Ed.), *Communication disorders in childhood cancer* (pp. 55–75). London, UK: Whurr.

Naidich, T. P., & Zimmerman, R. A. (1984). Primary brain tumors in children. *Seminars in Roentgenology, 19,* 100–114.

Neidhardt, M. K., Bamberg, M., & Riehm, H. (1986). Medulloblastoma: Strategies for therapy. In H. Riehm (Ed.), *Malignant neoplasms in childhood and adolescence* (Vol. 18, pp. 296–315). Basel, Switzerland: Karger.

Newcomer, P. L., & Hammill, D. D. (1982). Test of language development-primary. Austin, TX: Pro-Ed.

Nomura, S., Nishizaki, T., Tamashita, K., & Ito, H. (1998). Pediatric brain tumors in a 10-year period from 1986 to 1995 in Yamaguchi prefecture: Epidemiology and comparison with adult brain tumors. *Pediatric Neurosurgery, 28,* 130–134.

Ochs, J. J., Berger, P., Brecher, M. L., Sinks, L. F., Kinkel, W., & Freenam, A. I. (1980). Computed tomography brain scans in children with acute lymphoblastic leukaemia receiving methotrexate alone as central nervous system prophylaxis. *Cancer, 45,* 2274–2278.

Ochs, J. J., & Mulhern, R. K. (1988). Late effects of anti leukemic treatment. *Pediatric Clinics of North America, 35,* 815–833.

Ochs, J. J., Parvey, L. S., & Mulhern, R. (1986). Prospective study of central nervous system changes in children with acute lymphoblastic leukaemia receiving two different methods of central nervous system prophylaxis. *Neurotoxicology, 7,* 217–226.

Ochs, J. J., Rivera, G., Rhomes, J. A., Hustu, H. O., Berg, R., & Simone, J. V. (1985). Central nervous system morbidity following an initial isolated central nervous system relapse and its subsequent therapy in childhood acute lymphoblastic leukaemia. *Journal of Clinical Oncology, 3,* 622–626.

Packer, R. J., Nicholson, H. S., & Ryan, J. (1993). Chemotherapy of childhood posterior fossa tumors. In A. J. Raimondi, M. Choux, & C. Di Rocco (Eds.), *Posterior fossa tumors* (pp. 169–188). New York, NY: Springer-Verlag.

Palmer, S. L., & Leigh, L. (2009). Survivors of pediatric posterior fossa tumors: Cognitive outcome, intervention and risk-based care. *European Journal of Oncology Nursing, 13,* 171–178.

Parkin, D. M., & Stiller, C. A., Draper, G. J., & Bieber, C. A. (1988). The international incidence of childhood cancer. *International Journal of Cancer, 42,* 511–520.

Peylan-Ramu, N., Poplack, D. G., Pizzo, P. A., Adornato, B. T., & Di Chiro, G. (1978). Abnormal CT scans in asymptomatic children with acute lymphocytic leukaemia after prophylactic treatment of the central nervous system with radiation and intrathecal chemotherapy. *New England Journal of Medicine, 298,* 815–818.

Pfefferbaum-Levine, B., Copeland, D. R., Fletcher, J. M., Reid, H. L., Jaffe, N., & McKinnon, W. R. (1984). Neuropsychological assessment of long-term survivors of childhood leukemia. *American Journal of Pediatric Hematology/Oncology, 6,* 123–128.

Pieters, R., & Carroll, W. L. (2008). Biology and treatment of acute lymphoblastic leukemia. *Pediatric Clinics of North America, 55,* 1–20.

Pinkel, D. (1979). Treatment of acute lymphocytic leukaemia. *Cancer, 43,* 1128–1137.

Pizzo, P. A., Bleyer, W. A., Poplack, D. G., & Leventhal, B. G. (1976). Reversible dementia temporarily associated with intraventricular therapy with methotrexate in a child with acute myelogenous leukaemia. *Journal of Pediatrics, 88,* 131–133.

Pizzo, P. A., Poplack, D. G., & Bleyer, W. A. (1979). Neurotoxicities of current leukaemia therapy. *American Journal of Pediatric Hematology/Oncology, 1,* 127–140.

Plowman, P. N. (1992). Tumours of the central nervous system. In P. N. Plowman & C. R. Pinkerton (Eds.), *Paediatric oncology: Clinical practice and controversies* (pp. 240–267). London, UK: Chapman & Hall Medical.

Poplack, D. G., & Reaman, G. (1988). Acute lymphoblastic leukaemia in childhood. *Pediatric Clinics of North America, 35,* 903–932.

Prabu, R., & Bakhshi, S. (2009). Systematic reaction to leucovorin in a child with lymphoblastic lymphoma suggestive of hypersensitivity. *Pediatric Blood and Cancer, 52,* 148.

Price, R. A., & Birdwell, D. A. (1978). The central nervous system in childhood leukaemia: II. Mineralizing Microangiopathy and dystrophic calcification. *Cancer, 42,* 717–728.

Rekate, H. L., Grubb, R. L., Aram, D. M., Hahn, J. F., & Ratcheson, R. A. (1985).

Muteness of cerebellar origin. *Archives of Neurology, 42,* 697–698.

Riva, D. (2000). Cerebellar contribution to behavior and cognition in children. *Journal of Neurolinguistics, 13,* 215–225.

Riva, D., & Giorgi, C. (2000a). The cerebellum contributes to higher functions during development: Evidence from a series of children surgically treated for posterior fossa tumours. *Brain, 123,* 1051–1061.

Riva, D., & Giorgi, C. (2000b). The contribution of the cerebellum to mental and social functions in developmental age. *Human Physiology, 26,* 21–25.

Ross, G. W., & Rubinstein, L. J. (1989). Lack of histopathological correlation of malignant ependymomas with postoperative survival. *Journal of Neurosurgery, 70,* 31–36.

Rubenstein, C. L., Varni, J. W., & Katz, E. R. (1990). Cognitive functioning in long-term survivors of childhood leukemia: A prospective analysis. *Developmental and Behavioral Pediatrics, 11,* 301–305.

Said, J. A., Waters, B. G., Cousens, P., & Stevens, M. M. (1987). Neuropsychological after-effects of central nervous system prophylaxis in survivors of childhood acute lymphoblastic leukaemia. In G. R. Gates (Ed.), *Proceedings of the Twelfth Annual Brain Impairment Conference.* Armidale: Australian Society for the Study of Brain Impairment.

Salazar, O. M., Castro-Vita, H., VanHoutte, P., Rubin, P., & Aygun, C. (1983). Improved survival in cases of intracranial ependymoma after radiation therapy: Late report and recommendations. *Journal of Neurosurgery, 59,* 652–659.

Sands, S. A., van Gorp, W. G., & Finlay, J. L. (1998). Pilot neuropsychological findings from a treatment regimen consisting of intensive chemotherapy and bone marrow rescue for young children with newly diagnosed malignant brain tumors. *Child's Nervous System, 14,* 587–589.

Satz, P., & Bullard-Bates, C. (1981). Acquired aphasia in children. In M. T. Sarno (Ed.), *Acquired aphasia* (pp. 398–426). New York, NY: Academic Press.

Schatz, J., Kramer, J. H., Albin, A., & Matthay, K. (2000). Processing speed, working memory and IQ: A developmental model of cognitive deficits following cranial radiation therapy. *Neuropsychology, 14,* 189–200.

Semel, E. M., & Wiig, E. H. (1982). *Clinical evaluation of language functions.* Columbus, OH: Charles E. Merrill.

Silverman, C. L., & Thomas, P. R. M. (1990). Long-term neuropsychologic and intellectual sequelae in brain tumour patients. In M. Deutsch (Ed.), *Management of childhood brain tumors.* Boston, MA: Kluwer Academic.

Skullerud, L., & Halvorsen, L. (1978). Encephalomyelopathy following intrathecal methotrexate treatment in a child with acute leukemia. *Cancer, 42,* 1211–1215.

Smith, B. (1975). Brain damage after intrathecal methotrexate. *Journal of Neurology, Neurosurgery and Psychiatry, 38,* 810–815.

Southam, C. M., Craver, F. L., Dargeon, H. W., & Burchenal, J. H. (1951). A study of the natural history of acute leukemia with special reference to the duration of the disease and the occurrence of remissions. *Cancer, 4,* 39–59.

Stiller, C. A., & Bleyer, W. A. (2004). Epidemiology. In D. A. Walker, G. Perilongo, J. Punt, & R. E. Taylor (Eds.), *Brain and spinal tumors of childhood* (pp. 35–49). London, UK: Arnold.

Tait, D. M., Bailey, C. C., & Cameron, M. M. (1992). Tumours of the central nervous system. In P. A. Voute, A. Barrett, & J. Lemerle (Eds.), *Cancer in children: Clinical management* (pp. 184–206). Berlin, Germany: Springer-Verlag.

Tamaroff, M., Miller, D. R., Murphy, M. L., Salwen, R., Ghavimi, F., & Nir, Y. (1982). Immediate and long-term post-therapy neuropsychologic performance in children with acute lymphoblastic leukemia treated with central nervous system radiation. *Journal of Pediatrics, 101,* 524–529.

Taylor, H. G., Also, V. C., Phebus, C. K., Sachs, B. R., & Bierl, P. G. (1987). Postirradiation treatment outcomes for children with acute lymphocytic leukemia: Clarification of risks. *Journal of Pediatric Psychology, 12,* 395–411.

Tebbi, C. K. (1982). *Major topics in pediatric and adolescent oncology.* Boston, MA: Hall Medical.

Tew, J. M., Feibel, J. H., & Sawaya, R. (1984). Brain tumors: Clinical aspects. *Seminars in Roentgenology, 19,* 115–128.

Tivey, H. (1952). Prognosis for survival in the leukemias of childhood. *Pediatrics, 10,* 48–59.

Twaddle, V., Britton, P. G., Craft, A. C., Nobel, T. C., & Kernahan, J. (1983). Intellectual function after treatment for leukaemia or solid tumours. *Archives of Disease in Childhood, 58,* 949–952.

van Dongen, H. R., Loonen, M. C. B., & van Dongen, K. J. (1985). Anatomical basis for acquired fluent aphasia in children. *Annals of Neurology, 17,* 306–309.

van Eys, J. (1991). Malignant tumors of the central nervous system. In D. J. Fernbach & T. J. Vietti (Eds.), *Clinical pediatric oncology* (4th ed., pp. 409–426). St Louis, MO: Mosby-Year Book.

van Eys, J., Baram, T. Z., Cangir, A., Bruner, J. M., & Martinez-Prieto, J. (1988). Salvage chemotherapy for recurrent primary brain tumors in children. *Journal of Pediatrics, 113,* 601–606.

Van Lieshout, P., Renier, W., Eling, P., de Bot, K., & Slis, I. (1990). Bilingual language processing after a lesion in the left thalamic and temporal regions. *Brain and Language, 38,* 173–194.

Vietti, T. J. (1991). Cellular kinetics and cancer chemotherapy. In D. J. Fernbach & T. J. Vietti (Eds.), *Clinical pediatric oncology* (4th ed., pp. 173–212). St Louis, MO: Mosby-Year Book.

Volcan, I., Cole, G. P., & Johnston, K. (1986). A case of muteness of cerebellar origin (Letter to the Editor). *Archives of Neurology, 43,* 313–314.

von der Weid, N. (2001). Late effects in long-term survivors of ALL in childhood: Experience from SPOG late effects study. *Swiss Medical Weekly, 131,* 180–187.

von der Weid, N., Mosimann, I., Hirt, A., Wacker, P., Beck, M., Imbach, P., . . . Wagner, H. (2003). Intellectual outcome in children and adolescents with acute lymphoblastic leukaemia treated with chemotherapy alone: Age and sex-related differences. *European Journal of Cancer, 39,* 359–365.

Waber, D. P., Turek, J., Catania, L., Stevenson, K., Rodney, P., Romero, I., . . . Silverman, L. (2007). Neuropsychological outcomes from a randomized trial of triple intrathecal chemotherapy compared with 18 Gy cranial radiation as CNS treatment in acute lymphoblastic leukemia: Findings from Dana-Farber Cancer Institute ALL Consortium Protocol 95–01. *Journal of Clinical Oncology, 25,* 4914–4921.

Waber, D. P., Urion, D. K., Tarbell, N. J., Niemeyer, C., Gelber, R., & Sallan, S. (1990). Late effects of central nervous system treatment of acute lymphoblastic leukemia in childhood are sex dependent. *Developmental Medicine and Child Neurology, 32,* 238–248.

West, C. R., Bruce, D. A., & Duffner, P. K. (1985). Ependymomas: Factors in clinical and diagnostic staging. *Cancer, 56,* 1812–1816.

Wharam, M. D. (1983). Radiation therapy. In A. J. Altman, & A. D. Schwartz (Eds.), *Malignant diseases of infancy, childhood and adolescence* (2nd ed., pp. 96–110). Philadelphia, PA: W. B. Saunders.

Whitt, J. K., Wells, R. J., Lauria, M. M., Wilhelm, C. L., & McMillan, C. W. (1984). Cranial radiation in childhood acute lymphocytic leukemia: Neuropsychologic sequelae. *American Journal of Disease in Childhood, 138,* 730–736.

Wiig, E. H., & Secord, W. (1985). Test of language competence. Columbus, OH: Charles E. Merrill.

Wilson, C. B. (1975). Diagnosis and surgical treatment of childhood brain tumors. *Cancer, 35,* 950–956.

Yachnis, A. T. (1997). Neuropathology of pediatric brain tumors. *Seminars in Pediatric Neurology, 4,* 282–291.

Young, J. L., & Miller, R. W. (1975). Incidence of malignant tumors in U.S. children. *Journal of Pediatrics, 86,* 254–257.

Ziegler, D. S., Dalla Pozza, L., Waters, K. D., & Marshall, G. M. (2005). Advances in childhood leukaemia. Successful clinical trials research leads to individualized therapy. *Medical Journal of Australia, 182,* 78–81.

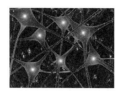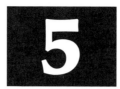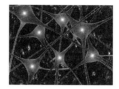

5

Language Disorders Associated with Childhood Metabolic Disorders

Introduction

Abnormal body metabolism can cause disturbances in brain development and function leading to a range of characteristic neurologic disorders. Systemic metabolic disorders for instance, such as inborn errors of metabolism, can lead to the accumulation of metabolites in the bloodstream and body tissues which may cause structural changes in the brain leading to a decline in intellectual function and, in some cases, speech and language disorders. Inborn errors of metabolism that have been reported to cause speech-language disorders include phenylketonuria (Ozanne, Krimmer, & Murdoch, 1990), galactosemia (Potter, Lazarus, Johnson, Steiner, & Shriberg, 2008; Waisbren, Norman, Schnell, & Levy, 1983), and Wilson disease (Berry, Darley, Aronson, & Goldstein, 1974). In addition to inborn errors of metabolism, speech-language disorders have been reported to occur in association with impaired intellectual function resulting from disruption of normal brain development in cases of congenital hypothyroidism (Dussault, Letarte, Glorieux, Morissette, & Guyda, 1980).

Inborn Errors of Metabolism Causing Speech-Language Disorders

Inborn errors of metabolism each result from a single mutant gene that codes for an enzymatic protein that in most instances is involved in a catabolic pathway. Although a large number of different inborn errors of metabolism have been recognized, not all lead to neurologic impairment and communication deficits. Three inborn errors of metabolism more frequently encountered by speech-language pathologists are phenylketonuria, galactosemia, and Wilson disease.

Phenylketonuria

Phenylketonuria is one of the most common inherited metabolic disorders. The condition represents an inborn error of metabolism that in most cases results from an absence of the hepatic (liver) enzyme phenylalanine hydroxylase that converts phenylalanine (an essential amino acid) into tyrosine, a process that is essential for the biosynthesis of specific neurotransmitters and the prevention of the neurotoxic accumulation of phenylalanine (Pietz, 1998). More rarely, deficiency of tetrahydrobiopterin (a cofactor of phenylalanine hydroxylase) is responsible. As a result of the deficiency in phenylalanine hydroxylase, phenylalanine (as well as other metabolites of phenylalanine such as phenylketones), normally present in only small amounts, accumulates in the blood as well as in the cerebrospinal fluid and tissues, and is excreted in the urine as phenylpyruvic acid in greater than normal amounts.

Phenylketonuria is inherited as an autosomal recessive disorder and occurs in approximately 1 in every 10,000 to 20,000 births. In past years, phenylketonuria has accounted for approximately 1% of institutionalized mentally deficient persons (Rosenberg & Pettegrew, 1980). The condition is most common in Caucasians and is rare in some racial groups, including the African, Jewish, and Japanese populations.

Clinical Manifestations

At birth, infants with phenylketonuria may appear normal although an increased frequency of vomiting and a poor appetite have been noted. In that melanin is formed from tyrosine, most children with phenylketonuria have reduced pigmentation in their skin, hair, and eyes. Consequently, the majority have fair skin, blond hair, and blue eyes. Phenylketonuria in the offspring of people with darker heritage may be red-haired or brunette. The occurrence of phenylketonuria is suspected on the basis of the presence of phenylpyruvic acid in the urine. A transient green color is produced when ferric chloride is added to urine containing excessive levels of phenylpyruvic acid. In that this test is not reliable until the infant is approximately 4 to 6 weeks of age, however, the early confirmation of phenylketonuria is dependent on the detection of elevated serum phenylalanine levels. The most commonly used screening test for phenylketonuria is the Guthrie technique. In this, a drop of the infant's blood is placed on a specific type of filter paper and the levels of various amino acids (including phenylalanine) determined by a microbiological method. With the worldwide practice of neonatal screening for phenylketonuria, the diagnosis is usually made during the first week of life, and consequently it is now rare to encounter an older infant or child with undiagnosed phenylketonuria.

Most, if not all, manifestations of phenylketonuria are accounted for by the disruption of normal body processes caused by the accumulation of phenylalanine and its metabolites. Although largely symptom-free at birth, children with phenylketonuria, if left untreated, eventually manifest a number of abnormal signs and symptoms including significant neuropathology and severe neurobehavioral impairments (Huttenlocher, 2000). The most important clinical characteristic of untreated phenylketonuria is severe mental retardation. Signs of mental retardation usually become evident clinically after the first

6 months of life, although the process may begin at an earlier stage and go undetected until this time. According to Rosenberg and Pettegrew (1980), when not treated, infants with phenylketonuria lose approximately five IQ points each 10 weeks and ultimately 96 to 98% of them have an IQ of less than 50. Even early and continuously treated children with phenylketonuria are at risk of developing subtle cognitive and behavioral impairments (Antshel & Waisbren, 2003; Channon, German, Cassina, & Lee, 2004).

The pathogenesis of mental retardation in phenylketonuria is not completely understood. No evidence exists that phenylpyruvic acid of any of the other phenylalanine metabolities are neurotoxic at concentrations in which they are seen in phenylketonuria. Probably no single factor is responsible. Rather, impairment of amino acid transport across the blood-brain barrier, disruption to the brain amino acid pool with consequent defective proteolipid protein synthesis, impaired myelination and low levels of neurotransmitters, such as serotonin are responsible to varying degrees (Hommes, 1991). Dopamine depletion has also been reported in early and continuously treated patients with phenylketonuria (Burlina et al., 2000) leading to the suggestion that reductions in executive functioning in children with early-treated phenylketonuria, at least to some extent, are the result of reduced activity of the prefrontal cortex due to mild depletion in dopamine (Welsh, Pennington, Ozonoff, Rouse, & McCabe, 1990). Both animal and human studies have demonstrated that dopamine depletion is associated with prefrontal dysfunction (Brozoski, Brown, Rosvold, & Goldman, 1979; Sawaguchi & Goldman-Rakic, 1991). Although the findings of some studies have offered some support for the suggestion that neuropsychological impairment in phenylketonuria are the result of dopamine depletion in the prefrontal cortex (Anderson, Wood, Francis, Coleman, Anderson, & Boneh, 2007) others have failed to support the executive deficit hypothesis (Channon et al., 2004).

Pathologic changes in the brain are nonspecific and diffuse. They involve both the gray and white matter and may be progressive with age. Brain growth is reduced and microscopic examination shows impaired cortical layering, delayed outward migration of neuroblasts, and heterotopic (displacement of parts) gray matter. Additionally, the amount of Nissl granules is markedly deficient, particularly in those areas of the brain that are not fully developed at birth. Dendritic arborization and the number of synaptic spikes are reduced within the cerebral cortex. These changes point to a period of abnormal brain development extending from the last trimester of gestation into postnatal life. Elevated phenylalanine and low tyrosine levels in the blood, which are characteristic of phenylketonuria, are thought to impair brain development, especially myelinization due to sensitivity of oligodendrocytes to high phenylalanine levels. Consequently, untreated phenylketonuria is associated with significant white matter loss. The lesions in the white matter range from irregular spongy degeneration (vacuolation) to profound demyelinization with accompanying gliosis. Areas of vacuolation are most commonly seen in the central white matter of the cerebral hemispheres and in the cerebellum. Brain lipids are reduced, especially the galactolipids associated with myelin.

In addition to mental retardation, other signs and symptoms often exhibited by children with untreated phenylketonuria include: eczematoid dermatitis (rash in the body folds), and aromatic, musty odor associated with the presence of phenylacetic acid in the sweat and urine, seizures, abnormal electroencephalographic activity, hyperactivity, erratic and unpredictable behavior, including temper tantrums, slowness in attaining motor milestones, motor performance habits (e.g., chewing on an arm), and insufficient head growth. Neurologic examination usually shows no specific abnormalities, although in some cases a little spasticity and hyperactivity may be evident without corticospinal signs. Seizures, common in the more severely retarded, usually start before 18 months of age and can cease spontaneously. During infancy, they often take the form of infantile spasms, later changing into tonic-clonic attacks. A variety of electroencephalographic abnormalities have been found; however, hypsarrhythmic patterns, recorded even in the absence of seizures, and single and multiple foci of spike and polyspike discharges are the most common. Magnetic resonance imaging is abnormal in almost every case, including children who have undergone early and continuous dietary treatment, with T2-weighted imaging demonstrating symmetrical increased signal intensity in the periventricular and subcortical white matter of the posterior cerebral hemispheres. The increased signal intensity can in more severe cases also extend to involve the deep white matter of the posterior cerebral hemispheres and the anterior cerebral hemispheres. The etiology of these white matter lesions is unknown but increased myelin turnover, elevated water content, and disturbed myelin synthesis have been proposed (Dyer, 1999). No signal abnormalities are seen in the brainstem, cerebellum, or cortex, although cortical atrophy may be present.

Medical Treatment of Phenylketonuria

Although the pathogenesis of phenylketonuria is not completely understood, treatment is required to prevent severe neurologic impairment, mental retardation, and behavioral difficulties. Treatment of phenylketonuria involves elimination from the diet of those foods that contain high concentrations of phenylalanine. This involves restriction of dietary protein intake and provision of phenylalanine-free amino acid supplements plus supplementation of the vitamins, minerals, and other micronutrients that are usually obtained from meat and dairy products (e.g., vitamin B_{12}, calcium and iron). Dietary management appears to be most effective when initiated shortly after birth. It has been suggested that in those cases where a phenylalanine-restricted diet is commenced early in infancy (before 3 months of age) and maintained during the period of most rapid myelinization, serious damage to the central nervous system is averted. Clinically, it has been observed that very young children with phenylketonuria who are placed on low phenylalanine diets while still normal (i.e., before onset of seizures, mental decline, etc.) and who have blood phenylalanine levels maintained at near-normal levels, appear to develop mentally at a normal rate. Despite their IQ measurements being within normal limits, however, there is evidence to suggest that the IQs of these children are significantly lower than those of their parents, siblings, or nonsibling controls (Berry et al., 1979; Netley, Hanley, & Rudner, 1984). Furthermore, as indicated previously, even children undergoing early and continuous treatment exhibit some pathologic changes in the brain as evidenced by magnetic resonance imaging as well as subtle cognitive and behavioral deficits.

Considerable uncertainty exists as to how long it is necessary to maintain the dietary treatment to ensure development of maximal intellectual capacity. There is a feeling that children with phenylketonuria should remain on a low-phenylalanine diet during the period when the brain is still undergoing myelinization and is, therefore, most susceptible to damage. Consequently, treatment may be required for the first 3 to 6 years of life or more. It is important, however, that intellectual and behavioral monitoring continue after the diet is discontinued. In that a decline in cognitive functioning and even language skills has been documented in some children who have been routinely taken off their low phenylalanine diet (Koch, Azen, Friedman, & Williamson, 1984; Seashore, Friedman, Novelly, & Bapat, 1985; Waisbren, Schnell, & Levy, 1980), dietary control in some countries is continued for the first 8 years of life. Evidence is available to suggest that children taken off a protein-restricted diet after 10 years of age will have IQ values in the normal range when tested later in life, implying that the brain becomes resistant to the toxic effects of phenylalamine as it matures. However, other studies have shown more subtle cognitive deficits in adult patients not on a protein-restricted diet when compared with those who have followed a diet throughout life. It is current practice in many countries to encourage patients to follow a protein restricted diet throughout childhood. Once they reach adulthood, however, many patients choose to resume a normal diet and their phenylalanine levels rise accordingly. There currently is no evidence that this poses any risk of irreversible neurologic damage. Based on a study of the effects of dietary management of phenylketonuria on long-term cognitive outcome, Channon, Goodman, Zlotowitz, Mockler, and Lee (2007) concluded that, although there were some disadvantages to discontinuing dietary treatment of the disorder in adolescence, any resulting deficits were relatively subtle. Internationally, there is no current consensus on what phenylalanine blood concentrations should be achieved in an adult patient following a protein restricted diet with targets ranging from <600 µmole per L in the United States to 1300 µmole per L in France.

In older children with phenylketonuria, initiation of a low phenylalanine diet has been found to reduce the occurrence of seizures and skin rashes and to improve the level of pigmentation. Only modest improvements in behavior, however, have been observed in these children. Furthermore, initiation of diets after brain damage has occurred does not reverse the process but may, if begun early enough, limit its progress. Therefore, it is important that phenylketonuria be detected early. The lack of symptoms in the neonatal period, however, makes this early detection difficult. Routine screening therefore is needed to detect affected infants.

Overall, with early neonatal diagnosis and appropriate dietary therapy, and with monitoring of behavior and intellectual abilities, the prognosis of children with phenylketonuria is good. Without early dietary treatment, however, the prognosis is very poor.

Linguistic Deficits Associated with Phenylketonuria

Little information regarding the linguistic skills of children with phenylketonuria is available. Early reports described the presence of speech and language disorders in children in association with intellectual handicap (Boehme & Theile, 1972). Since the introduction of low-phenylalanine diets, however, the speech and language skills of children with phenylketonuria have been assumed to be within normal limits, in line with their intellectual functioning. Given that numerous studies have identified that even early-treated children with phenylketonuria are at risk for developing subtle cognitive deficits (Anderson et al., 2007; Gassió et al., 2005), it could be assumed that subtle language impairments may also be present in these children.

Gross measures of language such as verbal IQ scores, in fact, have been found to be superior to performance IQ scores in some studies (Koff, Boyle, & Peuschel, 1977; Pennington & Smith, 1983), whereas in other studies no notable difference between the verbal and performance IQ scores of children with early treated phenylketonuria was evident (Koch, Azen, Friedman, & Williamson, 1982, 1984; Seashore et al., 1985). Studies utilizing neuropsychological assessments, aimed at detecting subtle cognitive defects in children with phenylketonuria and normal intelligence, have found deficits in visuospatial and conceptual tasks but minimal impairment on language tasks (Pennington,

van Doornick, McCabe, & McCabe, 1985). These conclusions, however, have been based on language assessment using neuropsychological tasks, such as word fluency tasks, rather than linguistic tests. Both types of findings would lead one to suspect that children with early-treated phenylketonuria do not present with language impairments.

Some authors have suggested, however, that speech and language disorders do occur in children with phenylketonuria. Vogel (1985) stated that, "diet-treated phenylketonuria homozygotes often show a slight weakness in verbal abilities" (p. 342), but provided no further details. To date, only two studies have reported on the speech and language skills in children with early-treated phenylketonuria using linguistic assessments. Melnick, Michals, and Matalon (1981) assessed 12 children with phenylketonuria between 4 months and 6 years of age. All children had normal intelligence. The children were assessed using the Bzoch-League Receptive-Expressive Emergent Language Scale (Bzoch & League, 1971), the Peabody Picture Vocabulary Test (Dunn, 1965), the Developmental Sentence Score (Lee, 1974a), mean length of utterance (Brown, 1973), the Northwestern Syntax Screening Test (Lee, 1974b), the Goldman-Fristoe Test of Articulation (Goldman & Fristoe, 1969), and the digit span subtest of the Stanford-Binet. Using the test percentile ratings for each child, Melnick et al. (1981) identified children who scored below the tenth percentile as having a speech and/or language disorder. By using this criterion, Melnick et al. (1981) found that 50% of their subjects showed a speech or language impairment; however, there was no particular pattern of linguistic deficit that appeared to be associated with phenylketonuria. Two of their subjects presented with articulation disorders four with receptive and six with expressive language problems. One child presented with all three areas of linguistic deficit; three subjects had both receptive and expressive language impairments, whereas one subject had expressive syntax and articulation deficits and one other had only expressive syntactic delays. After speech and language therapy, the one case with the expressive only problem was remediated, whereas two other cases had acquired age-appropriate receptive but not expressive skills. All other cases continued to exhibit persistent speech and/or language impairment. Despite the lack of commonality of presenting speech and language deficits, Melnick et al. (1981) did find that all the children who presented with linguistic deficits also had poor auditory memory skills.

A study by Ozanne et al. (1990) assessed a similar group to Melnick et al. (1981); the subjects were between 7 months and 3 years, 11 months of age, with normal intelligence. The subjects with phenylketonuria were assessed using the Sequenced Inventory of Communication Development (SICD) (Hedrick, Prather, & Tobin, 1978) with similar results to those reported by Melnick et al. (1981). Thirty-six percent (i.e., four of 11) of the subjects with phenylketonuria examined by Ozanne and co-workers were considered language-impaired. As the SICD does not use percentile scores or gives guidelines for the identification of language impairment, the authors used the criterion of a language age which was 75% or below of the subject's chronological age, to identify children whom they considered to have language impairment.

When the language skills of the subjects with phenylketonuria examined by Ozanne and co-workers were compared as a group, however, with a group of children matched for age and sex, no significant difference in language abilities was found between the two groups. The authors suggested that the wide variation in language skills observed in both groups of subjects accounted for this lack of a significant difference. The wide variation in language abilities in turn, was, attributed to the fact that all the children were in the period of maximum language growth when large individual differences may occur. In that both Melnick et al. (1981) and Ozanne et al. (1990) assessed children with normal intelligence, it could be said that the young children with phenylketonuria who presented as having a language impairment exhibited a specific language disorder rather than a language impairment as part of a general cognitive impairment, or that the language impairment was one of the first symptoms of a developing cognitive deficit. Longitudinal studies are required to investigate this further.

When a second group of 18 subjects with phenylketonuria, between 5 and 16 years of age, were studied by Ozanne et al. (1990), again no significant difference was noted between the subjects with phenylketonuria and their matched controls in the language scores, as measured on the Test of Language Development (TOLD) (Hammill, Brown, Larsen, & Weiderholt, 1987; Hammill & Newcomer, 1982; Newcomer & Hammill, 1987) series of language tests. This group of subjects was also assessed using the Fisher-Logemann Test of Articulation Competence (Fisher & Logemann, 1971) which also failed to distinguish the subjects with phenylketonuria from their control group. This time the criterion used by Melnick et al. (1981) (i.e., score below the tenth percentile) was used to identify any child who had a language impairment. No child in the study had an articulation/phonological disorder. Three children with phenylketonuria, but no control subjects, were identified as being language impaired. Like Mel-

nick et al.'s subjects there was no consistent pattern of linguistic deficit. When the language quotients of the subjects with phenylketonuria were ranked as shown in Table 5–1 a trend showing a relationship between language and intelligence quotient could be observed.

Table 5–1. Ranked Individual Language Quotients, Dietary Compliance Ratings and IQ Scores of Subjects with Phenylketonuria Studied by Ozanne et al. (1990)

Subject No.	LQ	DC	FIQ	VIQ	PIQ
1	123	good	126φ		
14	122	good	107	113	100
9	120	good	101	106	98
3	119	good	110φ		
6	116	fair	107	108	105
12	111	fair	109	114	102
11	105	good	91	108	80
18	103	good	91	95	91
7	98	fair	118	118	114
2	94	fair	95φ		
15	93	fair	105	105	106
5	92	fair	107φ		
8	92	fair	92φ		
10	92	poor	92	91	94
13	89	poor	85	90	78
16	74+	poor	88	90	88
17	68+	poor	75	81	72
4	56+	poor	65	65	67

LQ = Language quotient measured on TOLD tests.
+ = Language quotient measured below tenth percentile.
DC = Dietary compliance.
FIQ = Full IQ measure.
VIQ = Verbal IQ score.
PIQ = Performance IQ score.
φ = IQ assessed using Stanford-Binet.

A stronger trend, however, can be seen in the relationship between language quotient and dietary compliance. All subjects in both groups with phenylketonuria studied by Ozanne et al. (1990) were still currently on a low phenylalanine diet. Dietary compliance had been rated "good," "fair," or "poor" by the dietitian, at the clinic these subjects attended, based on serum phenylalanine levels in the blood measured on each visit to the clinic. All three subjects with language impairment had among the lowest IQ scores in this group of subjects and all had a poor dietary rating. Although the number of children with phenylketonuria with language impairment is too small to make definitive statements, individual data suggest that in older children, particularly those with poor dietary control, speech and language deficits may be part of a decline in cognitive functioning.

The clinical implications from the limited research data available suggest that as a group children with early-treated phenylketonuria do not have speech and language deficits, but rather that there are individual children with phenylketonuria (perhaps between 30 and 50%) who do present with specific language disorders before 5 years of age. As there is no common pattern of linguistic deficit each child must be assessed and treated on an individual basis. Therefore, regular monitoring of the speech and language skills of all young children with phenylketonuria and parent education programs by speech-language pathologists should become a routine part of the functioning of the clinic. For older children with phenylketonuria it appears that those most at risk may have difficulties maintaining their diet. Further studies of subjects with phenylketonuria present-

ing with language impairment are required to confirm this finding and to clarify the relationship between language abilities and cognitive functioning including auditory memory abilities.

Galactosemia

Galactosemia is an inborn error of carbohydrate metabolism in which, due to the absence or deficiency of enzyme galactose-1-phosphate uridyltransferase, the body is unable to utilize the sugars galactose and lactose (Bosch, 2006). Under normal circumstances, lactose (milk sugar) is broken down in the epithelium of the intestine to galactose and glucose. The galactose is then transported to the liver where it is converted into galactose-1-phosphate which, in turn, reacts with uridine diphosphate glucose (UDP-glucose) to form UDP-galactose. This substance is then transformed into glucose-1-phosphate. In galactosemia, the conversion of galactose-1-phosphate to UDP-galactose is blocked due to the enzyme deficiency. Consequently, galatose-1-phosphate accumulates in the body tissues. Diagnosis is made on the basis of galactosuria, increased levels of galactose in the blood or by demonstration of the absence or deficiency of galactose-1-phosphate uridyltransferase in the erythrocytes.

The disease is inherited as an autosomal recessive disorder and occurs with a frequency of 1 in 62,000 in the United States, and 1 in 72,000 in England (Menkes & Wilcox, 2006). The gene for galactosemia has been mapped to the small arm of chromosome 9 (9p13). As in phenylketonuria, infants with galactosemia may appear to be normal at birth. Symptoms tend to manifest, however, shortly after birth when the infant is exposed to large amounts of galactose derived from the lactose of the mother's milk. The toxic manifestations of galactosemia are thought to result from the accumulation of galactose-1-phosphate.

Clinical Manifestations

The major symptoms of the condition when the infant is exposed to galactose include cataract formation, hepatosplenomegaly (enlargement of the liver and spleen), nutritional failure, and, most importantly, mental retardatioin. In severe cases, symptoms develop in the first week of life including vomiting, listlessness, and failure to gain weight. Jaundice also may occur in some cases and the hepatosplenomegaly may progress to cirrhosis of the liver if galactose ingestion continues for a prolonged period. If galactosemia goes untreated growth failure becomes severe. Magnetic resonance imaging commonly shows multiple areas of increased signal in the cerebral white matter, predominantly in the periventricular region.

Medical Treatment of Galactosemia

Treatment of galactosemia involves the elimination of galactose from the diet (i.e., removal of all milk and galactose-containing foods). With the exception of mental retardation which is permanent once established, maintenance of a galactose-free diet may cause reversal of many of the other clinical symptoms of galactosemia or, in some cases, at least halt their progression. Maintenance of the galactose-free diet and avoidance of milk and milk products is recommended until at least after puberty. Even total exclusion of galactose from the diet, however, does not ensure the

absence of all pathology (Gitzelmann & Steinmann, 1984). Indeed, recent research findings indicate that the long-term outlook for children with galactosemia is not as good as initially believed, even when the diet is carefully monitored.

Speech, Language, and Cognitive Outcomes of Galactosemia: Early Studies

Newborn screening programs for galactosemia have been implemented in many parts of the world on the premise that early detection and treatment may reduce the occurrence of the negative outcomes of this condition (Hayes et al., 1986). As in the case of phenylketonuria, the screening process for galactosemia involves collection of a blood sample, via a heel-prick onto filter paper, from every newborn child during the first week of life.

Varying degrees of success for galactosemia screening programs have been reported in the literature. Prior to the introduction of screening programs, the presence of speech and language disorders were reported in a number of studies of children with galactosemia (Jan & Wilson, 1973; Komrower & Lee, 1970; Lee, 1972). Subsequent to the introduction of screening programs and the introduction of early treatment, it generally was believed that deficits of this kind would be either reduced or eliminated. Contrary to that belief, Gitzelmann and Steinmann (1984) reported that although early- and well-treated children with galactosemia show satisfactory general health and growth and make reasonable but suboptimal intellectual progress, they are, nonetheless, prone to developing speech deficits, ovarian failure, and visual perceptual difficulties, and in some cases exhibit social maladjustment. Similarly, the results of a study by Waisbren et al. (1983) showed that early-treated children with galactosemia are at risk for developing speech and language difficulties. They found that all eight of their early-treated galactosemic children exhibited delays or early speech difficulties and that all except one developed subsequent language problems. Waisbren et al. (1983) did not specify the tests used to assess the children's language. In addition, their criterion for a deficit has been questioned by some authors (Hayes et al., 1986). "A deficit is defined as one standard deviation below the mean on tests with standardized norms or 1 year below chronologic age on tests with age norms" (Waisbren et al., 1983, p. 76). Hayes et al. (1986) concluded that, "in the absence of information on the tests and the children's scores, there is insufficient information to support the authors' conclusions" (p. 238).

In contrast to the findings of Waisbren et al. (1983), Hayes, Bowling, Fraser, Krimmer, and Clague (1988) provided preliminary data indicating that neonatal screening and careful management results in improved outcomes for children with galactosemia. In particular these authors found that altough children with galactosemia diagnosed before the introduction of neonatal screening had intellectual development in the low average to moderately handicapped range, children with galactosemia diagnosed subsequent to the introduction of neonatal screening appeared to be developing normally. In addition, although most (5 of 7) of the children in their prescreening group presented with speech and language difficulties, only one child (1 of 6) in their screened

group presented with a speech and language deficit, this latter child showing mild expressive language and moderate articulation delays. The expressive language was reported to be characterized by immature syntax. In addition, Hayes et al. (1988) indicated that the speech of this child was affected by a phonological processing disorder that involved stopping and idiosyncratic palatization of fricatives.

Speech, Language, and Cognitive Outcomes of Galactosemia: Contemporary Studies

For many years the early impletation of a galactose-free diet was considered to be an effective intervention for the prevention of negative complications of galactosemia (Fridovich & Walter, 2008). Recent long-term follow-up studies of children treated for galactosemia, however, have shown that, although early medical intervention and dietary restrictions are necessary, they do not guarantee healthy cognitive, linguistic, and intellectual development (Brazeal & Farmer, 1999; Schweitzer-Krantz, 2003). Despite early diagnosis and compliance with galactose restrictions, structural changes to the cerebral white matter tracts (Brazeal & Farmer, 1999; Hughes et al., 2009), abnormal fine and gross motor development (Waggoner, Buist, & Donnell, 1990), developmental delays (Fridovich & Walter, 2008), intellectual impairment and declining IQ scores with age (Schweitzer, Shin, Jakobs, & Brodehl, 1993), speech and language difficulties (Nelson, Waggoner, Donnell, Tuerck, & Buist, 1991; Potter et al., 2008; Waggoner et al., 1990; Waisbren et al., 1983), significantly reduced academic outcomes, and cognitive and social dysfunction in adolescence (Bosch et al., 2004) have been reported in children and young adults with galactosemia.

Not all children or young adults with galactosemia present with intellectual and/or cognitive-linguistic deficits (Fridovich & Walter, 2008; Lambert & Boneh, 2004; Potter et al., 2008). Impaired cognitive development, including delayed developmental milestones and lowered IQ is evident in no more than 50% of children with the condition (Fridovich & Walter, 2008), and, based on findings from neuropsychological test batteries, not all children with the diagnosis experience receptive and expressive language deficits (Lambert & Boneh, 2004; Potter et al., 2008).

The relationship between intellectual/cognitive status and language outcomes in galactosemia currently is unclear. Kaufman, McBride-Chang, Manis, Wolff, and Nelson (1995) argued that the language deficits observed in the disorder are part of a more global set of cognitive impairments. In contrast, Waggoner et al. (1990) reported that language difficulties associated with galactosemia were more prevalent in, but not restricted to, children with borderline IQ scores. Potter et al. (2008), while identifying language deficits in children treated for galactosemia, suggested a dissociation exists between cognitive skill and language outcomes in the disorder.

Potter et al. (2008), in support of Waggoner et al.'s (1990) earlier findings, identified language impairments in 88% of the children treated for galactosemia and borderline-low intelligence investigated in their study. In addition, however, 56% of the children with galactosemia and average intelligence also presented with language deficits. Potter et al. (2008) described difficulties involving both receptive and expressive language as being more prevalent in the children with borderline-low IQ whereas difficulties restricted to expressive language only were more prevalent in the children with galactosemia with average IQ. The language difficulties (Kaufman et al., 1995; Potter et al., 2008; Waggoner et al., 1990) and cognitive deficits (Antshel, Epstein, & Waisbren, 2004; Kaufman et al., 1995; Schadewaldt et al., 2010) described in children treated for galactosemia do not appear to be related to age at diagnosis and restriction of galactose intake, severity of symptoms at diagnosis, and/or compliance with diet (Cleary, Heptinstall, Wraith, & Walter, 1995; Schadewaldt et al., 2010; Shield et al., 2000; Waggoner et al., 1990), suggesting other factors may contribute.

More than 150 mutations in the galactosemia gene have been associated with the enzyme deficiency in galactosemia, and of these mutations, the Q188R mutation is the most prevalent (Elsas & Lai, 1998). The Q188R mutation has been identified as increasing the risk of lower IQ and speech articulation disorders (Robertson, Singh, Guerrero, Hundley, & Elsas, 2000; Shield et al., 2000; Webb, Singh, Kennedy, & Elsas, 2003) and expressive but not receptive language disorders (Potter et al., 2008) in children with galactosemia. Potter et al.'s (2008) findings were based on superficial sampling of expressive and receptive abilities only, which is neither sufficiently sensitive nor comprehensive to adequately describe and define the language skills in children with the disorder. Assessments with language tests designed to tap into higher order cognitive-linguistic skills may be required in the future to adequately investigate the correlations between IQ, language skills, and genotype in children with treated galactosemia.

The acquisition and consolidation of skills during childhood is dependent on the integrity of white matter tracts within the brain (Anderson, 2007). White matter tracts facilitate high-speed transfer of information between networks linking the various parts of the brain, such as the ones involved in cognitive and language processing (Anderson, Northam, Hendy, & Wrennall, 2001). Disruption to nerve conduction along these network pathways, such as resulting from delayed or absent myelination as reported in children with galactosemia (Brazeal & Farmer, 1999; Hughes et al., 2009) impairs the efficient processing of information, which can manifest as cognitive-linguistic measures (Bernal & Ardila, 2009).

In summary, despite the introduction of screening programs and strict adherence to a galactose-free diet, intellectual and cognitive-linguistic deficits persist as long-term outcomes for 30-50% of children treated for galactosemia (Bosch et al., 2004; Fridovich & Walter, 2008; Hughes et al., 2009; Potter et al., 2008). As yet, however, the precise neuropathological basis of these disorders as well as their relationship to epigenetic and environmental factors such as compliance with dietary restrictions and genotype remains uncertain. Consequently speech-language pathologists should be aware of the need to monitor the development of these children over the long-term to enable early detection of any associated speech and/or language deficits and the implementation of appropriate management strategies to reduce long-term behavioral, academic, and social consequences of intellectual and cognitive-linguistic impairment.

Wilson Disease (Hepatolenticular Degeneration)

Wilson disease is a rare, inborn error of metabolism inherited as an autosomal recessive disorder. The condition is characterized by progressive degeneration changes in the brain and liver resulting from a deficiency in the body's ability to process dietary copper. As a consequence of this deficiency copper accumulates in the tissues of the body, especially in the brain, liver, and cornea of the eye. The basal ganglia are the most severely affected parts of the brain, although smaller amounts of copper may also be deposited in the cerebellum, brainstem, and parts of the cerebrum. Of the basal ganglia, the corpus striatum is involved most, with a greater degree of damage occurring in the putamen than in the caudate nucleus. Cirrhosis of the liver also occurs and the deposition of copper in the eye give a greenish-brown color to the cornea (Kayser-Fleisher rings).

Two separate neurologic pictures characterize Wilson disease, an acute form and a more chronic form. The acute form usually has an onset around puberty and is characterized by dystonia. It is the form of disorder that involves pediatric clinicians and, therefore, is described more fully here. The more chronic form, on the other hand, usually manifests around 19 to 35 years of age. It has a slowly progressive course and is characterized by a tremor and rigidity.

The initial symptoms of the acute form of Wilson disease vary from mild slowing of voluntary movements to dysarthria and mental changes. The latter includes problems with memory and concentration as well as mild personality changes such as increased irritability and emotional lability. In terms of the disturbances in speech, Berry et al. (1974) described a mixed ataxic-hypokinetic-spastic dysarthria as a feature of Wilson disease. Dystonia appears as a later symptom and serves to differentiate the acute form from the more chronic form. Ultimately, deterioration of intellectual function becomes evident. The face may become masklike and drooling is common. The degree of cognitive impairment increases with disease duration and severity of neurologic symptoms (Lauterbach, 2002). Portala, Levander, Westermark, Ekselius, and von Knorring (2001) reported that the pattern of neuropsychological deficits included impaired executive functions, specifically in dividing attention and slowed speed of processing. Lang (1989) reported that individuals treated for Wilson disease have mild deficits on divergent naming tasks and visuospatial/logical processing but not on auditory memory tasks. It is possible, therefore, that speech-language pathologists may be involved with patients with Wilson disease for the treatment of dysarthria as well as naming difficulties.

The course of the acute form is progressive unless treatment is provided. The rate of progress varies greatly and partial remissions and exacerbations may occur in some cases. Untreated Wilson disease is invariably fatal. In the past, the most common treatment was to recommend a restricted copper diet and anti-copper drug therapy, most commonly D-penicillamine (Rosselli, Lorenzana, Rosselli, & Vergara, 1987). Currently, treatment still focuses on the use of anti-copper drug therapy with the more successful zinc acetate, as this latter drug appears to be less toxic. Anti-copper drug therapy is a lifelong treatment for the disease, and dietary restrictions are not nearly as strict as once thought necessary (Brewer, 2001).

Other Metabolic Disorders Causing Speech-Language Disorders

Hypothyroidism

Thyroid hormones are important regulators of the metabolic activity of the body. An adequate supply of thyroid hormone is also necessary for the normal development of the nervous system, especially during the first few months after birth. Consequently, an absence or deficiency of thyroid hormone during this period has profound effect on brain development. In particular, thyroid deficiency in the first year of life leads to inadequate brain cell and dendritic development (Blasi et al., 2009; de Escobar, Ruiz-Marcos, & Escobar del Rey, 1983; Rovet & Brown, 2007) leading to a reduction in the intellectual potential of the affected child (Frost, 1986; Frost, Parkin, & Rowley, 1979; Salerno et al., 1999; Simons, Fuggle, Grant, & Smith, 1994). Speech-language disorders have been reported in association with the depressed intellectual abilities of hypothyroid children (Dussault et al., 1980; Marcheschi et al., 1997).

Congenital hypothyroidism can result from congenital absence of the thyroid gland, thyroid hypoplasia (underdevelopment of the thyroid gland) or, less commonly, from an enzymatic defect in the production of thyroid hormones. If left untreated, congenital hypothyroidism leads to cretinism, a historic clinical syndrome in which the affected individual exhibits marked mental retardation and deficiency in intellect as well as retarded skeletal growth and maturation. The child, termed a cretin, has a large head, short limbs, puffy eyes, a thick and protruding tongue, excessively dry skin, a lack of motor coordination (ataxia), and a low IQ (often below 75).

In recent years, early detection through neonatal screening and prompt treatment with replacement thyroid hormone in the first weeks of life has greatly improved the mental and physical prognosis of children with congenital hypothyroidism. As a consequence of such action, the incidence of historic cretinism has declined. Despite this several studies have shown that, especially in those cases where either the diagnosis and treatment was delayed for several weeks after birth or where the patients were negligent in adhering to the treatment program (i.e., neglected to take medication), the average IQ of children treated for hypothyroidism is one to two standard deviations below that of matched controls (Birrell, Frost, & Parkin, 1983; Hulse, 1984). In addition, these children may also exhibit a range of neurologic problems, including difficulties with coordination and balance, abnormal limb tone and reflexes, abnormal fine motor movement, speech problems, language delay, squints, and marked behavioral disturbances (Colombini et al., 2008; Frost, 1986; Hulse, 1984; Marcheschi et al., 1997).

It would appear, therefore, that amongst children with congenital hypothyroidism, speech and language disorders may be related to a child's intellectual ability and/or neurologic functioning.

Linguistic Deficits Associated with Hypothyroidism

As mentioned above, children who receive treatment for congenital hypothyroidism within the first three months of life develop intellectual functioning within the normal range (Frost, 1986; Glorieux et al., 1985; Moschini et al., 1986; Murphy et al., 1986; New England Congenital Hypothyroidism Collaborative, 1985). Yet, there still are some children who do not reach their full potential and present with less than average cognitive and/or neurologic functioning. This then has implications for the speech-language pathologist dealing with such children. In this section factors present in a child that relate to poor prognosis, and evidence for specific linguistic deficits outside of depressed intellectual ability is discussed as well as the implications of poor neurologic outcome.

Some studies (Glorieux et al., 1985; Rovet, Ehrlich, & Sorbara, 1987; Salerno et al., 1999) have shown that, despite IQ scores being within normal limits, children with hypothyroidism as a group have significantly lower IQ scores than their siblings or a group of matched controls. Such a difference, however, has not been found in the group of hypothyroid children studied by the New England Congenital Hypothyroidism Collaborative (1985). The distribution of the IQ scores obtained from children with congenital hypothyroidism reflects the distribution seen in the normal population (Frost, 1986). Some authors report an increase in IQ scores over time (Frost, 1986). One of the factors which relates to a poor prognosis for cognitive functioning in a child with congenital hypothyroidism is, as mentioned above, noncompliance with treatment. Other factors include perinatal and/or socioemotional problems (Moschini et al., 1986) such as socioeconomic status (Dussault et al., 1980); delay in treatment (Sack, Elicer, Sofrin, Theodor, & Cohen, 1986) although this effect has disappeared with the advent of neonatal screening procedures, and the absence of thyroid tissue in the child (Murphy et al., 1986; Sack et al., 1986). Children born without any thyroid tissue (athyrotic) have been found to have a poorer performance on intelligence tests than children who have reduced thyroid function (ectopic), even though there often is a delay in diagnosis in the ectopic group. Again, this effect seems to have disappeared since the introduction of neonatal screening (Glorieux et al., 1985; Sack et al., 1986).

Glorieux et al. (1988) examined pretreatment factors that could predict the consistently lower performance of certain children in a group of 150 children with congenital hypothyroidism included in their longitudinal study. Thirteen subjects who had IQ scores below or equal to 90 were found to differ from other subjects only on their initial thyroxine (T_4) values and their bone maturation score. Glorieux et al. (1988) then tested these parameters as predictive factors for cognitive development. They concluded that initial thyroxine values of less than 2 g per day, and bone maturation scores (calculated by measuring the surface areas of the ossification centers of the knee) of less than 0.05 cm^2, could be used for early identification of children with congenital hypothyroidism whose prognosis was poor.

The factors discussed above affect the cognitive abilities of children with congenital hypothyroidism. These same factors can be said to affect some speech and language skills as part of an overall cognitive delay in this same group of children. Information relating specifically to the speech and language skills seen in children with congenital hypothyroidism, however, is not readily available to clinicians because, to date, no study designed to specifically describe the linguistic abilities of children with congenital hypothyroidism has been reported. Although we can predict poor linguistic outcome associated with poor cognitive prognosis, an examination of cognitive profiles that include information on verbal abilities must be used to predict specific linguistic deficits until the results of appropriate research becomes available. The few studies, however, that do report separate verbal scores on the Wechsler Intelligence Scale for Children-Revised (WISC-R), the Gesell Developmental Test, or the Griffiths Mental Developmental Scales would indicate that most subjects with congenital hypothyroidism obtained verbal scores within a ten point range of either their global IQ or performance IQ scores (Frost & Parkin, 1986; Glorieux et al., 1988).

Moschini et al. (1986) noted that language scores of children with congenital hypothyroidism did not show any change over the ages of 6 months to 3 years as measured on the Brunet-Lezine Test (Brunet & Lezine, 1966). However, examination of individual scores show that although the group mean did not change, the range of scores did. At 18, 24, and 36 months of age the individual language scores showed the greatest range of scores of all developmental scales. Again in two cases of children with congenital hypothyroidism the verbal scores appeared to be lower than the global developmental quotient. Moschini et al. (1986) felt that perinatal risks and socioemotional conditions accounted for all children with congenital hypothyroidism who had low developmental quotients. Therefore, as in children with phenylketonuria there may be individual children who exhibit specific linguistic deficits. In some cases, however, this may relate to factors other than those directly resulting from congenital hypothyroidism.

Also like children with phenylketonuria it would appear that the majority of language impairments seen in children with hypothyroidism are associated with a decreased intellectual ability and as such are affected by those risk factors that have been documented as indicating a poor cognitive prognosis. Some studies are available to support this hypothesis. Glorieux et al. (1988) found a significantly lower verbal IQ score on the WISC-R and the Griffiths Mental Developmental Scales in a group of children with low T_4 values and retarded bone maturation before treatment. A study by Rovet et al. (1987) reported similar results in a group of children with congenital hypothyroidism, who had delayed skeletal maturity. In this study the children were assessed on a yearly basis and compared with another group of children with congenital hypothyroidism, but with normal skeletal maturity. At 12 months of age there was no difference between the two groups; however, by 2 years of age the children with delayed skeletal maturity scored significantly lower on all scales of the Griffiths Developmental Scales, including hearing and speech, even though all individual scores were within normal limits. There was no difference between groups at 2 years of age on the Receptive or Expressive Scales of the Reynell Developmental Language Scales (RDLS) (Reynell, 1977). At 4 years of age, the RDLS scores for both the receptive and expressive language scales were signif-

icantly lower for the children with congenital hypothyroidism with delayed skeletal development, as were the scores on the McCarthy Scales of Children's Abilities. By 5 years of age only the language comprehension scores on the RDLS and the motor subscore on the McCarthy Scales were significantly lower. The 5-year-old children with delayed skeletal development also scored significantly lower on the WISC-R quotients of full IQ and performance IQ (but not verbal IQ) and the WISC-R subtests, vocabulary geometric design and block design. Lower scores were also obtained on the Beery Buktenica Development Test of Motor Integration. This led Rovet et al. (1987) to conclude that children with congenital hypothyroidism who have delayed skeletal maturity have specific deficits in neuromotor, perceptual, and language aspects of intellectual functioning. As it was the RDLS comprehension score and the vocabulary subtest of the WISC-R that were significantly lower it may be that these language scores only represent a generalized cognitive deficit rather than a specific linguistic deficit. Therefore more research into the linguistic abilities of children with congenital hypothyroidism is required before definitive statements can be made about specific language deficits, even in the group of children with congenital hypothyroidism and delayed bone maturation.

The other aspect of congenital hypothyroidism that may result in communication disorders is neurologic impairments which are often noted in the literature. Several studies report motor impairments in children with congenital hypothyroidism when compared with matched controls (Murphy et al., 1986; New England Congenital Hypothyroidism Collaborative, 1985;

Rovet et al., 1987). As yet, no studies have assessed articulation or oromotor skills in children with congenital hypothyroidism.

Hypotonia was evident in 73% of the hypothyroid cases studied by Moschini et al. (1986) when examined at 33 ± 12 days of age. Nineteen percent of the cases studied by Moschini et al. (1986) also presented with feeding problems. Feeding problems were also reported by Thompson et al. (1986); 10% were in the ectopic gland group and 44% were in the athyrotic group.

Frost and Parkin (1986) listed the major neurologic problems in subjects with congenital hypothyroidism including: poor fine motor coordination, squints, and nystagmus and speech impairment in both children and adults. They reported that 22% of children and 18% of adults had received speech therapy, and 38% of children and 28% of adults presented with dysarthria. Furthermore, 37% of the children and 26% of adults with congenital hypothyroidism had three or more signs of cerebellar dysfunction (i.e., "intention tremor, dysdiadochokinesis, poor coordination, ataxia, abnormalities of balance and Romberg's sign, dysarthria, nystagmus") (Frost & Parkin, 1986, p. 483). Frost (1986) suggested that the cerebellum may be affected in utero by thyroxine deficiency causing motor coordination to be more affected than cognitive functioning even if early treatment is available.

Therefore, the role of the speech-language pathologist in cases of congenital hypothyroidism may be in monitoring language development and conducting parent education programs, especially for those children with risk factors for a poor prognosis. A greater involvement, however, may be required with the hypothyroid cases that present with impaired neurological functioning at the early stages in the area of feeding and later in the treatment of their dysarthria.

References

Anderson, P. J., Wood, S. J., Francis, D. E., Coleman, L., Anderson, V., & Boneh, A. (2007). Are neuropsychological impairments in children with early treated phenylketonuria (PKU) related to white matter abnormalities or elevated phenylalanine levels? *Developmental Neuropsychology, 32,* 645–668.

Anderson, V. (2007). Childhood white matter injuries: What are the issues? *Developmental Neuropsychology, 32,* 619–623.

Anderson, V., Northam, E., Hendy, E., & Wrennall, J. (2001). *Developmental neuropsychology: A clinical approach.* Philadelphia, PA: Taylor & Francis.

Antshel, K. M., Epstein, I. O., & Waisbren, S. E. (2004). Cognitive strengths and weaknesses in children and adolescents homozygous for the galactosemia Q188R mutation: A descriptive study. *Neuropsychology, 18,* 658–664.

Antshel, K., & Waisbren, S. (2003). Developmental timing of exposure to elevated levels of phenylalanine is associated with ADHD symptom expression. *Journal of Abnormal Child Psychology, 31,* 565–574.

Bernal, B., & Ardila, A. (2009). The role of the arcuate fasciculus in conduction aphasia. *Brain, 132,* 2309–2316.

Berry, H. K., O'Grady, D. J., Perlmutter, L. J., & Bofinger, M. K. (1979). Intellectual development and academic achievement of children early treated for phenylketonuria. *Developmental Medicine and Child Neurology, 21,* 311–320.

Berry, W. R., Darley, F. L., Aronson, A. E., & Goldstein, N. P. (1974). Dysarthria in Wilson's disease. *Journal of Speech and Hearing Research, 17,* 167–183.

Birrell, J., Frost, G. J., & Parkin, J. M. (1983). The development of children with congenital hypothyroidism. *Developmental Medicine and Child Neurology, 25,* 502–511.

Blasi, V., Longaretti, R., Giovanettoni, C., Baldoli, C., Pontesilli, S., Vigone, C., . . . Weber, G. (2009). Decreased parietal cortex activity during mental rotation in children with congenital hypothyroidism. *Neuroendocrinology, 89,* 56–65.

Boehme, G., & Theile, H. (1972). Speech disorders in phenylketonuria. *Deutsch Gesundheitsw, 27,* 561–563.

Bosch, A. M. (2006). Classical galactosaemia revisited. *Journal of Inherited Metabolic Disease, 29,* 516–525.

Bosch, A. M., Grootenhuis, M. A., Bakker, H. D., Heijmans, H. S., Wijburg, F. A., & Last, B. F. (2004). Living with classical galactosemia: Health-related quality of life consequences. *Pediatrics, 113,* e423–e428.

Brazeal, T. J., & Farmer, J. E. (1999). Natural course and treatment of neuropsychological deficits in a child with early-treated galactosemia. *Child Neuropsychology, 5,* 197–209.

Brewer, G. J. (2001). Overview of the disease for the clinician. In G. J. Brewer (Ed.), *Wilson's disease: A clinician's guide to recognition, diagnosis and management* (pp. 1–7). Boston, MA: Kluwer Academic.

Brozoski, T., Brown, R., Rosvold, H., & Goldman, P. (1979). Cognitive deficit caused by regional depletion of dopamine in prefrontal cortex of rhesus monkey. *Science, 205,* 929–932.

Brown, R. (1973). *A first language.* Cambridge, MA: Northwestern University Press.

Brunet, O., & Lezine, I. (1966). *Le développement psychologique de la premiere enfance. (Early infant psychomotor development scale)* (2nd ed.). Paris, France: Presses Universitaires de France.

Burlina, A., Bonafé, L., Ferrari, V., Suppiej, A., Zacchello, F., & Burlina, A. (2000). Measurement of neurotransmitter metabolites in cerebrospinal fluid of phenylketonuric patients under dietary treatment. *Journal of Inherited Metabolic Disease, 23,* 313–316.

Bzoch, K. R., & League, R. (1971). *Assessing language skills in infancy.* Tallahassee, FL: Anhinga Press.

Channon, S., German, C., Cassina, C., & Lee, P. (2004). Executive functioning, memory and learning in phenylketonuria. *Neuropsychology, 18,* 613–620.

Channon, S., Goodman, G., Zlotowitz, S., Mockler, C., & Lee, P. (2007). Effects of dietary management on phenylketonuria on long-term cognitive outcome. *Archives of Disease in Childhood, 92,* 213–218.

Cleary, M. A., Heptinstall, L. E., Wraith, J. E., & Walter, J. H. (1995). Galactosaemia: relationship of IQ to biochemical control and genotype. *Journal of Inherited Metabolic Disease, 18,* 151–152.

Colombini, M., Dall'Acqua, F., Vigone, M. C., Ciotti, F., Passoni, A., Maina, L., . . . Chiumello, G. (2008). Language development delay in early-treated congenital hypothyroidism affected children. *Hormone Research, 70* (Suppl. 1), 169.

de Escobar, G. M., Ruiz-Marcos, A., & Escobar del Rey, F. (1983). Thyroid hormone and the development brain. In J. H. Dassault, & P. Walker (Eds.), *Congenital hypothyroidism.* New York, NY: Marcel Dekker.

Dunn, L. M. (1965). Peabody picture vocabulary test. Circle Pines, MN: American Guidance Service.

Dussault, J. H., Letarte, J., Glorieux, J., Morissette, J., & Guyda, H. (1980). Psychological development of hypothyroid infants at age 12 and 18 months experience after neonatal screening. In G. N. Burrows (Ed.), *Neonatal thyroid screening.* New York, NY: Raven Press.

Dyer, C. A. (1999). Pathophysiology of phenylketonuria. *Mental Retardation and Development Disabilities Research Reviews, 5,* 104–112.

Elsas, L. J., II, & Lai, K. (1998). The molecular biology of galactosemia. *Genetics in Medicine, 1,* 40–48.

Fisher, H. B., & Logemann, J. A. (1971). The Fisher-Logemann test of articulation competence. Chicago, IL: Riverside.

Fridovich, J. L., & Walter, J. H. (2008). Galactosemia. In D. Valle, A. L. Beaudet, B. Vogelstein, K. W. Kinzler, S. E. Antonarakis, A. Ballabio, . . . Mitchell, G. (Eds.), *The online* metabolic and molecular bases of inherited disease. New York, NY: McGraw-Hill.

Frost, G. J. (1986). Aspects of congenital hypothyroidism. *Child Care, Health and Development, 12,* 369–375.

Frost, G. J., & Parkin, J. M. (1986). A comparison between the neurological and intellectual abnormalities in children and adults with congenital hypothyroidism. *European Journal of Pediatrics, 145,* 480–484.

Frost, G. J., Parkin, J. M., & Rowley, D. (1979). Congenital hypothyroidism. *Lancet, ii,* 1026.

Gassió, R., Fusté, E., López-Sala, A., Artuch, R., Vilaseca, M. A., & Campistol, J. (2005). School performance in early and continuously treated phenylketonuria. *Pediatric Neurology, 33,* 267–271.

Gitzelmann, R., & Steinmann, B. (1984). Galactosemia: How does long-term treatment change outcome. *Enzyme, 32,* 37–46.

Glorieux, J., Desjardins, M., Letarte, J., Morissette, J., & Dussault, J. H. (1988). Useful parameters to predict the eventual mental outcome of hypothyroid children. *Pediatric Research, 24,* 6–8.

Glorieux, J., Dussault, J. H., Morissette, J., Desjardins, M., Letarte, J., & Guyda, H. (1985). Follow-up at ages 5 and 7 years on mental development in children with hypothyroidism detected by Quebec Screening Program. *Journal of Pediatrics, 107,* 913–915.

Goldman, R., & Fristoe, M. (1969). Goldman Fristoe test of articulation. Circle Pines, MN: American Guidance Service.

Hammill, D. D., Brown, V. L., Larsen, S. C., & Wiederholt, J. L. (1987). Test of adolescent language-2: A multidimensional approach to assessment. Austin, TX: Pro-Ed.

Hammill, D. D., & Newcomer, P. L. (1982). Test of language development-intermediate. Austin, TX: Pro-Ed.

Hayes, A., Bowling, F. G., Fraser, D., Krimmer, H. L., Marrinan, A., & Clague, A. E. (1988). Neonatal screening and an intensive management programme for galactosaemia: Early evidence of benefits. *Medical Journal of Australia, 149,* 21–25.

Hayes, A., Elkins, J., Fraser, D., Bowling, F., Clague, A., Krimmer, H., . . . Marrinan, A. (1986). Galactosaemia: A preventable form of mental retardation? *Australia and New Zealand Journal of Developmental Disabilities, 12,* 235–241.

Hedrick, D. L., Prather, E. M., & Tobin, A. R. (1978). *Sequenced inventory of communication development.* Seattle, WA: University of Washington.

Hommes, F. A. (1991). On the mechanism of permanent brain dysfunction in hyperphenylalaninemia. *Biochemistry, Medicine, and Metabolic Biology, 46,* 277–287.

Hughes, J., Ryan, S., Lambert, D., Geoghegan, O., Clark, A., Rogers, Y., . . . Treacy, E. (2009). Outcomes of siblings with classical galactosemia. *Journal of Pediatrics, 154,* 721–726.

Hulse, J. A. (1984). Outcome for congenital hypothyroidism. *Archives of Disease in Childhood, 59,* 23–30.

Huttenlocher, P. R. (2000). The neuropathology of phenylketonuria: Human and animal studies. *European Journal of Pediatrics, 159* (Suppl. 2), S102–S106.

Jan, J. E., & Wilson, R. A. (1973). Unusual late neurological sequelae in galactosaemia. *Developmental Medicine and Child Neurology, 15,* 72.

Kaufman, F. R., McBride-Chang, C., Manis, F. R., Wolff, J. A., & Nelson, M. D. (1995). Cognitive functioning, neurologic status and brain imaging in classical galactosemia. *European Journal of Pediatrics, 154* (7, Suppl. 2), S2–S5.

Koch, R., Azen, C., Friedman, E. G., & Williamson, M. (1982). Preliminary report on the effects of diet discontinuation in PKU. *Journal of Pediatrics, 100,* 870–875.

Koch, R., Azen, C. Friedman, E. G., & Williamson, M. L. (1984). Paired comparisons between early treated PKU children and their matched sibling controls on intelligence and school achievement test results at eight years of age. *Journal of Inherited Metabolic Disorders, 7,* 86–90.

Koff, E., Boyle, P., & Peuschel, S. M. (1977). Perceptual-motor functioning in children with phenylketonuria. *American Journal of Diseases of Children, 131,* 1084–1087.

Komrower, G. M., & Lee, D. H. (1970). Long-term follow-up galactosemia. *Archives of Disordered Child, 45,* 367.

Lambert, C., & Boneh, A. (2004). The impact of galactosaemia on quality of life—A pilot study. *Journal of Inherited Metabolic Disease, 27,* 601–608.

Lang, C. (1989). Is Wilson's disease a dementing condition? *Journal of Clinical and Experimental Neuropsychology, 14,* 569–570.

Lauterbach, E. C. (2000). Wilson's disease. *Psychiatric Annals, 32,* 114–120.

Lee, D. H. (1972). Psychological aspects of galactosemia. *Journal of Mental Deficiency Research, 16,* 173.

Lee, L. (1974a). *Developmental Sentence Analysis.* Evanston, IL: Northwestern University Press.

Lee L. (1974b). The Northwestern syntax screening test. Evanston, IL: Harvard University Press.

Marcheschi, M., Bargagna, S., Dinetti, D., Giachetti, C., Millepiedi, S., & Nencioli, R. (1997). Neuropsychological follow-up for pre-school children with early-treated congenital hypothyroidism: A proposal for a methodological revision. *Giornale di Neuropsichiatria dell eta Evolutiva, 17,* 146–151.

Melnick, C. R., Michals, K. K. & Matalon, R. (1981). Linguistic development of children with phenylketonuria and normal intelligence. *Journal of Pediatrics, 98,* 269–272.

Menkes, J. H., & Wilcox, W. R. (2006). Inherited metabolic diseases of the nervous system. In J. H. Menkes, H. B. Sarnat, & B. L. Maria (Eds.), *Child neurology* (7th ed., pp. 29–141). Philadelphia, PA: Lippincott, Williams, & Wilkins.

Moschini, L., Costa, P., Marinelli, E., Maggioni, G., Sorcini Carta, M., Fazzini, G., . . . Brinciotti, M. (1986). Longitudinal assessment of children with congenital hypothyroidism detected by neonatal screening. *Helvetia Paediatricia Acta, 41,* 415–424.

Murphy, G., Hulse, J. A., Jackson, D., Tyrer, P., Glossop, J., Smith, I., . . . Grant, D. (1986). Early treated hypothyroidism: Development at 3 years. *Archives of Disease in Childhood, 61,* 761–765.

Nelson, C. D., Waggoner, D. D., Donnell, G. N., Tuerck, J. M., & Buist, N. R. M. (1991). Verbal dyspraxia in treated galactosemia. *Pediatrics, 88,* 346–350.

Netley, C., Hanley, E. B., & Rudner, H. L. (1984). Phenylketonuria and its variants: Observations on intellectual functioning. *Canadian Medical Association Journal, 131,* 751–755.

Newcomer, P. L., & Hammill, D. D. (1987). Test of language development-primary. Austin, TX: Pro-Ed.

New England Congenital Hypothyroidism Collaborative. (1985). Neonatal hypothyroidism screening: Status of patients at 6 years of age. *Journal of Pediatrics, 107,* 915–918.

Ozanne, A. E., Krimmer, H., & Murdoch, B. E. (1990). Speech and language skills in children with early treated phenylketonuria. *American Journal on Mental Retardation, 94,* 625–632.

Pennington, B. F., & Smith, S. D. (1983). Genetic influence on learning disabilities and speech and language disorders. *Child Development, 54,* 369–387.

Pennington, B. F., van Doornick, W. J., McCabe, L. L., & McCabe, E. R. B. (1985). Neurological deficits in early treated phenylketonuric children. *American Journal of Mental Deficiency, 89,* 467–475.

Pietz, J. (1998). Neurological aspects of adult phenylketonuria. *Current Opinions in Neurology, 11,* 679–688.

Portala, K., Levander, S., Westermark, E., Ekselius, L., & von Knorring, L. (2001). Pattern of neuropsychological deficits in patients with treated Wilson's disease. *European Archives of Psychiatry and Clinical Neuroscience, 251,* 262–268.

Potter, N. L., Lazarus, J-A. C., Johnson, J. M., Steiner, R. D., & Shriberg, L. D. (2008). Correlates of language impairment in children with galactosaemia. *Journal of Inherited Metabolic Disease, 31,* 524–532.

Reynell, J. (1977). Reynell developmental language scales-revised. Oxford, UK: NFER.

Robertson, A., Singh, R. H., Guerrero, N. V., Hundley, M., & Elsas, L. J. (2000). Outcomes analysis of verbal dyspraxia in classic galactosemia. *Genetics in Medicine, 2*, 142–148.

Rosenberg, R. N., & Pettegrew, J. W. (1980). Genetic diseases of the nervous system. In R. N. Rosenberg (Ed.), *Neurology* (Vol. 5). New York, NY: Grune & Stratton.

Rosselli, M., Lorenzana, P., Rosselli, A., & Vergara, I. (1987). Wilson's disease, a reversible dementia: Case report. *Journal of Clinical and Experimental Neuropsychology, 9*, 399–406.

Rovet, J., & Brown, R. (2007). Congenital hypothyroidism: Genetic and biochemical influences on brain development and neuropsychological functioning. In M. M. Mazzocco & J. L. Ross (Eds.), *Neurogenetic developmental disorders: Variations of manifestation in childhood* (pp. 265–295). Cambridge, MA: M.I.T. Press.

Rovet, J., Ehrlich, R., & Sorbara, D. (1987). Intellectual outcome in children with fetal hypothyroidism. *Journal of Pediatrics, 110*, 700–704.

Sack, J., Elicer, A., Sofrin, R., Theodor, R., & Cohen, B. (1986). Influence on psychological development of early treatment of congenital hypothyroidism detected by neonatal screening: A controlled study. *Israel Journal of Medical Sciences, 22*, 24–28.

Salerno, M., Militerni, R., Di Maio, S., Bravaccio, C., Gasparini, N., & Tenore, A. (1999). Intellectual outcome at 12 years of age in congenital hypothyroidism. *European Journal of Endocrinology, 141*, 105–110.

Sawaguchi, T., & Goldman-Rakic, P. (1991). D1 dopamine receptors in prefrontal cortex involvement in working memory. *Science, 251*, 947–950.

Schadewaldt, P., Hoffmann, B., Hammen, H-W., Kamp, G., Schweitzer-Krantz, S., & Wendel, U. (2010). Longitudinal assessment of intellectual achievement in patients with classical galactosemia. *Pediatrics, 125*, e374–e381.

Schweitzer, S., Shin, Y., Jakobs, C., & Brodehl, J. (1993). Long-term outcome in 134 patients with galactosaemia. *European Journal of Pediatrics, 152*, 36–43.

Schweitzer-Krantz, S. (2003). Early diagnosis of inherited metabolic disorders towards improving outcome: The controversial issue of galactosaemia. *European Journal of Pediatrics, 162*(Suppl. 1), S50–S53.

Seashore, M. R., Friedman, E., Novelly, R. A., & Bapat, V. (1985) Loss of intellectual function in children with phenylketonuria after relaxation of dietary phenylalanine restriction. *Pediatrics, 75*, 226–232.

Shield, J. P., Wadsworth, E. J., MacDonald, A., Stephenson, A., Tyfield, L., Holton, J. B., . . . Marlow, N. (2000). The relationship of genotype to cognitive outcome in galactosaemia. *Archives of Disease in Childhood, 83* , 248–250.

Simons, W. F., Fuggle, P. W., Grant, D. B., & Smith, I. (1994). Intellectual development at 10 years in early treated congenital hypothyroidism. *Archives of Disease in Childhood, 71*, 232–234.

Thompson, G. N., McCrossin, R. B., Penfold, J. L., Woodroffe, P., Rose, W. A., & Robertson, E. F. (1986). Management and outcome of children with congenital hypothyroidism detected on neonatal screening in South Australia. *Medical Journal of Australia, 145*, 18–22.

Vogel, F. (1985). Phenotypic deviations in heterozygotes of phenylketonuria (PKU). *Progress in Clinical and Biological Research, 177*, 337–349.

Waggoner, D. D., Buist, N. R. M., & Donnell, G. N. (1990). Long-term prognosis in galactosaemia: Results of a survey of 350 cases. *Journal of Inherited Metabolic Disease, 13*, 802–818.

Waisbren, S. E., Norman, T. R., Schnell, R. R., & Levy, H. L. (1983). Speech and language deficits in early-treated children with galactosaemia. *Journal of Pediatrics, 102*, 75–77.

Waisbren, S. E., Schnell, R. R., & Levy, H. L. (1980). Diet termination in children with phenylketonuria: A review of psychological assessments used to determine outcome. *Journal of Inherited Metabolic Diseases, 3,* 149–153.

Webb, A. L., Singh, R. H., Kennedy, M. J., & Elsas, L. J. (2003). Verbal dyspraxia and galactosemia. *Pediatric Research, 53,* 396–402.

Wechsler, D. (1974). The Wechsler intelligence scale for children-revised. New York, NY: Psychological Press.

Welsh, M., Pennington, B., Ozonoff, S., Rouse, B., & McCabe, E. (1990). Neuropsychology of early-treated phenylketonuria: Specific executive function deficits. *Child Development, 61,* 1697–1713.

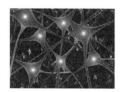  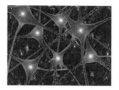

6

Language Disorders in Childhood Infectious Diseases

Introduction

Many different pathogens may invade the developing central nervous system (CNS) and are usually associated with high morbidity and mortality. Most varieties of intracranial infection have a diffuse effect and hence produce rather widespread neurologic symptomatology and any associated language disorder is nonspecific (i.e., does not fit into any of the historic aphasia syndromes) in nature and, therefore, liable to be lost among other neurobehavioral and cognitive dysfunctions. Occasionally, however, speech-language pathologists do encounter a child who presents with a significant aphasia in association with focal brain lesions of infectious origin. For example, localized bacterial infections in the frontal or temporal lobes may give rise to the formation of an intracerebral abscess leading to disrupted language function. Aphasia syndromes in children also, on occasion,

have been reported in association with specific CNS infections (e.g., herpes simplex encephalitis).

Infectious diseases of the CNS are classified according to the type of infecting organism and by the major site of involvement. Infections of the nervous system can be caused by viruses, bacteria, protozoa, and fungi. They may affect the lining of the brain (meninges), cerebrospinal fluid (CSF), brain parenchyma, spinal cord, nerve roots, peripheral nerves, or muscles. Infections of the CNS can be divided into meningitis, encephalitis, focal suppernation, or inflammation. Meningitis involves inflammation of the leptomeninges (pia and arachnoid mater) and the subarachnoid space. Encephalitis is infection and inflammation within the brain parenchyma. Focal infection causes abscess formation within or immediately adjacent to the brain or spinal cord. Occasionally infections involve multiple sites such as the brain, meninges, spinal cord, nerve roots, and so forth. In such cases descriptive compound names are used (e.g., meningoencephalitis, meningomyelitis, encephalomyelitis, meningoencephalomyelitis). Neurologic disturbances may also arise as a consequence of direct infection or from a secondary parainfectious immune-mediated mechanism.

The clinical presentation of infections of the nervous system can be highly variable, ranging from acute, rapidly developing meningitis or encephalitis leading to death within hours, to the development of disease many years after the initial infection. The spectrum of neurologic manifestation is also highly variable, ranging from signs of meningeal infection such as fever, headache, neck stiffness and impaired consciousness, to signs of cortical and subcortical dysfunction, or involvement of the spinal cord, peripheral nerves, or muscles. The diagnosis of infectious disorders of the CNS requires laboratory analysis, including isolation and molecular detection of the specific pathogen and the identification of organism-specific serologic or pathologic abnormalities. In recent years, new techniques of molecular diagnosis, in particular wider availability of polymerase chain reaction assay to detect bacterial and viral nucleic acid in CSF and improved neuroimaging of the brain and spinal cord have enhanced the detection and diagnosis of neurologic infections. Furthermore, there have been important developments of new therapies targeted toward specific pathogens such as antiretrovirus therapy.

Meningitis

Inflammation of the leptomeninges can be caused by bacteria, viruses, parasites, and fungi as well as by noninfectious conditions including inflammatory disorders (e.g., systemic lupus erythematosis or Kawasaki disease) and neoplasia (e.g., leukemic meningitis) (Saez-Llorens & McCraken, 2003). Historically, meningitis due to viruses and certain other nonbacterial pathogens has been designated "aseptic meningitis."

Clinical Presentation

Meningitis may evolve as a sudden onset and rapidly developing illness over a few hours, particularly in children, but progression is variable and less commonly can be a progressive subacute infection worsening over several days. The leptomeninges should be suspected as a site of infection in childhood illnesses whenever the child's presenting signs and symptoms include fever, headache, altered states of consciousness ranging from drowsiness to coma, irritability, a high-pitched cry in infants, neck stiffness (especially inability to touch chin to chest), back stiffness (inability to sit normally), positive Kernig's sign (inability to extend knee when the leg is flexed anteriorly at the hip), positive Brudzinski's sign (flexion of the lower extremity with the head bent forward), projectile vomiting, and shock. Other CNS signs may include bulging fontanelles, increased diplopia, increased CSF pressure, constriction of visual fields, papilledema, slow pulse rate, and irregular respiration. Seizures may be focal or generalized and may occur at presentation or at any time during the course of bacterial meningitis in up to 40% of patients. They may arise from focal arterial or venous infarction, hemorrhage, localized cerebral edema, or as a consequence of systemic features including pyrexia, septicemia, shock, toxicity, or other metabolic derangement. Meningitis may lead to vascular occlusion and subsequent brain infarction, progressive cranial nerve lesions, and hydrocephalus secondary to impaired CSF absorption and obstruction.

Clinically, pathologic signs of meningeal infection depend on the underlying etiology and may include petechial or purpuric rashes, conjunctivitis, arthritis, myocarditis, a history of upper respiratory tract infection or otitis, urinary tract or other localized infection, jaundice, abluminuria, and oliguria. Laboratory findings are required to establish an accurate diagnosis of CNS infections, especially meningitis. Examination of the CSF will include cultures, glucose levels (decreased), lactic acid content (increased), protein (increased), and white blood count (increased). Results of these laboratory investigations provide the best indication of neurologic damage and help to determine prognosis as well as final diagnosis.

Bacterial Meningitis

Bacterial meningitis is the most common CNS infection in childhood and is caused by a primary infection within the subarachnoid space that causes acute inflammation of the pia and arachnoid mater. It may present with few or many of the signs and symptoms indicated above, depending on the specific causative organism and the severity of the infection.

The pathogens causing pediatric bacterial meningitis vary according to the age of the child. The organisms which are most frequently responsible for bacterial meningitis among children and adolescents include *Haemophilus influenzae* type b (HIB), *Neisseria meningitidis* (meningococcal

meningitis) a gram-negative diplococcus, and *Streptococcus pneumoniae* (pneumococcal meningitis) a gram-positive diplococcus. In those countries with active immunization programs for HIB, however, the incidence of HIB meningitis has declined dramatically. Prior to the development of a HIB vaccine, it was estimated that as many as 1 in every 400 children between 1 and 4 years of age experienced meningitis due to this organism, with HIB meningitis accounting for 75 to 80% of pediatric cases of bacterial meningitis (Sell, 1987). In newborns *Streptococcus agalactiae* (group B streptococcus), *Escherichia coli*, *Staphylococcus* species, *Listeria monocytogenes*, and *Pseudomonas aeruginosa* are the most frequent causes of bacterial meningitis.

Neisseria Meningitidis (Meningococcal Meningitis)

Currently this is the most commonly identified cause of meningitis in children and young adults with an incidence of 1 to 1.5 per 100,000. In many countries, meningococcal disease remains the leading infectious cause of death in childhood with a mortality of approximately 10%. It is the only type of meningitis that may occur in larger community-wide outbreaks and hence is a notifiable disease in many countries. Transmission of pathogenic bacteria occurs by respiratory droplet spread, particularly through close contact with the carrier. Approximately 5 to 10% of all adults are asymptomatic nasopharyngeal carriers of these pathogenic bacteria. There is a high risk of family members developing the disease and all household close contacts should be treated to eradicate nasopharyngeal carriage.

Clinical manifestations of meningococcal infection may develop within minutes or hours. In approximately 40% of patients there is isolated meningitis; 10% develop septicemia alone and the remainder a mixed pattern. Isolated meningococcal meningitis carries a better prognosis than when occurring in combination with septicemia. Clinically, sudden onset meningococcal meningitis is characterized by pyrexia, headache, and signs of meningeal infection such as nausea, vomiting, photophobia, and progressive lethargy. In early meningococcal meningitis there is a diffuse erythematous macular papular rash which eventually develops into the characteristic petechiae found across the trunk and lower extremities in the mucous membranes, conjunctiva, and occasionally on the palms and soles. The development of meningococcal septicemia is associated with progressive vasomotor disturbance culminating in profound hypotension, tachycardia, and a rising respiratory rate indicating pulmonary edema or raised intracranial pressure resulting from cerebral edema. The mortality associated with meningococcal meningitis rises to 40% in those with meningococcal septicemia. Up to 20% may have neurologic sequelae including hearing loss, loss of limbs secondary to large vessel vasculitis and neurologic disability (including cognitive and linguistic deficits) resulting from cerebral ischemia.

Streptococcus Pneumoniae (Pneumococcal Meningitis)

This is the most common cause of meningitis in adults over the age of 18 years, although child cases do occur. Fatality rate is approximately 20%. As in meningococcal meningitis, the primary site of colonization is the nasopharynx with spread occurring via respiratory droplet infection. Pneumococcal meningitis is also commonly caused by local extension from otitis media, or a paranasal source of infection, following a skull base fracture or sinus injury with dural tear. Other predisposing features include pneumonia, alcoholism, diabetes, immunodeficiency states (e.g., splenectomy, hypogammaglobulinemia, HIV). Clinical presentation is similar to other forms of pyogenic (pus-forming) meningitis although a coexisting pneumococcal pneumonia may be present. Residual neurological sequelae are common, with approximately 35% of children surviving pneumococcal meningitis exhibiting negative neurologic sequelae including hearing loss among other neurologic complications.

Haemophilus Influenzae

HIB is a small gram-negative coccabacillus. Although, as indicated above, prior to HIB vaccination this was the most common cause of meningitis in children, the incidence has declined since the introduction of widespread vaccination. Currently HIB meningitis occurs almost exclusively in unimmunized children younger than 6 years of age, although cases have been described in neonates or apparently healthy adults. The condition occurs as a consequence of respiratory droplet spread. Risk factors include otitis media, head trauma, previous neurosurgery or a CSF leak. Presentation may be with acute meningitis although vasculitis may also occur leading to focal signs.

The most common neurologic sequelae of HIB meningitis is hearing loss which affects approximately 11% of surviving children. Hearing deficits range from mild to profound hearing loss and are more common in children who began treatment 24 hours or more after onset of symptoms. Approximately 15% of survivors of HIB meningitis also exhibit other negative neurologic sequelae such as learning disability, focal neurologic deficits, epilepsy, cortical blindness, and mental retardation.

Pathogenesis

The fundamental pathologic process in bacterial meningitis is inflammation of the leptomeninges. Bacteria can reach the leptomeninges in several different ways including: Passage through the choroid plexus and/or cerebral capillaries to the CSF; hematogenous spread (via the bloodstream); rupture of superficial cortical abscesses; or contiguous spread from an adjacent infection (e.g., osteomyelitis of the cranial bones).

In most instances bacterial meningitis begins with bacterial colonization of the nasopharynx by attaching to epithelial cells. The bacteria pass across the epithelium cells into the intravascular space. Those that survive in the bloodstream then gain access to the CSF via the choroid plexus epithelium or cerebral capillaries by disrupting intercellular tight junctions or causing endothelial cell injuries. Once in the CSF the bacteria rapidly multiply inducing inflammation of the leptomeninges. This, in turn, increases the permeability of the blood-brain barrier allowing plasma proteins to enter the CSF enhancing the inflammatory response and contributes purulent exudates to the subarachnoid space. Worsening exudates penetrate arterial walls leading to intimal thickening and large vessel constriction, eventually culminating in cerebral ischemia and possible infarction. Finally, the purulent exudate can reduce resorption of CSF by the arachnoid villi or obstruct the flow of CSF through the ventricular system leading to hydrocephalus and interstitial cerebral edema.

Hematogenous spread involves the passive transfer of bacteria by infected leukocytes. Organisms can also enter the CNS from damaged blood vessels, via neurosurgical procedures or via compound fractures of the skull. Risk factors for the development of bacterial meningitis therefore include: Penetrating cranial trauma; foreign bodies within the CNS (e.g., CSF shunts); defects in the mucocutaneous barrier (e.g., skull base fractures); and defects in the immune system (e.g., splenectomy, HIV, etc.)

Treatment

The life-threatening nature of bacterial meningitis and the potential for permanent neurodevelopmental sequelae demands that antibiotic therapy be instituted as soon as diagnosis is suspected. The specific antibiotics used are dependent on the nature of the pathogen as well as on factors such as any known allergies (e.g., the child may be allergic to penicillin) the child may have to certain antibiotics. In addition, the treatment of certain types of meningitis has recently been complicated by the development of antibiotic resistant strains of pathogens. For example, penicillin-resistant strains of pneumococcal infection have now been identified requiring the use of alternative antibiotics such as vancomycin in the treatment of pneumococcal meningitis (for detailed reviews of the treatment of bacterial meningitis see Saez-Llorens & McCracken, 2003; Wubbel & McCracken, 1998). Adjunctive management of infants and children with suspected or proven bacterial meningitis includes control of increased intracranial pressure, treatment of seizures, correction of electrolyte disturbances, treatment of fever, and close monitoring of subdural effusions and severe systemic complications such as hemorrhagic purpura or renal failure.

Prognosis

Three principal factors influence the outcome of pediatric bacterial meningitis. These include: The age of the child; the species of the bacterial pathogen; and the duration of the disease before the initiation of appropriate antibiotic therapy. In general, neonates have a less favorable prognosis regardless of the pathogen, as do older children with pneumococcal meningitis. Most, but not all, studies also indicate that negative sequelae are more likely in children who diagnosis and treatment are delayed.

The advent of antibiotics (e.g., penicillin, chloramphenicol, etc.) has greatly reduced the mortality rate of bacterial meningitis from about 90% to less than 10% (Dodge, 1986; Sell, 1987). Despite this reduction in the mortality rate, there is, however, a body of research to indicate that bacterial meningitis is associated with a high incidence of permanent neurologic sequelae, including speech, language, and hearing disorders, in those children who survive the disease. Therefore, as noted by Tejani, Tobias, and Sambursky (1982), the reduction in mortality rate has not been matched with a decrease in morbidity. The most common negative outcome of bacterial meningitis is sensorineural hearing loss which has been observed in 8.5% of surviving children. In addition children who survive bacterial meningitis may also exhibit learning disabilities, motor problems, and speech and language delay, hyperactiv-

ity, blindness, obstructive hydrocephalus, and recurrent seizures.

Viral Meningitis (Aseptic Meningitis)

Viral meningitis in children is characterized by fever, abrupt onset of frontal headaches, vomiting, irritability, and physical findings of meningeal irritation such as Kernig and Brudzinski signs. Although pyrexia, neck stiffness, and meningeal signs are present, children with this condition are generally less unwell than those with bacterial meningitis and long-term negative sequelae, including cognitive and language impairments much less likely. Nonpolio enteroviruses by far are the most common cause of viral meningitis including coxsackie and echovirus strains. Symptoms of viral meningitis usually resolve spontaneously within 2 weeks regardless of the causative agent. Treatment, therefore, primarily involves supportive care once appropriate tests have been conducted to rule out the possibility of bacterial meningitis.

Encephalitis

Encephalitis involves acute infection of the parenchyma of the brain, usually caused by a virus, which results in a diffuse inflammatory process, often also involving the meninges. The annual incidence of viral encephalitis in the United States has been estimated to be between 3.5 to 7.4 per 100,000 of the population. Viral infections can affect the CNS in three ways: hematogenous (blood-borne) dissemination of a systemic viral infection (e.g., arthropod-borne viruses); neuronal spread of the virus by axonal transport (e.g., herpes simplex, rabies); and autoimmune post-infectious demyelination (e.g., varicella, rubella, influenza). The presenting signs of encephalitis include lethargy, coma, seizures, headache, nausea, vomiting, and cerebral edema.

A wide spectrum of etiologic agents may cause viral encephalitis, and diagnosis and management are dependent on identifying specific causative agents. In children, viral encephalitis is most commonly caused by childhood exanthems (mumps, varicella, measles, rubella), arthropod-borne agents (e.g., eastern equine encephalitis, Lyme disease, West Nile encephalitis), and herpes simplex.

Herpes Simplex

Herpes simplex encephalitis is the most common acute encephalitis seen in most western countries with an annual incidence of 1 in 250,000 to 1 in 500,000. It affects all ages and both sexes equally. Early antiviral treatment (usually high-dose aciclovir) significantly reduces mortality (from around 70 to 20%), but morbidity remains unacceptably high. Most cases of herpes simplex encephalitis are caused by oral herpes (herpes simplex virus—type 1) but genital herpes (herpes simplex virus—type 2) is more common in neonates with disseminated disease. The condition may occur during primary infection or, more commonly, recurrent infection. Primary infection usually develops in the oropharyngeal mucosa before the virus is transported via retrograde transneuronal spread via the olfactory or trigeminal nerves.

The herpes virus leads to inflammation, infection, and necrotizing lesions particularly in the inferior and medial temporal lobes which also may involve the orbital frontal cortex and limbic structures. The onset of herpes simplex encephalitis involves fever, headache, and alteration of consciousness which may develop gradually or rapidly over a matter of hours. The most common manifestations are personality change, aphasia (usually a Wernicke-type aphasia) with progressive behavioral disturbance and occasionally psychotic features. Less typical features include the development of hemiparesis or a visual field defect (particularly superior quadrantic). Focal or generalized seizures are often associated with olfactory or gustatory hallucinations.

Arthropod-Borne Viruses (Arboviruses)

Arthropod-borne (arbo) viruses are RNA viral agents transmitted between susceptible vertebrate hosts by means of blood-sucking arthropods (e.g., mosquitoes, ticks). Approximately 200 viruses have been tentatively classified into this group with at least 51 having been associated with human disease. These infections show considerable geographic variation and their epidemiology is largely determined by the nature and lifestyle of the vector. Most of the infections are sustained in wild animals, with transmission through humans and domestic animals being usually incidental and insignificant in the natural history of the virus.

Arboviruses of particular relevance in the United States include among others: eastern equine encephalitis, western equine encephalitis, St. Louis encephalitis, Colorado tick fever, West Nile virus, and Lyme disease. In Australia, Murray Valley encephalitis is representative of endemic arbovirus infections. Given the increase in international travel, clinicians need also to take into account potential arbovirus infections endemic to countries visited by their clients such as dengue virus in South East Asia, South America, and the Indian subcontinent.

Childhood Exanthems (Mumps, Varicella, Rubella, etc.)

The establishment of effective immunization programs in many countries has seen a major decline in the incidence of these childhood disorders. Consequently, their importance as potential causes of viral encephalitis has declined. For example, mumps was once the most common cause of CNS involvement by any of the contagious diseases of childhood prior to the widespread use of mumps immunization.

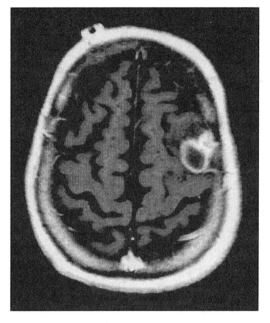

FIGURE 6-1. MRI scan showing the presence of a brain abscess in the left parietal lobe.

Focal CNS Infections: Brain Abscess

Although relatively uncommon, brain abscess represents a life-threatening infection in children. A brain abscess arises from a focal pyogenic (pus-forming) infection occurring within the cerebral parenchyma and consists of localized free or encapsulated pus within the brain substance (Figure 6–1). It develops as a result of contiguous spread of infection from paranasal sinuses, mastoiditis, otitis media, osteomyelitis, or following postoperative and post-traumatic infections. Less commonly, it may arise as a result of hematogenous spread from distant sites including the teeth and lungs, or in association with a cardiopulmonary malfunction, most commonly cyanotic congenital heart disease.

Abscesses resulting from hematogenous spread can be localized within any part of the brain, but most commonly occur in the distribution of the middle cerebral artery at the junction of gray and white matter of the cerebral hemispheres. By contrast, abscesses derived from contiguous sources tend to be superficial and close to the infected bone or dura. Multiple abscesses may occur in children where sepsis or congenital heart disease is the predisposing cause. Brain abscesses that arise from dental, frontal, or ethmoid sinuses tend to involve the frontal lobe whereas those arising from the sphenoid sinuses or otitic infection particularly involve the temporal lobes. Cerebral abscesses resulting from hematogenous spread tend to occur as multiple rather than single abscesses, often in the region of greatest blood flow, within the basal ganglia.

The onset of clinical features in most cases of brain abscess is gradual and in the initial stages the clinical picture may be nonspecific. The first signs often include a complex of fever, headache, vomiting, and seizures. As the abscess progresses more focal neurologic signs including papilledema, lateralizing signs such as hemiparesis or homonymous hemianopia and, depending on the location of the abscess, aphasia become more evident. Furthermore, more obvious indications of increased intracranial pressure develop. On occasion, a more rapid onset of neurological symptoms suggestive of a space-occupying lesion or cerebral infarction is present.

Untreated brain abscess is usually fatal, either as a consequence of decompensated increased intracranial pressure or from rupture of the abscess into the ventricular system. Sudden rupture is marked by a sudden high fever, meningeal signs, and deterioration of consciousness. Treatment involves the use of antibiotics and surgical evacuation of the abscess.

Parasitic Infections of the CNS

A large number of protozoal and helminthic infections are important causes of CNS disease, particularly in immunosuppressed individuals. These disorders also show considerable geographical variation, their incidence varying greatly in different regions of the world.

Protozoal Infections

Protozoal infections constitute some of the most important causes of childhood mortality and morbidity worldwide. These disorders include diseases such as malaria and toxoplasmosis among others. Malaria is the most important parasitic disease of humans with estimates that greater than 5% of the world population has been infected. Malaria is caused by the protozoan *Plasmodium falciparum* or another *Plasmodium* species that is transferred to humans by the female *Anopheles* mosquito. Clinical features include fever, chills, myalgia, nausea and vomiting, anemia, renal failure, hypoglycemia, and pulmonary edema. The vast majority of deaths from malaria and long-term neurologic impairments are caused by cerebral malaria, which is the most common, severe, and potentially fatal complication of the infection.

The clinical severity of malaria is highly dependent on the malaria-specific immune status of the infected individual. In malaria-endemic countries, cerebral malaria most commonly affects young children. However, in nonendemic areas and in nonimmune travelers who acquire malaria, cerebral malaria can occur at any age. Although in the past it was assumed that individuals who recover from acute cerebral malaria had no negative sequelae, it is now recognized that a significant proportion of survivors are left with long-term negative neurologic sequelae. Cerebral malaria, therefore, is an important cause of long-term childhood neurologic disability in many countries.

Toxoplasmosis results from ingestion of *Toxoplasma gondii*, an intracellular protozoan whose definitive hosts include members of the cat family with humans acting as intermediate hosts. Human infection occurs by ingestion of oocytes in cat feces and the ingestion of tissue cysts in undercooked meat. In healthy individuals the condition is usually asymptomatic although an acute mononucleosis-like illness develops occasionally. Unfortunately, the protozoan has the capacity to cross the placenta to cause intrauterine infection of the developing fetus. The majority of infants with intrauterine infection lack symptoms at birth but later develop ophthalmologic or neurologic sequelae. Symptomatic neonates exhibit jaundice, splenomegaly, hepatomegaly, fever, anemia, chorioretinitis, hydrocephalus, or microcephaly and petechiae secondary to thrombocytopenia. Furthermore, toxoplasmosis may also manifest as a severe disease in immunocompromised individuals.

Helminthic Infections

This group of parasitic infections produce symptoms of space-occupying lesions or damage to the CNS caused by the migration of worm larvae through the substance of the brain. Some of the more important helminthic infections that can cause neurologic dysfunction in children are neurocysticercosis, echinococcosis (hydatid disease), and angiostrongyliasis among others. Of these only neurocysticercosis is relatively common in western countries, including the United States and Europe.

Neurocysticercosis is caused by infection of the human brain by the larvae of the pork tapeworm (*Taenia solium*) through the ingestion of eggs from contaminated water, food or by spread from food handlers who harbor the adult parasites in their intestines. Once ingested the larvae undergo hematogenous dissemination, forming cysts in various organs of the body, including the CNS. In particular cysts may develop in the brain parenchyma, subarachnoid space, ventricular system or spinal cord. Parenchymatous cysts develop in the cerebral cortex or the basal ganglia due to the relatively high blood flow to these areas of the brain. Neurologic manifestations of neurocysticercosis result from the space-occupying mass effect of the intraparenchymal cysts as they develop, obstruction of CSF flow by intraventricular cysts, or inflammation that causes basilar meningitis. They include seizures, headache, focal neurologic signs including cognitive and language impairments, hydrocephalus, myelopathy, and subacute meningitis.

Congenital and Perinatal Infectious Diseases Affecting the CNS

The capacity to cross the placental barrier has long been recognized as a characteristic of the TORCH group of infections: toxoplasmosis, rubella, cytomegalovirus (CMV), herpes simplex, hepatitis B, syphilis, and others. Such maternal infections are well known causes of CNS disorders in the infant. Hearing loss is common in affected infants and mental retardation, blindness, and less severe forms of CNS involvement are possible sequelae. The TORCH syndromes occur as a result of intrauterine infection generally in the first trimester. However, the CMV appears to have the potential to affect the fetus beyond the first trimester. Other infections may also occur relatively late in pregnancy and affect the fetus. Table 6–1 lists infections known to affect the human fetus or neonates.

ual functional disability and long-term monitoring is necessary. In many cases cause and effect relationships are difficult to ascribe with any degree of certainty or statistical reliability.

Long-Term Sequelae of CNS Infections in Childhood

In all types of CNS infection residual impairment of CNS function may range from nil to subtle to severe. Children may have peripheral hearing loss or central auditory processing dysfunction leading to varying degrees of learning disability. In some instances selective attention problems may occur and children may be hyperactive with significant behavioral problems. Pragmatic skills may be disordered or language development may be delayed. In the extreme instance intellectual retardation will result. Disturbances in equilibrium may lead to delays in motor skill development. The apparent severity of CNS infection does not correlate with resid-

Linguistic Disorders in Childhood Infectious Diseases of the CNS

Linguistic Deficits Associated with Childhood Encephalitis

No study to date has systemically evaluated the linguistic outcome of a group of children who had suffered encephalitis. Such cases, however, have often been included in studies of acquired childhood aphasia of mixed etiology (Cooper & Flowers, 1987; Van Hout, Evrard, & Lyon, 1985). In such studies, however, the specific outcomes attributable to the encephalitis are usually lost in the group results. The few individual case studies reported in the literature in combination with the case descriptions included within the group data, however,

Table 6-1. Infections Able to Produce Disease in the Human Fetus or Neonate (ranging from subclinical to severe multifacet CNS involvement)

Arboviruses	Toxoplasmosis (protozoal)
Coxsackie B virus	Syphilis
Cytomegalovirus	Echovirus
Herpes simplex	Coxsackie A virus
Varicella zoster	Measles
Influenza	*Streptococcus*
Polioviruses	*Escherichia coli*
Rubella	Hepatitis B

do give some idea of the prognosis after encephalitis. In most reported cases the encephalitis associated with the occurrence of linguistic deficits has resulted from the herpes simplex virus.

From these case descriptions we can see the effects of encephalitis in the acute and recovery stages and then judge the outcome by assessing long-term deficits. For the sake of discussion the acute stage is taken to represent the period while the child is still hospitalized. One deficit frequently described in the acute stages of encephalitis is impaired comprehension. This has been described as a severe comprehension deficit similar to that seen in global aphasia. Two cases described by Cooper and Flowers (1987) presented initially as mute. One with meningoencephalitis presented with global aphasia following this mutism, whereas the other case who only had suspected encephalitis presented with poor receptive language skills, paragrammaticism, and naming difficulties when the mute period ended. Other aphasic symptoms described in the acute stage following an attack of encephalitis include paraphasias, poor repetition skills, stereotypes, and perseveration (Cooper & Flowers, 1987; Van Hout et al., 1985).

Van Hout and co-workers described two cases of acquired childhood aphasia resulting from infectious disease in terms of adult aphasic syndromes. The first case had an infection of unknown type and presented with an apparent conduction aphasia, as comprehension remained relatively intact in the presence of marked naming problems, slight paragrammaticism, and phonemic paraphasias noted in spontaneous speech but more prominent on repetition tasks (Van Hout et al., 1985). A second case with herpes simplex encephalitis was described in detail by Van Hout and Lyon (1986). They described their case, a 10-year-old boy, as presenting with a Wernicke aphasia. His comprehension was severely affected and initially he presented in a perseverative state that lasted for 5 weeks. He then became anosognosic when he presented with logorrhea. Initially, stereotypic behavior that varied daily was also noted. As he became more fluent alliterative behavior was evident in his spontaneous speech, his reading and on repetition tasks. Neologisms increased during this fluent period from 15% on day 6 (after the perseverative period) to 65% on day 16. Verbal paraphasias were absent on day 8 but up to 30% on day 16, also showing an increase in the acute stage. In the recovery phase, however, there was a decrease in neologisms together with an increase in verbal paraphasias and circumlocutions. This change in the number of paraphasias, was observed between 2 and 8 months after the perseverative period. After 2 months the comprehension abilities of the case described by Van Hout and Lyon (1986) also showed some improvement.

The length of time children stayed in a paraphasic phase postonset was used by Van Hout et al. (1985) to separate their 11 subjects with acquired childhood aphasia into three groups. It is of importance to note that four of the five children in whom paraphasias were evident months after onset had suffered from herpes simplex encephalitis. In this group phonemic paraphasias disappeared before the semantic ones and generally the overall number of paraphasias was greater than in the other two groups. This group had severe comprehension and aphasic symptoms and tended to have had longer coma periods, although the period of mutism did not differ from the other two groups. The second group, although comprising only two cases, had paraphasias lasting weeks, moderate comprehension deficits but no history of mutism or coma. The etiology for this group was also infectious in nature, one from measles and one from an infection of unknown origin.

The pattern of language deficits and strengths seen during this recovery phase, as measured on the Gaddes and Crockett (1975) norms of the Neurosensory Center Comprehensive Examination of Aphasia (NCCEA) (Spreen & Benton, 1969), was similar for the two groups although generally more severe for those children who had had herpes simplex encephalitis. Generally, the pattern was as follows: poor on visual and tactile naming tasks, sentence repetition, identification by sentence, good performance on naming by description of use, and moderate performance on digit repetition and word fluency. The greatest individual variation was on the tasks of sentence construction, identification by name and the number of words produced per minute.

During this recovery period (in this discussion taken to be up to 1 year postonset) some individual cases were described as regaining functional communication skills within 1 month postonset (Cooper & Flowers, 1987). One case had regained functional communication 4 months postonset yet, at chronologic age 12 years, her language skills were 6 to 7 years delayed. Specific deficits described in individual cases during this phase included: word-finding and naming difficulties, difficulties associating and integrating verbal information, slow rate of speech and articulation difficulties, poor verbal memory, and difficulties with written language (Cooper & Flowers, 1987; Van Hout et al., 1985).

One case of acquired childhood aphasia associated with encephalitis, described by Cooper and Flowers (1987) did not regain basic communication skills until 6 months postonset. At that time he presented with impairments in both receptive and expressive language skills. This same case when assessed almost 4 years postonset, presented with a delay in the language and academic areas tested. In addition, he was the only subject assessed by Cooper and Flowers (1987) who was intellectually handicapped and who had pragmatic deficits. Of all the cases of acquired childhood aphasia resulting from encephalitis reported in the literature, the prognosis for this latter case was the worst.

Another case of acquired aphasia occurring in a child following encephalitis was assessed by Cooper and Flowers (1987) as having a borderline intellectual handicap with poor performance on all language and academic skills assessed except reading ability. In the other cases described by these authors, intellectual functioning was within normal limits but specific language deficits were found on certain syntactic constructions and receptive vocabulary, and academic problems in the areas of arithmetic, reading, and spelling. Although Van Hout et al. (1985) did not give information on the intellectual functioning of their cases, they did describe long-term linguistic deficits. These included naming difficulties, poor verbal memory, written language problems, and paralexia.

Therefore, it would appear from the few case descriptions outlined above that the prognosis is poor for linguistic and academic abilities of children who have suffered encephalitis. This particularly appears to be so when the outcome of these cases is compared with cases of acquired childhood aphasia from other causes (Cooper & Flowers, 1987; van Dongen & Visch-Brink, 1988; Van Hout et al., 1985). This generally poor prognosis may be due to bilateral brain damage, for while some cases of acquired childhood aphasia associated with encephalitis reported in the literature showed unilateral lesions, and indeed others presented with normal CT scans, it would seem that infections are likely to involve both cerebral hemispheres. In view of the severe comprehension deficits displayed by a number of the cases described and the presence of two cases where intellectual functioning has been affected, it is imperative that linguistic functioning is evaluated in the light of cognitive functioning. It is important that clinicians publish detailed longitudinal case studies of children with encephalitis.

Neurologic Problems Associated with Childhood Meningitis

A number of researchers have reported neurologic sequelae after an episode of meningitis. These sequelae include ataxia, paralysis, elevated muscle tone, clinically significant hearing deficits, seizures, visual disturbances, depressed IQ, behavioral changes (Feigin & Dodge, 1976), learning problems (Taylor, Michaels, Mazur, Bauer, & Liden, 1984), social adjustment deficit (Sell, 1987), receptive and expressive language delays (Jadavji, Biggar, & Gold, 1986), and "soft" neurologic signs.

Although some of these researchers have noted the presence of speech and language deficits among the sequelae of meningitis (Feldman et al., 1982; Jadavji et al., 1986; Taylor et al., 1984) there is a paucity in the literature of detailed linguistic outcome subsequent to recovery from bacterial meningitis. In the following general review of the literature on the neurological sequelae of childhood meningitis emphasis is given to studies that have highlighted speech and language deficits as specific sequelae.

Bacterial Meningitis

Bacterial meningitis in childhood may result in neurologic sequelae of varying types and degree. Jadavji et al. (1986) looked at neurologic sequelae in children (4 days to 18 years) after bacterial meningitis. These children were treated with ampicillin or chloramphenicol. The pathogens responsible for the meningitis in the study group included *H. influenzae* type B (HIB; 70%), *Strep. pneumoniae* (20%), and *N. meningitidis* (10%). Of the 171 follow-up assessments performed on the subjects, 20% had mild to severe handicaps. Children recovering from meningitis caused by *Strep. pneumoniae* had a 57% frequency of handicap. HIB resulted in 14.5% handicap and there were no subsequent handicaps noted in the children with *N. meningitidis* meningitis.

It is particularly important to note that 5% of the group studied by Jadavji et al. (1986) had a disorder of language (i.e., 8 of the 171 subjects). Over 16% of the children with *Strep. pneumoniae* meningitis had receptive and/or expressive language delay in comparison to 2.4% of children with HIB meningitis with language delays. An identifiable developmental delay was present in 5.3% of the children. Jadavji et al. (1986) did not specify the speech and language tests used in the analysis. Long-term assessment of the children was carried out by an infectious disease consultant, neurologist, audiologist, ophthalmologist, and psychologist.

Haemophilus Influenzae Type B (HIB) Meningitis. Many studies have detailed the incidence and type of sequelae due to HIB meningitis. The incidence of sequelae noted in subjects varies among researchers. Of the 75 subjects monitored by Sell, Merrill, Doyne, and Zimsky (1972a), 29% had severe or significant handicaps and 14% had possible neurological sequelae. Sproles, Azarrad, Williamson, & Merrill (1969) indicated that 55% of the subject group of 45 children with influenza meningitis had permanent effects. Eight per cent of the subject group of a study by Feigin and Dodge (1976) had neurologic or intellectual deficits.

Sell et al. (1972a) looked at the long-term sequelae of HIB meningitis. Significant handicaps included mild spastic hemiparesis, moderately/severe mixed type hearing loss, hyperactivity, slow learning, poor speech, and left spastic hemiplegia. These authors highlighted that prevention of this disorder should be of a primary concern, because of the long-term neurologic sequelae.

In another study Sell, Webb, Pate, and Doyne (1972b) reported on two controlled studies of the psychological sequelae subsequent to bacterial meningitis. The first considered the WISC scores for HIB survivors. The second compared children's performances following meningitis with those of their classroom peers. The children were assessed on the Illinois Test of Psycholinguistic Abilities (ITPA) (McCarthy & Kirk, 1961), the Frostig Developmental Test of Visual Perception (Frostig, 1963), and the Peabody Picture Vocabulary Test (PPVT) (Dunn, 1965). The first study showed that the post-meningitis group had a mean IQ of 86, while the control group had an IQ of 97. The second group of children, who had had meningitis, was selected because it was considered that there were no apparent sequelae from their meningitis. The results of the PPVT indicated that the vocabulary quotient for the post-meningitis group was 90.96%, with the control group at 12.60%. This was significantly different at the 0.35 level. In both cases the subject group performed at a significantly lower intellectual level than the control group.

Feldman et al. (1982) attempted to ascertain if the concentrations of *H. influenzae* type B in the CSF before treatment had any relationship to later sequelae. The results of the study showed that patients who had 1×10^7 CFU (colony forming units) of *H. influenzae* type B per mL of CSF were significantly more likely to have abnormalities of speech and hearing and more severe neurologic sequelae than those with a lower concentration at the acute stage. Forty-five subjects were evaluated in the study, with 12 subjects having a speech delay and three with expressive speech defects. Five subjects had a bilateral and sensorineural hearing loss, with three having a unilateral sensorineural hearing loss. The results of the study indicated that the concentration of HIB in the CSF prior to treatment was predictive of the sequelae. This study indicated that further research was needed to ascertain whether pretreatment concentrations of *H. influenzae* is an indicator of intellectual ability.

Taylor et al. (1984) investigated the neurologic sequelae of HIB meningitis in 24 children 6 to 8 years after recovery. They tested the children for intellectual, neuropsychological and achievement outcomes using a test battery which included among others the Wechsler Intelligence Scale for Children-Revised (WISC-R) (Wechsler, 1974), the Token Test for Children (DiSimoni, 1978), and the Expressive One-Word Picture Vocabulary Test (Gardner, 1979). The performance of the HIB children was compared with an appropriately matched control group. The HIB subjects performed more poorly than the control subjects on tests that required verbal comprehension and memory, verbal list learning, and visuomotor dexterity. Academic achievement, however, was not adversely affected in the HIB subjects. It was suggested by Taylor et al. (1984) that a further study should monitor the performances of the HIB children through the school years. Although the morbidity of meningitis is measurable, Taylor et al. (1984) suggested other factors must be considered when predicting the long-term effects on the child.

Feldman and Michaels (1988) looked at academic achievement in children several years after an episode of HIB meningitis. Using specific academic tests, they showed that the children continued to perform well academically 10 to 12 years after recovery from the episode. The only test that showed any statistically significant difference was in reading accuracy (i.e., the fluency of reading paragraphs).

In contrast to the findings of the studies outlined above, Emmett, Jeffery, Chandler, and Dugdale (1980) were unable to find any major neurologic sequelae in children who had had HIB meningitis. Based on the findings of a range of psychological tests, which included the WISC–R and the Frostig and Bender Psychological tests they concluded that children promptly diagnosed and treated for HIB have no detectable residual deficits. Emmett et al. (1980), however, did note that prolonged fever during the meningitis was associated with poorer results in psychological tests.

Streptococcal Meningitis. Incidence figures vary on the neurologic sequelae of Group B streptococcal meningitis. Chin and Fitzhardinge (1985) reported that 36 to 44% of survivors of streptococcal meningitis in their study had long-term sequelae. Others authors, however, such as Baker and Edwards (1983), Barton, Feigin, and Lins (1973) and Edwards et al. (1985) have found that up to 50% of survivors of Group B streptococcal meningitis show long sequelae. In their study of 38 infants with bacteriologically proven Group B streptococcal meningitis, Edwards et al. (1985) identified 29% as having major sequelae and 21% with mild to moderate deficits. In particular they noted that subtle deficits in cognitive abilities and language or learning deficits may not be manifest until later years.

Wald et al. (1986) also looked at the performance of children subsequent to Group B streptococcal meningitis. They found the mortality rate to be 27%, with another 12% of the subjects having major neurological sequelae. The study, however, did indicate that there was no significant difference between the subject group and a control group in communication behavior, if the children with major neurologic sequelae were excluded.

Aseptic Meningitis

The term aseptic meningitis refers to a clinical syndrome characterized by signs of meningeal inflammation, fever and pleocytosis (presence of a greater than normal number of cells) of the CSF with bacteriological sterility of the CSF. Although most frequently associated with viral infections, other agents may also cause this disorder. Fee, Marks, Kardash, Reite, and Seitz (1970) evaluated the long-term effects of aseptic meningitis by following the neurologic, behavioral, and visuomotor perceptual development and electroencephalographic changes in a group of 18 children for a period up to 10 years after meningitis. Based on their findings, Fee et al. (1970) concluded that the majority of children with aseptic meningitis showed only mild abnormalities in the long term, although no definite pattern of deficit was identified. It was noted, however, that behavior and school performance of children following aseptic meningitis should be monitored, especially in those cases where seizures accompany the original illness.

Implications of Childhood Meningitis for Speech and Language Function

The information in the literature on speech and language deficits subsequent to meningitis is inconsistent. Although some researchers have indicated a deficit in communicative abilities as one neurologic sequelae, others have not. One reason for this discrepancy may lie in the different types of research designs used by different authors to investigate the long-term outcomes of meningitis. Tejani et al. (1982) stressed the need to carefully evaluate the control group used in particular studies. The use of a sibling control group, for instance, may lend weight to the conclusion that a neurologic deficit observed in the subject group is the result of the meningitis rather than the outcome of some environmental or educational factor. In addition, the failure of some specific linguistic test to indicate the presence of a linguistic deficit may not in itself signal that communication skills are appropriate. Furthermore, when considering speech and language deficits it is important to note that these deficits may not

fully manifest themselves until later years. Haslam et al. (1977) acknowledged that, although they observed no significant differences in language testing of their subject group after recovery from meningitis, the children had not progressed to the 3rd and 4th grades where learning difficulties become evident. Similarly, Edwards et al. (1985) indicated that it is difficult to identify neurodevelopmental disorders at an early age. They recommended a 3-year follow-up period to assess linguistic delay or mild/moderate mental retardation.

Although discrete speech and language tests may highlight specific deficits in the younger child, as the child matures and academic skills are monitored, further deficits may become obvious. High-level speech and language deficits that impinge on the child's abilities may also become evident and these deficits may then pervade other aspects of the child's learning. Swartz (1984) discussed the need for more information to define factors that may be responsible for neurological damage and to design strategies beyond prompt administration of appropriate medication to alleviate such factors after meningitis.

Overall, more information is needed on linguistic aspects of meningeal complications including: (1) an examination of the onset time of the meningitis (pre- or postlinguistic) and its effect, and (2) the etiology of the meningitis (viral or bacterial). Linguistic skills need to be analyzed thoroughly and patterns detailed if present. Ongoing monitoring, with assessment at critical academic stages, needs to be instituted. These issues need to be considered in relation to the implications for long-term management of speech-language pathology. They also are vital in considering long-term academic programming.

Summary

Communicative disorders following childhood infectious diseases represent a significant area in which available knowledge in the literature is sparse and fragmented. The CNS diseases occurring in children are variable in onset, manifestation, and outcome. The incidence of handicapping sequelae documented in the literature and the severity of such sequelae suggests the need for clinical surveillance well beyond the normal medical regimen in order to detect residual deficits that range from hearing impairment to subtle cognitive dysfunction and possible speech-language disturbances.

References

Baker, C. J., & Edwards, M. S. (1983). Group B streptococcal infections. In J. S. Remington & J. O. Klein (Eds.), *Infectious diseases of the fetus and newborn infant*. Philadelphia, PA: W. B. Saunders.

Barton, L. L., Feigin, R. D., & Lins, R. (1973). Group B beta-hemolytic streptococcal meningitis in infants. *Journal of Pediatrics, 82*, 719.

Chin, K. C., & Fitzhardinge, P. M. (1985). Sequelae of early-onset Group B haemolytic streptococcal neonatal meningitis. *Journal of Pediatrics, 106*, 820–823.

Cooper, J. A., & Flowers, C. R. (1987). Children with a history of acquired aphasia: Residual language and academic impairments. *Journal of Speech and Hearing Disorders, 52*, 251–262.

DiSimoni, F. G. (1978). The token test for children. Boston, MA: Teaching Resources.

Dodge, P. R. (1986) Sequelae of bacterial meningitis. *Pediatric Infectious Diseases, 5*, 618–620.

Dunn, L. M. (1965). Peabody picture vocabulary test. Circle Pines, MN: American Guidance Service.

Edwards, M. S., Rench, M. A., Haffar, A. A. M., Murphy, M. A., Desmond, M. M., & Baker, C. J. (1985). Long-term sequelae of Group B streptococcal meningitis in infants. *Journal of Pediatrics, 106*, 717–722.

Emmett, M., Jeffery, H., Chandler, D., & Dugdale, A. (1980). Sequelae of Haemophilus influenzae meningitis. *Australian Paediatric Journal, 16*, 90–93.

Fee, W., Marks, M., Kardash, S., Reite, M., & Seitz, C. (1970). The long-term prognosis of aseptic meningitis in childhood. *Developmental Medicine and Child Neurology, 12*, 321–329.

Feigin, R. D., & Dodge, P. R. (1976). Bacterial meningitis: Newer concepts of pathophysiology and neurologic sequelae, Symposium on Pediatric Neurology. *Pediatric Clinics of North America, 23*, 541–556.

Feldman, H., & Michaels, R. (1988). Academic achievement in children 10 to 12 years after haemophilus influenzae meningitis. *Paediatrics, 81*, 339–344.

Feldman, W., Ginsburg, C. M., McCracken, & G. H., Allen, D., Ahmann, P., Graham, J., Graham, L. (1982). Relation of concentration of Haemophilus influenzae type B in cerebrospinal fluid to late sequelae of patients with meningitis. *Journal of Pediatrics, 100*, 209–212.

Frostig, M. (1963). Developmental test of visual perception. Palo Alto, CA: Consulting Psychologists Press.

Gaddes, W. H., & Crockett, D. J. (1975). The Spreen-Benton aphasia tests, normative data as a measure of normal language development. *Brain and Language, 2*, 257–280.

Gardner, M. F. (1979). Expressive one-word picture vocabulary test. Novato, CA: Academic Therapy Publications.

Haslam, R., Allen, J., Dorsen, M., Kanofsky, D., Mellits, D., & Norris, D. (1977). The sequelae of Group B haemolytic streptococcal meningitis in early infancy. *American Journal of Diseases of Children, 131*, 845–849.

Jadavji, T., Biggar, W., & Gold, R. (1986). Sequelae of acute bacterial meningitis children treated for 7 days. *Pediatrics, 78,* 21–25.

McCarthy, J. J., & Kirk, S. A. (1961). Illinois test of psycholinguistic abilities. Urbana, IL: Institute for Research on Exceptional Children.

Saez-Llorens, X., & McCracken, G. H. (2003). Bacterial meningitis in children. *Lancet, 361,* 2139–2148.

Sell, S. (1987). Haemophilus influenzae type B meningitis: Manifestations and long-term sequelae. *Pediatric Infectious Diseases Journal, 8,* 775–778.

Sell, S., Merrill, R., Doyne, E., & Zimsky, E. (1972a). Long-term sequelae of Haemophilus influenzae meningitis. *Pediatrics, 49,* 206–211.

Sell, S., Webb, W., Pate, J., & Doyne, E. (1972b). Psychological sequelae to bacterial meningitis: Two controlled series. *Pediatrics, 49,* 212–216.

Spreen, O., & Benton, A. L. (1969). *Neurosensory Center Comprehensive Examination for Aphasia: Manual for directions.* Victoria, B.C.: University of Victoria.

Sproles, E. T., Azarrad, J., Williamson, C., & Merrill, R. E. (1969). Meningitis due to Haemophilus influenzae: Long-term sequelae. *Journal of Pediatrics, 75,* 782.

Swartz, M. (1984). Bacterial meningitis: More involved than just the meninges. *New England Journal of Medicine, 310,* 912–914.

Taylor, H. G., Michaels, R., Mazur, P., Bauer, R., & Liden, C. (1984). Intellectual, neuropsychological and achievement outcomes in children 6–8 years after recovery from Haemophilus influenzae meningitis. *Pediatrics, 74,* 198–205.

Tejani, A., Tobias, B., & Sambursky, J. (1982). Long-term prognosis after H. influenzae meningitis: Prospective evaluation. *Developmental Medicine and Child Neurology, 24,* 338–343.

van Dongen, H. R., & Visch-Brink, E. G. (1988). Naming in aphasic children: Analysis of paraphasic errors. *Neuropsychologia, 26,* 629–632.

Van Hout, A., Evrard, P., & Lyon, G. (1985). On the positive semiology of acquired aphasia in children. *Developmental Medicine and Child Neurology, 27,* 231–241.

Van Hout, A., & Lyon, G. (1986). Wernicke's aphasia in a 10-year-old boy. *Brain and Language, 29,* 268–285.

Wald, E. R., Bergman, I., Taylor, H. G., Chiponis, D., Porter, C., & Kubek, K. (1986). Long-term outcome of Group B streptococcal meningitis. *Pediatrics, 77,* 217–221.

Wechsler, D. (1974). *Manual for the Wechsler Intelligence Scale for Children-Revised.* New York, NY: Psychological Corporation.

Wubbel, L., & McCracken, G. H. (1998). Management of bacterial meningitis. *Pediatric Review, 19,* 78–84.

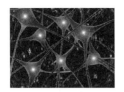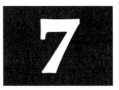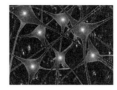

7

Language Outcomes Following Acute Cerebral Anoxia in Childhood

Introduction

A continuous and adequate supply of oxygen to the brain is essential for the maintenance of normal brain function. According to Bell and Lastimosa (1980), although the brain constitutes only about 2% of the total body weight of the adult, it accounts for approximately 20% of the oxygen consumption of the entire body. In the nursing infant and in children up to 4 years of age, the proportion of the total body oxygen consumption accounted for by the brain rises to over 30% (McIlwain, 1955). To provide the necessary oxygen, approximately 15% of the cardiac output is received by the adult brain, equivalent to around 45 mL of blood per 100 g per minute. In children, the cerebral perfusion rate is even higher, being about twice that of the adult brain (Auer & Sutherland, 2002; McIlwain, 1966). Furthermore, oxygen pressure is not uniform throughout the brain, being higher in gray matter than in white matter (Auer & Sutherland, 2002).

Anoxia is the condition in which the oxygen levels in the body tissues fall below physiological levels (i.e., below the level required to maintain normal function) as a result of either an absence or deficiency of oxygen. The supply of oxygen to the brain is dependent on two factors, the level of cerebral blood flow and the oxygen content of the blood. Anything causing a drop in either of these two factors may lead to cerebral anoxia. Nerve cells or neurons are particularly susceptible to anoxia as they have an obligatory, aerobic, glycolytic metabolism. Consequently, any period of prolonged cerebral anoxia can lead to permanent brain damage (anoxic encephalopathy) which, in turn, may be associated with the production of a range of neurologic disorders, among which speech and language deficits may be included.

The neurologic deficits that may occur following cerebral anoxia are determined to a large extent by the length of the anoxic period. These deficits may range from no deficit, to mild intellectual impairment, to a pure vegetative state, and at worst, death. The eventual degree of clinical recovery is determined by whether or not satisfactory resuscitation can be achieved before permanent brain damage ensues. Patients with acute cerebral anoxia have been reported to recover without clinical functional sequelae if tissue oxygenation is restored with 1 to 2 minutes (Bell & Lastimosa, 1980). It should be noted, however, that the exact duration of anoxia that separates recovery of the neural tissue on the one hand and extensive permanent brain damage on the other, has not been critically defined in man (Plum, 1973). According to Bell and Lastimosa (1980), under normal circumstances, anoxia lasting more than 4 minutes causes destruction of neurons in the brain, especially in the cerebral cortex, hippocampus, and cerebellum. Similarly, Brierley (1972) stated that in cases of cardiac arrest, under normal conditions complete clinical recovery is unlikely if the period of arrest is more than 5 to 7 minutes. Neuronal death has been reported to follow cerebral anoxia lasting more than 10 minutes (Weinberger, Gibbon, & Gibbon, 1940).

Certain parts of the brain are selectively vulnerable to the effects of cerebral anoxia. Consequently, the maximum period of anoxia compatible with recovery varies in different areas of the brain. Neurons are more vulnerable than glial cells to anoxia and oligodendrocytes generally are more vulnerable than astrocytes (Petito, Olarte, Roberts, Nowak, & Pulsinelli, 1998). Neurons in certain areas of the brain such as the basal ganglia and hippocampus appear particularly vulnerable whereas spinal cord neurons are more tolerant of periods of anoxia. The factors that determine selective vulnerability of certain neuronal populations are still incompletely understood. The most vulnerable areas of the brain are the so-called "watershed" or "border-zone" regions of the cerebral hemispheres in that they receive their vascular supply from the most distal branches of the cerebral arteries. More specifically, areas most sensitive to anoxia, as occurs after sudden cardiac arrest, are the middle cortical layers of the occipital and parietal lobes, the hippocampus, amygdala, caudate nucleus, putamen, anterior and dorsomedial nuclei of the thalamus, and cerebellar Purkinje cells (Brierley, Graham, Adams, & Simpsom 1971). In contrast, those regions of the brain concerned with autonomic (vegetative) functions, such as the lower brainstem, appear to be the most resistant areas to anoxic damage, although brainstem nuclei are more likely to be involved in infants than older children.

Anoxic encephalopathy may result from any condition that causes the oxygen supply to the brain to become inadequate. It therefore is a potential outcome in any person subjected to general anesthesia, a severe episode of hypotension (low blood pressure), cardiac arrest, suffocation, near-drowning, status epilepticus, carbon monoxide poisoning, barbiturate intoxication, and hypoglycemic coma.

Types of Anoxia

Four different major causes of anoxia are commonly recognized in the literature including: anoxic (hypoxic) anoxia; anemic anoxia, stagnant anoxia, and metabolic, or toxic, anoxia. In that all of these four type of anoxia may occur in children and are known to cause brain damage (see Sites of Anoxic Brain Damage below), it is conceivable that any of them might also lead to the production of acquired speech and language disorders.

Anoxic anoxia involves an absence or reduction (hypoxic anoxia) of oxygen in the lungs as a result of either respiratory insufficiency or a lack of oxygen in the inhaled air. This type of anoxia may result from events which include, among others, accidental suffocation, strangulation, near-drowning, exposure to high altitudes, accidents in anesthesia, and exposure to places with inadequate ventilation. Respiratory insufficiency may occur, especially in children, from spasm of the respiratory muscles in status epilipticus. This condition, involving a rapid succession of epileptic fits without intervals of consciousness, may cause brain damage as a result of the cerebral anoxia that arises from the respiratory insufficiency. Although many individuals make an uneventful recovery from status epilepticus, others who survive may be left with permanent intellectual or neurological deficits resulting from the associated anoxic encephalopathy.

Anemic anoxia is caused by a reduction in the oxygen-carrying capacity of the blood which, in turn, results in an insufficient amount of oxygen carried to the brain. The reduction on oxygen-carrying capacity may be the result of either an insufficient level of hemoglobin in the blood (e.g., in pernicious anemia) or carbon monoxide poisoning. Hemoglobin has a much higher affinity for carbon monoxide than for oxygen. Consequently, the presence of carbon monoxide in the inhaled air reduces the oxygen levels in the blood by more

effectively competing with oxygen for the binding sites on the hemoglobin molecule.

Both anemic anoxia and anoxic anoxia lead to a deficiency in the oxygenation of the blood (hypoxemia) which in turn causes problems in the intracellular oxidation of glucose for energy by the brain cells (hypoxidosis). Schwedenberg (1959) referred to this condition as hypoxemic hypoxidosis.

Any interruption to the blood supply to the brain causes stagnant anoxia. This type of anoxia is divided into two subtypes: ischemic and oligemic. Ischemic cerebral anoxia results from either localized or generalized arrest of the blood supply to the brain, as may occur following cerebrovascular accidents involving blockage or rupture of one of the cerebral arteries or following cardiac arrest. Oligemic anoxia is caused by either a localized or generalized reduction in cerebral blood flow, as may occur, for instance, in association with systemic arterial hypotension (i.e., a generalized drop in blood pressure).

Factors that interfere with oxygen consumption by brain cells or which have direct toxic effects on nervous tissue lead to metabolic, or toxic, anoxia. These factors include, among others, hypoglycemia (low blood glucose levels) and cyanide poisoning. Hypoglycemia occurs idiopathically in some infants or also may occur as a result of an excess of insulin administered for the treatment of diabetes mellitus. Cyanide poisoning severely reduces the energy state of the brain in the presence of normal supplies of oxygen by interfering with the oxidative enzymes of the nerve cells. In addition, however, it also induced respiratory failure. Consequently, the brain damage resulting from exposure to cyanide not only occurs as a result of its direct effects on the brain tissues but also form secondary effects on respiration and circulation.

Sites of Anoxic Brain Damage

As indicated earlier, some parts of the brain have been reported to be more susceptible to the damaging effects of anoxia than others (Adams, 1963; Brierley et al., 1971; Graham, 1977; Petito et al., 1998). Studies based on either pathologic examination of the brains of victims of anoxia at post mortem or the findings of computed tomographic (CT) scans have shown that brain lesions resulting from cerebral anoxia may involve both the gray and the white matter of the brain (Brierley, 1972; Brucher, 1967; Graham, 1977). Gray matter involvement may include damage to the cerebral and cerebellar cortex, the hippocampus, the basal ganglia, the thalamus, and various brainstem nuclei. Damage to the white matter (anoxic leucoencephalopathy) may take the form of both diffuse changes in the white matter including demyelination, as well as circumscribed areas of total necrosis. The diffuse white matter changes occur predominantly in the centrum semiovale (Brucher, 1967).

According to studies of cases of anoxia of different origins, such as those reported by Brucher (1967) and Richardson, Chambers, and Heywood (1959), the clinical signs and the anatomic location of anoxic brain lesions are fundamentally the same for all type of anoxia. Although to a large extent this appears to be true, some subtle differences in the topography of lesion sites associated with the different types of cerebral anoxia have been reported. These subtle differences become evident in the following discussion.

Anoxic lesions involving the cerebrum most commonly involve the border-zones of the cerebral cortical and subcortical arterial circulation (Adams, Brierley, Connor, & Treip, 1966; Graham, 1977), with damage often being most severe in the parieto-occipital region, which represents the common border-zone between the territories of the anterior, middle, and posterior cerebral arteries. Although anoxic lesions of the cerebral cortex are usually bilateral, they may be asymmetric and, especially where the anoxia is the result of systemic arterial hypotension, even unilateral in some cases, the pattern of anoxic damage often being determined in such cases by the presence of atheroma and variations in the caliber of the vessels comprising the circle of Willis (Graham, 1977).

Involvement of the basal ganglia in lesions induced by cerebral anoxia is variable. Several CT studies of patients with anoxic lesions, including those resulting from accidental suffocation (Murdoch, Chenery, & Kennedy, 1989), carbon monoxide poisoning (Murray, Stensaas, Anderson, & Matsuo, 1987; Zeiss & Brinker, 1988) cardiorespiratory arrest (Murray et al., 1987), and hydrogen sulphide inhalation (Matsuo, Cummins, & Anderson, 1979) have shown the presence of symmetric lesions involving the lenticular nucleus bilaterally. In some reports, concomitant bilateral involvement of the head of the caudate nucleus has also been demonstrated. For example, in the case of anoxic brain damage following accidental suffocation reported by Murdoch et al. (1989), the CT scan showed a bilateral symmetric decrease in attenuation in the head of the caudate nucleus in addition to bilateral damage to the lenticular nucleus (Figure 7–1).

Graham (1977) reported variations in the involvement of the basal ganglia depending on the type of anoxia involved. In cases of ischemic cerebral anoxia following cardiac arrest, Graham (1977) noted that the associated basal ganglia lesions most commonly involved the outer halves of the head and body of the caudate nucleus and the outer portions of the putamen with occasional damage to the globus pallidus. In patients with oligemic anoxic brain damage resulting from a major and abrupt drop in blood pressure followed by a rapid return to normal blood pressure, how-

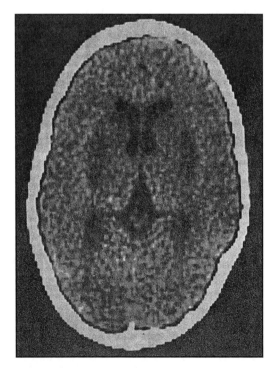

FIGURE 7–1. CT scan showing bilateral hypodense changes in the head of the caudate nucleus and lenticular nucleus consistent with cerebral anoxia in a 13-year-old boy 5 weeks after accidental suffocation.

ever, Graham (1977) reported that the components of the basal ganglia that were damaged most frequently involved the head of the caudate nucleus and the upper parts of the putamen. Although the globus pallidus may be damaged by any type of cerebral anoxia, there is a particular predilection for infarction of this structure in carbon monoxide poisoning.

As in the case of the cerebrum, anoxic damage to the cerebellum most frequently involves the border-zones between the distributions of the major cerebellar arteries (e.g., between the superior and posterior-inferior cerebellar arteries). Damage to the cerebellum appears to be a common finding in all types of cerebral anoxia (Graham, 1977).

Adams et al. (1966) reported that, although anoxic damage to the brainstem nuclei may occur following an episode of ischemic anoxia (e.g., cardiac arrest), it usually is not present subsequent to oligemic anoxia. Furthermore, these investigators reported that anoxic damage to the brainstem nuclei is more severe in young children and infants that adults.

Not all types of cerebral anoxia appear to cause damage to the thalamus. Thalamic lesions induced by cerebral anoxia appear to be most severe following oligemic anoxia resulting from a drop in blood pressure, with a slow onset but of long duration (Adams et al., 1966; Graham, 1977). Although present in most cases, involvement of the hippocampus in anoxic brain damage is also variable.

Clearly, the lesions identified in cases of anoxic encephalopathy are in a position to cause speech and language problems. In adults, lesions in the arterial border-zone of the dominant cerebral cortex have been linked to the occurrence of transcortical aphasia (Benson, 1979;

Murdoch, 2010). The term "transcortical aphasia" is used to describe a group of aphasic syndromes characterized by retention of repetition out of all proportion compared with other language functions. Furthermore, lesions of the striatocapsular region have been reported to be associated with the occurrence of speech and language disorders in adults (Alexander & LoVerme, 1980; Murdoch, 2010; Murdoch, Thompson, Fraser, & Harrison, 1986; Murdoch & Whelan, 2009) and children (Aram, Rose, Rekate, & Whitaker, 1983).

Aram et al. (1983) documented the presence of language difficulties, but not dysarthria, in a 7-year-old girl who had an acquired vascular lesion in the putamen, anterior limb of the internal capsule and the lateral aspect of the head of the caudate nucleus. After an initial period of mutism, oral apraxia, and moderate comprehension difficulties, the child gradually regained expressive language by going through the stages of using phrases, short sentences, and simple sentences until 6 months after the cerebrovascular accident (CVA) she had fully regained her verbal language abilities. Severe anomia, in that she was unable to name on confrontation, was also present in the early stages, but it too resolved after passing through a stage of semantic paraphasias and word-finding difficulties. Her written language skills at 6 months after the accident showed reading to be at her appropriate grade level, although minor spelling difficulties were noted. Five years after the accident, however, she presented with major learning problems including reading difficulties.

Four other children with subcortical lesions studied by Aram, Ekelman, and Gillespie (1989) also presented with reading problems. All four children had lesions involving the head of the cau-

date nucleus and the anterior limb of the internal capsule and three of them also showed speech and language problems. One of the three children presented with global language problems in auditory comprehension, word retrieval, and expressive syntax. The presence of a motor speech impairment was indicated by his impaired articulation skills and slow diadochokinetic rate and a memory problem was noted. A second subject reported by Aram et al. (1989) presented with similar language problems; however, his speech was described as having a mild dysarthric quality. Again, verbal memory was poor. The third subject presented with only a persistent word-retrieval problem and a mild to moderate fluency disorder, which only became evident after the CVA. The findings in these three cases led Aram et al. (1989) to hypothesize a relationship between language and reading function and left subcortical structures in children. Such subcortical structures (e.g., the head of the caudate nucleus) have also been noted as a site of anoxic damage.

Mechanisms of Anoxic Brain Damage

The pathologic mechanisms involved in the genesis of anoxic brain lesions are complex. Brucher (1967) identified four principal factors that may be involved including: hypoxidosis, edema, circulatory disorders, and histotoxic action.

Hypoxidosis refers to the basic disruption to intracellular metabolism that occurs in neurons as a result of cerebral anoxia. One theory proposed to explain the topography of focal anoxic brain lesions that has gained some acceptance in the literature suggests that the pattern of lesions observed in patients who have suffered anoxia is determined by a process of selective cellular vulnerability (pathoclisis). According to this theory, tissue hypoxidosis induces the necrosis of neurons in certain susceptible regions of the brain where the nerve cells are more vulnerable to the effects of anoxia. The basis of this vulnerability is not clear. Some authors have suggested that it is metabolically mediated (Helgason, Caplan, Goodwin, & Hedges, 1987). Others, however, such as Környey (1963), believe that the areas of the brain most sensitive to anoxia present a particular type of arterial irrigation that makes them more susceptible to ischemia. In particular, the susceptible areas tend to lie at the ends of arterial distributions or in arterial border-zones.

It has been suggested that focal anoxic brain lesions are caused by compression of the cerebral arteries against the cranium as a result of cerebral edema (Lindenberg, 1955). Anoxia causes disruption of the walls of the brain capillaries, leading to an increase in the permeability of the blood-brain barrier. Consequently, fluid and macromolecules pass from the blood into the parenchyma of the brain leading to cerebral edema. As a result of the increased volume that it produces, it has been suggested that the resulting cerebral edema causes an intracranial hypertension which in turn leads to compression of various cerebral blood vessels (Lindenberg, 1955, 1963). Lindenberg (1955) proposed compression of the anterior choroidal artery as a result of cerebral edema as a possible mechanism to explain basal ganglia necrosis secondary to cerebral anoxia. According to Lindenberg, therefore, the determining factor in the topography of anoxic lesions is

not a selective cellular vulnerability but rather a capillary stasis caused by arterial compression.

In recent years Lindenberg's proposal has been refuted by the findings of several studies that have shown that the distribution of brain lesions following anterior choroidal artery occlusion are not entirely consistent with the distribution of lesions observed in patients who have suffered an anoxic episode (Helgason et al., 1987; Murray et al., 1987). For one thing, although the posterior limb of the internal capsule is damaged in cases of anterior choroidal artery occlusion (Helgason, Caplan, Goodwin, & Hedges, 1986), it usually is not involved in anoxic encephalopathy. Furthermore, as pointed out by Helgason et al. (1987), anoxic brain damage usually involves the thalamus and other structures distant to the distribution of the anterior choroidal artery. As a consequence of their findings, Helgason et al. (1987) and Murray et al. (1987) concluded that the mechanism of damage to the basal ganglia in cases of anoxic brain damage probably is not related to compression of the anterior choroidal artery, but rather may be metabolically mediated and due to selective cellular vulnerability. Finally, as further evidence against Lindenberg's proposal, a number of investigators have reported that many patients with anoxic brain damage do not show evidence of brain swelling with associated intracranial hypotension, particularly those patients whose vital signs become stabilized after the anoxic event (Adams et al., 1966; Edstrom & Essex, 1956).

The oxygen needs of the cerebral white matter are five times less than those of the gray matter (Gänshirt, 1957). Consequently, factors other than hypoxidosis are probably responsible for the production of anoxic white matter lesions. Brucher (1967) suggested that cerebral edema following breakdown of the blood-brain barrier caused by hypoxemia is the probable cause of the diffuse lesions of the cerebral white matter observed in patients following anoxia.

In addition to causing disorders in the permeability of the vascular walls, anoxia also has a number of other effects on the circulation that might exert secondary influences on the distribution of anoxic brain lesions. These include vasoparalysis, vasostasis, and obstructions in small blood vessels either by swelling of the endothelium or possibly by vasospasms. Edema of the endothelial cells of the cerebral capillaries has been found to result from severe and prolonged ischemia (De Reuck & Vander Eecken, 1978). Following correction of the ischemia (e.g., by resuscitation), the presence of capillary edema is responsible for the production of a "no-reflow" phenomenon (Ames, Wright, Kowada, Thurston, & Majno, 1968) whereby restoration of circulation to the affected area of the brain is prevented, thereby leading to infarction of that area. De Reuck and Vander Eecken (1978) proposed that focal infarctions associated with cerebral anoxia result from the "no-reflow" phenomena rather than from arterial compression secondary to brain swelling as proposed by Lindenberg (1955).

In addition to the above mechanisms, in cerebral anoxia induced by chemical agents such as carbon monoxide or anesthetic products it is possible that the agents, in addition to causing anoxia, also have a direct toxic action on the neurons of the brain.

Although the majority of the evidence suggests that selective cellular vulnerability represents the principal pathologic mechanism underlying the genesis of anoxic brain lesions, it is possible that under different circumstances all of the mechanisms described above may contribute to the pattern of brain damage observed in patients who have experienced an anoxic episode.

Delayed Postanoxic Encephalopathy

The histologic manifestations of anoxic brain damage take time to become evident (Auer & Sutherland, 2002). Partial recovery after anoxic events is sometimes followed by dramatic clinical deterioration. This syndrome occurs with strangulation (Dooling & Richardson, 1976) and with many forms of anoxia, including near-drowning (Ginsberg, Hedley-Whyte, & Richardson, 1976; Plum, Posner, & Hain, 1962). It is most dramatic after carbon-monoxide poisoning. Most cases with delayed deterioration, whether their initial injury was due to anoxia or carbon monoxide poisoning develop extensive deep white matter injury, "Grinker's myelinopathy" (Kim et al., 2002). However, some patients are reported to have only gray matter lesions (Dooling & Richardson, 1976). A postanoxic dystonic syndrome has also been recognized in children. It appears 1 week to 36 months after the anoxic insult and tends to worsen for several years. Dysarthria and dysphagia are common. Neuroimaging studies reveal putaminal lesions in the majority of these cases. The pathophysiologic mechanism underlying this condition and the reason for its progression remain unknown (Bhatt, Obeso, & Marsden, 1993).

Speech and Language Disorders Associated with Anoxic Encephalopathy in Children

In children, speech and language disorders have been reported to occur in association with anoxic encephalopathy resulting from near-drowning (Reilly, Ozanne, Murdoch & Pitt, 1988), accidental suffocation (Murdoch et al., 1989), cardiac arrest resulting from cardiac surgery (Cooper & Flowers, 1987), and respiratory arrest (Cooper & Flowers, 1987).

Neurologic and Linguistic Status Subsequent to Near-Drowning in Childhood

Although speech and hearing impairments, including dysarthria and mild dysphasia, have been reported to occur in near-drowned children secondary to anoxic encephalopathy (Pearn, 1977; Pearn, De Buse, Mohay, & Golden, 1979b), only one study has been reported that has specifically investigated the effects of immersion and its associated intracranial pathophysiology on speech and language skills (Reilly et al., 1988). The morbidity of immersion is both pulmonary and neurologic in origin (Peterson, 1977). The neurologic morbidity following immersion injury is of particular interest to speech-language pathologists in that it is known to be associated with the occurrence of speech and language deficits. In order to comprehend the basis of the neurologic morbidity following immersion, and hence the basis of any associated speech

and language deficits, it is important that the process and physiology of the near-drowning incident be understood, with particular reference to anoxia.

During the initial period of immersion, the child panics and struggles. Apnea or breath holding occurs and the victim gasps and swallows quantities of water which enter the larynx and trachea. At this point tachycardia and arterial hypoxemia occur, due to the presence of high carbon dioxide levels and low oxygen concentrations in the blood. Blood pressure at this time increases. A phase of secondary apnea occurs followed by involuntary gasping under water and eventually by respiratory arrest. Arrhythmias are inevitable and, in the absence of ventilation, lead to death within minutes. Consciousness is lost within 3 minutes of involuntary submersion, almost always because of cerebral anoxia (Pearn, 1985).

Neurologic Deficits Following Immersion

Specific neurologic morbidity reported to occur secondary to childhood immersion includes spastic quadriplegia (Frates, 1981), truncal ataxia, strabismus and optic atrophy (Peterson, 1977), tetraplegia (Eriksson, Fredin, Gerdman, & Thorsan, 1973), upper motor neuron lesions (Fleetham & Munt, 1978), peripheral neuromuscular paralysis (Pearn, Bart, & Yamaoka, 1979a), and athetosis (Kruus, Bergstrom, Suutarinen, & Hyvonen, 1979). Although some children exhibit persistent neurologic deficits following immersion, in most studies reported in the literature, the majority of near-drowning cases have been described as showing a good recovery of neurologic function (Table 7–1).

Table 7–1. Neurologic Deficits Reported in Children Following Immersion

Study	Number of Subjects	Follow-up Period	Assessment	Neurologic Outcome		Clinical Features of Impaired Group
Eriksson et al. (1973)	36	2–7 years	(a) Hospital records examined; (b) Parents interviewed by phone	Serious disablement Normal	= 2 = 34	• Occasional reaction to light or pain • Tetraplegic syndrome with general rigidity and dystonia
Fandel and Bancalari (1976)	34	ND	Records reviewed	Without neurologic sequelae With neurologic sequelae Death	= 24 = 4 = 6	Defined as persistent coma or vegetative state
Pearn (1977)	54	3–60 months	• Neurologic examination • 3 years assigned development quotient • Psychometric tests	Normal Severe brain deficit The remaining case had complications from a head injury	= 52 = 1	Spastic quadraplegic
Peterson (1977)	72	NS	Review of records	No detectable neurologic deficit Severe anoxic encephalopathy Moderate anoxic encephalopathy	= 57 = 13 = 1	Truncal ataxia strabismus, optic atrophy

Study	Number of Subjects	Follow-up Period	Assessment	Neurologic Outcome		Clinical Features of Impaired Group
Kruus et al. (1979)	30	6–58 months	• Interview with parents • EEG recording • Clinical neurologic examination • Psychometric tests	Complete recovery (to preaccident level) Slight neurologic signs (coordination failure) Mental retardation and tetraplegic Death	= 8 = 5 = 4 = 13	Decrease in IQ; no movement or speech, difficulty in swallowing, slowing in EEG, muscle hypotomia, spastic tetraplegic
Pearn et al. (1979a)	104	6–58 months	Review of case history	No significant neurologic damage Neurologic deficit Death	= 98 = 0 = 6	—
Modell et al. (1980)	64	—	Retrospective review	Normal survival Severe brain deficit Death	= 53 = 3 = 8	ND
Frates (1981)	42	—	Retrospective review of case studies	Death Normal Profound cerebral injury	= 10 = 27 = 5	Spastic quadraplegia
Oakes et al. (1982)	40	Mean = 11.4 months	Review hospital	Full recovery Severe neurologic impairment Death	= 23 = 7 = 10	ND

continues

Table 7–1. *continued*

Study	Number of Subjects	Follow-up Period	Assessment	Neurologic Outcome		Clinical Features of Impaired Group
Conn and Barker (1984)	140	ND	ND	Abnormal	= 9	ND
				Normal	= 105	
				Death	= 26	
Frewen et al. (1985)	28	6 months	Neurologic examination	Good recovery	= 15	ND
				Impaired, severe	= 4	
				Impaired, mild-moderate	= 1	
				Death	= 8	
Nussbaum (1985)	51	—	ND	Complete recovery	= 19	Mental deterioration, spasticity
				Brain damage	= 14	
				Death	= 18	

NS = Not stated.

ND = No details provided.

Unfortunately, with the exception of the studies reported by Kruus et al. (1979) and Pearn (1977), none of the investigations listed in Table 7–1 provided details of the specific procedures used to assess the neurologic status of the victims of near-drowning. In most instances to determine the incidence of neurological sequelae following immersion, the authors either reviewed hospital records retrospectively or administered the subjects an unspecified neurologic examination. In one study, the presence or absence of neurologic deficit following immersion was determined by obtaining, by way of a telephone conversation, the parents' perception of whether their child had recovered or not (Eriksson et al., 1973). As a result of their failure to use detailed and specific neurological assessment procedures, it is possible that many researchers who have investigated the neurologic sequelae of near-drowning may have missed the presence of subtle or mild neurologic deficits. Towbin (1971) suggested that mild hypoxia results in focal or diffuse neuronal damage with consequent neurologic symptoms of a minimal or latent nature. If present it is possible that subtle neurologic changes occurring secondary to immersion could influence the high-level language performance of victims of near-drowning.

Pearn (1977) investigated the possible existence of subtle neurologic deficits following immersion. In a large ($n = 54$) population study, he examined the neurologic and psychologic outcome of all childhood survivors of freshwater immersion accident who lost consciousness in the water. Pearn's subjects were neurologically examined and psychologically tested between 3 months and 60 months after immersion by means of a full specific neurologic assessment

and a range of psychometric tests. Neurologic examination revealed that 52 of the 54 immersion cases had no clinically detectable evidence of motor, cerebellar, extrapyramidal, sensory (tactile), or cranial nerve dysfunction (i.e., they were neurologically normal). However, comparison of the verbal intelligence quotient scores with the performance intelligence quotient scores that were achieved on the Wechsler Preschool and Primary Scale of Intelligence (Wechsler, 1967) by 16 of the immersion cases yielded a significant difference ($p < 0.05$) of 11 points or more in five subjects. Three of the 16 children showed disparities between verbal and performance scores of greater than 15 IQ points: the term "minimal cerebral dysfunction" is sometimes applied to this (Pearn, 1977). Also, such a discrepancy between performance IQ and verbal IQ is said to be indicative of a specific language impairment and/or a language-learning disability (Wechsler, 1974).

The presence of coma following immersion has been shown to be prognostically indicative of neurologic impairment in victims of near-drowning (Modell, Graves, & Kuck, 1980). Modell et al. (1980) retrospectively reviewed 121 cases of near-drowning and compared their neurologic outcome with their neurological status on admission to hospital as determined by the neurologic classification scale for victims of near-drowning (Conn & Barker, 1984). According to this scale, victims of immersion can be placed into one of three different neurological classifications: A (awake), alert and fully conscious; B (blunted), obtunded, stuporous but rousable with purposeful response to pain and abnormal respiration; and C (comatose), not rousable with abnormal response to pain and abnormal respiration. Modell et al. (1980) reported that neurologic deficit was apparent only in Group C cases. Allman, Nelson, Pacentine, and McComb (1986) stated that no near-drowned child presenting as flaccid and comatosed on admission to hospital recovers normal neurologic functioning. Reports from several other centers are similar, indicating that children who have experienced near-drowning who still require cardiopulmonary resuscitation on arrival at the hospital experienced permanent, severe anoxic encephalopathy. In a Hawaiian study, all children who ultimately survived intact made spontaneous respiratory efforts within 5 minutes of rescue, and the majority of those did so within 2 minutes (Fandel & Bancalari, 1976). None of the children still comatose in 15 to 30 minutes after their rescue survived without major neurologic sequelae, and 60% of children in this latter group died. Fields (1992) listed the following factors that predict poor outcome after near-drowning: (1) submersion for more than 5 minutes; (2) serum pH below 7.0 at time of admission to emergency room; (3) the need for cardiopulmonary resuscitation in the emergency room; (4) a delay before the first postresuscitation gasp; and (5) poor initial neurologic evaluation on resuscitation. Immersion in cold or icy water appears to give a better chance for survival (DeNicola, Falk, Swanson, Gayle, & Kissoon, 1997).

Linguistic Deficits Following Immersion

The findings of several studies have either indicated or suggested the presence of speech and language disorders in children who have experienced near-drowning. Pearn et al. (1979b) identified dysarthria and aphasia as potential

sequelae of near-drowning incidents. In addition, as discussed earlier, the findings of Pearn (1977) were suggestive of the presence of a language impairment in children following immersion. Reilly et al. (1988), however, are the only authors to date to have specifically investigated and documented the linguistic abilities of near-drowned children. These researchers investigated the linguistic abilities of two groups of children who had been involved in near-drowning incidents, one group 12 months after immersion ($n = 25$) and the second group 5 years after immersion ($n = 9$). Reilly et al. (1988) compared the performances of the two groups on standardized language tests with the performances of appropriate controls matched for age, sex and socioeconomic status. In addition Reilly and co-workers assigned each of their immersion subjects to one of the categories A, B, or C of the neurologic classification for victims of near-drowning (Conn & Barker, 1984) and correlated their neurologic status with their language abilities.

The findings of Reilly et al. (1988) showed that the 12-month after immersion group was language delayed, as determined by their performance on the Sequenced Inventory of Communicative Development (Hedrick, Prather, & Tobin, 1975) compared with their control group. In particular, Reilly et al. (1988) found that the near-drowned children had significantly lower scores than their controls for expressive language age and receptive language age when these scores were calculated as percentages of the child's chronologic age.

Reilly et al. (1988) also reported that all their subjects in the 12-months after immersion group who were categorized as either Group A or B according to the Conn and Barker (1984) neurologic scale at the time of their admission to hospital, exhibited language abilities within normal limits. In contrast, however, four of the five near-drowned cases from the 12-month after immersion group categorized as Group C did exhibit some degree of language impairment (Table 7–2).

The low level of performance of subject 5 would be anticipated from the findings of Allman et al. (1986), as he was the only child in the study who presented on admission to hospital in a flaccid comatose condition. Reilly et al. (1988) also noted that all of the Group C children, with the exception of subjects 3 and 5, had been described as "neurologically normal" except for drooling from the mouth and the presence of a mild speech problem.

No significant differences were found by Reilly et al. (1988) between the language scores achieved by the immersion subjects assessed 5 years after the near-drowning incident and their controls, although it was noted by the authors that the majority of the immersion subjects in this group were categorized as Group A on the Conn and Barker (1984) scale.

Two subjects in the 5-year after immersion group were comatose at the time of their admission to hospital and were therefore categorized as Group C. One of the Group C subjects exhibited a linguistic impairment when assessed 5 years later, his performance being below the 20th percentile for the receptive vocabulary, sentence-imitation and articulation subtests of the Test of Language Development-Primary (Newcomer & Hammill, 1982). The other Group C child, however, did not exhibit a linguistic problem when assessed 5 years later. This child was assessed initially by a speech-language pathologist 4 weeks after the immersion incident. At that time he presented with auditory processing difficulties and word-finding problems. Three months after the near-drowning incident, the child was reported as functioning within normal limits on all speech and language tests. Despite this, he presented at the hospital outpatient clinic 5 years later for investigation of suspected learning difficulties. His parents, at this time, reported that they had noted that the child was slow to learn, had a poor concentration span and exhibited auditory inattention.

Table 7–2. Speech and Language Outcome in Group C Subjects in the 12-Month-Following Immersion Study by Reilly et al. (1988)

Subject No.	Age (months)	Receptive language age (months)	Expressive language age (months)
1	40	32	36
2	37	40	40
3	22	16	16
4	47	36	40
5	45	12	8

Subsequent assessments of the child showed normal performance on neurological examination, psychometric IQ testing and speech and language assessment. However, in the light of the presenting symptoms, Reilly et al. (1988) were unable to rule out the presence of an auditory processing deficit, as at that time a comprehensive audiologic assessment had not been carried out. Both of these subjects had been described as "neurologically normal" within 3 months of the near-drowning incident.

Reilly et al. (1988) concluded that children who are victims of near-drowning incidents, and who initially present at hospital as comatose, form a population that is at risk for impaired development of linguistic abilities.

Motor Speech Disorders in a Case of Accidental Childhood Suffocation

Murdoch et al. (1989) described the case of a 13-year-old boy who had suffered anoxic encephalopathy as a result of being accidentally buried under sand for approximately 20 minutes. A CT scan taken 5 weeks after the injury demonstrated the presence of bilateral striatocapsular lesions involving the lenticular nucleus and head of the caudate nucleus in each hemisphere (see Figure 7–1). The topography of the lesions was consistent with the pattern observed in cases of cerebral anoxia (De Reuck & Vander Eecken, 1978). Administration of a series of speech and language tests, including the Frenchay Dysarthria Assessment (Enderby, 1983), the Apraxia Battery for Adults (Dabul, 1979) and the Western Aphasia Battery (Kertesz, 1982) over a 3-month period starting at 6 weeks

postonset revealed that the subject displayed a range of symptoms typical of aphemia (Schiff, Alexander, Naeser, & Galaburda, 1983) including a progression from initial mutism to syntactically intact verbalizations with retained ability to write and comprehend spoken language. Murdoch et al. (1989) concluded that the aphemia was best explained by either a disruption of the subcortical connections of the perirolandic region of each hemisphere or alternatively by an impairment in speech motor planning due to direct involvement of the basal ganglia.

At the time of the initial assessment some 6 weeks after the injury, Murdoch et al. (1989) described their patient as being mute but able to communicate by means of a letter board. No receptive language disturbance was evident at this time. Although his intelligibility was poor, the subject was able to vocalize in single words 7 weeks after the injury and could use short sentences by 8 weeks after his accidental burial. Murdoch et al. (1989) noted that when examined 12 weeks postonset, the patient's speech contained some elements typical of hypokinetic dysarthria. In particular, an increase in speech rate reminiscent of that seen in Parkinson disease was reported to be present during speech production. Furthermore, the patient also showed difficulty in initiating speech movements.

A Western Aphasia Battery administered 14 weeks postonset showed the presence of intact receptive language abilities, with only a minor expressive problem being evident, probably resulting from the above mentioned concomitant dysarthria. Written language was described as being syntactically appropriate and orthographically correct, although the motor aspects of writing were abnormal. Certainly, no overt aphasia was evident. The authors noted, however, that they were unable to rule out with certainty the possible presence of subtle language problems, in that the Western Aphasia Battery does not assess high-level language function. Murdoch et al. (1989) also noted that the subject may have shown a transient language disorder in the acute stage following suffocation which could have resolved during the 6 weeks before their initial assessment of the patient.

The findings in the above case of anoxic encephalopathy led Murdoch et al. (1989) to suggest that if striatocapsular structures do have a role in language, as suggested by evidence from the adult literature and in children by Aram et al. (1983), this role may be assumed by other brain structures in children following damage to the striatocapsular region.

Linguistic Deficits Following Cardiac Arrest and Respiratory Arrest

Two cases of acquired childhood aphasia resulting from anoxic encephalopathy were described by Cooper and Flowers (1987). One case (subject 1) was a boy who suffered a cardiac arrest following cardiac surgery while the second case (subject 11) was a girl who developed anoxic encephalopathy subsequent to respiratory arrest at 8 years 4 months of age. Both children were described as being mute in the initial period postonset. In the case of subject 11, verbal communication did not return until 6 months postonset, whereas in subject 1, at the time of his discharge from hospital 2 months postonset, no comment on the presence of communication difficulties was noted.

When assessed with a range of speech-language assessments just over 6 years postonset, subject 1 was reported to show deficits in receptive and expressive single-word vocabulary. Cooper and Flowers (1987) also noted that, during the course of the language assessment, subject 1 appeared reticent to talk, spoke rarely, and did not initiate conversation. Subject 1 scored only 29 of a possible 85 correct responses on the Boston Naming Test (Kaplan, Goodglass, & Weintraub, 1983) with the errors being described by Cooper and Flowers (1987) as being primarily semantically related, phonological or misperceptions of the picture stimulus. Word fluency was also disturbed and subject 1 was reported to have problems with arithmetic computation. His intellectual function, however, was reported to be normal although it was noted that he did attend full-time special education.

Unlike subject 1, hospital and school reports indicated that subject 11 had persistent language difficulties from the time of onset until assessed by Cooper and Flowers (1987), almost 7 years later. Based on her performance on the various language tests administered, Cooper and Flowers (1987) reported that subject 11 had deficits in receptive single-word vocabulary and production and completion of syntactic constructions. Impaired performance on the Token Test was also noted; subject 11 scoring more than two standard deviations below the mean for her peer age category. As in subject 1, problems with arithmetic computation were also present. Indeed, all areas of academic performance were said to be impaired, with the exception of reading comprehension. In terms of intellectual functioning, subject 11 was reported to fall in the low-average to borderline range and she attended special education.

The two anoxia cases described by Cooper and Flowers (1987) clearly demonstrate that anoxic encephalopathy may be associated with the occurrence of long-term linguistic deficits, even in those cases where apparent recovery of speech and language abilities occurs in the acute stage postonset.

Summary

Although there are few reports in the literature that have related anoxic encephalopathy to the occurrence of speech and language deficits in childhood, the evidence available suggests that anoxic brain damage can cause linguistic deficits in both the acute and chronic stages post-onset. To date, speech and language disorders in childhood have only been described subsequent to anoxia resulting from events such as near-drowning, accidental suffocation and cardiac arrest. In that all types of anoxia cause fundamentally the same distribution of lesions in the brain, it could be expected, however, that anoxia resulting from any cause has the potential to induce linguistic deficits in children.

It is important, therefore, that speech-language pathologists recognize that any child who has experienced some type of anoxic episode, and especially those cases that initially present at hospital as comatose, are at risk of developing speech and language disorders. Although in some cases the long-term linguistic deficits that result from the anoxic encephalopathy may be sufficiently overt to be detected by parents, teachers, and so forth, in many cases these deficits are of a subtle, subclinical or latent nature and are only evidenced by an extensive and detailed speech and language examination. However, despite their subtle nature, these subclinical linguistic problems may manifest as impaired academic performance in later life, with affected subjects in some cases presenting many years after the anoxic injury for investigation of suspected learning difficulties. The need for speech-language pathologists to monitor the development of the speech and language of children who have had an anoxic episode is imperative.

References

Adams, J. H., Brierley, J. B., Connor, R. C. R., & Treip, C. S. (1966). The effects of systemic hypotension upon the human brain: Clinical and neuropathological observation in 11 cases. *Brain, 89,* 235–268.

Adams, R. (1963). General discussion. In J. P. Schadé & W. H. McMenemey (Eds.), *Selective Vulnerability of the brain in hypoxaemia.* Oxford, UK: Blackwell Scientific Publications.

Alexander, M. P., & LoVerme, S. R. (1980). Aphasia after left hemispheric intracerebral hemorrhage. *Neurology, 30,* 1193–1202.

Allman, F. D., Nelson, W. B., Pacentine, G. A., & McComb, G. (1986). Outcome following cardiopulmonary resuscitation in severe pediatric near-drowning. *American Journal of Disorders in Children, 140,* 571–575.

Ames, A., Wright, R. L., Kowada, M., Thurston, J. M., & Majno, G. (1968). Cerebral ischaemia: The no-reflow phenomenon. *American Journal of Pathology, 52,* 437–453.

Aram, D. M., Ekelman, B. L., & Gillespie, L. L. (1989). Reading and lateralized brain lesions in children. In K. von Euler (Ed.),

Developmental dyslexia and dysphasia. Basingstoke, UK: Macmillan.

Aram, D. M., Rose, D. F., Rekate, H. L., & Whitaker, H. A. (1983). Acquired capular/striatal aphasia in childhood. *Archives of Neurology, 40,* 614–617.

Auer, R. N., & Sutherland, G. R. (2002). Hypoxic brain damage. In D. I. Graham & P. L. Lantos (Eds.), *Greenfield's neuropathology* (7th ed., pp. 33–280). London, UK: Arnold.

Bell, R. D., & Lastimosa, A. C. B. (1980). Metabolic encephalopathies. In R. N. Rosenberg (Ed.), *Neurology* (pp. 115–164). New York, NY: Grune & Stratton.

Benson, D. F. (1979). *Aphasia, alexia and agraphia.* New York, NY: Churchill Livingstone.

Bhatt, M. H., Obeso, J. A., & Marsden, C. D. (1993). Time course of postanoxic akinetic-rigid and dystonic syndromes. *Neurology, 43,* 314–317.

Brierley, J. B. (1972). The neuropathology of brain hypoxia. In M. Critchley, J. L. O'Leary, & B. Jennett (Eds.), *Scientific foundations of neurology.* London, UK: Heinemann.

Brierley, J. B., Graham, D. I., Adams, J. H., & Simpsom, J. A. (1971). Neocortical death after cardiac arrest: A clinical, neurophysiological, and neuropathological report of two cases. *Lancet, 298,* 560–565.

Brucher, J. M. (1967). Neuropathological problems posed by carbon monoxide poisoning and anoxia. *Progress in Brain Research, 24,* 75–100.

Conn, A. W., & Barker, G. A. (1984). Fresh water drowning and near-drowning—an update. *Canadian Anaesthetists' Society Journal, 31,* 538–544.

Cooper, J. A., & Flowers, C. R. (1987). Children with a history of acquired aphasia: Residual language and academic impairments. *Journal of Speech and Hearing Disorders, 52,* 251–262.

Dabul, B. (1979). Apraxia battery for adults. Tigard, OR: C. C. Publications.

DeNicola, L. K., Falk, J. L., Swanson, M. E., Gayle, M. O., & Kissoon, N. (1997). Submersion injuries in children and adults. *Critical Care Clinics, 13,* 477–502.

De Reuck, J. L., & Vander Eecken, H. M. (1978). Periventricular leukomalacia in adults. *Archives of Neurology, 35,* 517–521.

Dooling, E. C., & Richardson, E. P. (1976). Delayed encephalopathy after strangling. *Archives of Neurology, 33,* 196–199.

Edstrom, R. F. S., & Essex, H. E. (1956). Swelling of the brain induced by anoxia. *Neurology, 6,* 118–124.

Enderby, P. M. (1983). Frenchay dysarthria assessment. San Diego, CA: College-Hill Press.

Eriksson, R., Fredin, H., Gerdman, P., & Thorsan, J. (1973). Sequelae of accidental near-drowning in childhood. *Scandinavian Journal of Social Medicine, 1,* 3–6.

Fandel, I., & Bancalari, E. (1976). Near drowning in children: Clinical aspects. *Pediatrics, 58,* 573–579.

Fields, A. I. (1992). Near-drowning in the pediatric population. *Critical Care Clinics, 8,* 113–129.

Fleetham, J. A., & Munt, P. W. (1978). Near-drowning in Canadian waters. *Canadian Medical Association Journal, 118,* 914–917.

Frates, R. C. (1981). Analysis of predictive factors in the assessment of warm water near-drowning in children. *American Journal of Diseases in Childhood, 135,* 1006–1008.

Frewen, T. C., Sumabat, W. O., Han, V. K., Amacher, A. L., Del Mastro, R. F., & Sibbald, W. J. (1985). Cerebral resuscitation therapy in pediatric near-drowning. *Journal of Pediatrics, 104,* 615–617.

Gänshirt, H. (1957). *Die Sauerstroffversorgung des Gehirns und ihre Störung bei der Liquordrucksteigerung und beim Hirnödem.* Berlin, Germany: Springer.

Ginsberg, M. D., Hedley-Whyte, T., & Richardson, E. P. (1976). Hypoxic-ischemic leukoencephalopathy in man. *Archives of Neurology, 33,* 5–16.

Graham, D. I. (1977). Pathology of hypoxic brain damage in man. *Journal of Clinical Pathology, 30* (Suppl. 11), 170–180.

Hedrick, D. L., Prather, E. M., & Tobin, A. R. (1975). Sequenced inventory of communication development. Seattle, WA: University of Washington Press.

Helgason, C., Caplan, L. R., Goodwin, J. A., & Hedges, T. (1986). Anterior choroidal artery—territory infarction. *Archives of Neurology, 43,* 681–686.

Helgason, C., Caplan, L. R., Goodwin, J. A., & Hedges, T. (1987). Bilateral basal ganglia necrosis following diffuse hypoxic-ischemic injury—a reply. *Archives of Neurology, 44,* 897.

Kaplan, E., Goodglass, H., & Weintraub, S. (1983). *Boston Naming Test.* Philadelphia, PA: Lea & Febiger.

Kertesz, A. (1982). The western aphasia battery. New York, NY: Grune & Stratton.

Kim, H. Y., Kim, B. J., Moon, S. Y., Kwon, J. C., Shon, Y. M., Na, D. G., . . . Na, D. L.(2002). Serial diffusion-weighted MR imaging in delayed postanoxic encephalopathy: A case study. *Journal of Neuroradiology, 29,* 211–215.

Környey, S. (1963). Patterns of CNS vulnerability in CO, cyanide and other poisoning. In J. P. Schadé & W. H. McMenemey (Eds.), *Selective vulnerability of the brain in hypoxaemia.* Oxford, UK: Blackwell Scientific Publications.

Kruus, Bergstrom, L., Suutarinen, T., & Hyvonen, R. (1979). The prognosis of near-drowned children. *Acta Paediatrica Scandinavica, 68,* 315–322.

Lindenberg, R. (1955). Compression of brain arteries as pathogenetic factor for tissue necrosis and their areas of predilection. *Journal of Neuropathology and Experimental Neurology, 14,* 223–243.

Lindenberg, R. (1963). Patterns of CNS vulnerability in acute hypoxaemia, including anaesthesia accidents. In J. P. Schadé & W. H. McMenemey (Eds.), *Selective vulnerability of the brain in hypoxaemia.* Oxford, UK: Blackwell Scientific Publications.

McIlwain, H. (1955). *Biochemistry and the central nervous system.* London, UK: Churchill Livingstone.

McIlwain, H. (1966). *Biochemistry and the central nervous system* (3rd ed.). London, UK: Churchill Livingstone.

Matsuo, F., Cummins, J. W., & Anderson, R. E. (1979). Neurological sequelae of massive hydrogen sulfide inhalation. *Archives of Neurology, 36,* 451–452.

Modell, J. H., Graves, S. A., & Kuck, E. J. (1980). Near-drowning: Correlation of level of consciousness and survival. *Canadian Anaesthetists' Society Journal, 27,* 211–215.

Murdoch, B. E. (2010). *Acquired speech and language disorders: A neuroanatomical and functional neurological approach* (2nd ed.). Oxford, UK: Wiley Blackwell.

Murdoch, B. E., Chenery, H. J., & Kennedy, M. (1989). Aphemia associated with bilateral striato-capsular lesions subsequent to cerebral anoxia. *Brain Injury, 3,* 41–49.

Murdoch, B. E., Thompson, D., Fraser, S., & Harrison, L. (1986). Aphasia following nonhaemorrhagic lesions in the left striato-capsular region. *Australian Journal of Human Communication Disorders, 14,* 5–21.

Murdoch, B. E., & Whelan, B-M. (2009). *Speech and language disorders associated with subcortical pathology.* Oxford, UK: Wiley Blackwell.

Murray, R. S., Stensaas, S. S., Anderson, R. E., & Matsuo, F. (1987). Bilateral basal ganglia necrosis following diffuse hypoxic-ischaemic injury. *Archives of Neurology, 44,* 897.

Newcomer, P. L., & Hammill, D. D. (1982). Test of language development-primary. Austin, TX: Pro-Ed.

Nussbaum, E. (1985). Prognostic variables in nearly-drowned comatose children. *American Journal of Diseases in Childhood, 139,* 1058–1059.

Oakes, D. D., Sherck, J. P., Maloney, J. R., & Crane-Chaters, A. (1982). Prognosis and management of victims of near drowning. *Journal of Trauma, 22,* 544–548.

Pearn, J. H. (1977). Neurologic and psychometric studies in children surviving freshwater immersion accidents. *Lancet, i,* 7–9.

Pearn, J. H. (1985). Pathophysiology of drowning. *Medical Journal of Australia, 142,* 586–588.

Pearn, J. H., Bart, R. D., & Yamaoka, R. (1979a). Neurologic sequelae after childhood near-drowning: A total population study from Hawaii. *Pediatrics, 64,* 187–191.

Pearn, J. H., De Buse, P., Mohay, H., & Golden, M. (1979b). Sequential intellectual recovery after near-drowning. *Medical Journal of Australia, 1,* 463–464.

Peterson, B. (1977). Morbidity of childhood drowning. *Pediatrics, 59,* 364–365.

Petito, C. K., Olarte, J-P., Roberts, B., Nowak, T. S. Jr., & Pulsinelli, W. A. (1998). Selective glial vulnerability following transient global ischemia in rat brain. *Journal of Neuropathology and Experimental Neurology, 57,* 231–238.

Plum, F. (1973). The clinical problem: How much anoxia-ischemia damages the brain? *Archives of Neurology, 29,* 359–360.

Plum, F., Posner, J. B., & Hain, R. F. (1962). Delayed neurological deterioration after anoxia. *Archives of Internal Medicine, 110,* 18–25.

Reilly, K., Ozanne, A. E., Murdoch, B. E., & Pitt, W. R. (1988). Linguistic status subsequent to childhood immersion injury. *Medical Journal of Australia, 148,* 225–228.

Richardson, J. C., Chambers, R. A., & Heywood, P. M. (1959). Encephalopathies of anoxia and hypoglycemia. *Archives of Neurology, 1,* 178–190.

Schiff, H. B., Alexander, M. P., Naeser, M. A., & Galaburda, A. M. (1983). Aphemia: Clinical anatomic correlations. *Archives of Neurology, 40,* 720–727.

Schwedenberg, T. H. (1959). Leukoencephalopathy following carbon monoxide asphyxia. *Journal of Neuropathology and Experimental Neurology, 18,* 597–608.

Towbin, A. (1971). Organic causes of minimal brain dysfunction. *Journal of American Medical Association, 217,* 1207–1214.

Wechsler, D. (1967). Wechsler pre-school and primary scale of intelligence. New York, NY: Psychological Corporation.

Wechsler, D. (1974). Wechsler intelligence scale for children. New York, NY: Psychological Corporation.

Weinberger, L. M., Gibbon, M. H., & Gibbon, J. H. (1940). Temporary arrest of the circulation to the central nervous system: 1. Physiological effects. *Archives of Neurology and Psychiatry, 43,* 615.

Zeiss, J., & Brinker, R. (1988). Role of contrast enhancement in cerebral CT of carbon monoxide poisoning. *Journal of Computer Assisted Tomography, 12,* 341–343.

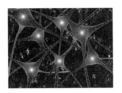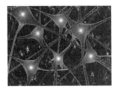

8

Language Impairments in Neural Tube Disorders

During the early weeks of pregnancy, the central nervous system (CNS), including both the brain and spinal cord, develops from a hollow cylinder of cells called the neural tube. Congenital malformations of the nervous system that arise from defective formation of the neural tube in the embryo are referred to as neural tube disorders. In that failure of the neural tube to form properly also causes disruption of supportive tissues such as bone, muscle, and connective tissue, as well as producing abnormalities in the central nervous system, neural tube disorders also cause defects in overlying structures such as the vertebrae and cranium. The etiologic factor or factors that cause neural tube disorders in humans clearly have not been defined, although both genetic and environmental factors have been implicated (Simpson, 1976). Overall, the incidence of neural tube disorders is approximately 2.6 per 1,000 total single births with this incidence declining in recent

years. Supplementation of the maternal diet with folic acid or with a multivitamin preparation that contains folic acid even prior to conception has been shown to reduce the recurrence rate of neural tube defects (Czeizel & Dudas, 1992) leading the government in some countries to mandate the supplementation of bread with folate. The reason for the apparent effect of folic acid is unclear. Although the decline in the incidence of neural tube disorders partly may be explained by the introduction of mandatory vitamin and folic acid supplementation programs, it also probably reflects the outcome of widespread use of antenatal screening.

Neural tube disorders can involve anatomical deformities in either the brain or spinal cord. The major types of neural tube disorders include anencephaly, encephalocele and spina bifida. The more severe types of neural tube disorders, such as anencephaly, are incompatible with extrauterine life. Consequently, children with this disorder do not form part of the clinical caseloads of speech-language pathologists and, is mentioned only briefly here. Less severe neural tube disorders, however, such as several forms of spina bifida are compatible with extra-uterine life. Although extrauterine life is possible, some of these less severe neural tube disorders may cause functional disabilities manifest as a variety of neurologic problems which may include, among others, impaired intellectual abilities and communication deficits.

Brain Abnormalities

Anencephaly

Anencephaly is a severe condition that occurs in approximately 1 in every 1,000 births and results from a failure of the neural tube to close at the cranial end. The condition has been reported to occur 37 times more frequently in female than in male newborns (Nakano, 1973). Anencephaly is not compatible with sustained extrauterine life and therefore is not related to the occurrence of communication deficits. The presence of anencephaly or other open neural tube defects can be predicted by measuring α-fetoprotein (AFP) in amniotic fluid or maternal serum. Because of a substantial leak of fetal blood components directly into amniotic fluid, AFP concentrations in amniotic fluid and maternal serum AFP levels are elevated in anencephaly and in open spina bifida (myeloschisis) or cranium bifidum (encephalocele) (Brock, 1977).

Encephalocele

Encephalocele occurs in approximately 1 in every 2,000 births and involves the protrusion of a portion of the brain and meninges through a defect in the skull (cranium bifidum). The defect is always in the midline and occurs most commonly in the occipital region. The condition is often accompanied by hydrocephalus.

If the protruding meningeal sac contains only cerebrospinal fluid (CSF), the brain remaining within the cranium, the condition is called cranial meningocele. In some cases the cranial defect may be repaired.

Spina Bifida

Spina bifida, which literally translated means "bifid spine," is a term used to refer to a number of different neural tube disorders involving defective fusion of structures dorsal to the spinal cord. Females are affected more commonly than males in a ratio of approximately 1.3 to 1 (Anderson & Spain, 1977). Overall, the incidence of spina bifida varies from 1 to 2 per 1,000 live births (Anderson & Spain, 1977; Knowlton, Peterson, & Putbrese, 1985). Although spina bifida may occur anywhere along the length of the vertebral column, it is most common in the lower thoracic, lumbar, and sacral regions.

Depending on the involvement of the underlying meninges and spinal cord, several different types of spina bifida are recognized. These include: spina bifida occulta and spina bifida cystica (including meningocele and spina bifida with meningomyelocele, and myeloschisis). Of the different types of spina bifida, occulta is the most common followed by myeloschisis. Many of the infants with the latter condition, however, are born dead or die within a few days of birth from infection of the spinal cord.

In its simplest form (spina bifida occulta), spina bifida involves a failure of the bilateral dorsal lamina of the vertebrae to fuse in the midline to form a single spinous process. As a result of this failure, two unfused halves of the vertebral arch remain as short spines on either side of the midline. The defect may not, however, be limited to abnormal growth of the neural arches, but also may involve the meninges, especially in those cases where the defect in the vertebral column is large. In such cases the meninges may herniated through the defect in the vertebral column to form a large fluid-filled cyst on the child's back. Such a condition is called spina bifida cystica.

Spina Bifida Occulta

Spina bifida occulta, the most common but least serious form of spina bifida, involves an absence of the spinous process of one or more vertebrae. The vertebral defect, usually located in the lumbosacral region, is covered by postvertebral muscles and skin and in most cases is not evident from the surface. Occasionally, however, a small tuft of hair or fatty tumor may be present over the defect (Figure 8–1).

In that the spinal cord and nerve roots lie in their normal position in the vertebral canal and are therefore not damaged, spina bifida occulta usually is symptomless, with no neurologic or

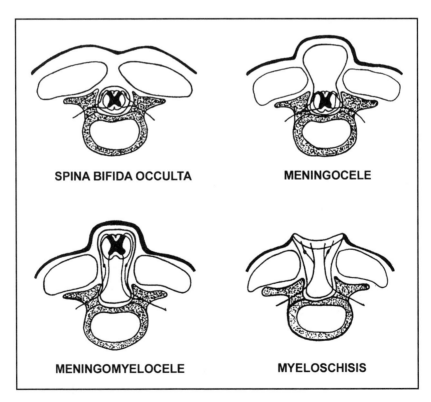

SPINA BIFIDA OCCULTA

MENINGOCELE

MENINGOMYELOCELE

MYELOSCHISIS

FIGURE 8–1. Diagrammatic sketches showing the major types of spina bifida and the commonly associated malformations of the nervous system.

musculoskeletal abnormalities being present. Consequently, spina bifida occulta also is not usually associated with the occurrence of speech-language or hearing deficits. Often, the condition is only detected by chance when radiographs are taken of the vertebral column.

Meningocele

In this type of spina bifida the meninges protrude through the defect in the vertebral column to form a cystic swelling covered by skin, usually in the lumbosacral region of the child's back. The spinal cord and cauda equina, however, remain in their normal position in the vertebral canal (see Figure 8–1) and therefore function normally. As a result there may be no abnormal neurologic signs present in children with spina bifida with meningocele and, as in the case of spina bifida occulta, communication disorders are an unlikely occurrence. The meningocele can be repaired surgically.

Myeloschisis (Myelocele)

This type of spina bifida results from a failure of the neural tube to close, usually in the lumbosacral region (see Figure 8–1). Consequently, the spinal cord appears on the surface of the child's back as a raw area in the configuration of the wide-open neural plate. CSF discharges from the central canal of the spinal cord onto the surface of this raw patch. In that microorganisms have easy access to the exposed CNS, the chance of survival of infants with this condition is slight.

Meningomyelocele

Meningomyelocele is the most complex congenital malformation of the CNS that is compatible with extrauterine life and represents the most common severely disabling birth defect in North America (Fletcher, Barnes, & Dennis, 2002). The condition results from incomplete neural tube closure in the first 5 to 6 weeks of gestation. It differs from meningocele in that in addition to the meninges the spinal cord or cauda equina also protrude through the defect in the vertebral column and adhere to the inner surface of the meningeal cyst (see Figure 8–1). The cystic swelling in this case is covered by a thin membrane which is easily ruptured and is present in most cases in the lumbar and lumbosacral regions.

The postdietary fortification rate of meningomyelocele has been reported to be 0.3 to 0.6 per 1,000 live births (Williams, Rasmussen, Flores, Kirby, & Edmunds, 2005). Unlike spina bifida occulta and meningocele, meningomyelocele is associated with a range of neurologic impairments, including motor, cognitive, and language difficulties and consequently will represent the primary focus for discussion in the present chapter. Characteristically, meningomyelocele is associated with varying degrees of paralysis or paresis of the lower limbs, sensory loss (anesthesia), and autonomic disturbances including bladder and bowel incontinence and urine retention associated with damage to the spinal cord. However, meningomyelocele is a disorder of both the spine and brain. In addition to abnormalities in spinal cord development, the condition is also associated with profound disturbances of brain development that include abnormal formation and maturation of the posterior cerebral cortex and white matter, midbrain, cerebellum, and corpus callosum (Fletcher, Dennis, & Northrup, 2000; Hannay, 2000). About 80 to 90% of children with meningomyelocele also experience subsequent hydrocephalus that required shunt diversion (Reigel & Rothstein, 1994). As a result, children with meningomyelocele often have difficulties, as well as relative strengths, with the development of cognitive, language, and adaptive behavior skills (Barnes & Dennis, 1992; Barnes et al., 2006; Brewer, Fletcher, Hiscock, & Davidson, 2001; Dennis, Landry, Barnes, & Fletcher, 2006; Yeates, Fletcher, & Dennis, 2005).

The segmental level of the lesion determines the area of anesthesia and which muscles are affected. In general, a child with meningomyelocele will be unable to move the muscles receiving their nerve supply from the spinal cord below the level of the lesion. The most severely physically handicapped children with meningomyelocele are those with lesions at or above the third lumbar vertebra who are totally paraplegic (Anderson & Spain, 1977; Smith, 1965). Cases with lesions at or below the fourth lumbar vertebra suffer from paralysis of some, but not all, muscles of the hips, knees, and feet. Children with lesions at the first and second sacral vertebrae may have adequate function of the hips but have paralysis of the feet. Least handicapped are children with lesions at or below the third sacral vertebra. Although these latter children may have normal function of the lower limbs, they may be incontinent (Smith, 1965). Overall, between 30 to 50% of all children with a meningomyelocele show a total paraplegia whereas most others have significant locomotor problems (Anderson & Spain, 1977). Children with severe functional impairment may require a wheelchair for mobility.

In addition to motor problems, damage to the spinal cord in cases of meningomyelocele results in anesthesia in parts of the body receiving their nerve supply from the spinal cord below the level of the lesion (Anderson & Spain, 1977). Anesthesia of the lower limbs may lead to the development of pressure sores and increases the child's susceptibility to burns and frostbite because the child feels no discomfort for extremes of temperature.

Menelaus (1980) reported that only 7% of persons with meningomyelocele have normal urinary and bowel control. Urinary control generally is achieved through intermittent self-catheterization or urinary diversion. Management of bowel incontinence is achieved through developing regular habits of elimination with the use of suppositories. Urinary incontinence increases the risk of urinary tract infection and kidney damage.

Some of the neurologic deficits shown by children suffering from spina bifida with meningomyelocele are the direct consequence of the spinal cord defect, whereas others arise from brain anomalies or deformities. As indicated above, meningomyelocele is associated with corpus callosum malformations, most commonly in the posterior regions (Hannay, 2000), which are important for interhemispheric transfer (Klaas, Hannay, Caroselli, & Fletcher, 1999). The extent of corpus callosum dysmorphology varies in children with meningomyelocele with some children having an intact but hypoplastic corpus callosum whereas other exhibit corpus callosum hypoplasia or agenesis as part of the primary neuroanatomic malformations associated with their disorder. Importantly, hypoplasia or agenesis of the corpus callosum disrupts the integration of information between the two cerebral hemispheres.

One complication often associated with meningomyelocele that has important clinical consequences is hydrocephalus. Approximately 80 to 90% of children with meningomyelocele develop hydrocephalus (Reigel & Rothstein,

1994). In infants the bones of the skull are not fused. Consequently, as a result of the accumulation of CSF, the heads of infants with untreated hydrocephalus expand without necessarily causing much damage to the brain itself. In older children, however, where the skull bones have fused increased intracranial pressure resulting from the increase in volume of CSF causes compression and damage to the brain, and if not relieved leads to impaired control of the movements of the upper and lower limbs, ocular defects, and progressive loss of sight and eventually to cognitive and communication impairments. Apart from death in the first few weeks of life, of which hydrocephalus is a major cause, the major significance of the presence of hydrocephalus is that the long-term problems of meningomyelocele, including impaired communicative and intellectual abilities, in part are likely caused by the effects of hydrocephalus on the brain. For instance, research suggests that hydrocephalus and its complications are the primary associated features of children with meningomyelocele who show evidence of decreased cognitive skills (Knowlton et al., 1985).

The occurrence of hydrocephalus in children with meningomyelocele is largely accounted for by two structural anomalies: the Arnold-Chiari hindbrain malformation and stenosis of the aqueduct of Sylvius. In some children with meningomyelocele both of these abnormalities may occur. Arnold-Chiari malformation often coexists with meningomyelocele. The malformation consists of a caudal displacement of the hindbrain involving projection of components of the medulla oblongata, cerebellum, choroid plexus and fourth ventricle through the foramen magnum into the spinal canal. As a consequence of this caudal displacement, the circulation of CSF is blocked at the foramina of the fourth ventricle leading to the accumulation of fluid in the ventricular system of the brain.

As in the case of meningocele, children with meningomyelocele can be treated surgically. The cyst is opened and the spinal cord or nerves are freed and carefully replaced in the vertebral canal. Full recovery of function, however, rarely if ever occurs. Associated hydrocephalus, if present, may be controlled by insertion of either a ventriculoperitoneal shunt or a ventriculoatrial shunt which reduce the abnormally high cerebrospinal fluid pressure and maintain normal intracranial pressure by draining fluid away from the ventricles of the brain. Complications of shunting procedures include occasional obstruction of the catheter due to growth of the child, infection, blockage of the shunt and disconnection of the shunt (Anderson & Spain, 1977). Not every child with hydrocephalus, however, requires surgical treatment. In some cases the hydrocephalus becomes "arrested" in that the amount of CSF produced becomes balanced with the amount of CSF absorbed. In such children, the head stops growing at an abnormal rate.

Children with meningomyelocele usually do not experience mental retardation, despite the severity and nature of their CNS anomalies. However, they do often exhibit domain-specific strengths and weaknesses by the time they reach school age. Specifically, although they are able to sustain attention, they do have problems with focus and shifting attention (Brewer et al., 2001; Dennis et al., 2005). Furthermore, their action-based visual perception is weak, but categorical perception is not (Dennis, Fletcher, Rogers, Hetherington, & Francis, 2002).

Rule-based problem solving and performance that relies on the assembly of meaning from context is difficult, but rote learning is preserved (Barnes, Faulker, Wilkinson, & Dennis, 2004; Dennis & Barnes, 2002). Although problems with word recognition are infrequent, approximately two-thirds of the children with meningomyelocele develop problems in academic areas such as reading comprehension and math (Barnes & Dennis, 1992; Barnes et al., 2006; Fletcher et al., 2005). The language disorders exhibited by a child with meningomyelocele are discussed further below.

Cognitive Deficits in Children with Meningomyelocele

A large number of studies show that the normal distribution of IQ is not seen in the spina bifida population. Instead, the distribution curve is skewed toward the lower end of the IQ range with a peak of scores below average (Anderson & Spain, 1977; Badell-Ribera, Schulman, & Paddock, 1966; Mapstone et al., 1984; Ruchert, Hansel-Freidrich, & Wolff, 1986; Shurtleff, Kronmal, & Foltz, 1975; Spain, 1974; Tew & Laurence, 1975). Several factors have been related to this decreased cognitive functioning. These include: the complications of shunting (Mapstone et al., 1984); the presence of seizures (Dennis et al., 1981); the level of the lesion (Hunt & Holmes, 1975), social class (Scherzer & Gardner, 1970); and ventriculitis and meningitis (Billard, Santini, Gillet, Nargeot, & Adrien, 1986; Hunt & Holmes, 1975; Lorber & Segall, 1961; Mc-Clone, Czyzewski, Raimondi, & Somers, 1982). The most significant factor, however, is the presence of hydrocephalus (Badell-Ribera et al., 1966; Billard et al., 1986; Hagberg & Sjorgen, 1966; McClone et al., 1982; Spain, 1974).

Studies of cognitive deficits in children with meningomyelocele and hydrocephalus have reported a 10- to 20-point difference between verbal and performance IQ scores (Anderson & Spain, 1977; Billard et al., 1986; Dennis et al., 1981). The performance IQ score is the lower because of poor visuospatial skills (Billard et al., 1986; Ruchert et al., 1986).

Linguistic Abilities of Children with Meningomyelocele

Poor cognitive functioning is only one of the factors affecting the communication skills of children with meningomyelocele. Other factors that may predispose these children to impairments in speech and/or language skills include: poor attending behaviors; hypersensitivity to auditory, tactile, and visual stimuli; difficulties in visual-motor coordination, spatial orientation and figure-ground perception; limitations in gross and fine motor skills; and long illnesses or hospitalizations (Williamson, 1987). Therefore, any assessment or treatment procedure for communication skills used with children with spina bifida must take into account the individual child's level of functioning in each of these areas.

Children with meningomyelocele exhibit a characteristic language profile, with their language abilities often described as appearing to be well functioning on the surface. Indeed, basic language processes appear to be relatively well preserved in children with meningomyelocele (Barnes & Dennis, 1998; Dennis, Jacennik, & Barnes, 1994; Fletcher et al., 2002), with basic structural language and single-word skills such as picture vocabulary and grammar remaining intact (Brookshire et al., 1995; Byrne, Abbeduto, & Brooks, 1990;

Fletcher et al., 2002). In contrast, children with meningomyelocele exhibit relative impairment of context-dependent language with significant difficulties in the construction of meaning and in pragmatic communication, both of which require flexible language processing in real time (Barnes & Dennis, 1998; Dennis et al., 1994; Fletcher et al., 2002). Their specific impairments are in discourse coherence, inferencing, suppressing contextually irrelevant meaning, and deriving meaning from context (Barnes & Dennis, 1998; Dennis et al., 1994; Fletcher et al., 2002).

Phonology. In general, most authors report a low incidence of phonological disorders in children with spina bifida (Brookshire et al., 1995; Byrne et al., 1990; Fletcher et al., 2002; Spain, 1974). In a number of studies, Tew found less than 10% of children with meningomyelocele and hydrocephalus had difficulties with speech production (Tew, 1979; Tew & Laurence, 1972, 1975, 1979). In contrast to this low incidence, Khan and Soare (1975) reported phonological impairment in 65% of their hydrocephalic subjects. Henderson, Murdoch, and Ozanne (1989) studied the linguistic abilities of children with meningomyelocele and hydrocephalus, most of whom had intellectual handicaps and all of whom lived in residential care, and reported that five of the nine subjects had phonological impairment. In two of these cases the level of phonological development was consistent with their language and cognitive skills whereas in two more cases phonological development was only comparable with their language level and was below their cognitive level. In one case phonological skills were in advance of other language skills. All phonological processes used by these nine children with meningomyelocele were reported by Henderson et al. (1989) to be developmental rather than disordered in nature.

Receptive Language. A number of researchers have reported receptive language deficits in children with meningomyelocele (Anderson & Spain, 1977; Billard et al., 1986; Menelaus, 1980). In several studies receptive language scores were in advance of expressive language scores but both were below chronological age (Tew, 1979; Tew & Laurence, 1979; Spain, 1974). This pattern was also found in five of the eight children with meningomyelocele with language impairment studied by Henderson et al. (1989). Two other cases studied by these latter authors, however, had the reverse pattern (i.e., expressive skills in advance of receptive skills) and one case presented with both skills at the same level.

Very little information is presented relating receptive language skills to intellectual functioning, in children with meningomyelocele. Khan and Soare (1975), however, reported scores of receptive vocabulary as measured on the Peabody Picture Vocabulary Test (Dunn, 1965) were commensurate with IQ scores. This was not the case with the children studied by Henderson et al. (1989) as all of their meningomyelocele subjects with language impairment scored in the range +1 to −1 percentile ranks on the Peabody Picture Vocabulary Test-Revised (Dunn & Dunn, 1981) irrespective of their intellectual functioning. Other factors such as occular deficits, attentional deficits, visuospatial impairments, and the effect of hospitalization and institutionalization must be considered in these subjects. Horn, Lorch, Lorch, and Culatta (1985), however, reported that their subjects performed as well as controls on vocabulary comprehension tasks until irrelevant background stimuli were introduced. Although some children with meningomyelocele may perform well on picture vocabulary tasks, according to Swisher and Pinsker (1971) they perform more poorly on comprehension and reasoning tasks.

Dennis, Hendrick, Hoffman, and Humphreys (1987) suggested that poor comprehension and reasoning may not be directly related to the condition of meningomyelocele but rather to the hydrocephalus and factors related to that. In their study of 75 hydrocephalic children between 5 and 22 years of age, Dennis and coworkers assessed five domains of language and compared the performance of the hydrocephalic children with that of a control group. Thirty were children with meningomyelocele. Fourteen had intraventricular hydrocephalus associated with meningomyelocele, two had extraventricular hydrocephalus also associated with meningomyelocele, whereas the remaining 14 had an unspecified type of hydrocephalus associated with meningomyelocele. Thirty-four medical variables and verbal (VIQ) and performance intelligence quotients (PIQ) were then related to the performance of the hydrocephalic subjects on the language tests. From this Dennis et al. (1987) concluded that the hydrocephalic brain provided "an adequate but not ideal substrate for the acquisition of language" (p. 614), and that all language domains were not equally affected.

For both comprehension tasks (comprehension of grammar and metalinguistic awareness) assessed by Dennis et al. (1987), hydrocephalic subjects improved less well with increasing age than the normal control group. On the comprehension of grammar task this

delayed improvement with age was true for both the number of items correct and the response time taken. The presence of intraventricular hydrocephalus particularly disrupted the development of the language skill measured by the number of items correct on this task. Metalinguistic awareness was measured on a number of features but only the detection of surface structure anomalies developed less well in the hydrocephalic subjects as age increased. This test score was found to relate to both verbal and performance IQ scores. This was particularly so for the Lexical Anomaly Identification and Optional Anomaly Identification scores which were accounted for by moderate amounts of variability in the VIQ scores. On this test the best predictor of a poor performance was being female. As stated before, there are a larger number of females who have meningomyelocele. Therefore, the receptive language deficits reported in children with meningomyelocele may be multifactorial in etiology stressing the need for assessment of the individual child with meningomyelocele on a number of different aspects of comprehension, and with regard to the medical, cognitive, social, and perceptual factors operating within that child.

Expressive Language. Contrary to the majority of children with developmental language disorders, Parsons (1968) found no difference in morphemic development in a group of children with meningomyelocele when compared with a group of controls. This apparent morphological ability would be in line with statements that children with meningomyelocele have well-developed syntax compared with other language skills (Anderson & Spain, 1977; Swisher & Pinsker, 1971; Tew, 1979) in that their syntactic skills are within normal limits for chronologic age (Schwartz, 1974; Spain, 1974; Tew & Laurence, 1979). Anderson and Spain (1977) suggested that it was this ability to use complex syntax that was one of the reasons that children with meningomyelocele appear to have normal verbal ability. An imitation task, for different grammatical constructions, given to hydrocephalic children by Dennis et al. (1987) demonstrated that intraventricular and extraventricular hydrocephalus both predicted a poor sentence imitation score. This score also appeared to be related to VIQ but not PIQ. Although a poor performance score was predicted by hydrocephalus, this poor performance did not occur if shunt treatment had been implemented.

Some researchers also state that expressive vocabulary is generally well developed in children with meningomyelocele (Billard et al., 1986; Spain, 1974). Tew (1979) reported that the vocabulary score on the Wechsler Preschool and Primary Scale of Intelligence (WPPSI) (Wechsler, 1989) was the highest of all the subtest scores, whereas Ingram and Naughton (1962) found their hydrocephalic subjects to have vocabulary scores superior to their "general psychometric status." Normal vocabulary acquisition and normal performance on a vocabulary learning task have also been reported (Parsons, 1968; Schwartz, 1974). The presence of shunts was shown by Anderson and Spain (1977) to adversely affect vocabulary scores, with only one-third of the group with shunts having vocabulary scores within normal limits.

Despite these reports of normal vocabulary development, descriptions of the language of children with meningomyelocele and hydrocephalus have been described as meaningless and lacking content (Hadenius, Hagberg, Hyttnas-Bensch, & Sjorgen, 1962; Ingram & Naughton, 1962; Swisher & Pinsker, 1971; Tew & Laurence, 1975, 1979). Below average scores for the content subtests of the Reynell Developmental Language Scales (Reynell, 1977) have been reported (Spain, 1974; Tew, 1979). Dennis et al. (1987) also found that semantic lexical access measured on the Word-Finding Test (Wiegel-Crump & Dennis, 1986) improved less with age in the children with hydrocephalus than in the control group. This lexical access ability appeared to relate moderately to VIQ. Poor scores on both the semantic and visual lexical accessing conditions of the Word-Finding Test were reported in children with intraventricular hydrocephalus.

Shunt treatment in children with hydrocephalus, moreover, predicted a poor performance on the automaticity of language as assessed on the Automatized Naming Test (Denckla & Rudel, 1974). Errors made by the children with hydrocephalus studied by Dennis et al. (1987) on this test were Serial Order errors such as perseveration, anticipation, and incorrect sequencing of items. The only language skill that was specifically affected by the presence of meningomyelocele, in the hydrocephalic subjects studied by Dennis et al. (1987), was verbal fluency as measured on Automatized Naming Test (i.e., the time it took the subject to name the 300 items).

Therefore, some expressive language deficits have been identified in children with meningomyelocele; however, in some cases this relates to the presence of hydrocephalus, the type of hydrocephalus or the treatment of the hydrocephalus. In that different language skills were related to VIQ and PIQ in varying amounts and that the level of relationship was only moderate,

Dennis et al. (1987) considered that any cognitive deficits produced by hydrocephalus could not fully account for all language deficits, as it appeared "that the language tests tapped functions other than those involved in intelligence" (p. 615). Therefore, hydrocephalus was shown to produce some specific linguistic deficits but the only one specifically related to the condition of meningomyelocele was poor verbal fluency. As stated by a number of authors, however, despite what appears to be good development of expressive language in children with meningomyelocele, they lack the ability to use language appropriately (Anderson & Spain, 1977; Billard et al., 1986; Horn et al., 1985; Schwartz, 1974; Spain, 1974; Swisher & Pinsker, 1971; Tew & Laurence, 1979).

Pragmatic Language Skills. Although a number of studies have highlighted the relative preservation of language skills based on formal language assessments at the word and sentence level, many authors have reported the presence of deficits in the social and pragmatic communication abilities of children with meningomyelocele and associated hydrocephalus.

The term "cocktail party syndrome" refers to the use of language that has been noted in some children with hydrocephalus, both with and without the presence of meningomyelocele. It is described as a chatty, superficial quality of the children's discourse. Various labels have been used to try to capture the essence of this inappropriate language usage. Some terms used in the literature are: chatterboxes and blethers (Ingram & Naughton, 1962), shallow intellect (Laurence & Coates, 1962), dysverbal (Badell-Ribera et al., 1966), and hyperverbal (Spain, 1974). The term most frequently used in the literature, however, is "cocktail party syndrome," a term coined by Hadenius et al. (1962). Some definitions of "cocktail party syndrome" commonly cited are, "a good ability to learn words and talking without knowing what they are talking about" (Hadenius et al., 1962, p. 118); "their spontaneous verbal behavior is superficial and lacking in appropriateness to the situation at hand" (Fleming, 1968, p. 74); "they show a characteristic pattern for language with good syntax but poor comprehension and inability to use language creatively" (Spain, 1974, p. 779). This characteristic pattern of language abilities was refined into two sets of criteria to aid in the diagnosis of "cocktail party syndrome." One set of criteria was developed by Tew (1979) and the other by Schwartz (1974) (Table 8–1).

The prevalence of "cocktail party syndrome" reported in the literature has ranged from 0% (Khan & Soare, 1975) to 40% (Tew & Laurence, 1979). The most commonly reported figure, however, is around 28%. This figure stands whether the children have meningomyelocele (Diller, Paddock, Badell-Ribera, & Swinyard, 1966; Spain, 1974) or meningomyelocele with and without hydrocephalus (Tew & Laurence, 1972). Several factors appear to influence the presence of "cocktail party syndrome." These factors include: low intellectual functioning (Tew & Laurence, 1972, 1979; Spain, 1974), multiple physical handicaps (Tew & Laurence, 1979), younger age group (Tew & Laurence, 1979), shunted hydrocephalus (Spain, 1974), and female sex (Tew & Laurence, 1972, 1979).

Likewise, many explanations of the underlying cause of "cocktail party syndrome" have been postulated. These include: subtle brain damage (Laurence

TABLE 8–1. Criteria for Identification of Cocktail Party Syndrome

Tew (1979)

- perseveration of response
- an excessive use of social phrases in conversation
- an overfamiliarity in manner
- irrelevant introduction of personal experience into conversation
- fluent and normally well-articulated speech

[four of these criteria must be met]

Schwartz (1974)

- excessive verbalization
- performance IQ lower than verbal IQ
- inflection and stress patterns resembling adult speech
- spontaneous utterances out of context
- use of automatic phrases and cliches
- utterances often in the form of verbal commands and inappropriate questions
- good articulation

& Coates, 1962), self-stimulation (Diller et al., 1966), reinforcement of hyperverbal behavior by parents (Diller et al., 1966; Swisher & Pinsker, 1971; Tew, 1979; Tew & Laurence, 1979), attention-seeking behavior to gain adult attention in hospital (Tew, 1979; Tew & Laurence 1979), or poor ability at monitoring verbal output (Dennis et al., 1987).

Despite the development of behavioral descriptions and criteria as described earlier to diagnose "cocktail party syndrome," few empirical studies have been able qualitatively or quantitatively to demonstrate its true nature. Those studies that have addressed the issue of hyperverbality have measured the number of words per turn per response (Diller et al., 1966; Fleming, 1968), the total number of words (Fleming, 1968; Swisher & Pinsker, 1971),

and type token ratio (Henderson et al., 1989; Swisher & Pinsker, 1971). The study by Swisher and Pinsker (1971) was the only one to find an increase in the number of words used by children with meningomyelocele when compared with a group of controls or normative data. All of the above authors, however, commented on the inappropriateness of the language usage observed in their group of subjects. Billard et al. (1986) found their subjects not to be too excessive but merely irrelevant, whereas Fleming (1968) felt that the "personal and socially aggressive nature of their spontaneous conversation" (p. 81) made her hydrocephalic subjects appear more verbose.

It would be expected that the inappropriateness of the language observed in children with meningomyelocele could be demonstrated using a pragmatic language assessment, most of which have been developed since the publication of the studies cited. In addition, such a pragmatic analysis should identify behaviors described in the literature as being associated with "cocktail party syndrome" such as: irrelevant responses, difficulty staying on topic, overfamiliarity of manner, prosodic features and superficiality of output (Diller et al., 1966; Fleming, 1968; Schwartz, 1974; Tew, 1979). Based on this assumption Henderson et al. (1989) assessed a group of children with meningomyelocele who were most likely to exhibit "cocktail party syndrome" (i.e., they had intellectual handicaps, lived in residential care, had moderate to severe physical disabilities, and had hydrocephalus) using the Pragmatic Protocol (Prutting & Kirchner, 1987). The children all were between 6 and 13 years of age. Pragmatic deficits were found in seven of the nine subjects studied (Figure 8–2). Subject 1, who had pragmatic skills within normal limits, did not present with a language disorder and had normal intellectual functioning.

As can be seen from Figure 8–2 the notion that some of the children with meningomyelocele exhibit inappropriate language behavior is supported by this study, as between 4 and 14 inappropriate pragmatic behaviors were identified in each of the subjects presenting with pragmatic deficits. Some of these behaviors would have been predicted from the literature, for example, speech pair act analysis, topic selection, topic introduction, topic maintenance, turn-taking response, and prosody. The difficulties noted on specificity and accuracy would support Dennis et al.'s (1987) findings re. poor verbal fluency in children with meningomyelocele or poor word-finding skills in children with intraventricular hydrocephalus. It may also relate to the low receptive vocabulary scores also found in the Henderson et al. (1989) subjects. Despite confirmation of the descriptive symptoms of "cocktail party syndrome" seen in this group of subjects, no individual subject met the criteria of either Tew (1979) or Schwartz (1974) for the identification of "cocktail party syndrome." Further research is required to refine these descriptive terms and to ascertain the pragmatic profiles of children with comparable linguistic and/or cognitive skills, and to utilize that information for the purpose of evaluating the underlying mechanisms operating in hydrocephalic children.

Both microscopic and macroscopic level procedures have been used to analyze the discourse abilities of children with meningomyelocele. Analysis at the microscopic level includes factors such as the amount of discourse produced, fluency of production, and the use of personal pronouns or conjunctions that provide cohesion to the discourse by connecting semantic relations within the narrative. On the other hand, macroscopic analysis assesses semantic-pragmatic aspects of language, such as the quality of information conveyed, text organization, and comprehension (Halliday & Hanson, 1976). Overall these techniques have revealed that children with meningomyelocele are not impaired on factors such as the quantity and fluency of language output, syntactic complexity and simple measures of cohesion. For example, children with meningomyelocele can produce narratives with the same number of words as controls (Dennis et al., 1994; Huber-Okrainec, Dennis, Brettschneider, & Spiegler, 2002). In contrast,

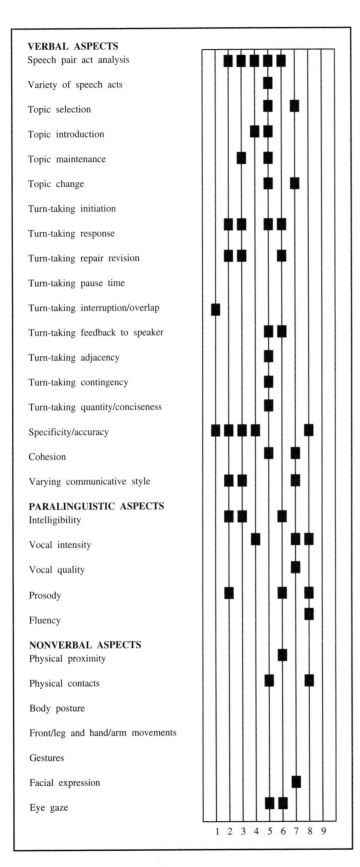

FIGURE 8–2. Inappropriate pragmatic parameters on the pragmatic protocol for individual subjects with meningomyelocele (from Henderson et al., 1989).

at the macroscopic level, the discourse abilities of these children are impaired with their oral narratives tending to be verbose and convoluted and lacking cohesion and coherence (Dennis et al., 1994). Even though they are able to produce the same amount of discourse as normally developing peers, children with meningomyelocele communicate less of the actual core semantic content of a story. The discourse deficits involving core semantic content in children with meningomyelocele do not appear to be due to general intellectual impairment. Content-poor discourse has been observed in children with meningomyelocele with average intelligence (Barnes & Dennis, 1998; Dennis et al., 1994). They have poor discourse coherence, impoverished semantic content, and difficulty deriving the gist of discourse (Barnes & Dennis, 1998; Dennis et al., 1994; Fletcher et al., 2002).

According to Barnes and Dennis (1998) children with meningomyelocele also have difficulties evidenced by standardized tests of discourse comprehension, especially those involving inference making. Furthermore, these children also have problems with meaning suppression. Although they can activate meaning they are less able than normally developing peers to suppress contextually irrelevant meanings (Barnes et al., 2004). Barnes and Dennis (1998) suggested that difficulties in using context to understand meaning may underlie many of the discourse deficits associated with meningomyelocele. This suggestion is supported by the findings of Huber-Okrainec, Blaser, and Dennis (2005) that compared to age-matched peers, children with meningomyelocele are able to understand decomposable idioms (which they suggest are processed more like literal language) but not nondecomposable idioms (which require contextual analyses for acquisition). Furthermore, Huber-Okrainec et al. (2005) suggested that the noted impairment in comprehension of non-decomposable idioms was related to congenital agenesis of the corpus callosum and hence represent the outcome of impaired interhemispheric communication.

Summary of Linguistic Abilities and Clinical Implications

Despite the presence of brain malformations involving the cerebellum, corpus callosum and hydrocephalus, in the minds of clinicians and educators meningomyelocele is often considered to represent a purely spinal cord disorder. This, combined with the fact that these children often have relatively intact surface language and can read words, often results in clinicians and educators failing to recognize problems with discourse production and listening/reading comprehension that can impair the affected child's academic performance and social skills. Most children with meningomyelocele show adequate development of language at the level of form and content (grammar and lexicon). In contrast, regardless of their cognitive status, the majority of these children show difficulties in construction of meaning and in pragmatic communication as evidenced by their performance on discourse tasks. The narrative discourse of children with meningomyelocele is characterized by impoverished semantic content and verbosity. Listening and reading comprehension assessments further demonstrate that these children also have difficulties making inferences because of problems learning and accessing both textual information and general knowledge. According to Fletcher et al. (2002), assessment and intervention should focus on the development of meaning construction and semantic-pragmatic communication.

References

Anderson, E. M., & Spain, B. (1977). *The child with spina bifida*. London, UK: Methuen.

Badell-Ribera, A., Shulman, K., & Paddock, N. (1966). The relationship of nonprogressive hydrocephalus to intellectual functioning in children with spina bifida cystic. *Pediatrics, 37,* 787–793.

Barnes, M. A., & Dennis, M. (1992). Reading in children and adolescents after early onset hydrocephalus and in their normally developing age peers: Phonological analysis, word recognition, word comprehension and passage comprehension skill. *Journal of Pediatric Psychology, 17,* 445–465.

Barnes, M. A., & Dennis, M. (1998). Discourse after early onset hydrocephalus: Core deficits in children of average intelligence. *Brain and Language, 61,* 309–334.

Barnes, M. A., Faulkner, H., Wilkinson, M., & Dennis, M. (2004). Meaning construction and integration in children with hydrocephalus. *Brain and Language, 89,* 47–56.

Barnes, M. A., Wilkinson, M., Boudousquie, A., Khemani, E., Dennis, M., & Fletcher, J. M. (2006). Arithematic processing in children with spina bifida: Calculation accuracy, strategy use, and fact retrieval fluency. *Journal of Learning Disabilities, 39,* 174–187.

Billard, C., Santini, J. J., Gillet, P., Nargeot, M. C., & Adrien, J. L. (1986). Long term intellectual prognosis of hydrocephalus with reference to 77 children. *Paediatric Neuroscience, 12,* 219–225.

Brewer, V. B., Fletcher, J. M., Hiscock, M., & Davidson, K. C. (2001). Attention processes in children with shunted hydrocephalus versus attention deficit-hyperactivity disorder. *Neuropsychology, 15,* 185–198.

Brock, D. J. (1977). Biochemical and cytological methods in the diagnosis of neural tube defects. *Progress in Medical Genetics, 2,* 1–37.

Brookshire, B. L., Fletcher, J. M., Bohan, T. P., Landry, S. H., Davidson, K. C., & Francis, D. J. (1995). Verbal and non-verbal skill discrepancies in children with hydrocephalus: A five-year longitudinal follow-up. *Journal of Pediatric Psychology, 20,* 785–800.

Byrne, K., Abbeduto, L., & Brooks, P. (1990). The language of children with spina bifida and hydrocephalus: Meeting task demands and mastering syntax. *Journal of Speech and Hearing Disorders, 55,* 118–123.

Czeizel, A. E., & Dudas, I. (1992). Prevention of the first occurrence of neural tube defects by preconceptional vitamin supplementation. *New England Journal of Medicine, 327,* 1832–1835.

Denckla, M. B., & Rudel, R. (1974). Rapid "automatized" naming of pictures, objects, colors, letters and numbers by normal children. *Cortex, 10,* 186–202.

Dennis, M., & Barnes, M. A. (2002). Numeracy skills in adults with spina bifida. *Developmental Neuropsychology, 21,* 141–156.

Dennis, M., Edelstein, K., Copeland, K., Frederick, J., Francis, D. J., Hetherington, R., . . . Humphreys, R. P.. (2005). Space-based inhibition of return in children with spina bifida. *Neuropsychology, 19,* 456–465.

Dennis M. E., Fitz, L. R., Netley, C. T., Sugar, J., Harwood-Nash, D. C. F., Hendrick, E. B., . . . Humphreys, R. (1981). The intelligence of hydrocephalic children. *Archives of Neurology, 38,* 607–615.

Dennis M., Fletcher, J. M., Rogers, S., Hetherington, R., & Francis, D. (2002). Object-based and action-based visual perception in children with spina bifida and hydrocephalus. *Journal of the International Neuropsychological Society, 8,* 95–106.

Dennis, M. E., Hendrick, B., Hoffman, H. J., & Humphreys, R. P. (1987). Language of hydrocephalic children and adolescents. Journal of Clinical and Experimental Neuropsychology, 9, 593–621.

Dennis, M., Jacennik, B., & Barnes, M. A. (1994). The content of narrative discourse in children and adolescents after early-onset hydrocephalus and in normally developing age peers. Brain and Language, 46, 129–165.

Dennis, M., Landry, S. H., Barnes, M., & Fletcher, J. (2006). Neurocognitive functioning in spina bifida over the lifespan. Journal of the International Neuropsychological Society, 12, 285–298.

Diller, L., Paddock, N., Badell-Ribera, A., & Swinyard, C. A. (1966). Verbal behavior in spina bifida children. In C. A. Swinyard (Ed.), Comprehensive care of the child with spina bifida manifesta, Rehabilitation Monograph No. 31. New York, NY: Institute of Rehabilitation.

Dunn, L. M. (1965). Peabody Picture Vocabulary Test. Circle Pines, MN: American Guidance Service.

Dunn, L. M., & Dunn, D. M. (1981). Peabody Picture Vocabulary Test-Revised. Circle Pines, MN: American Guidance Service.

Fleming, C. P. (1968). The verbal behavior of hydrocephalic children. Developmental Medicine and Child Neurology, 10, 74–82.

Fletcher, J. M., Barnes, M., & Dennis, M. (2002). Language development in children with spina bifida. Seminars in Pediatric Neurology, 9, 201–208.

Fletcher, J. M., Copeland, K., Frederick, J. A., Blaser, S. E., Kramer, L. A., Northrup, H., . . . Dennis, M. (2005). Spinal lesion level in spina bifida: A source of neural and cognitive heterogeneity. Journal of Neurosurgery (Pediatrics 3), 102, 268–279.

Fletcher, J. M., Dennis, M., & Northrup, H. (2000). Hydrocephalus. In K. O. Yeates, M. D. Ris, & H. G. Taylor (Eds.), Pediatric neuropsychology: Research, theory and practice (pp. 25–46). New York, NY: Guilford.

Hadenius, A., Hagberg, B., Hyttnas-Bensch, K., & Sjorgen, I. (1962). The natural prognosis of infantile hydrocephalus. Acta Pediatrics Scandinavica, 51, 117–118.

Hagberg, B., & Sjorgen, I. (1966). The chronic brain syndrome of infantile hydrocephalus: A follow-up study of 63 spontaneously arrested cases. American Journal of Diseases of Children, 112, 189–196.

Halliday, M., & Hanson, R. (1976). Cohesion in English. London, UK: Longman.

Hannay, H. J. (2000). Functioning of the corpus callosum in children with early hydrocephalus. Journal of the International Neuropsychological Society, 6, 351–361.

Henderson, S., Murdoch, B., & Ozanne, A. (1989). Speech and language disorders in children with spina bifida. Paper presented at the Annual Conference of the Australian Association of Speech and Hearing, Perth, Australia.

Horn, D. G., Lorch, E. P., Lorch, R. F., & Culatta, B. (1985). Distractibility and vocabulary deficits in children with spina bifida and hydrocephalus. Developmental Medicine and Child Neurology, 27, 713–720.

Huber-Okrainec, J., Blaser, S. E., & Dennis, M. (2005). Idiom comprehension in relation to corpus callosum agenesis and hypoplasia in children with spina bifida meningomyelocele. Brain and Language, 93, 349–368.

Huber-Okrainec, J., Dennis, M., Brettschneider, J., & Spiegler, B. (2002). Neuromotor speech deficits in children and adults with spina bifida and hydrocephalus. Brain and Language, 80, 57–63.

Hunt, G. M., & Holmes, A. E. (1975). Some factors relating to intelligence in treated children with spina bifida cystica. Developmental Medicine and Child Neurology, 17, (Suppl. 35), 65–70.

Ingram, T. T. S., & Naughton, J. A. (1962). Paediatric and psychological aspects of cerebral palsy associated with hydrocephalus. Developmental Medicine and Child Neurology, 4, 287–291.

Khan, A. V., & Soare, P. (1975). Intelligence, speech and language development of hydrocephalic children. Developmental Medicine and Child Neurology, 17, 116–117.

Klaas, P. A., Hannay, H. J., Caroselli, J. S., & Fletcher, J. M. (1999). Interhemispheric transfer of visual, auditory, tactile and visuomotor information in children with hydrocephalus and partial agenesis of the corpus callosum. *Journal of Clinical and Experimental Neuropsychology, 21,* 837–850.

Knowlton, D. D., Peterson, K., & Putbrese, A. (1985). Team management of cognitive dysfunction in children with spina bifida. *Rehabilitation Literature, 46,* 259–263.

Laurence, K. M., & Coates, S. (1962). The natural history of hydrocephalus: Detailed analysis of 182 inoperated cases. *Archives of Disease in Childhood, 37,* 345–362.

Lorber, J., & Segall, M. (1961). Bacterial meningitis in spina bifida cystica. *Archives of Disease in Childhood, 37,* 300–308.

Mapstone, T. B., Rekate, H. L., Nulsen, F. E., Dixon, M. S., Glaser, N., & Jaffe, M. (1984). Relationship of CSF shunting and IQ in children with myelomeningocele: A retrospective analysis. *Child's Brain, 11,* 112–118.

McClone, D. G., Czyzewski, D., Raimondi, A. J., & Somers, R. C. (1982). Central nervous system infections as a limiting factor in the intelligence of children with myelomeningocele. *Pediatrics, 70,* 338–342.

Menelaus, M. B. (1980). *The orthopaedic management of spina bifida cystica* (2nd ed.). New York, NY: Churchill Livingstone.

Nakano, K. K. (1973). Anencephaly: A review. *Developmental Medicine and Child Neurology, 15,* 383–400.

Parsons, J. G. (1968). An investigation into the verbal facility of hydrocephalic children with special reference to vocabulary, morphology and fluency. *Developmental Medicine and Child Neurology, 10,* (Suppl. 16), 109–110.

Prutting, C. A., & Kirchner, D. M. (1987). A clinical appraisal of the pragmatic aspects of language. *Journal of Speech and Hearing Disorders, 52,* 105–119.

Reigel, D. H., & Rothstein, D. (1994). Spina bifida. In W. R. Cheek (Ed.), *Pediatric neurosurgery* (3rd ed., pp. 51–76). Philadelphia, PA: W. B. Saunders.

Reynell, J. (1977). *Reynell Developmental Language Scales-Revised.* Oxford, UK: NFER.

Ruchert, N., Hansel-Friedrich, G., & Wolff, G. (1986). Assessment of intelligence of school-aged children with spina bifida under hospital supervision. In D. Voth & D. Glees (Eds.), *Spina bifida—neural tube defects* (pp. 283–291). New York, NY: De Gruyter.

Scherzer, A. L., & Gardner, G. G. (1970). Studies of the school age child with meningomyelocele: 1. Physical and intellectual development. *Pediatrics, 47,* 424–430.

Schwartz, E. R. (1974). Characteristics of speech and language development in the child with myelomeningocele and hydrocephalus. *Journal of Speech and Hearing Disorders, 39,* 465–468.

Shurtleff, D. B., Kronmal, R., & Foltz, E. L. (1975). Follow-up comparison of hydrocephalus with and without myelomeningocele. *Journal of Neurosurgery, 42,* 61–68.

Simpson, D. (1976). Congenital malformations of the nervous system. *Medical Journal of Australia, 1,* 700–702.

Smith, E. D. (1965). *Spina bifida and the total care of spinal myelomeningocele.* Springfield, IL: Charles C. Thomas.

Spain, B. (1974). Verbal and performance ability in preschool children with spina bifida. *Developmental Medicine and Child Neurology, 16,* 773–780.

Swisher, L. P., & Pinsker, E. J. (1971). The language characteristics of hyperverbal, hydrocephalic children. *Developmental Medicine and Child Neurology, 13,* 746–755.

Tew, B. (1979). The "cocktail party syndrome" in children with hydrocephalus and spina bifida. *British Journal of Disorders of Communication, 14,* 89–101.

Tew, B., & Laurence, K. (1972). The ability and attainments of spina bifida patients born in South Wales between 1956–1962. *Developmental Medicine and Child Neurology, 14,* (Suppl. 27), 124–131.

Tew, B., & Laurence, K. M. (1975). The effects of hydrocephalus on intelligence, visual perception and school attainment.

Developmental Medicine and Child Neurology, 17, (Suppl. 35), 129–134.

Tew, B., & Laurence, K. M. (1979). The clinical and psychological characteristics of children with the "cocktail party" syndrome. *Zeitschrift für Kinderchirurgie und Grenzbegiete, 28,* 360–367.

Wechsler, D. (1989). *The Wechsler Preschool and Primary Scale of Intelligence-Revised.* New York, NY: Psychological Corporation.

Wiegel-Crump, C. A., & Dennis, M. (1986). Development of word finding. *Brain and Language, 27,* 1–23.

Williams, L. J., Rasmussen, S. A., Flores, R. S., Kirby, R. S., & Edmunds, L. D. (2005). Decline in the prevalence of spina bifida and anencephaly by race/ethnicity: 1995–2002. *Pediatrics, 116,* 580–586.

Williamson, G. C. (1987). *Children with spina bifida.* Baltimore, MD: Paul H. Brookes.

Yeates, K. O., Fletcher, J. M., & Dennis, M. (2005). Spina bifida and hydrocephalus. In J. E. Morgan, & J. H. Ricker (Eds.), *Handbook of neuropsychology* (pp. 61–75). New York, NY: Taylor & Francis.

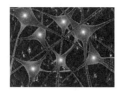 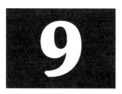 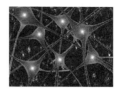

Language Dysfunction Associated with Childhood Convulsive Disorder (Landau-Kleffner Syndrome)

Introduction

Landau-Kleffner syndrome is a rare epileptic condition marked by an acquired aphasia in children who have previously had normal language and motor development. First described by Landau and Kleffner (1957), in this condition the child's language deteriorates in association with epileptiform discharges seen in their electroencephalogram (EEG). Although clinical seizures do not occur in all cases, the EEG abnormalities are diagnostic, showing paroxysmal unilateral or bilateral spike-and-wave discharges maximal over the temporal regions during wakefulness and becoming almost continuous during slow-wave sleep. In some cases the language deterioration is either preceded, accompanied, or fol-lowed by a series of convulsive seizures (van de Sandt-Koenderman, Smit, van Dongen, & van Hest, 1984).

Onset of Landau-Kleffner syndrome is usually between 2 and 13 years of age, with initial loss of language function occurring between 3 and 7 years of age. The condition has also been referred to by several other names including "acquired epileptic aphasia," "acquired aphasia with convulsive disorder," "acquired receptive aphasia," and "acquired verbal agnosia" (Deonna, Beaumanoir, Gaillard, & Assal, 1977; Lees, 1993). Most authors agree that males are affected twice as often as females (Cooper & Ferry, 1978; Msall, Shapiro, Balfour, Niedermeyer, & Capute, 1986). The most common aphasic feature is a moderate to severe deficit in auditory comprehension which, in many cases, is the first symptom preceding epileptic manifestations and expressive language impairments. Other aspects of higher cortical function are preserved. Landau-Kleffner syndrome is of particular interest to speech-language pathologists because it combines two elements of language development not commonly seen in clinics, that is, a moderate to severe auditory comprehension deficit in the presence of preserved cognitive abilities and regression of language skills.

Neuropathology

Although the cause of Landau-Kleffner syndrome is unknown, several hypotheses on the pathogenesis of this disorder have been proposed. Landau and Kleffner (1957) together with Sato and Dreifuss (1973) postulated that the language regression may be the result of a functional ablation of the primary cortical language areas by persistent electrical discharges. Gascon, Victor, Lombroso, and Goodglass (1973) suggested that the electrical discharges in the brain displayed by these children occur secondary to a lower level subcortical deafferenting process and that the discharges are not directly responsible for the aphasia. As for the actual cause of the convulsive disorder, the data on which several hypotheses are based were obtained from pathoanatomic studies (Miller, Campbell, Chapman, & Weismer, 1984). One hypothesis proposes that there exists a pathogenic mechanism related in an unknown way to the convulsive disorder (Gascon et al., 1973). For instance, there may be an unusual genetic pattern of cerebral organization that makes a child particularly sensitive to brain damage or seizure activity as far as lan-

guage is concerned (Deonna et al., 1977). Another hypothesis suggests that the convulsive disorder and language loss is caused by an active low-grade selective encephalitis (or inflammatory process) that affects the temporal lobes (McKinney & McGreal, 1974; Worster-Drought, 1971). It also has been suggested that Landau-Kleffner syndrome may be caused by vascular disorders. A diminished vascular supply in the territory of the left middle cerebral artery was found in one individual with this disorder examined by Rapin, Mattis, Rowan, and Golden (1977). Dulac, Billard, and Arthuis (1983) concluded that the aphasia in Landau-Kleffner syndrome is the result of functional disorganization of the language centers due to important intercortical EEG abnormalities. Based on an examination of six children with what they call "aphasia with convulsive disorder, Deonna et al. (1977) concluded that the Landau-Kleffner syndrome is not a homogeneous syndrome but rather appears to result from a heterogeneous group of pathologic processes that selectively involve the primary language areas of the brain. This latter proposal is discussed more fully under the heading of subgroups of Landau-Kleffner syndrome.

Structural neuroimaging based on computed tomography (CT) or magnetic resonance imaging (MRI) provide no evidence of anatomic brain lesions. Likewise other clinical measures, such as arteriography and cerebrospinal fluid (CSF) examination usually yield completely normal results. However, functional brain imaging using positron emission tomography (PET) has revealed a focal increase of cerebral glucose utilization over one temporal lobe during the active phase of epilepsy (Maquet et al., 1995). Electrophysiologic studies based on evoked response potentials

(ERPs) have provided evidence that focal epileptic activity in Landau-Kleffner syndrome may lead to permanent dysfunction in the associative auditory cortex of the temporal lobe (Wioland, Rudolf, & Metz-Lutz, 2001).

Medical Treatment of Landau-Kleffner Syndrome

Treatment of Landau-Kleffner syndrome largely involves administration of anticonvulsant drugs and in some rare cases surgical intervention. Valproate, ethosuximide, and the benzodiazepines can improve the condition whereas phenobarbital and carbamazepine generally are ineffective (Marescaux et al., 1990). Adrenocorticotrophic hormone or corticosteroids can also be partially effective. Other therapeutic approaches include the use of immunoglobulins, which can be effective in some patients and multiple subpial transections (Grote, van Slyke, & Hoeppner, 1999; Morrell, Whistler, & Bleck, 1989). Subpial transection represents a surgical approach to the treatment of epilepsy and involves selective severing of certain horizontal intercortical neural fibers while preserving vertical fibers. The objective of the surgery is to reduce the possibility of the occurrence of synchronized neuronal discharge in a way that does not disrupt the major functional capacity of the tissue. Morrell et al. (1989) reported 10 cases where this procedure had been carried out directly to Broca's and Wernicke areas, all of whom continued to be verbal language users postsurgery. As a rule, the EEG abnormalities regress with time, leaving the child with a moderate to severe receptive and expressive aphasia.

Clinical Features of Landau-Kleffner Syndrome

Landau-Kleffner syndrome is characterized by an initial deterioration of language comprehension followed by disruption of the child's expressive abilities. In some cases the onset of language deterioration is abrupt whereas in others the language disturbance develops gradually. Twenty-five percent of cases show a gradual onset, with language regression taking place over a period of more than 6 months. In the remaining cases, the language regression may occur within hours or days. Comprehension may be totally lost or reduced to understanding only short phrases and simple instructions (Worster-Drought, 1971). Cooper and Ferry (1978) found 42% of their children with Landau-Kleffner syndrome had a severe comprehension deficit, 24% had a moderate to mild comprehension impairment, whereas the other 34% recovered their receptive abilities. One major difficulty in assessing comprehension skills in children with Landau-Kleffner syndrome is the fluctuating performance of some of these children from day to day or even within one session.

In numerous cases of Landau-Kleffner syndrome, the inability to identify auditory information, which extends to nonverbal stimuli, has been classified as an auditory agnosia involving language as well as environmental sounds. Often due to the reduced comprehension ability the presence of a hearing loss is suspected in the early stages of the disorder and many of the subjects are initially thought to be deaf. However, in the majority of cases their audiogram in the early stages is within normal limits (Cooper & Ferry, 1978; van Harskamp, van Dongen, & Loonen, 1978; van de Sandt-Koenderman et al., 1984). In association with the reduction in comprehension, the spontaneous speech of the child also changes.

These receptive deficits have been interpreted in various ways. Most authors consider them to be a specific deficit in phonological decoding, that is, the child has difficulty at the phonemic identification and discrimination levels (Denes, Balliello, Volterra, & Pellegrini, 1986; Pearce & Darwish, 1984; Rapin et al., 1977). The poorer prognosis for children who have not learned language (i.e., those under 5 years of age) is offered as support for a phonemic decoding deficit (Bishop, 1985). The fact that children with Landau-Kleffner syndrome perform on a comprehension test like hearing-impaired children and not like normal control or children with a developmental expressive language disorder is also presented as evidence for a deficit at phonemic discrimination level (Bishop, 1982). The comprehension deficits noted in both the Landau-Kleffner and the hearing-impaired subjects were shown to occur whether the input was oral, signed, or written. Bishop (1982) hypothesized that both groups of children fail to develop the hierarchical interpretation of sentences because they have to learn language through a signing system that fosters a more sequential interpretation of sentence meaning.

Comprehension abilities in Landau-Kleffner syndrome cases have also been shown to improve if the rate of presentation is slowed. Interestingly, when a first instruction is presented at a slower rate but a second instruction is presented at a normal rate, both instructions were more readily comprehended. Campbell and McNeil (1985) explained this phenomenon in terms of Kahneman's model of attention capacity which would indicate that children with the Landau-Kleffner syndrome may have difficulty decoding rapid speech because of an inefficient allocation of attention from a finite attentional capacity. More research obviously is required before a complete understanding of the comprehension deficits in children with Landau-Kleffner syndrome and their recovery over time is forthcoming.

In most reported cases expressive language impairments succeed the onset of auditory comprehension deficits, with either a progressive loss of vocabulary and/or phonological disturbances. Expressively, the child may become mute, use jargon or produce odd sounds, exhibit misarticulations, inappropriate substitution of words and anomia, or resort to gestures and grunts (Cooper & Ferry, 1978). Unlike acquired childhood aphasia following focal unilateral lesions, in Landau-Kleffner syndrome jargon aphasia with paraphasia and neologisms are often observed before the complete loss language function that may last several months or even years. Over the course of the condition the degree of language impairment often fluctuates, with periods of transient recovery after the introduction or change of an anticonvulsant drug.

Voice quality changes have also been noted in children with Landau-Kleffner syndrome. Some authors report a "deaf-like" voice, whereas others note a high pitch. A case reported by Deonna, Chevrie, and Hornung (1987) presented with only a prosodic disturbance after partial complex seizures. The prosodic features observed were marked slowness and irregularity with prolonged pauses and hesitations and lack of intonation and were not due to motor speech disorders or emotional disturbance. Therefore, what is predominantly a phonemic deficit presents as a wide range of expressive speech and language impairments.

Preceding, co-occurring with, or following the language deterioration there may be a series of convulsive seizures (van de Sandt-Koenderman et al., 1984). Although seizures do occur often, they are not the defining feature of the syndrome. Miller et al. (1984) reported that of those cases that exhibit seizures, 43% experience the seizures before the language regression, 16% display co-occurrence of seizures and language regression, and 41% experience seizures sometime after the language regression. Regardless of whether or not there are clinically observable seizures, however, all patients with the syndrome exhibit epileptiform discharges in their electroencephalograms (Deonna, Fletcher, & Voumard, 1982). The electroencephalographic abnormalities usually take the form of bilateral synchronous disturbances, frequently with a temporal predominance (Gascon et al., 1973; Deonna et al., 1982).

In addition to the language disorder, a number of other associated problems may also occur in acquired epileptic aphasia. Emotional problems have been reported in a number of cases (Miller et al., 1984) and behavioral problems such as aggressiveness, temper outbursts, refusing to respond, inattention, withdrawal, and hyperactivity occur frequently (Campbell & Heaton, 1978; Deonna et al., 1977; Gascon et al., 1973). One surprising feature of this syndrome is that the child's nonverbal intelligence usually remains unimpaired (Miller et al., 1984).

Subgroups of Landau-Kleffner Syndrome

Based on their observation of differences in the course of the disease, individual characteristics of the aphasia and the long-term prognosis, Deonna et al. (1977) proposed that Landau-Kleffner syndrome is not a homogeneous disorder. From examination of their own cases and a review of the literature they proposed three subgroups of Landau-Kleffner syndrome. The first group they felt was similar to the cases of epileptic aphasia described in the adult population. The children in this group showed rapid deterioration of language skills or fluctuating performance usually associated with seizures. Likewise, the recovery of language in this group is rapid. The second group showed progressive aphasic symptoms after a seizure or repeated episodes of aphasia. Recovery in this group may take months or years. The third group is made up of children who gradually develop marked auditory comprehension deficits. This group has no or few seizures. Deonna et al. (1977) noted variable rates and degrees of recovery of language skills in this last group. The differences in onset and recovery of language skills lead them to postulate different mechanisms underlying the aphasic symptoms for the three groups.

Miller et al. (1984), however, noted that the recovery of language skills in each of Deonna et al.'s groups was still variable and as such their groupings of cases with the Landau-Kleffner syndrome could not be used to predict language recovery. Instead, they proposed another method of grouping children with the Landau-Kleffner syndrome based on their language profiles collected over a 2-year period. Again, three subgroups emerged. The first group consisted of two children, aged 6;10 and 11;8 years who presented with complete loss of auditory comprehension and expressive language abilities after a period of normal language development. Seizures were present. Nonverbal cognitive functioning was age appropriate. Their ability to discriminate linguistic stimuli and their performance on auditory comprehension tasks was at chance levels. Some ability to discriminate nonspeech sounds was evident until these sounds were a less familiar form. This performance on auditory task lead Miller et al. (1984) to diagnose a verbal auditory agnosia. No improvement in auditory comprehension was observed over the 2-year follow-up. Better performance on comprehension tasks, however, was noted in both children when signs, gestures, comprehension strategies, and written language were used. Expressive language was very restricted on initial assessment in both cases. After 18 months, the 6-year-old subject was using one or two word utterances with good intelligibility. The 11-year-old subject, however, showed little change over a 2-year period. His expressive language consisted of consonant vowel combinations and his voice quality was similar to that of a deaf child. In addition, some apraxic like movements of the articulators were noted on the production of isolated phonemes.

The second subgroup described by Miller et al. (1984) presented with variable comprehension abilities, delayed expressive language and a word-finding problem. These children also had normal language development prior to onset, and they also presented with seizures. Receptive language was described as variable because the children responded to the same words or strings of words differently from moment to moment. Particular difficulty was noted in processing conversational speech. Expressive language impairments were demonstrated to be similar to those seen in children with developmental language disorders. Miller et al. (1984) reported that this group of children with the Landau-Kleffner syndrome was able to function in a normal educational setting, though spelling and reading problems were encountered. If speech and language skills improved, however, this improvement was rapid.

The third subgroup of children with Landau-Kleffner syndrome described by Miller et al. (1984) never had a history of normal language development. Two of the cases described did not show a regression of language skills. Both children presented with language deficits similar to those described above in the second subgroup. In one of these cases a cognitive delay was present. The third case belonging to this third subgroup did show language regression at 4 years of age. At this stage the subject's language development was delayed, being at a two- to three-word level. In association with seizures this child's receptive and expressive language as well as cognitive skills regressed to below the 1-year level. The language skills were similar to those described in the children with verbal auditory agnosia (i.e., the first subgroup described above) except that cognitive skills also were affected. Children with Landau-Kleffner syndrome who have never had a normal language history have been described by Rapin et al. (1977) and Maccario, Hefferen, Keblusek, and Lipinski (1982), leading to the notion of a developmental form of the syndrome.

Therefore, whether based on the onset or recovery of aphasic symptoms or the linguistic profiles shown by children with the Landau-Kleffner syndrome, it is clear that a range of language skills are present in this population.

Prognosis of Landau-Kleffner Syndrome

The prognosis of aphasia with convulsive disorder is unclear. Van de Sandt-Koenderman et al. (1984) caution that many reports concentrate on the medical aspects of the syndrome, whereas the aphasia is poorly described. Consequently, the many contradictory statements about the prognosis may be due to the variation in the particular aspect of the disorder being described as recovering. A medical examination of children may declare them "completely recovered" when there still may be demonstrable aphasic characteristics evidenced if sufficiently sensitive testing is carried out. Most studies emphasize a better outcome for epilepsy than for language disorders. Indeed, complete recovery from epilepsy occurs at the beginning of adolescence whereas language remains impaired. In many cases the language recovery in Landau-Kleffner syndrome is very limited. Miller et al. (1984) stated that over 80% of cases reported in the literature have receptive and expressive deficits that persist for longer than six months. Long-term follow-up studies have shown that persisting verbal impairments result from phonological short-term memory deficit (Metz-Lutz, Seegmuller, Kleitz, de Saint Martin, Hirsch, & Marescaux, 1999).

In general it appears that the prognosis for recovery is poor if there has been no progress within one year post-onset. As indicated above some children with this disorder go through periods of exacerbations and remissions. Mantovani and Landau (1980) found that children who exhibit this latter type of course have a relatively good prognosis. However, as a rule, the younger the age when symptoms start, the worse the prognosis in terms of language function (Paquier, van Dongen, & Loonen, 1992). Bishop (1985) reported that children younger than 5 years of age at the time of onset of symptoms showed a very poor prognosis for language outcomes. The relationship between the recovery of language skills, changes in EEG recordings and seizures, however, is still unclear. Therefore, predicting which children will recover completely their language skills without language intervention cannot readily be based on changes in EEG data.

Differential Diagnosis of Landau-Kleffner Syndrome

In many cases the differential diagnosis of Landau-Kleffner syndrome is difficult. As noted above, 80% of children with the Landau-Kleffner syndrome have behavioral disturbances such as aggression, withdrawal, inattention, hyperactivity, and temper outbursts. Organic bases and a reaction to sudden loss of comprehension have been put forward to explain these behavioral problems. Whatever the causes, these behaviors together with the loss of communication skills are often thought to reflect a psychiatric problem. Consequently, the differential diagnosis of Landau-Kleffner syndrome is crucial. Sometimes, the sudden loss of language skills are mistaken for elective mutism. Similarly the sudden or gradual loss of comprehension is often attributed to a hearing loss. The authors warn against using behavioral measures of audiologic status because of the nature of the syndrome.

Any regression of language skills should be assessed by a neurologist for if the acquired aphasia is not due to any of the other causes of aphasia (e.g., tumors, vascular lesions, infections, or head injury) an EEG is necessary for the diagnosis of Landau-Kleffner syndrome. The gradual regression of language skills makes the diagnosis of the syndrome particularly difficult as it takes longer to identify the loss of language skills and alternative explanations for the observed behavior may be given. This is even more so if the aphasic symptoms precede seizures or if seizures are not present. Diagnosis is even more difficult in those cases where a period of normal language development was not present. Therefore, it would seem important to get EEG information on any child who presents with a moderate to severe developmental receptive language disorder particularly if cognitive skills are age appropriate.

Clinical Management of Language Disorder in Landau-Kleffner Syndrome

Due to the complex nature of Landau-Kleffner syndrome, management of children with this condition necessitates the involvement of a multidisciplinary team. Ideally, this team should comprise a speech-language pathologist, a special education teacher (or educational psychologist), a pediatric neurol-

ogist, and an audiologist. In the early stages of diagnosis the pediatric neurologist is essential to rule out other potential causes of the language impairment such as brain tumor, cerebrovascular accident, and so forth Likewise, at this time, it is critical to establish the child's audiologic status. Given the frequent confusion of Landau-Kleffner syndrome with deafness, the audiologist is vital to rule out conductive hearing loss as a cause of the deterioration in language skills and to monitor the hearing status of the child on an ongoing basis. Any future hearing loss would further compound the existing language deficit thereby exacerbating problems with both communication and behavior.

Bishop (1982) determined that children with Landau-Kleffner syndrome have a similar pattern of difficulty in comprehending language to that of deaf children. Furthermore, Bishop (1982) suggested that this similarity is the result of an auditory processing difficulty in Landau-Kleffner syndrome that forces the child to rely on the visual modality to learn the grammar of the language as in the case of deaf children. The object of language intervention in children with Landau-Kleffner syndrome is to bypass the phonemic decoding deficit by using alternative methods to access the language skills that are still preserved. For children with severe receptive language deficits placement in special classes for either the language disordered or the hearing impaired is important to provide a signing environment. Using the visual system either through signing or written language also helps children with less severe impairment. Bishop (1982), however, warns that signing or written language helps children with less severe impairments, but that signing is not to be considered as a "panacea" for children with Landau-Kleffner syndrome for the reasons stated earlier. Children who do not have oral language skills still learn to read. Some children with the Landau-Kleffner syndrome, however, present only with written language deficits. Therefore, the type of speech and language intervention will depend on the child's age at onset and therefore the language skills already developed and the extent of recovery.

There is little information available in the literature relating to language therapy and educational rehabilitation programs applied to children with Landau-Kleffner syndrome. Two examples are the programs developed by De Wijngaert (1991) and Vance (1991). The program outlined by De Wijngaert (1991) involved the integration of speech and language therapy into a classroom program to provide a comprehensive approach for educational needs. Centered on the creation of the right environment for learning and engendering of enthusiasm in the children, this program was essentially oral in nature and advocated the teaching of oral and written skills in a staged manner. Unfortunately no outcome measures as to the success of this program were provided.

Vance (1991) reported a detailed case study of a boy who exhibited a slow deterioration in his language abilities at the age of 3 years 6 months and which lasted over 8 months. Initially, this child was introduced to signing through the Makaton Vocabulary (Walker, 1980) and subsequently to the Paget-Gorman Sign System (Paget, Gorman, & Paget, 1976). By age 7 years the child was able to produce strings of 7 or more signs. The child was also introduced to Cued Articulation (Passy, 1990), a system that uses a series of hand shapes to identify each English consonant. These methods were used in individual therapy and in the classroom where other educational techniques included a daily picture diary to help develop the concept of time and a color pattern scheme for literacy skills (Lea, 1965, 1979). Other communication skills taught included auditory training and interaction skills. Vance (1991) noted that the boy eventually attended a unit for the partially hearing where signing was used.

References

Bishop, D. V. M. (1982). Comprehension of spoken, written and signed sentences in childhood language disorders. *Journal of Child Psychology and Psychiatry, 23*, 1–20.

Bishop, D. V. M. (1985). Age of onset and outcome in acquired aphasia with convulsive disorder (Landau-Kleffner syndrome). *Developmental Medicine and Child Neurology, 27*, 705–712.

Campbell, T. F., & Heaton, E. M. (1978). An expressive speech program for a child with acquired aphasia: A case study. *Human Communication (Summer), 89*, 102.

Campbell, T. F., & McNeil, M. R. (1985). Effects of presentation rate and divided attention of auditory comprehension in children with an acquired language disorder. *Journal of Speech and Hearing Research, 28*, 513–520.

Cooper, J. A., & Ferry, P. C. (1978). Acquired auditory verbal agnosia and seizures in childhood. *Journal of Speech and Hearing Disorders, 43*, 176–184.

Denes, G., Balliello, S., Volterra, V., & Pellegrini, A. (1986). Oral and written language in a case of childhood phonemic deafness. *Brain and Language, 34*, 252–267.

Deonna, T., Beaumanoir, A., Gaillard, F., & Assal, G. (1977). Acquired aphasia in childhood with seizure disorder: A heterogeneous syndrome. *Neuropaediatric, 8*, 263–273.

Deonna, T., Chevrie, C., & Hornung, E. (1987). Childhood epileptic speech disorder: Prolonged isolated deficit of prosodic features. *Developmental Medicine and Child Neurology, 29*, 96–109.

Deonna, T., Fletcher, P., & Voumard, C. (1982). Temporary regression during language acquisition: A Linguistic analysis of a two-and-one-half year old child with epileptic aphasia. *Developmental Medicine and Child Neurology, 24*, 156–163.

De Wijngaert, E. (1991) The Landau-Kleffner syndrome: Rehabilitation. In I. P. Martins, A. Castro-Caldas, H. R. van Dongen, & A. Van Hout (Eds.), *Acquired aphasia in children: Acquisition and breakdown of language in the developing brain*. Dordrecht, the Netherlands: Kluwer Academic.

Dulac, O., Billard, C., & Arthuis, M. (1983). Aspects electrocliniques et evolutifs de l'epilepsie dans le syndrome aphasie-epilepsie. *Archives Francaises de Pediatrie, 40*, 299–308.

Gascon, G., Victor, D., Lombroso, C. T., & Goodglass, H. (1973). Language disorder, convulsive disorder and electroencephalographic abnormalities. *Archives of Neurology, 28*, 156–162.

Grote, C. L., van Slyke, P., & Hoeppner, J. A. (1999). Language outcome following multiple subpial transection for Landau-Kleffner syndrome. *Brain, 122*, 561–566.

Landau, W. M., & Kleffner, F. R. (1957). Syndrome of acquired aphasia with convulsive disorder in children. *Neurology, 10*, 915–921.

Lea, J. (1965). A language scheme for children suffering from receptive aphasia. *Speech Pathology and Therapy, 8*, 56–68.

Lea, J. (1979). Language development through the written word. *Child Care Health and Development, 5*, 69–74.

Lees, J. (1993). *Children with acquired aphasia.* London, UK: Whurr.

Maccario, M., Hefferen, S. J., Keblusek, S. J., & Lipinski, K. A. (1982). Developmental dysphasia and electroencephalographic abnormalities. *Developmental Medicine and Child Neurology, 24*, 141–155.

Mantovani, J. F., & Landau, W. M. (1980). Acquired aphasia with convulsive disorder: Course and prognosis. *Neurology, 30*, 524–529.

Maquet, P., Hirsch, E., Metz-Lutz, M. N., Motte, J., Dive, D., Marescaux, C., . . . Franck, G. (1995). Regional cerebral glucose metabolism in children with deterioration of one or more cognitive functions and continuous spike-and-wave discharge during sleep. *Brain, 118*, 1497–1520.

Marescaux, C., Hirsch, E., Finck, S., Maquet, P., Schlumberger, E., Sellal, F., . . . Franck, G. (1990). Landau-Kleffner syndrome: A pharmacological study of five cases. *Epilepsia, 31*, 768–777.

McKinney, W., & McGreal, D. A. (1974). An aphasic syndrome in children. *Canadian Medical Association Journal, 110*, 637–639.

Metz-Lutz, M. N., Seegmuller, C., Kleitz, C., de Saint Martin, A., Hirsch, E., & Marescaux, C. (1999). Landau-Kleffner syndrome: A rare childhood epileptic aphasia. *Journal of Neurolinguistics, 12*, 167–179.

Miller, J. F., Campbell, T. F., Chapman, R. S., & Weismer, S. E. (1984). Language behavior in acquired aphasia. In A. Holland (Ed.), *Language disorders in children*. Baltimore, MD: College-Hill Press.

Morrell, F., Whisler, W. W., & Bleck, T. P. (1989). Multiple subpial transection: A new approach to the surgical treatment of focal epilepsy. *Journal of Neurosurgery, 70*, 231–239.

Msall, M., Shapiro, B., Balfour, P. B., Niedermeyer, E., & Capute, A. J. (1986). Acquired epileptic aphasia: Diagnostic aspects of progressive language loss in preschool children. *Neurology, 25*, 248–251.

Paget, R., Gorman, P., & Paget, G. (1976). *The Paget Gorman sign system*. London, UK: Association for Experiment in Deaf Education.

Paquier, P. F., van Dongen, H. R., & Loonen, M. C. B. (1992). The Landau-Kleffner syndrome or acquired aphasia with convulsive disorder: Long-term follow-up of six children and a review of the recent literature. *Archives of Neurology, 49*, 354–359.

Passy, J. (1990). *Cued articulation.* London, UK: Australian Council for Educational Research.

Pearce, P. S., & Darwish, H. (1984). Correlation between EEG and auditory perceptual measures in auditory agnosia. *Brain and Language, 22,* 41–48.

Rapin, I., Mattis, S., Rowan, A. J., & Golden, G. S. (1977). Verbal auditory agnosia in children. *Developmental Medicine and Child Neurology, 19,* 192–207.

Sato, S., & Dreifuss, F. E. (1973). Electroencephalographic findings in a patient with developmental expressive aphasia. *Neurology, 23,* 181–185.

Vance, M. (1991). Educational and therapeutic approaches used with a child with acquired aphasia with convulsive disorder (Landau-Kleffner syndrome). *Child Language, Teaching and Therapy, 7,* 41–60.

van de Sandt-Koenderman, W. M. E., Smit, I. A. C., van Dongen, H. R., & van Hest, J. B. C. (1984). A case of acquired aphasia and convulsive disorder: Some linguistic aspects of recovery and breakdown. *Brain and Language, 21,* 174–183.

van Harskamp, F., van Dongen, H. R., & Loonen, M. C. B. (1978). Acquired aphasia with convulsive disorder in children: A case study with a seven year follow-up. *Brain and Language, 6,* 141–148.

Walker, M. (1980). *The Revised Makaton Vocabulary.* London, UK: Walker.

Wioland, N., Rudolf, G., & Metz-Lutz, M. N. (2001). Electrophysiological evidence of persisting unilateral auditory cortex dysfunction in the late outcome of Landau-Kleffner syndrome. *Clinical Neurophysiology, 112,* 319–323.

Worster-Drought, C. (1971). An unusual form of acquired aphasia in children. *Developmental Medicine and Child Neurology, 13,* 563–571.

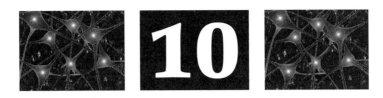

Assessment and Treatment of Acquired Childhood Language Disorders

Little research has been published regarding the efficacy and utility of various approaches to the assessment and treatment of language disorders in children with acquired brain injury. Consequently, the literature provides little advice and support to clinicians in their selection and application of appropriate assessment and treatment techniques for use with children with brain injuries under their care. To a large extent this lack of research stems from a long held, but now disproven, assumption that if a child made an excellent physical recovery after brain injury then their recovery of language function also was complete. Consequently, for many years the presence of persistent cognitive linguistic impairments in these children were not suspected and their language abilities not subjected to a comprehensive and in-depth analysis. However, for some years now clinicians have been aware that many children who were declared fully recovered from their brain lesion have subtle underlying language problems which may affect their later academic performance, vocational opportunities, and social interaction. More specifically, as highlighted in a number of earlier chapters in this book, since the early 1990s a number of reports in the literature have demonstrated the presence of chronic subtle language disorders in children following traumatic brain injury (TBI) (Docking, Murdoch, & Ward, 2003; Jordan & Murdoch, 1993; Jordan, Murdoch, Buttsworth, & Hudson-Tennent, 1995) and brain tumor (Hudson & Murdoch, 1992; Murdoch & Hudson-Tennent, 1994).

Assessment of Acquired Childhood Aphasia

Prior to initiation of any treatment for acquired language disorders the clinician must complete a detailed case history and comprehensive assessment of the language disorder. The case history provides essential background information to aid the clinician in determination of the specific assessments and treatments required for the individual child with acquired brain injury and provides an understanding of the client's perspective on their disorder. A comprehensive case history should provide details of the client's age, education level, academic abilities and status, and prior history of speech-language impairments. In addition, the case history should determine the onset and course of the condition. Details of any prior treatment and management regimens should be recorded and the client's awareness and understanding of the disorder determined. The effects and consequences of the disorder on the client's daily life (e.g., disruption to school, social activities, and family life) from the client's perspective needs to be documented and details of any reports documenting the findings of neurologic and neuroimaging examinations together with reports from any other professionals involved in the child's care recorded.

There are a number of concomitant problems associated with acquired aphasia which must be recognized if accurate assessment results are to be obtained and realistic treatment goals formulated. Dyspraxia, dysarthria, and occasionally an agnosia may coexist with the aphasia. Visual and hearing acuity should be tested so that the child is not further disadvantaged by being unable to hear or see clearly. It also is important for differential diagnosis that peripheral problems are not mistaken for central difficulties.

Motor problems such as hemiplegia, quadriplegia, and paraplegia, along with a variety of dyspraxias, may hinder the child's ability to respond appropriately to assessment instructions, even though the individual's language skill necessary for carrying out the instructions is intact. For example, the quadriplegic child, particularly if there is an accompanying dysarthria or dyspraxia, may have difficulty responding to test stimuli by pointing or moving tokens and is certainly disadvantaged when there is a time limit on the subtest. A child with a limb dyspraxia and a right hemiplegia may have difficulty carrying out instructions if asked to pantomime an action with his or her left hand. For example, "Show me what you would do with scissors." If the child failed to respond, his or her failure could be interpreted wrongly as a comprehension problem rather than as a motor planning difficulty. Perseveration may also be confused as incorrect responses (e.g., the child continues to point to a picture in the same place on each page).

Many language tests use visual stimuli. If children with visual deficits, such as a homonymous hemianopsia, have not learned to compensate using good visual scanning, then they can miss stimuli placed too far to the right or left of the focal point. Visual perceptual problems may cause an individual to fail because they cannot effectively discriminate between the visual cues. For example, one child with severe figure-ground problems could not manage any subtest which had a visual stimulus because he could not discriminate the line drawing from the rest of the page. This difficulty also prevented any testing of his reading or writing skills. Double vision and nystagmus may also cloud the child's real linguistic abilities, particularly reading skills. For example, as the child moves from line to line in a paragraph, he or she may lose his or her place and then forget the content of the passage in the effort of finding his or her place again.

Behavioral problems, including personality changes, egocentricity, depression, and mood swings, can influence both day-to-day treatment sessions and long-term goals. Also, the child is usually an integral member of a family unit so that the changes in family life and structure brought about by the child's injury must be addressed. For example, one father, who previously had had a close relationship with his daughter found it difficult to make regular hospital visits to his child after her injury. The girl was extremely upset and believed that her father no longer loved her. Consequently, she was unmotivated in therapy and it was not until the situation was rectified that she regained her motivation.

Underlying all assessment procedures and treatment plans must be an awareness of children's cognitive abilities. In particular, memory may mask the child's linguistic skills (e.g., the child cannot remember the instructions and therefore cannot respond correctly). Also, children's susceptibility to fatigue and any medical conditions such as seizures which could affect assessment and remediation must be taken into consideration.

In the early stages postinjury, a bedside examination often constitutes the initial type of assessment. Most often the bedside examination is based largely on observation by the clinician rather than administration of formal language tests. As part of the bedside assessment the speech-language pathologist should consider factors such as: the patient's ability to comprehend spoken language (e.g., do they follow the conversation, can they follow one-, two-, or three-stage commands such as, "point to the floor then to the ceiling"); naming abilities; and the patient's ability to repeat words of increasing complexity and sentences.

Once a client is medically stable, observation can then be supplemented with a range of formal tests. In general these tests fall into one of two major categories: tests that evaluate basic language skills; and tests of functional and pragmatic language abilities. A summary of the recommended assessment process for children with acquired language disorders is presented in Figure 10–1.

Language Assessments

Most clinicians use three methods for assessing the communication of the child with a brain lesion: formal tests (standardized tests), informal procedures (i.e., nonstandardized tests), and observation. Each method is important but it is the integration and interpretation of information obtained from all areas which allows the clinician to diagnose the child's difficulties, effect the appropriate treatment, and measure subsequent progress.

Formal Tests (Standardized Tests)

Standardized tests play an important role in assessment, especially when progress needs to be measured objectively. In the acute stage of recovery, however, informal testing and observation are usually adopted because these two methods are less threatening to anxious children and their parents. If the clinician persists in using standardized tests and other formal procedures in their entirety when the child is not ready or able to cope with the demands, then the child/clinician relationship and the child's progress in therapy may be put at risk.

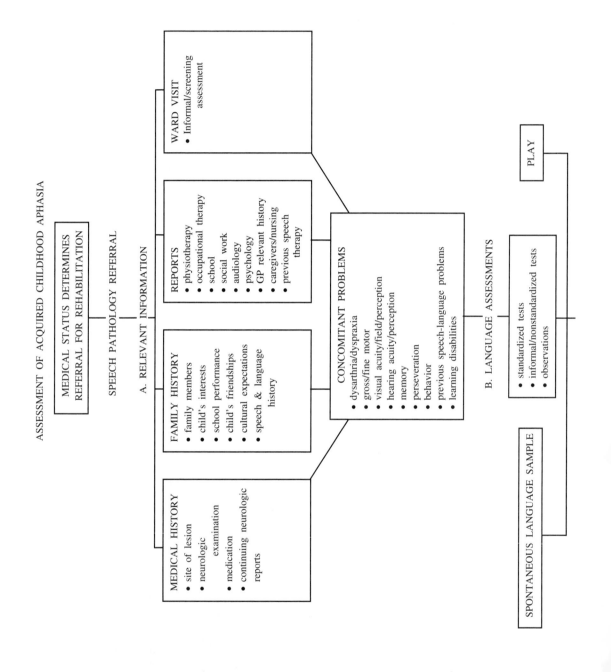

ASSESSMENT OF ACQUIRED CHILDHOOD APHASIA

MEDICAL STATUS DETERMINES
REFERRAL FOR REHABILITATION

SPEECH PATHOLOGY REFERRAL

A. RELEVANT INFORMATION

MEDICAL HISTORY
- site of lesion
- neurologic
  examination
- medication
- continuing neurologic
  reports

FAMILY HISTORY
- family members
- child's interests
- school performance
- child's friendships
- cultural expectations
- speech & language
  history

REPORTS
- physiotherapy
- occupational therapy
- school
- social work
- audiology
- psychology
- GP relevant history
- caregivers/nursing
- previous speech
  therapy

WARD VISIT
- Informal/screening
  assessment

CONCOMITANT PROBLEMS
- dysarthria/dyspraxia
- gross/fine motor
- visual acuity/field/perception
- hearing acuity/perception
- memory
- perseveration
- behavior
- previous speech-language problems
- learning disabilities

B. LANGUAGE ASSESSMENTS
- standardized tests
- informal/nonstandardized tests
- observations

SPONTANEOUS LANGUAGE SAMPLE

PLAY

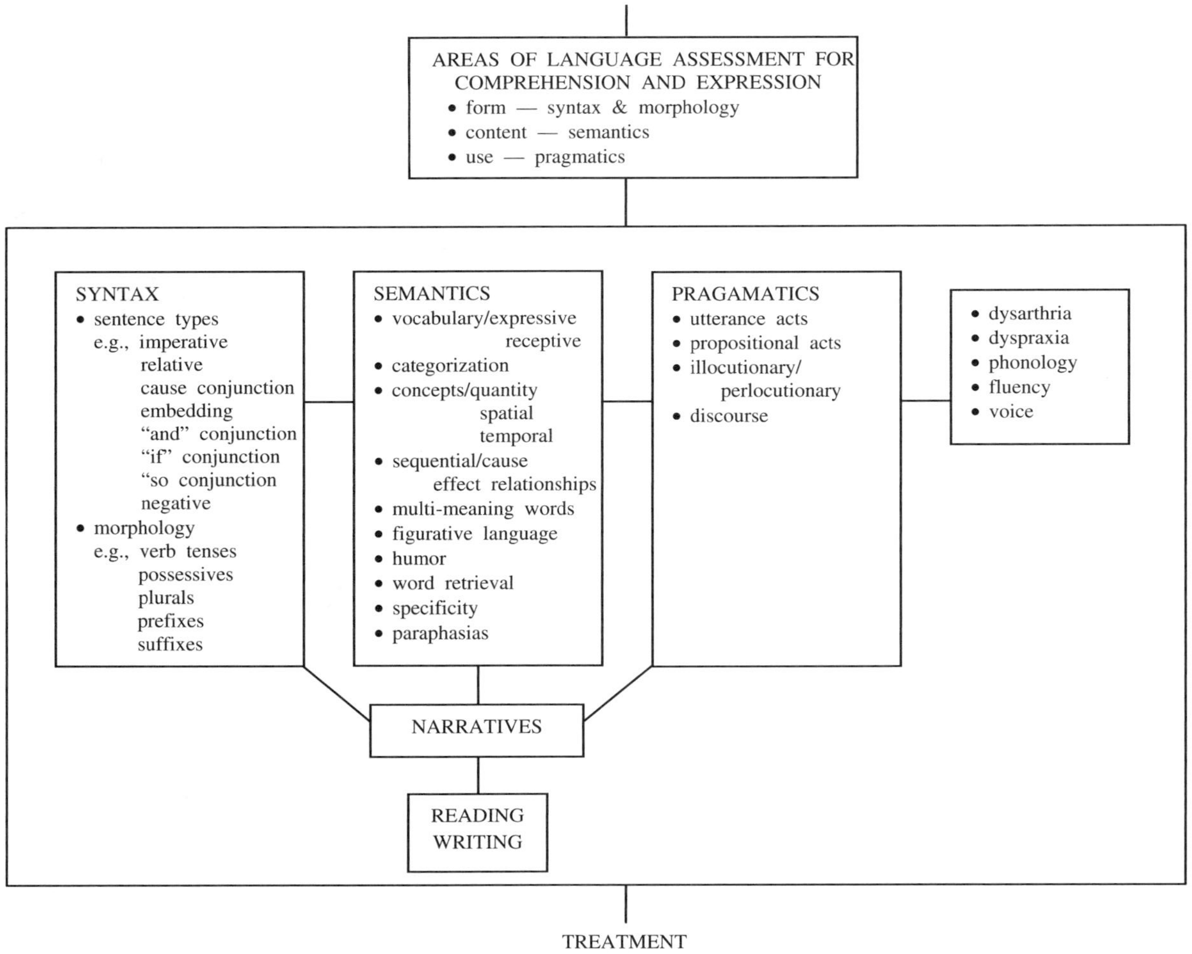
AREAS OF LANGUAGE ASSESSMENT FOR COMPREHENSION AND EXPRESSION
• form — syntax & morphology
• content — semantics
• use — pragmatics
SYNTAX
• sentence types
e.g., imperative
relative
cause conjunction
embedding
"and" conjunction
"if" conjunction
"so conjunction
negative
• morphology
e.g., verb tenses
possessives
plurals
prefixes
suffixes
SEMANTICS
• vocabulary/expressive
receptive
• categorization
• concepts/quantity
spatial
temporal
• sequential/cause
effect relationships
• multi-meaning words
• figurative language
• humor
• word retrieval
• specificity
• paraphasias
PRAGAMATICS
• utterance acts
• propositional acts
• illocutionary/
perlocutionary
• discourse
• dysarthria
• dyspraxia
• phonology
• fluency
• voice
NARRATIVES
READING
WRITING
TREATMENT

FIGURE 10–1. Summary of assessment of acquired childhood aphasia.

There are a number of excellent tests of child language development that can be used in the assessment of children with acquired childhood aphasia, for example, Clinical Evaluation of Language Fundamentals–Fourth Edition (CELF–4) (Semel, Wiig, & Secord, 2003), Clinical Evaluation of Language Fundamentals Preschool–Second Edition (CELF–Pre) (Wiig, Secord, & Semel, 2006), Test of Language Development Series (TOLD) (Hammill & Newcomer, 1997a, 1997b), Preschool Language Assessment Instrument (Blank, Rose, & Berlin 1978), Porch Index of Communicative Ability in Children (PICAC) (Porch, 1974), and the Reynell Developmental Language Scales–III (RDLS–III) (Edwards et al., 1977), plus tests that assess specific linguistic abilities for example, Peabody Picture Vocabulary Test–Fourth Edition (PPVT–4) (Dunn & Dunn, 2007), Token Test for Children (DiSimoni, 1978), Test of Auditory Comprehension of Language–Revised (TACL–R) (Carrow-Woolfolk, 1985), and Hundred Pictures Naming Test (HPNT) (Fisher & Glenister, 1992). Adult aphasic tests can also provide valuable information when used with the older child or adolescent, for example, the Boston Naming Test (Kaplan, Goodglass, & Weintraub, 1983), the Neurosensory Center Comprehensive Examination for Aphasia (NCCEA) (Spreen & Benton, 1977), or the Communicative Abilities in Daily Living–Revised (CADL) (Holland, Frattali, & Fromm, 1999). The increasing use of these adult tests with children has prompted the development of childhood norms for the Boston Naming Test (Guilford & Nawojczyk, 1988) and the NCCEA (Gaddes & Crockett, 1975).

Some of the more common tests used for assessing children with acquired aphasia are listed in Table 10–1.

Table 10–1. Formal Tests and Analyses Commonly Used in the Assessment of Children with Acquired Aphasia

Test	Author(s)
General	
Clinical Evaluation of Language Fundamentals-Fourth Edition (CELF-4)	Semel, Wiig, & Secord, 2003
Clinical Evaluation of Language Fundamentals-Preschool Second Edition (CELF-3)	Wiig, Secord, & Semel, 2006
Test of Early Language Development, 3rd ed. (TELD-3)	Hresko, Reid, & Hammill, 1999
Test of Language Development-Primary, 3rd ed. (TOLD-P3)	Hammill & Newcomer, 1997b
Test of Language Development-Intermediate, 3rd ed. (TOLD-I3)	Hammill & Newcomer, 1997a
Test of Adolescent and Adult Language, 4th ed. (TOAL-4)	Hammill, Brown, Larsen, & Weiderholt, 2007
Pre-school Language Assessment Instrument (PLAI)	Blank, Rose, & Berlin, 1978
Test of Auditory Comprehension of Language-Revised (TACL-R)	Carrow-Woolfolk, 1985
The Token Test for Children (TT)	DiSimoni, 1978

Table 10–1. *continued*

Test	Author(s)
Porch Index of Communicative Ability in Children (PICAC)	Porch, 1974
Reynell Developmental Language Scales-III (RDLS-3)	Edwards et al., 1997
Test of Language Competence-Expanded (TLC-E)	Wiig & Secord, 1989
Test of Problem Solving-Third Edition	Bowers, Huisingh, & LoGiudice, 2005
Test of Problem Solving-Adolescent	Zachman, Barrett, Huisingh, Orman & Blagden, 1991
Test of Problem Solving-Elementary	Zachman, Huisingh, Barrett, Orman, & LoGiudice, 1994
Wiig-Semel Test of Linguistic Concepts (WSTLC)	Wiig & Semel, 1974
Semantics	
Peabody Picture Vocabulary Test-Fourth Edition (PPVT-4)	Dunn & Dunn, 2007
Boehm Test of Basic Concepts-3rd Edition	Boehm, 2000
Double Administration Naming Technique (DANT)	Fried-Oken, 1987
The Word Test: A Test of Expressive Vocabulary and Semantics (TWT)	Jorgensen, Barrett, Huisingh, & Zachman, 1981
WORD-Test 2: Elementary	Bowers, Huisingh, LoGiudice, & Orman, 2004
WORD-Test 2: Adolescent	Huisingh, Bowers, LoGiudice, & Oman, 2005
Boston Naming Test (BNT)	Kaplan, Goodglass, & Weintraub, 1983
Content/Form Analysis	Bloom & Lahey, 1978
Test of Word Knowledge (TOWK)	Wiig & Secord, 1992
Syntax	
Language Assessment, Remediation and Screening Procedure (LARSP)	Crystal, Fletcher, & Garman, 1982
Phonological Awareness	
Test of Phonological Awareness (TOPA)	Torgesen & Bryant, 1994
Pragmatics	
Let's Talk Inventory for Adolescents	Wiig, 1982
Clinical Discourse Analysis	Damico, 1985
Communicative Abilities in Daily Living-Revised (CADL)	Holland, Frattali, & Fromm, 1999

Although the provision of a detailed description of each of the assessments listed in Table 10–1 is beyond the scope of the present chapter, in order to demonstrate the range of language tasks covered by these types of assessments, further details of representative examples of the various categories shown in Table 10–1 are provided below.

Neurosensory Center Comprehensive Examination for Aphasia (NCCEA). The NCCEA constitutes a detailed assessment of language functions, incorporating subtests that evaluate primary as well as high-level linguistic abilities. Principally designed for the assessment of aphasic adults, the NCCEA is comprised of 20 language tasks which specifically evaluate the status of immediate verbal memory, verbal production and fluency, receptive language, reading, writing, and basic articulatory proficiency. Overall, the assessment provides a descriptive versus taxonomic classification of linguistic abilities (Table 10–2 provides a description of individual NCCEA subtests).

Clinical Evaluation of Language Fundamentals–4th Edition (CELF–4). The CELF–4 was designed to identify, diag-nose, and follow-up language skill deficits in school-age children and adolescents aged 6 to 21 years. It identifies children who lack the basic foundations of content and form that characterize mature language use, including knowledge or word meanings (semantics), word and sentence structure (morphology and syntax), and recall and retrieval (memory). Within the CELF–4, two age levels are accommodated. Four of the core subtests have been designed for administration to children aged 6 years and older. Two subtests are appropriate only for older children 9 years and above, and two are appropriate only for younger children aged 6 to 8 years, 11 months. A related test, the CELF–Preschool, was designed as a clinical tool to identify, diagnose, and follow-up language deficits in preschool age children aged 3 years to 6 years, 11 months.

Boston Naming Test (BNT). The BNT is a reliable measure of confrontation naming abilities and provides information about the effectiveness of semantic and phonemic cues in facilitating word retrieval. Clients are instructed to name 60 constituent black and white line drawings of various objects ranging in frequency from *bed* to *abacus* and are

Table 10–2. Description of Individual Neurosensory Center Comprehensive Examination for Aphasia Subtests

1. Visual object naming (VN): requires subjects to verbally label objects presented on a tray.

2. Description of object use (DOU): requires subjects to provide a description of use pertaining to a range of presented objects following the probe, "What do you use this for?"

3. Tactile naming right hand (TNR): a range of objects are individually placed into the subject's right hand under a covering screen, and the subject is instructed to name the objects accordingly.

Table 10–2. *continued*

4. Tactile naming left hand (TNL): as per TNR, however, objects are placed in left hand.

5. Sentence repetition (SR): requires subjects to repeat spoken sentences of increasing length but of minimal grammatical complexity.

6. Repetition of digits (REPD): requires subjects to repeat a series of spoken digit strings ranging from 3 to 7 numbers.

7. Reversal of digits (REVD): subjects are instructed to reverse a series of spoken digit strings ranging from 3 to 7 numbers.

8. Phonemic fluency (WF): requires subjects to generate as many words as possible beginning with the letters F, A and S, each within 60-second time intervals.

9. Sentence construction (SC): subjects are instructed to produce grammatically correct sentences incorporating 2 or 3 stimulus words provided by the examiner.

10. Object identification by name (IDNAME): subjects are instructed to point to a range of objects on command.

11. Token (TT): subjects are required to point to or move a number of colored tokens relative to a series of spoken instructions of increasing length and grammatical complexity.

12. Oral reading of names (ORNAME): subjects are instructed to read object names from a series of flash cards.

13. Oral reading of sentences (ORSENT): subjects are instructed to read sentences of increasing difficulty extracted from the token test, from a series of flash cards.

14. Reading names for meaning (RNM): typically administered after subtest 12 (ORNAME), subjects are required to point to range of objects corresponding to written names on a series of flash cards.

15. Reading sentences for meaning (RSM): typically administered after subtest 13 (ORSENT), subjects are required to follow simple commands written on a series of flash cards.

16. Visual graphic naming (VGN): subjects are instructed to write the names of a range of presented objects.

17. Written naming (WN): relates to performance on the VGN task. Items are scored according to accuracy of writing and spelling.

18. Writing to dictation (WD): subjects are required to write their name and 2 dictated sentences.

19. Writing to copy (WC): subjects are instructed to copy 2 sentences presented on flash cards.

20 Articulation (ART): subjects are required to repeat a series of real words and non-words containing a variety of consonant-vowel blends.

Source: Spreen & Benton (1977).

permitted up to 20 seconds to respond to each item. A semantic cue is given if the subject provides a response that represents a misinterpretation of the target or a lack of recognition. A phonemic cue is provided subsequent to any failure to respond or incorrect response to a semantic cue, or in the event of recognition of the item but an inability to produce its name.

The Test of Language Competence–Expanded Edition (TLC–E). The TLC-E is an assessment of language proficiency and metalinguistic ability, consisting of a range of subtests that probe the semantic system, semantic–syntactic interfaces and pragmatics. Designed and standardized on two levels (i.e., Level 1: children 5 to 9 years and Level 2: preadolescents and adolescents age 9 to 18+ years), the TLC–E assesses language competence by way of complex tasks that demand divergent language production, cognitive–linguistic flexibility and planning for production. Subtests included in the TLC–E Level 2 include: Ambiguous Sentences (AS), Listening Comprehension: Making inferences (MI), Oral Expression: Recreating Sentences (RS), Figurative Language (FL), and Remembering Word Pairs (RWP) subtests.

The AS subtest assesses the ability to identify and interpret the alternative meanings of lexical and structural ambiguities. Lexically, ambiguous sentences contain lexical elements with more than one possible meaning (e.g., *He bought the glasses*, where glasses may refer to *eyeglasses* or *drinking glasses*). Structural ambiguities may be classified as either surface or deep subtypes. Surface structure level ambiguities contain adjacent words that may be grouped in two or more distinct ways (e.g., *Mary likes small dogs and cats*, where *small dogs and cats*

may refer to *all small dogs* and *small cats* or rather *small dogs* and *cats in general* [regardless of size]). Deep structure level ambiguities contain more than one logical relationship between words and phrases (e.g., *The turkey is ready to eat*, where the *turkey* may *be ready to eat something* or *ready to be eaten*). Subjects are presented with a series of ambiguous sentences in both spoken and written form and instructed to provide two distinct interpretations for each item. Responses are scored quantitatively according to essential meaning criteria.

The MI subtest assesses a client's ability to utilize causal relationships or chains in short paragraphs to make logical inferences. Clients are provided with a series of paired propositions including a lead-in (e.g., *Jack went to a Mexican restaurant*) and concluding sentence (e.g., *He left without giving a tip*). On the basis of this information they are then instructed to make logical inferences pertaining to the event chain, by selecting two plausible intervening clauses from four possible choices (e.g., (a) *The restaurant closed when he arrived*, (b) *He only had enough money to pay for the meal*, (c) *The food and service were excellent*, or (d) *He was dissatisfied with the service*). All test stimuli are provided in spoken as well as written form. The correct responses for the above example would be (b) and (d).

The RS subtest evaluates the ability to formulate grammatically complete sentences utilizing key semantic elements within defined contexts. Clients are provided with a situational context (e.g., *At the ice-cream store*) and three words (e.g., *some, and, get*) in spoken and written/pictorial form, and instructed to generate a complete sentence that reflects the relevant situational context, utilizing all three words. Responses are scored according to holistic scoring rules pertaining to semantic, syntactic, and pragmatic accuracy, as well as the number of target words successfully used.

The FL subtest evaluates the ability to interpret metaphorical expressions and to correlate structurally related metaphors according to shared meanings. Clients are provided with a series of metaphorical expressions (e.g., *She sure casts a spell over me*) accompanied by defined situational contexts (e.g., *A boy talking about a girl at a school dance*), and instructed to provide a novel verbal interpretation of the metaphor. Once clients have explained the metaphor in their own words, they are then instructed to identify a match for the sample metaphor from four possible choices. Response choices include: a metaphoric match (e.g., *She is totally bewitching to me*), an oppositional foil (e.g., *I am out from under her spell*), a literal foil (e.g., *She spells much better than I*), and a nonrelated foil (e.g., *In her life, every day is Halloween*). All test stimuli are presented in spoken as well as written form. Metaphorical explanations are recorded verbatim and scored according to specified interpretation rules. The final score represents a composite of the verbal interpretation score and the matched selection score.

The RWP supplemental subtest assesses the ability to recall paired word associates. Associations are classified as one of four possible categories, including: paradigmatic (e.g., *coat–sock*), spatial (e.g., *plane–cloud*), temporal (e.g., *moon–bed*), and unrelated (e.g., *antler–egg*). Clients are provided with two presentations (i.e., elicitation lists A and B) of 16 spoken word pairs, considered to be representative of common and familiar vocabulary. Subsequent to the oral presentation of each elicitation list, the ex-

aminer provides one of the words from each pair. Clients are then instructed to recall its associate. The sum of correctly recalled pairs relative to elicitations list A and B represents the total score.

The Word Test–Revised (TWT–R). The Word Test–Revised (TWT–R) represents an assessment of expressive vocabulary and semantics, originally designed for use with school age children. The TWT–R specifically probes the ability to identify and express critical semantic features of the lexicon by way of tasks that involve categorization, definition, verbal reasoning, and lexical selection. Subtests of the TWT–R include: Associations (ASS), Synonyms (SYN), Semantic Absurdities (SEMAB), Antonyms (ANT), Definitions (DEF), and Multiple Definitions (MULDEF).

The ASS subtest requires clients to identify a semantically unrelated word within a group of four spoken words and to provide an explanation for the selected word in relation to the category of semantically related words. For example, from the group of words *knee, shoulder, bracelet*, and *ankle* the word *bracelet* is considered semantically unrelated *because it is not a body part*. Responses are scored according to word choices as well as criteria pertaining to acceptable and unacceptable explanations.

The SYN subtest requires clients to generate synonyms for verbally presented stimuli. Answers are again scored in reference to acceptable and unacceptable response criteria. For example, in response to the stimulus *donate*, acceptable responses include words with similar sets of semantic features such as *give/contribute*, whereas unacceptable responses include *offer/fund*.

The SEMAB subtest evaluates a client's ability to identify and repair semantic incongruities. Clients are presented orally with a series of semantically absurd sentences (e.g., *My grandfather is the youngest person in my family*) and instructed to repair the evident incongruity by generating a semantically appropriate sentence. Scoring is again based on acceptable response criteria. Acceptable responses demand the simultaneous identification of the resident semantic incongruity, the replacement of inappropriate with appropriate vocabulary, and the maintenance of the integrity of essential elements within the generated sentence (e.g., *My grandfather is the oldest person in my family*). Incorrect repairs (e.g., *My grandfather is the biggest person in my family*), explanation of the semantic absurdity despite prompting (e.g., *My grandfather can't possibly be the youngest person in my family*), or semantic negation (e.g., *My grandfather is not the youngest person in my family*), are all classified as unacceptable responses.

The ANT subtest requires clients to generate antonyms for verbally presented stimuli. Answers are scored in reference to acceptable and unacceptable response criteria. In response to stimulus *first*, *last* would be classified as an acceptable response as it encapsulates reversible critical semantic dimensions of the stimulus word, whereas *second* would be classified as an unacceptable response.

The DEF subtest evaluates a client's ability to identify and describe the critical semantic features of a word. Subjects are provided with a series of stimulus words and instructed to explain their meaning. Answers are again scored according to acceptable and unacceptable response criteria, in relation to specific critical semantic elements. For example, in providing a definition of the word *house*, the attributes *person* + *lives* are

defined as critical semantic elements. *Where my family lives* therefore, would be classified as a complete/acceptable definition, however, *Where you play* would be classified as an incomplete/unacceptable response.

The MULDEF subtest requires clients to provide two distinct meanings for a series of spoken homophonic words in relation to specific referents, probing flexibility in vocabulary use. Scoring is again based upon acceptable and unacceptable response criteria. For example, germane definition references pertaining to the word *rock* include *stone*, *music*, or an *action*. Acceptable task responses would include, *It's a hard piece of earth*, *Music you play* or *Moving back and forth*. *A hard thing* or *A thing you throw*, however, would be classified as unacceptable responses, as they fail to incorporate specified semantic referents.

Wiig–Semel Test of Linguistic Concepts (WSTLC). The WSTLC assesses the auditory comprehension of complex linguistic structures. Consisting of 50 yes/no questions, correct responses are contingent upon the undertaking of logical semantic operations in the manipulation of a range of complex linguistic relationships, including passive, comparative, temporal, spatial, and familial structures.

Tests of Functional and Pragmatic Language Abilities. A primary limitation of tests of basic language function is that they primarily focus on the evaluation of language abilities from an impairment perspective (i.e., identify the presence of language deficits but fail to ascertain the impact of these deficits on the functional communication skills). Alternatives or adjuncts to the assessments outlined above include measures of communication activity limitation and participation restriction. Assessments of communication activity limitation encompass measures of functional and pragmatic communication abilities, which enable the evaluation of a client's ability to plan, deliver, and understand communication content within a range of interactive contexts. Pragmatic assessments typically appraise the ability to use language within natural contexts, including knowledge of language structure, knowledge of the environment and social rules, as well as the ability to adapt to changing environmental demands (Penn, 1999). In contrast, functional communication assessments largely aim to evaluate the quality of communication attempts (Manochiopining, Sheard, & Reed, 1992), or the impact of communication disorders on social and vocational roles, otherwise referred to as participation restrictions. Although a more in-depth discussion of these assessment tools is beyond the scope of this chapter, the incorporation of such measures is considered critical to any thorough clinical evaluation of language dysfunction, as opposed to an exclusive impairment-driven approach. The reader is referred to Table 10–1 for some suggested functional and pragmatic assessments that may be used with children.

Selection and Modification of Standardized Language Tests. The battery of standardized tests selected by clinicians varies from child to child and the choice of which tests to use is based on careful observation of the child's communicative behavior. For example, if a child appears to be operating at a younger level than his chronologic age then a test for younger children, even though he is outside the age range, may be chosen.

When a child is unable to cope with the entire age-appropriate standardized test then the clinician may have to omit or modify a number of subtests. For example, if the child appears to have significant word-retrieval problems then the subtest involving confrontation naming might not be administered in full or could be adapted to allow the child some success. Modification of standardized tests can include the simplification of instructions for administration, allowing different methods of responding (e.g., written instead of verbal) and the use of a variety of cues to help elicit a response (e.g., semantic or phonemic prompts).

Many standardized test results, unless they are language samples, only yield information about the child's abilities in comparison with his peers. Although this information is important and necessary, it is not descriptive enough to assist the clinician with the development of therapy aims. Information gleaned when tests have been modified is mostly descriptive and can contribute greatly to a clinician's understanding of a child's abilities and help in the formulation of treatment goals. For example, what cues best assisted the child to retrieve words or what level of language or linguistic complexity enhanced the child's comprehension or caused a breakdown in understanding? It is important, though, that all modifications of standardized tests be noted and reported. As the child recovers, test modifications are often no longer necessary and this in itself is a measure of progress.

Informal Tests (Nonstandardized Tests)

Informal testing may serve a number of functions when working with a child with acquired aphasia. Such testing may be used to: quickly assess children who fatigue easily, measure the rapid recovery of language skills, assess children who fail on standardized procedures because of concomitant problems, followup on deficits noted by the child's family or by other professionals, and allows the clinician flexibility of assessment when limited resources of standardized tests are available.

Informal testing, as already stated, is often used in the early stages of recovery. Individual improvement can be so rapid that a test administered on a Friday can be invalid on the Monday (e.g., a child may begin to say single words one day and over a weekend may progress to using sentences). An informal test, devised by the clinician himself or herself can have a similar framework to and be based on a standardized test. An example of an informal test for acquired childhood aphasia is presented in Appendix 10–A. These informal tests are usually shorter with only a few items used to sample a wide range of semantic and syntactic abilities. They primarily are designed to give the clinician an indication of a child's linguistic and functional abilities soon after onset of the aphasia. Most often it is suitable for use at the child's bedside. For example, such a test may be a selection of doll's house furniture with matching photos that can be used receptively and expressively for activities such as naming, functions and associations. Another informal assessment might be a set of "yes/no" questions specific to the child's environment or a checklist of pragmatic behaviors.

Structured but nonstandardized procedures that are often based on the results obtained from standardized tests or suggested from colleagues' comments can be devised for extension testing. For example, the teacher may report that the aphasic child is having problems when the teacher is explaining or discussing school work, thereby indicating the need to assess further the child's ability to recall and retain varying amounts of information presented verbally. In addition, tasks experimenting with different linguistic variables, such as the complexity of semantic content in an utterance or the length of instructions given, can be used to further probe the child's comprehension skills. Although these forementioned tasks are nonstandardized they can yield highly specific linguistic information (e.g., the individual's ability to comprehend 'where' questions of varying syntactic difficulty).

Observation

Observation of the child in a number of different settings will yield necessary information on how that child functions in various social situations, such as with his peers in the school playground, in class discussions or with his parents and siblings. Careful note should be taken of how the child receives and gives a message. Did the listener understand? If not, why not? Where did the breakdown occur? Was it the child's inability to encode the message syntactically or his unintelligible speech which appeared to be the main difficulty? If the message was understood, why was it understood? Did the accompanying nonverbal behaviors enable the listener to decode the message?

It is best to have some framework (i.e., a mental or written checklist) from which to base an observation so that the behaviors seen are not random observations and are easily interpreted when all information is gathered and analyzed. (An example of an observational checklist is presented in Appendix 10–B.) A knowledge of Bloom and Lahey's Content Categories (Bloom & Lahey, 1978), Brown's

14 grammatical morphemes (Wiig & Semel, 1984), or some behaviors from the Pragmatic Protocol developed by Prutting and Kirchner (1987) may form part of such an observation checklist. If possible, audiotape and videotape recordings of these observation and assessment sessions should be made. These can be analyzed later and specific information, which could have been missed during the session, extracted.

During assessment or treatment sessions the clinician may observe children using strategies to help them decode or remember information, for example, mouthing the words after the clinician before giving a response, counting on their fingers or writing letter cues on their legs to help them remember and repeating the instructions. Many children may discover their own strategies and it is important for the clinician to identify them and bring them to the child's awareness. These strategies may be used consistently in later treatment sessions and may become part of the repertoire which the child adopts to assist him in his day-to-day living. Information about those strategies which proved useful in their treatment sessions (e.g., the complexity of language to use with the child when giving instructions) should be made available to other team members.

Areas of Language Assessment for Comprehension and Expression

Language is the knowledge of how content/form/use integrate and this knowledge underlies the behaviors of speaking and understanding (Bloom & Lahey, 1978). Therefore, to assess the language of a child with acquired aphasia, as with any child with a language impairment, it is difficult, if not impossible, to treat semantics, syntax, morphology and pragmatics as discrete areas of language without being aware of the influence each has on the other. There is no doubt that children with acquired aphasia may have greater difficulty in one language area than in another, for example, the child with word-retrieval problems has more difficulty in the semantic area, the child with telegrammatic-type communication may have the greatest difficulty with morphology and syntax, whereas the child with frontal lobe damage appears to have significant problems with pragmatic language skills. However, the goal of language assessment of a child with a brain lesion is to discover how well that child integrates content/form/use for understanding and speaking. The assessment procedures outlined below are not intended to be definitive but rather to offer suggestions and avenues for the clinician to pursue and explore.

Spontaneous Language Sample

A spontaneous language sample gives the clinician the best indication of how well the child with acquired aphasia is integrating content/form/use for communication. It provides a detailed description of the child's language abilities, both receptive and expressive, particularly when samples are taken in a number of natural settings (e.g., in the classroom, with a peer in play, with parents or siblings and with the clinician). Each sample can be analyzed semantically, syntactically or pragmatically, the choice of analysis depending on what specific information the clinician may wish to gather. For example, Bloom and Lahey Content/ Form analysis (Bloom & Lahey, 1978), Prism–L/Prism–G (Crystal, 1982) for semantics, the Language and Remediation Screening Procedure (LARSP) (Crystal, 1982) for syntax and morphology, and the Clinical Discourse Analysis (Damico, 1985), Graphic Conversational Profile (Wilks & Monaghan, 1988) in the pragmatic area. From analyses of the samples hypotheses may be formed about the child's language skills and these hypotheses then tested using elicited language samples or informal assessment procedures (e.g., asking "why" questions to test the child's skill at coding and encoding cause-effect relationships). Also, particular formal tests that the clinician thinks best suit the type and level of the child's abilities may be chosen to further explore and test these hypotheses.

In the early stages of a child's recovery, however, it may not be an appropriate assessment tool. The child may have little language to sample or his or her expressive language may be changing so rapidly that by the time a representative sample may be gathered and analyzed it may not truly reflect the child's language abilities. Concomitant problems such as a dysarthria or dyspraxia may also prevent the accurate transcription of the child's expressive language and so limit its use for diagnostic and treatment purposes. It is in such situations that an audiotape or preferably a videotape of the child's communicative abilities should be made. This can serve as a record of the child's recovery or may be analyzed later if the comparison of specific behaviors (e.g., eye contact, turn-taking skills, word retrieval difficulties) in different recovery phases becomes important. As noted in the literature, it is necessary for clinicians to remember, when collecting a language sample, that many children with acquired aphasia are reluctant to communicate and so a representative

language sample may not be obtained. However, as trust and rapport grow between the clinician and the child this reluctance may be overcome. Also, much depends on the setting of the language sample. For example, in a play setting with a small group of peers where the emphasis is not on language the child may feel free to communicate.

In the middle and late stages of recovery from acquired aphasia, the spontaneous language sample is a necessary assessment tool, complementing standardized testing procedures. A subtest involving confrontation naming may show that a child is having word-retrieval problems, the language sample then may reveal the types of naming errors that the child uses, which in turn is important for the formulation of treatment goals. Information on children's use and comprehension of complex syntactic structures or their ability to maintain a topic of conversation also may be obtained from the spontaneous language sample. Time constraints in a busy clinic may limit the size and representative quality of the sample but being pressed for time should not be used as an excuse for not taking one. The information obtained from a spontaneous language sample is too valuable for it to be omitted from an assessment battery. Short supplementary observations (hand subscribing of utterances and context) in particular situations, seeking information on one or two language behaviors (e.g., Are the child's responses to "wh" questions, single words, simple or complex sentences? Does the child use negative structures and if so, what are they?) may enhance or clarify the information already obtained from the spontaneous language sample. The teacher or parent, if given specific instructions, may be the transcriber in such situations.

Comprehension

Most of the standardized tests mentioned previously (e.g., CELF–4, TOLD–I3, TOLD–P3) have subtests which are specifically designed to sample and measure different aspects of auditory comprehension. The literature documenting adult aphasic problems as well as the literature relating to the learning disabled child has relevance to the child with acquired aphasia. The literature on both adult aphasia and learning disabilities detail examples of auditory comprehension nonstandardized tasks (Chapey, 1981, 1986; Simon, 1985; Wiig & Semel, 1984). In some circumstances the tasks used with adult clients may be modified for the child with acquired aphasia (e.g., "yes/no" questions about school may replace questions about occupations). Often, it needs only the topic to be changed for the activity to be suitable for the child (e.g., activities that involve newspaper articles may be changed to information for school projects).

Conversation. The assessment of auditory comprehension in a child with acquired aphasia should include a judgment of the child's ability to understand unstructured spontaneous language such as "yes/no" questions about the individual's family, school and interests or general conversation among peers and caregivers about what is happening, has happened or will happen in daily living situations. The age and interests of the child should not be forgotten (e.g., a young child may have had difficulty before his brain lesion with certain time concepts).

Word Meanings. Assessing the child's knowledge of the meaning of words and their relationship to one another is important. Testing this knowledge may include evaluations of a child's:

receptive vocabulary

semantic categories of words ("lights" may include "light bulb," "torch," and "candle")

antonyms ("big"—"little")

synonyms ("rabbit"—"bunny"—"hare")

homonyms ("blew"—"blue")

reciprocity ("give"—"take")

multimeaning words ("walk" as a verb or as a noun, in expressions such as "take a walk" meaning "go away" or "walk away" meaning "ignore")

spatial terms ("under"—"next"—"against")

temporal terms ("first"—"after"—"before")

comparative ("bigger"—"biggest")

familial ("sister"—"grandmother")

cause-effect relations ("why/because")

relational terms ("if/then"—"all/except")

Nonstandardized testing needs to take into account the child's age and what he or she is expected to know and use in school.

With the older child, the clinician can assess the child's understanding of figurative language such as idioms ("sharp tongued"), similes and metaphors ("the hours creep by"), adages ("still waters run deep"), colloquialisms ("pulling your leg"), and verbal analogies ("a key is to a door as a dial is to a telephone"). Normal everyday communication abounds with figurative language but for the child returning to high school and who will be studying literature (poetry is full of similes and metaphors) it is of particular importance that these areas are assessed.

Recall of Verbal Information. When assessing the amount of verbal information that a child can process it is often beneficial to use material from the child's own schoolwork (e.g., science or social studies information which the teacher is likely to use when teaching the subject matter to the class). This may serve a twofold purpose. First, the clinician is able to make an objective judgment of how much semantic content the child can manage and comprehend before his or her understanding breaks down, and second, as a meaningful example to the teacher of his or her comprehension problems. Part of this assessment may include the child's ability to recall detail and make inferences from the information presented. The clinician needs to be aware that with some children memory difficulties may affect their performance as the information load increases.

Morphology and Syntax. Assessment should involve the evaluation of a child's understanding of morphology and syntax. Can the child demonstrate comprehension of plurals, tenses, cases, comparatives, superlatives, adjectival and adverbial forms, or auxiliary verbs? What sentence structure helps or hinders the child's understanding of language (e.g., questions, negation or passive transformations)? Literature, detailing the normal development of morphology and syntax (e.g., Crystal, 1982) may help in formulating systematic nonstandardized tasks to test certain linguistic forms. Much of this information on form may

be obtained from a representative spontaneous language sample (e.g., if a child uses plurals consistently, then generally they must understand them).

Pragmatics. A child's auditory comprehension difficulties may influence his or her pragmatic abilities, particularly those skills dependent on linguistic competence (e.g., semantics and syntax must be intact for cohesion, sequencing skills for clarification). Comprehension of a communicative act involves not only the understanding of language but also the ability to perceive situational cues (e.g., facial expressions or the fact that two people are speaking privately and would not appreciate being interrupted). It seems that some children with a brain lesion, particularly frontal lobe damage, have difficulty perceiving or understanding body language and situational cues. They often are the children that people label as "strange" although these people cannot always describe the specific behavior that warranted the label. These "strange" children may be able to respond appropriately given a picture to explain (e.g., What will this girl say when she sees her friend?) but fail to act appropriately when they are in the actual situation. Assessment of pragmatic skills involving the understanding of nonverbal language may be done by using a picture format as in some items of "Let's Talk Inventory for Adolescents" (Wiig, 1982), from a videotaped recording of the child's social interactions or from observations.

Extension testing like many of the subtests in standardized tests can take the form of a choice between a number of pictures. However, judgment tasks may prove the easiest to design and can be used to test semantic, syntactic, and pragmatic knowledge. For example, the child is shown the picture of a girl running and asked if what the clinician says ("He is running.") is correct or incorrect. As another example the child may be given two sentences, "I ate an apple and a pear" and "I ate the fruit" and then asked if the two sentences are the same or different? Alternatively, pictures of a child talking to a teacher and to her friend may be shown and the child asked, "In which one would she say, "Hi, Jan"?" Individual assessment procedures can be designed. However, it may save time if records of any assessment procedures are kept because parts of them may be relevant for another child. If judgment tasks are stored on computer then it is a simple matter to create new tasks by cutting and pasting from other established files.

Humor. The appreciation of humor and its use by children with acquired aphasia is frequently neglected by researchers and clinicians. Yet parents frequently comment that their brain-injured child does not joke any more, that the good-natured teasing in the family is taken too seriously by the child with acquired aphasia and may lead to outbursts of anger or frustration on the child's part and fights amongst the siblings. For example, one 11-year-old girl's father had a teasing, joking-type of affectionate relationship with his daughter. This relationship suffered after the child's brain lesion and although her difficulty with language was explained the relationship continued to suffer. Two years after the insult the first comment that the father made to the clinician when the child was brought in for a review was, "She's got her dry wit back again."

Many verbal jokes are resolved on the basis of lexical, semantic or phonological ambiguity (e.g., "shaggy dog" stories with the punch line being interpreted two ways: "The Pirates of Penzance" to "the pie rates of Penzance"). The riddle also seems to involve an appreciation of jokes as well as a type of problem solving. A question is asked and the answer is incongruous and the listener has the task of solving how the answer does make sense in terms of the original question.

Obviously, humor in the infant and young child is different from that of the older child and adult. Shultz (1976), however, reported findings that suggested that laughter at word plays begins as early as 3 years of age. Humor not only involves appreciation of verbal language but also an awareness of non-verbal and situational cues, in fact, an appreciation of pragmatic, semantic, and syntactic areas of communication. Therefore, it would seem valuable to observe how a child with acquired aphasia appreciates and uses humor. Knowledge gained from these observations may help design probes and formulate goals in all areas of communication.

Reading. Children with acquired aphasia, particularly those who have an auditory comprehension problem, often exhibit difficulties with reading, either in recognizing letters and words or in comprehending the written material. The assessment of reading must take into account the level of the child's ability before his or her brain lesion, and the expertise of the occupational therapist, the teacher and the guidance officer/psychologist in the assessment is desirable. Their collective knowledge of perceptual problems, the process of normal reading development and of reading problems in the normal population helps with the differential diagnosis of the reading difficulty.

Assessment of reading may include matching of letters, matching of letters to sounds, matching words and sentences to pictures, and graded reading tests. Reading problems appear to reflect deficits apparent in the child's semantic, syntactic and pragmatic systems. Difficulties understanding the meanings of multi-meaning words, complex syntactic structures, figurative language, and inferences are problems common to many children with acquired aphasia.

Assessment of the reading abilities of children with acquired aphasia should involve some measure of the amount of written material that the child is able to assimilate and the nature of the details that the child may recall (e.g., names and ages of persons mentioned, directions given or the sequence of events leading to the climax). The recovery of reading ability in a child with acquired aphasia appears to follow similar stages to that of his or her oral language recovery, although this seems to depend on the child's age at the time of his or her brain lesion and its severity. If the child was under school age at the time of the insult then it is possible that the child will have difficulty acquiring the skills of reading. The comprehension of written material often poses the greatest problem for the child with acquired aphasia who has recovered many of his or her other reading skills (i.e., his ability to read words and sentences).

Little has been documented about the problems a child with acquired aphasia has with mathematics but undoubtedly a difficulty often exists. This problem may be language related (e.g., the child is confused with the meaning of mathematical words, "divide," "multiply," or is unable to read the instructions which introduce the mathematical problem). The speech and language clinician can assist other professionals by assessing the child's ability to understand the mathematical terms and the underlying concepts related to mathematics (e.g., few, some, many, half, etc.) which he or she is expected to know in the classroom.

Expression

Most standardized tests (see Table 10–1) which can be used with the child with acquired aphasia have a number of subtests which evaluate the child's expressive language abilities.

Syntax. The literature reports that children with acquired aphasia often used simplified syntax and telegraphic language, as well as being reluctant to communicate. This reluctance to speak may influence the complexity of their language which in turn may affect any spontaneous language sample taken. For example, a 6-year-old girl with acquired aphasia examined by the author enjoyed a game after the therapy activities and would ask the clinician, "Game?" using a rising intonation and appropriate facial expression. In the initial period following her brain lesion, resulting from a cerebrovascular accident, she used telegraphic language but was, at that time, able to produce complex sentences. When the clinician prompted her, "Kate, can you ask me in a longer sentence?" she would reply, "Can we play a game now, please?" with no apparent difficulty in generating the sentence structure.

Assessment, then, of morphology and syntax in children with acquired aphasia needs to include information from a spontaneous language sample, standardized tests and elicited tasks. Areas probed may involve activities such as the following:

plurals (regular and irregular)

case (use of the possessive "s," nominative pronouns)

tenses (regular and irregular, past, present, future)

comparative and superlative forms

production in a sentence of all parts of speech (nouns, verbs, adjectives, adverbs, prepositions, pronouns, conjunctions)

noun and adverb derivations ("er," "ly")

prefixes and suffixes

use of articles

use of different sentence structures (passive, negative, interrogative, "wh" questions)

ambiguous sentences

Mean length of utterance (MLU)

the types of complex sentences (co-ordination, relative clauses "subordination" embedded)

the percentage of complex sentences attempted and the percentage correct

the proportion of simple to complex sentences

(The last two areas often can be used as an index of improvement in children who are more fluent in the acute stage.)

Assessment tasks may include the use of visual stimuli (pictures of a cat and cats), sentence completion (e.g., She is teaching, She is a . . .), production of sentences (e.g., Make up a sentence with the word "farm," "beneath," "sadly") and the manipulation of given words to make sentences (e.g., "is," "hat," "the," "red." Can the child make a statement

and a question with the words?). The imitation of sentences of increasing complexity by the child (e.g., The boy hit the dog. The boy who was wearing a red cap hit the little dog.) may be useful to the clinician to evaluate the structures the child is able to imitate and possibly to produce spontaneously. Semantic understanding and short-term memory may influence the child's results. Short-term memory problems seen in the child with acquired aphasia are similar to those observed in the learning disabled child (Wiig & Semel, 1984). The literature discussing the learning disabled child reports in more detail the effects of short-term memory problems on imitation tasks and syntactic structures (Wiig & Semel, 1984; Wallach & Butler, 1984).

Semantics. As with acquired aphasia in adults, a deficit in the ability to produce language content is also a characteristic of acquired aphasia in childhood. This lack of content is similar to that heard in the expressive language of many learning-disabled children although the child with acquired aphasia may have a more pronounced problem, especially in the early stages of recovery. Spontaneous or elicited language samples give some indication of the deficits experienced by the child with semantic language problems. Semantic analyses (e.g., Bloom & Lahey, 1978; Prism–L/Prism-G analysis, Crystal, 1982) may be used to detail the presence of content categories or the usage of specific parts of speech.

Word-retrieval difficulties, dysfluency, and semantic and literal paraphasias are common symptoms heard in the expressive language of a child with acquired aphasia. Word-retrieval problems and dysfluency characteristics need to be recorded when transcribing the sample. Qualitative analysis of a child's naming errors (Wiig & Semel, 1984) will give some indication of what types of semantic or literal paraphasias are used mostly by the child or whether many of his or her word retrieval problems are camouflaged by circumlocution. For example, when shown a picture of a boy writing and asked "What is the boy doing?," one child replied, "He's using a pencil. It's something to do with school." When a phonetic cue was given the same child replied correctly, "Writing." The analysis of dysfluency characteristics may help the clinician decide whether the child has a comprehension difficulty and needs time to process the information, or whether there is a word-retrieval problem. The Double Administration Naming Technique (Fried-Oken, 1987) assists the clinician in determining whether the child has word-retrieval problems or expressive vocabulary limitations and further describes what cues (e.g., the object's function, its category, a description of the object or the sound at the beginning of the word) are best used for helping the child recall specific words.

Semantic and literal paraphasias should be noted and the percentage of occurrence in the sample calculated. The compilation of these percentages at intervals during recovery phases may be used as an objective measure of progress for, as recovery occurs, the percentage of paraphasias decreases.

Further assessment tasks should involve confrontation naming (e.g., body parts, colors, shapes, animals, common objects, and actions), and automatic-sequential naming (e.g., the days of the week, the months of the year, counting). Expressive tasks similar to those proposed for assessing receptive skills may form part of the assessment, particularly with the older child when metalinguistic

skills become important for classroom success. The child is asked to respond when given a verbal stimulus consisting of either a single word or short sentence. For example, these expressive tasks may include:

antonyms ("up"—"down")

synonyms ("happy"—"glad"—"elated")

homonyms ("meet—"meat")

rhyming words ("cat"—"hat"—"fat")

definitions of words (What does "jump" mean?)

categorization tasks (Tell me as many things as you can think of that we eat?)

figurative language (What does it mean if someone has a "green thumb"?)

similarities and differences (How are wind-surfing and sailing alike and how are they different?)

convergent semantic tasks (Finish the sentence, "I dig with a . . . ")

divergent semantic tasks (If you can't use sugar in your tea to make it sweet, what (ingredients) could you use instead?)

sentence formulation using different parts of speech (Make me a sentence with the word "emu" or "beside" or "except")

definition of mathematical terms ("divide," "subtract," "plus")

The choice of tests and tasks depends on the child's stage of recovery and their age and is greatly influenced by the clinician's knowledge of a child's normal language development. For example, metalinguistic tasks would neither be appropriate for the preschool child nor the older child with severe expressive language difficulties.

Pragmatics. Behavioral changes in children who have sustained a brain lesion have been noted and reported in the literature. Parents frequently comment that their child's personality has changed (e.g., "She is not a leader anymore."). However, as the child recovers, parents frequently report that the child is more like his or her previous personality.

It is commonly acknowledged that frontal lobe damage may contribute to disinhibited behavior in adults. Similar behavior has been observed in adolescents with known frontal lobe damage. Also, it seems that most children who sustain brain damage show some behavioral change. It is doubtful whether behavioral changes can be attributed solely to the brain lesion. Other influences such as the impact of the brain lesion on the child and his or her family must be considered. It would appear, in some cases, that the injury may exacerbate already existing problems. However, more research is needed in this area before conclusive statements can be made.

Regression of behavior is known to be a coping mechanism that some children adopt when they have suffered any type of trauma. Also, while in hospital and particularly if their stay is lengthy, children's inappropriate behaviors are often reinforced by anxious parents and concerned hospital staff. This would seem a natural reaction on the part of the caregivers in these circumstances. The child most probably was dangerously ill and perhaps not expected

to live. As the child recovers, the full extent of his or her injuries becomes apparent and parents and staff often "spoil" the individual and accept behaviors that in normal circumstances would have been unacceptable to them.

When assessing the pragmatic behaviors of a child with acquired aphasia the clinician must be aware of the hospital and family situation before deciding whether some pragmatic behaviors are inappropriate and need specific treatment. As the child recovers and the family situation stabilizes the child's behavior may also change without any direct treatment simply because normal expectations are placed on the child again.

There are acquired aphasic children, however, who continue to exhibit inappropriate behaviors and these behaviors persist even as their semantic and syntactic skills improve. Concomitant problems, particularly dysarthric symptoms such as disturbances in the rate of speech, prosody, volume, and facial expression frequently influence pragmatic behaviors.

The children with persistent pragmatic problems appear to have significant difficulties in the social domain of pragmatics. They have difficulty in perceiving the social situation and in reading nonverbal cues. Consequently, they fail to read that a person may be teasing, or is angry or in a hurry. They may address adults, persons in authority, strangers and friends in the same casual manner, they often invade personal space, make embarrassing personal comments, fail to turn-take, or interrupt appropriately. For example, an 11-year-old girl with acquired aphasia used to tell strangers after only a few minutes conversation that she loved them and often would try to kiss or hold their hand. It transpired that in the hospital she had been making statements such as, "If you come here, I'll punch you in the face." Her mother had told her that she was not to say that even as a joke because she must love everyone because they were helping her. The girl then told everyone indiscriminately that she loved them. Reports from the school she attended before her injury did not indicate any previous problem with social skills.

Children with acquired aphasia usually have difficulties in the linguistic and cognitive domains of pragmatics. Their deficits in semantics and syntax decrease their ability to clarify or explain a statement, to use language imaginatively or to be specific. These disabilities impinge on their conversational skills and prevent them meeting the obligations of discourse. They often have difficulty with topic coherence, turn-taking, repair and revision, and role adjustment.

Assessment of pragmatic skills is best done from observation or from a videotape of the child with another speaker. A spontaneous language sample will assist the clinician with the evaluation of discourse skills. The literature on the normal development of pragmatic skills is relevant to the assessment of the child with acquired aphasia. Several descriptions of pragmatic behaviors are to be found in tests on the normal development of language and in the literature describing the learning-disabled child (Miller, 1981; Prutting & Kirchner, 1983, 1987; Ripich & Spinelli, 1985; Simon, 1985; Wiig & Semel, 1984). Procedures such as the Pragmatic Protocol by Prutting and Kirchner (1987), the Clinical Discourse Analysis (Damico, 1985), and the Graphic Conversational Profile (Wilks & Monaghan, 1988) may be used.

Narratives. Narratives are midway between oral and literate language and require planning and the dynamic integration of content, form and use. In recent years a significant amount of research has accumulated on the difficulties experienced by learning disabled students on producing narratives and the implications this has on their education. Children with acquired aphasia appear to be similar in many respects to learning-disabled individuals so that it is logical to assume that they too may encounter problems with narratives.

The literature on reading and writing skills of the child with acquired aphasia states that difficulties persist in these two areas of language. Specific help with narrative skills may then facilitate the recovery of reading and writing abilities. Therefore, in the latter stages of recovery when the child with acquired aphasia is using complex language, the narrative abilities of the individual should be assessed. Westby (1984) stated that the more traditional testing methods used with the learning-disabled child will not detect the language difficulties that become apparent on narrative analysis.

It also has been noted that children who have made a good recovery from acquired aphasia continue to have problems with academic learning although on traditional language tests, the same that are used with the learning-disabled students, their scores are within the normal range. Westby (1984) believed that this discrepancy arises because language tests are concerned with the components of language (i.e., vocabulary, morphology and syntax) rather than the integrative process. Narrative analysis, therefore, may be one way of tapping the higher abstract learning skills that are often difficult to assess in the child with acquired aphasia. Further research is needed to determine whether children with acquired aphasia and learning-disabled students do have similar difficulties with narrative tasks and whether specific intervention will improve their skills and facilitate reading and writing abilities.

Writing. In the early stage of recovery of a child with acquired aphasia concomitant problems such as visual perceptual deficits and hemiplegia or sensory deficits of the dominant hand may prevent the assessment of writing skills. The literature reports that writing deficits tend to persist and are in most cases certainly slower at recovering than oral language abilities. The recovery of writing skills appears to follow similar stages to those of reading skills. The older child who already has some written language ability will regain his or her skills along with oral abilities but the young child who has never learned to spell may have difficulty acquiring these new skills. Word-retrieval difficulties may affect the child's ability to write words and sentences. As with reading the assessment of writing skills requires a team approach.

The child may be asked to copy letters or words, write letters and words from dictation, and construct sentences and paragraphs. Phoneme to grapheme relationships may also be evaluated. Dysorthographic errors need to be noted and consideration even to how the child made them (e.g., Was the phoneme-grapheme relationship correct? Did the child sound out the word correctly?). As with adult aphasic clients the small abstract words such as "was," "saw," or "the" appear to pose persistent prob-

lems. For example, the author observed a 9-year-old girl who was making an excellent recovery in other language areas but her spelling of abstract words remained poor. When asked to spell "this" she might write "there" or "that" and then comment that she knew it looked something like the word she had written. She did not appear to use any strategy to help her spell the words correctly.

Play. Observation of the play of children who have had a brain lesion may help in the assessment of their language abilities. Imaginative or pretend play, particularly when interacting with peers, requires a child to organize events, sequence the events, take roles, and distance themselves from the "here and now." Researchers have suggested that pretend play and narratives are closely linked (Westby, 1984).

There is an interdependent relationship between language and play and gains in both areas are related to cognitive development. The three processes seem inextricably interwoven. Play appears to serve as preparation for children to live in society whereas language allows children to master their environment, which in turn contributes to their cognitive development (Irwin, 1975). Through play a child learns to use many pragmatic functions (regulatory, permission, imaginative). Assessment of the child with a brain lesion should involve some evaluation of the child's play skills. Observations (depending on the age of the child) may include: transcriptions of the complexity of language used (in play situations a child often uses more complex structures than when in "formal" situations), a judgment on whether the child understands the group rules of the game, whether he or she contributes ideas, protests over the role allotted him or her, uses verbal reasoning skills for compromising or collaborating, and whether the child seems to be part of the group or just an observer tolerated by the other children.

A child's ability to play is often compromised by concomitant problems and it is interesting to note what strategies the child may use to circumvent these difficulties, strategies that may be adapted for use in daily living situations. For example, one quadriplegic boy had a talking tracheostomy tube (consequently the volume of his voice was soft and he required frequent breaths) and a loud whistle on his chair. When he wanted to contribute anything to the group discussion he whistled and the group would quieten and listen to him. His pragmatic skills were good (e.g., He waited for a break in the conversation before he whistled.). This whistle has now become his way of interrupting appropriately and he uses it with discretion, a soft whistle to let you know he is there or a loud, long whistle if the message is urgent.

Summary of Assessment Procedures

The assessment of a child with acquired aphasia is an ongoing process and continues as part of treatment activities. Ideally, the assessment should be comprehensive and include a selection of standardized and nonstandardized tests and observations. The team approach to assessment of a child with a brain lesion is the only method that will provide all persons concerned with the child's welfare with an adequate understanding of the child's problems.

Formal tests used in assessing the child with acquired aphasia may include those shown in Table 10–1. The steps taken in assessing children with acquired aphasia are summarized in Figure 10–1.

Treatment of Acquired Childhood Aphasia

General Considerations

The clinician when formulating treatment goals for the child with acquired aphasia should be cognizant of the normal development of speech and language skills and the treatment procedures applicable to children with developmental language delays. As previously stated, many of the treatment techniques used with the learning-disabled child and those used with adult aphasic clients have relevance to the child with acquired aphasia.

Children with acquired aphasia although exhibiting similar difficulties to both learning-disabled children and adult aphasic clients do differ in a number of ways and the clinician must be aware of these differences. For example, although some children with a severe head injury may be unable to learn new material or strategies to compensate for their disability, others may learn rapidly. Such a range of learning ability is not seen in the learning-disabled population. Also, a child with acquired aphasia may have a wide scattering of abilities, some skills being severely depressed while others are near the norm for his or her age. This range of abilities within the one child is usually not so great in the child with a learning disability. Memory problems also may be far greater in the aphasic child than those exhibited by learning-disabled children. One major difference between adults with acquired aphasia and children with acquired aphasia that needs to be taken into account when developing treatment strategies is the fact that language skills are still developing in children. This development process with all the environmental ramifications which influence the normal acquisition of language should not be forgotten when planning remediation.

When treatment goals are selected they should take into account the child's age, his or her interests, and the concomitant problems that may affect his or her performance (e.g., short-term memory deficits, visual perceptual problems, or the presence of primitive reflex patterns such as the asymmetric tonic neck reflex). Goals formulated by other health professionals should be reinforced in the speech and language sessions whenever possible (e.g., transferring from a wheelchair to a chair for the session, correct postural positioning, and use of the affected arm when performing activities).

Treatment sessions with children with acquired aphasia, when they are in the period of spontaneous recovery, should be frequent and occur at the time of day when the child is alert. In most cases this occurs in the morning. The clinician must remain aware that children with a brain lesion fatigue easily and that this tiredness may continue for many months. The duration of time that fatigue continues to be an important consideration in therapy seems to be highly variable among children (e.g., Parents reported that their 13-year-old daughter was still going to bed at 7 p.m. or 7.30 p.m. 12 months after the injury and that

by the weekend she was "absolutely exhausted" and would sleep even longer).

The length of treatment sessions may need to be kept short initially (15 minutes, twice a day) and then gradually lengthened when the child is able to cope better with increased demands. While the child continues to show good progress the frequency of therapy should be maintained (not less than three times per week in most instances). Clinicians in busy general clinics may need to decide which clients have priority and timetable accordingly. The child with a brain lesion is usually considered a priority particularly if the child is still improving his or her communication skills.

Other professionals who are concerned with the child's rehabilitation may also wish to treat the child when he or she is fresh and alert. Unfortunately, this may not be possible and in such a situation a cooperative team approach is vital. Priorities, agreed on by all persons concerned with the care of the child, should be established and taken into account by each professional when deciding daily treatment goals. For example, a demanding language task may not be advisable after the child has just finished a difficult physiotherapy session. Instead, at this time the child might be better placed in a language group where other children would share the workload. Perhaps, if the physiotherapist wishes to have the child stand at various times during the day she or he can do so in the language session. A committed team approach is essential if the child is to gain maximum benefit from his or her rehabilitation program.

Activities and materials used in the session should be functional and interesting to the child although making all activities into games is not usually necessary for school-age children. Close liaison between the teacher and the clinician helps the clinician formulate language goals that are pertinent to the child and reinforces the communicative and academic skills required in the classroom. School reading texts, spelling lists, and other general English activities may be incorporated into many treatment sessions (e.g., An activity that requires the child to rearrange words to make a satisfactory sentence may include words which the child is reading in school or those that he or she is learning to spell).

A child's strengths and weaknesses should be considered when structuring tasks for treatment sessions. For example, if a child is helped by visual cues, either pictures or written words, when given a verbal task then these should be used and gradually faded as the child is better able to cope with the task. A hierarchy of steps may need to be devised so that only one variable is introduced at any one time. For example, short-term memory activities would use familiar materials initially. When the child is able to respond consistently at one level then the task is made more demanding by either adding another familiar item or keeping the same number of items but adding a word or object that has not been used previously. As the child progresses, steps may be missed (e.g., more items as well as unfamiliar ones may be added) but the clinician must always be ready to return to an easier step if the child is unable to cope.

The first sessions may need to have behavioral rather than linguistic goals. Children may be uncooperative (which is understandable considering the trauma that has occurred) in the new setting and try the limits. These goals may include, besides cooperation with activities, increased attention to a task and the completion of a set task in a given time. Often some activity which the child is capable of doing (e.g., a simple puzzle or matching of objects or pictures) may be used which will allow him or her to succeed and be positively reinforced. This same type of task may also be used to gain the child's cooperation. Operant conditioning principles may be used effectively in these situations. Children may respond best and be cooperative if they know exactly what is expected of them. For example, "John, you have these (indicating the number of picture cards) to do then you may play a game" or using a cardboard clock face and showing the child how long he has before the activity changes, "John, when the big hand reaches this point, then you may choose a game to play." The clinician moves the hand of the clock after the completion of each activity. When a child is transferred to another rehabilitation facility these goals may need to be restated because the child may again try the limits of the new staff involved with his or her treatment. Also, contributing factors to uncooperative behavior are the fact that emotional ties he or she has forged with the staff in the former facility have to be cut and that frequently the therapy and behavioral demands in the new setting have been increased to keep pace with his or her recovery.

In each treatment session the clinician must be alert to any situation in which pragmatic behaviors may be encouraged. For example, when the child first comes into the treatment room, he or she can be expected to give eye contact and greet the clinician appropriately (the expected behavior would be dependent on the child's abilities) and then use appropriate leave-taking skills. If the clinician is working on some particular concept then a situation may be engineered in the session. Most children love actively participating in the session (e.g., taking the game from a box, choosing which color token to have and which to give the clinician or going to the cupboard to collect the game). The clinician may tell the child, "Get the game on top of the cupboard," "Find the game in the cupboard on the bottom shelf." The complexity of the oral directions may be increased or the concept chosen be more advanced each session in line with the child's abilities. The integration of form/content/use would be a goal in each treatment session.

As children with acquired aphasia who appear to have recovered have been shown to have subtle problems, particularly in the areas of syntax and lexical retrieval, it would appear that strategies to help the child in these areas need to be given to the parents before the child's discharge.

Treatment Goals

Treatment goals may be formulated when relevant information has been gathered and priorities formulated. The treatment of morphologic, syntactic, semantic, and pragmatic problems would be based on the interpretation of test results, information gleaned from non-standardized tests and from observation. Activities used in treatment sessions may include tasks similar to those previously employed to assess the child's communicative skills. These tasks should consist of both comprehension and expressive activities and should use the developmental order of acquisition of morphemes, sentence structures, content categories, and pragmatic behaviors as guidelines when selecting treatment goals.

Syntax

Content/form/use interact and are inseparable, but when introducing new morphemes and sentence structures, content and use must be controlled. The semantics of the task need to be restricted (e.g., use words that are simple and familiar to the child) and initially only require the child to use the structure in one functional context (e.g., in a game format, "Does your mystery person have . . . ?"). Immediate auditory memory problems may require consideration when more complex sentence structures are introduced and the sentence length restricted as much as possible.

Visual material, in most instances, assists the child with comprehension or expressive tasks. Children enjoy seeing photographs of themselves or friends so pictures of them doing various activities may be used for eliciting certain sentence structures. For example, subject-verb-object, "I am eating a banana" or subject–verb–object–adverbial, "I am eating my banana under the tree." An activity such as cooking which the child may have done in her or his occupational therapy session can be photographed and used successfully in a language session to facilitate the use of "after" or "before" (e.g., After I put butter on my toast, I ate it). The clinician, when playing games such as "Fish" or "Memory" may require the child to use certain grammatical question structures (e.g., "Have you got the . . . ? Will you give me the . . . ?").

Children learn by doing. Activities which involve the child doing an action (provided the child's physical problems do not restrict her or him too much) may be used to help the child understand and express tenses. For example, the child walks around the room. The clinician asks, "What are you doing?" The expected reply is, "Walking." The child sits down. "What did you do?" The reply, "Walked." Past, present and future tenses may be elicited in this manner as well as prepositions and adverbial phrases (e.g., "climbing under the table").

Imaginative play situations, if the child is capable, may be enjoyable for the child and be designed to help facilitate more complex sentence structures. For example, she or he could pretend to be a fireman, going to a fire, fighting the fire and returning to the station. The child may use "ing" endings while describing the activities she or he is playing and then past tense with complex sentence structures to tell what she or he did (e.g., After I put the ladder up I climbed to the top and hosed the fire.)

Other treatment activities may include judgment tasks which require the child to decide on whether some structure or morpheme is correct or incorrect and may involve tense, case and any part of speech. For example, the child is shown a picture of a man walking. The clinician says, "The man is walking. She is walking. Is that right or wrong?" or "Yesterday, I am walking. Correct or incorrect?" Activities comprising scrambled sentences, sentence completion, sentence formulation and sentence correction, may be designed for individual children. These activities should include morphemes and complex sentences of differing structures.

Semantics

Semantic tasks must be functional for the child with acquired aphasia, for example, the preschool child may find attributes such as "dirty" or "sticky" more functional in her or his environment than the names of colors. The clinician needs to investigate what is meaningful for each child in the child's home and school environments and allow this information to direct the choice of materials and content in treatment sessions.

Simple comprehension activities may consist of asking the child to choose the correct object by name or function from a set number, perhaps only a choice of two or three in the early stages of recovery. This activity may be varied using a variety of semantic categories (e.g., "Show me the dirty car. Which dog is under the table?"). Categorization and association tasks may vary from the simple to the more complex as the child progresses. For example, the child may be required to place the pictures of animals and clothes in their correct piles or for a more difficult task, to distinguish between wild animals and farm animals or things made of plastic and those made of glass. Sorting by function or attribute (e.g., "Put all the things you read together," or "Find all the big objects.") may be used and increased in complexity when necessary to make the task more demanding (e.g., "Show me all the big blue things in this picture".). A variation on a categorization or association that may ask the child to choose, "Which picture (or word) does not belong: apple, chair, or orange?" Comprehension and expressive tasks are often combined (e.g., the categorization task may involve confrontation naming or require the child to describe why pictures go together or why one object does not belong).

Judgment tasks involving the meaning of two sentences (e.g., Are these two sentences similar in meaning? "Jim bought the table and chairs. Jim bought the fruit.") are useful and children seem to enjoy them, particularly if some nonsense sentences are also added (e.g.,

"I ate the cake and the ice cream. I ate the furniture."). Judgment of meaning can also involve antonyms, synonyms and homonyms (e.g., synonym—"He yelled at the boys. He shouted at the boys. Same or different?").

Expressive tasks may require the child to explain the similarities and differences between two objects (e.g., "glasses and a microscope"). Variations of the game of "Twenty Questions" may be played where the clinician and the child take turns in giving short descriptions of some item in a designated category. For example, "It is an animal. It has four legs. It lives on a farm. It gives us milk." The child may choose from among four animal pictures in front of him or her: a horse, a cow, an elephant and a lion. A visual cue may not be needed as the child becomes more proficient in understanding and expressing language. The game of "Twenty Questions" itself or an association game where the child has to guess what goes with some object (e.g., "shoes and . . . ?") facilitates comprehension and expression.

The adult literature discusses convergent and divergent semantic tasks and their place in aphasia therapy to aid problem solving and pragmatic tasks such as getting and giving information (Chapey, 1981). These tasks are similar to examples of verbal elaboration (Wiig & Semel, 1984) used in therapy for learning-disabled children. Convergent tasks require the individual to give a specific commonly used response (e.g., You drink from a . . . "cup" or "glass" would be the usual response but not "shoe" or "hose"). Divergent production includes tasks that call for a variety of logical responses (e.g., "Can you think of all the things that may be yellow?"). Many language stimulation activities used in the classroom with normal children to enhance their language abilities (e.g., Peabody Development Kits [Dunn & Smith, 1965]) contain similar suggestions to divergent semantic activities and may be adapted for use with children with acquired aphasia. Adaptation primarily is by controlling the semantic and syntactic aspects of the tasks.

The use of riddles and jokes may be employed to assist the child with multi-word meanings and phonological plays on words. For example, "Why did the tomato blush? Because it saw the salad dressing." What word has a double meaning and what are those two meanings? "When do astronauts eat? At launch time." What word was changed to make the joke? Selections from children's commercial joke and riddle books are a valuable and enjoyable resource for treatment activities. Also, the clinician may make use of children's favorite television programs. The child is asked to identify what was funny about a situation, particularly if irony is involved. Homework, which includes watching a favorite television program, is usually willingly done. This task may also involve narrative skills or the clinician may only choose to ask specific questions about the program ("Why was it funny when . . . ?"). These types of activities are particularly useful with the older child who has a good understanding of oral language.

The older child may also be given activities that require him or her to define words, formulate sentences which show that he or she understands the meaning of the words (e.g., "steak," "stake") or explain figurative language. For example, explain these sayings: "Her skin was as white as snow, Too many cooks spoil the broth, I am pulling your leg." Care should be taken when giving instructions to children that figurative language is not used with a child who has problems understanding colloquial and multimeaning words (e.g., A child may seem to be uncooperative because he or she does not comply when asked, "Hop up on the table." He cannot "hop" that far!).

Many children with acquired aphasia have significant word retrieval problems. The strategies used to facilitate word recall may be brought to the child's awareness during confrontation naming and rapid automatic naming tasks so that he or she may trigger the specific word himself or herself. These strategies may include:

> sentence completion—I cut with a . . .
>
> opposite cues—old and . . .
>
> association cues—It goes with shoes. Shoes and . . .
>
> descriptions of object—It's found in the bathroom. You wash your hands in it
>
> category cues—It's an animal
>
> syllable or sound cues—"pot" for potato, /f/ for fire
>
> rhyming cue—It sounds like "rain" for train
>
> pantomime cue—Pretending to bounce the ball for ball

Teaching strategies may involve taking the child through the "thinking" process. For example, picture the object in your mind. What do you do with it? Make a sentence in your mind about the function (e.g., I cut with the . . .). Can you think of what sound it starts with? Some children, as they recover their language skills, may become proficient in using synonyms although this is not a common occurrence and these children have usually had excellent vocabularies before their brain lesion.

Reading and Writing

Treatment in these areas may mostly involve the clinician in a supportive role to the teacher. Many of the activities used in the treatment of auditory comprehension and expressive skills may be adapted to the written mode (e.g., sentence correction and sentence formulation). Liaison with the teacher about the child's difficulties in oral language will help the teacher decide on her/his expectations for the child in reading, spelling, sentence formulation, and essays. Reading and spelling may be used as visual cues in oral language tasks and this in turn reinforces written skills. In a group situation in the classroom the teacher may also be able to reinforce narrative and metalinguistic treatment goals.

Pragmatics

Pragmatic problems may be best treated in a group situation. With older children (10 years and over), specific pragmatic or social skills groups can be successful particularly if video recording equipment is available. Younger children seem to respond best in situations where pragmatic situations occur naturally and the clinician can facilitate the appropriate behavior. This approach is discussed further in the section on group therapy.

Individual work on pragmatic skills in the linguistic domain may be done in language sessions when they occur naturally in context (e.g., repair/revision skills may be facilitated if the child is explaining). Work on a child's narrative skills also provides an opportunity for teaching pragmatic abilities (e.g., requesting and giving specific information).

In recent years, clinicians in many disciplines have addressed the issue of social skills and how they can be taught (Foxx, 1985). An awareness of group dynamics and how to structure the group is an important consideration before deciding to work directly on social skills. In a pragmatic or social skills group, ideally involving another team member such as the occupational therapist, the teacher, the social worker or the psychologist, a target behavior (e.g., a greeting) is selected and task analyzed by the group members. It is useful if the team members involved role play the appropriate speech act before any discussion takes place. Each group member is then given the chance to role-play the situation while it is video-recorded. The group then can discuss whether the behavior was appropriate or inappropriate and decide if a breakdown occurred and if so how to correct it (e.g., "Did the child fail to make eye contact? Did the child call out when the person was too far away to hear? Did the child fail to say the person's name or use an appropriate greeting?") Besides analyzing various speech acts it is also useful to discuss nonverbal behavior and what facial expressions or various tones of voice mean, as well as to assist the children to read social situations, start or finish conversations, decide on what the main topic of conversation was, and what they could contribute to the discourse. Once the child has become proficient in the group then the behavior needs to be transferred into other situations.

In groups such as this it is the responsibility of the speech-language clinician to decide on what is appropriate linguistically for each individual. For example, eye contact, a smile, and "Hello, Chris" may be all that a child with dysarthria can manage whereas a child with good language skills may have the same nonverbal goals but say, "Hello, Chris, how are you today?"

Group Treatment

Backus and Beasley (1951) advocated that group instruction form the core of speech and language treatment. They believed that it was the forces operating in the interpersonal relationships between the child and the clinician and among children as a group that brought about the appropriate changes in their speech and language behavior. Since 1951 these forces have been identified and analyzed and the importance of these pragmatic aspects of language realized. Language allows us to master and manipulate our environment to our advantage and competence in communicating is important for social, educational, and personal development.

Children with acquired aphasia benefit from group treatment. It allows these children to put into practice the language behaviors that they have learned in their individual sessions (e.g., Asking permission using a particular syntactic structure, "Can I have the glue, please?"), and gives them the opportunity for interacting naturally in a controlled learning situation.

Group treatment sessions with the child with acquired aphasia may take many forms and include both homogeneous and heterogeneous populations. Language groups directed by the speech-language clinician may involve engineered tasks. For example, in a group addressing mostly pragmatic behaviors, something may be placed in the doorway so that a child in a wheelchair is unable to enter. The clinician can remain close and prompt the child, if necessary, to ask for specific help (e.g., "Helena, would you move the chair please?"). Different tasks are devised for each child so as the child learns the appropriate behavior, the prompts decrease in the language group situation. Generalization of this behavior is helped by engineering similar situations in different contexts (e.g., going with the physiotherapist to another room and something is placed in the child's way). Other team members are aware of the behavioral goals and can prompt if necessary.

In other language groups the emphasis of the activities may be on semantics and syntax. Divergent semantic tasks are particularly successful in group situations because an idea given by one child may stimulate further ideas from other children (e.g., "Think of all the things you could do with a box." "What would happen if we did not have water?"). Their ideas may be written or drawn on the board so that revision may take place. Turn-taking and repair/revision skills may also be reinforced. Barrier games facilitate specific word usage and aid organizational skills. For example, the children have a number of objects in front of them and arrange them in some way. The clinician has the same objects behind a barrier and the children must tell her how to arrange the objects. It is helpful to have two team members involved, one behind the barrier and the other to facilitate specific instructions.

Interdisciplinary or transdisciplinary groups, where the emphasis is not primarily communication skills, provide numerous pragmatic situations and facilitate the generalization of skills learned in individual language sessions. A fine motor control group directed by the occupational therapist may involve cutting and pasting skills. It also provides the children with an opportunity for learning requesting behaviors (e.g.,

"Chris, may I have the scissors please?" or "Chris, scissors please."). Care must be taken in such groups that the language demands do not overshadow the other activities. It is best to focus on only one communication skill (e.g., The goal for each child might be to give eye contact and say the name of the person they are addressing.). Other team members ensure that this occurs whereas the speech-language clinician may help individual children to frame their present request in the most appropriate language depending on their language abilities.

Creative dramatics is a group activity that is closely linked to the dramatic play of children and is a technique that, when adapted, offers the clinician another treatment procedure. It is an informal spontaneous drama situation which allows a leader to structure and give form to the imaginative play of children. Because of the nature of the activities it provides numerous pragmatic opportunities for the children involved as well as stimulating divergent semantic behavior.

The guided activities used in creative dramatics give children a chance to examine life in a more concrete form through the development of replica-of-life situations. This allows them to gain insight into their own and others' feelings and learn to understand and adapt to a variety of situations because they can experience present and future events and re-examine past ones.

There are several aspects to creative dramatics and each step may be successfully adapted for use with children with acquired aphasia. Simple activities such as "Simon says," action songs, finger plays, or a simple, "Guess what I am doing" activity may serve to introduce children to the imaginative situation. As they become more confident sensory awareness activities incorporating all senses may be suggested (e.g., concentrate on a real or imaginary object and discuss everything about it or listen to all the sounds in the room and name them. Pretend you are bush walking. What sounds can you hear?).

Movement activities (e.g., pretend to be raking leaves, reading a book, picking apples from a tree) follow sensory awareness tasks. Because the situations are imaginary it does not matter whether the children can actually do the physical actions well. Some severely disabled children use only small arm or finger movements yet enjoy the activity and make suggestions for further activities. Characterization and improvisation are more demanding imaginary tasks but often facilitate the use of spontaneous language. Before beginning characterization or improvisation activities, discussion takes place. For example, How would you know whether someone was a fireman or a policewoman? What do they do? How do you know someone is old? Improvisation involves dialogue. Again discussion centers on what a person would say if they were: buying an ice-cream, calling a puppy, or selling tickets on a wheel of fortune; situations that some children would find difficult, such as asking for help or information, may be included in the imaginative situation. Children never play themselves in creative dramatics and so the demands to produce language correctly are lessened.

The final stage in creative dramatics is the dramatization of a chosen theme or story and this is excellent for improving children's narrative and sequencing skills. Stories chosen for dramatization may be those that are the children's current favorites or the "classics" such as, "The Three Billy Goats Gruff" or "The Ginger Bread Man." For younger children stories with repetition are excellent because the more able child

may serve as a model for another child. Discussion plays an important role in deciding what and how the actions are to be played. Children need to have a firm idea of the sequence of the story, what is to happen in each scene, where and why it happens, what characters are involved and how they react. A scene or the story is played and an evaluation of the playing takes place immediately (e.g., The character or action is discussed but the children's names are never used. "Was the king angry enough when . . . " not "Was Alex angry enough when . . . "). The story, with improvements, may be played again with a further evaluation.

Initially, older children may be inhibited but these barriers gradually disappear as they become more secure in the group situation and with the activities. Older children particularly enjoy problem-solving situations. For example, they are members of a company and because of a strike by the pilots they cannot send their goods by air. What will they do? They play out the situation and the solutions. Many children with a brain lesion may not be able to cope with the final stage of creative dramatics but find enjoyment and benefit in short improvisation situations and other earlier stages. The speech-language clinician may direct creative dramatic activities but if the school the children attend has access to a drama specialist then her or his expertise is extremely valuable and the sessions may be jointly planned with all team members involved and goals for each child established.

Summary of Treatment of Acquired Childhood Aphasia

The steps to be taken during the treatment of acquired childhood aphasia are summarized in Figure 10–2.

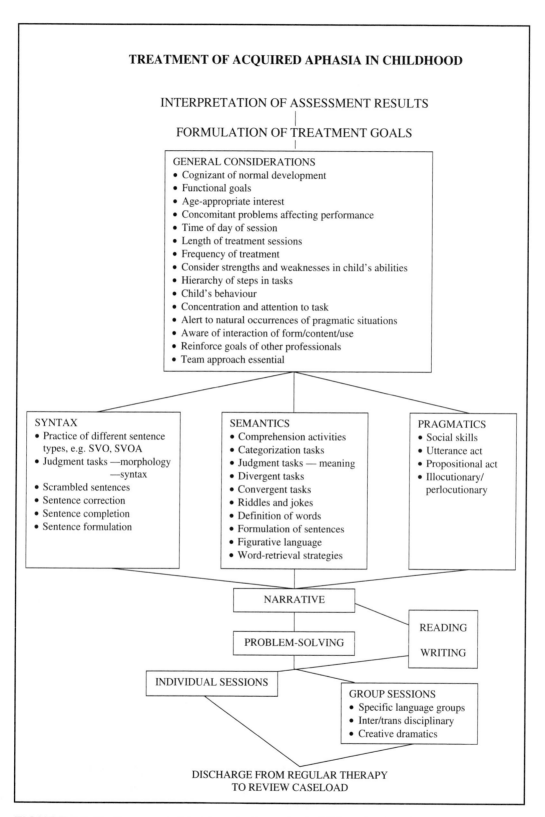

FIGURE 10–2. Summary of treatment of acquired childhood aphasia.

Both reports of practicing clinicians and descriptions of children with acquired aphasia documented in the literature seem to suggest that children with a brain lesion may present with communicative difficulties similar to those problems experienced by learning-disabled children and the adult aphasia population. Assessment and treatment procedures may be successfully adapted for the child with acquired aphasia from techniques used with both learning disabled and adult aphasic clients. Although many treatment ideas used with aphasic adults can be successfully adapted for children, clinicians must remember that the process of rehabilitation in children is entirely different. In both adults and children treatment goals are influenced by the various stages of the recovery process. However, children, unlike adults, are still acquiring speech and language skills. Consequently, developmental processes that influence the normal acquisition of language need to be taken into account in planning treatment strategies for children with acquired aphasia.

Case Example

The following case is presented to illustrate the major features of the assessment and treatment of children with acquired aphasia.

The client, Jane, was a 10-year-old, right-handed girl who had suffered a severe brain injury as a result of being knocked off her bicycle by a motor vehicle. She remained unconscious after the injury, and while being transported to hospital first the left and then the right pupil dilated. Prior to a computed

tomography (CT) scan examination she underwent an urgent craniotomy. She remained in intensive care for 3 weeks during which time she underwent surgery for removal of the extensive fragmented fracture and the repair of her dura. Two weeks after admission extubation was attempted but was unsuccessful because her vocal folds had developed extensive granulation tissue. A tracheostomy had to be performed.

Neurologic Examination

A month after her injury Jane's neurologic status was assessed. Although she was conscious and alert the examining neurologist reported severe expressive dysphasia and a moderate receptive dysphasia. Visual acuity in both eyes was poor, with the left eye in particular being virtually blind. Also present was a complete left third cranial nerve palsy and a temporal hemianopia in the right eye. All other cranial nerves appeared normal although her tongue deviated to the right. She had a dense right hemiparesis but was able to walk with assistance.

Neuroradiologic Examination

The CT scan performed after the craniotomy showed extensive left temporoparietal fracture complex with extensive contusion of the underlying left temporal lobe. The following day a further CT scan showed hemorrhagic contusion in the left temporal region with considerable blood and some dilation of the lateral ventricles. A month later a CT scan showed significantly advanced ventricular dilation and a ventricular peritoneal shunt was inserted. The CT scan taken

4 months after the injury showed that the catheter was in a good position and there was some reduction in the size of the lateral, third and fourth ventricles. The left cerebellar–pontine subdural collection no longer was apparent.

Concomitant Problems

Jane made a good recovery of movement and strength in her right side. Although the initial dense hemiparesis in her right upper limb resolved to near normal motor functioning, she exhibited marked sensory deficits particularly on the palmar surface. These deficits hampered her functional ability but she continued to be right hand dominant in most activities except writing. Her visual acuity improved but the visual field deficit persisted and caused some minor motor incoordination of the eye- and figure-ground difficulties but she compensated by good visual scanning. Perceptually, she scored within the average range.

Speech and Language Recovery

A month after her admission Jane had no meaningful vocalization and her responses to "yes/no" questions were inconsistent. Oral feeds were commenced and she tolerated a soft diet. Two weeks later her responses to "yes/no" questions were consistent and she had some automatic expressive language such as "no" and "bye." She was able to imitate some vowels and consonants with effort. Feeding was no problem. Seven weeks after the accident, Jane was able to understand some complex sentences (e.g., "The boy is running and the girl is jumping" but not, "Show me all of the

red lines except the last one"), and responded to social language appropriately. Her expressive skills were grammatically correct at this time but lacked content words.

Eight weeks after injury, when her irritability had decreased, an informal but systematic speech and language assessment was attempted. Receptively she could identify objects by name, color, function, size and position, and could follow simple instructions. When sentences were semantically and syntactically complex she failed to comprehend. Her reading abilities were also severely affected. She could match letters and some letters to phonemes. She also was able to recognize some simple words (e.g., "dog," "cat").

Severe difficulties in using semantically important words in utterances and verbal and literal paraphasias characterized her expressive language. Her sentences were grammatically correct but with few content words. She usually required a sentence completion or a phonemic cue before she could produce a content word. Articulation was characterized by problems sequencing phonemes in complex words and exacerbated by literal paraphasias.

Written expression was complicated by fine motor deficits. She was able to write from dictation some letters of the alphabet, her name, and some simple sentences that she initiated (e.g., "The cat is black").

Language Evaluation

Jane was discharged from speech therapy 14 months after injury because her family were moving to another state. During the period before her discharge, Jane made significant gains in the comprehension and expression of oral language. Three months after her accident the CELF–4 was attempted. The production subtests of the CELF–4 were not administered because Jane could not cope with these subtests and became distressed. She only managed to produce one name for each category on the Word Associations subtest and then only when prompted (e.g., At breakfast we eat bacon and . . .). Literal paraphasias were numerous during the Word Series subtest and she refused to continue because she was aware of her failures. Her Processing Score was below the 5th percentile with a language age of 5 years 5 months (chronologic age = 10 years, 3 months). All subtests were below criterion level. Significant problems were noted on the Processing Spoken Paragraphs subtest. She was unable to answer any of the questions correctly. On the PPVT–4 she scored at the 30th percentile. Visual field deficits negatively influenced her PPVT–4 score.

Seven months after her injury her Processing Score on the CELF–4 was at the 5th percentile with a language age of 6 years 9 months (chronologic age = 9 years, 1 month). Linguistic Concepts, Relationships and Ambiguities subtests were above the criterion level and her performance on the Word Classes subtest was borderline. She was still having significant problems with expressive tasks and most of the production subtests of the CELF–4 were not attempted. However, she was willing to attempt Word Associations and the Formulated Sentences subtests. Her sentences were simple when given the stimulus word (e.g., "car": "I can see a car" or "children": "I like children") but sentences requiring conjunctions or adverbs were incorrect (e.g., "because": "because I said so" and "slowly": "My friend is slow

at running."). Her word associations tended to consist of broad categories (i.e., "fruit," "vegetables," or "meat") and the animals named were mostly farm animals. Word-retrieval problems had decreased since her previous assessment. On the PPVT–4 she scored at the 50th percentile, compensating well for her visual field deficit.

Twelve months after the accident her Processing Score on the CELF–4 was at the 30th percentile and her Production Score at the 10th percentile yielding language ages of 9 years for processing and 7 years 3 months for Production (chronological age = 11 years 0 months). The subtest giving her the greatest problems was Processing Spoken Paragraphs. Her score on the PPVT–4 at this time was at the 90th percentile.

Spontaneous Speech

Jane's spontaneous speech recovered quickly. Within 7 weeks of injury her communication progressed from no meaningful vocalization to grammatically correct sentences lacking content words. She had severe word-retrieval difficulties. When she was asked specific questions she would often pantomime her reply (e.g., getting on the floor and doing exercises to denote physiotherapy). Her language was circumlocutory with numerous literal paraphasias and some verbal paraphasias. Because her communication lacked content her listeners often did not understand her message.

There was gradual decrease in paraphasias and circumlocution over the 14-month period of speech and language therapy. Literal and verbal paraphasias disappeared first from her spontaneous speech. Content words specific to the "here and now" seemed to be the easiest for Jane to recall, followed by recall of the immediate past (e.g., the activities she had just completed at school before coming to therapy). Word retrieval was particularly difficult when she was required to explain or clarify her meaning. Memory did not appear to play a significant part in these problems. On discharge, 14 months after her injury, Jane had few problems if the linguistic demands of conversational speech were minimal. Literal and verbal paraphasias were rarely heard and word-retrieval problems were few. Difficulties with word retrieval still persisted, however, when she was required to clarify or explain her meaning she gave her listeners enough content (often a context clue, e.g., "beach" or "holidays") for them to understand her message. Two years after the injury, when speaking with Jane on the phone, the clinician noted that Jane had no apparent problems in conversation and could explain logically what had happened at school and in her family life since her discharge.

Humor

Initially, Jane could only understand humor when it was concrete (i.e. "slapstick comedy"). If a joke or riddle was dependent on a word having two or more meanings, Jane could neither understand the joke nor retell it (e.g., "How do you stop a herd of rhinoceroses from charging?" Answer, "Take away their credit cards."). Furthermore, she could not answer riddles even when presented with options from which to choose (e.g., "What goes up but never comes down?" Answer, "Smoke"). Jane also had problems in accepting good-natured teasing from her peers. She failed

to read their nonverbals or understand the incongruities in their language. This would often lead to frustration and arguments. However, as her language comprehension improved so did her ability to cope in these situations.

Narrative

Jane's written stories before the accident were well above average for her age. After the injury, as her written language recovered her narrative was a series of short simple sentences in a sequence (e.g., The family is at the beach. The boy is swimming. The girl is making a sand castle.). As her recovery continued her narratives appeared to progress through the normal developmental stages even though therapy did not stress these steps. Her main difficulty in the latter stages of recovery was the lack of specificity and organization. Verbal difficulties were mirrored in her written work, for example, her stories contained a predominance of simple sentences or complex sentences with "and then" as the conjunction rather than coordinators such as "before," "after," "but," "when," or "because" which she had used before her injury. Nine months after her injury, a narrative, the story of Cinderella which she knew well, was analyzed. It was cohesive, sequenced correctly, and used a variety of conjunctions and syntactical structures. Word-retrieval problems, however, were still in evidence and seemed to be the cause of pauses, often two to three seconds in duration, and false starts and repetitions. However, the organizational framework (i.e., a beginning, middle, and end with specific descriptions of the characters and their relationship to one another), was apparent.

Play

From observation Jane was able to play imaginatively as soon as she was physically able. However, her play involved much pantomime and action with little verbal reasoning skills required (e.g., pop-stars singing on stage or mothers and fathers). When her class was involved in drama sessions with a visiting drama specialist Jane initially was unable to cope because her comprehension and verbal reasoning skills were inadequate; she became extremely frustrated during these sessions.

In one imaginative situation the children in her class pretended to be a group of scientists who were concerned about pollution on Earth. The scenario was as follows. The scientists had decided to escape from Earth and had discovered another planet which was similar to their world. Unfortunately, it was inhabited by a few survivors of a superior race who did not want the Earth people to settle there. The aliens were scared that the scientists would bring pollution to their planet. The same things that were happening to Earth had happened on their planet eons ago and virtually destroyed their civilization. The alien planet had few trees, flowers, birds, or animals and over the centuries fewer and fewer children were being born so that now the survivors were unable to have children.

These drama sessions continued for 17 hours for 10 weeks during which time the children had to decide what action they could take. Following their decision the children then had to negotiate with rather hostile aliens (played by the speech-language pathologists). As part of this negotiation the children had to convince the aliens that they had skills and resources that would help the planet.

Toward the end of the 10 weeks Jane was able to contribute ideas and understand the reasoning process. Both her mother and previous teacher reported that Jane would have had no difficulty participating in such an activity before the accident. By observing her difficulties in these sessions further therapy goals were formulated. This situation provided an excellent opportunity to sample a number of Jane's linguistic and pragmatic skills and to observe her progress. The standardized tests used with Jane failed to identify this verbal reasoning difficulty. However, extrapolation of her standardized test results would seem to suggest the probability of problems in this area. Also, a normal language sample may not have provided the same information because most samples do not place the child in such a demanding linguistic situation. This imaginative scenario required a high level of cognitive, comprehensive and expressive abilities. As yet, there is little information in the literature about verbal reasoning skills in acquired childhood aphasia.

Reading

Before her accident, Jane had been an excellent reader and read for recreation. Her reading skills improved almost daily after the injury, progressing from matching letters and words to choosing the correct sentence for a picture. Her written difficulties mirrored her verbal difficulties but were slower recovering. It was the amount of information that she was required to process rather than specific syntactic or semantic elements that gave her problems; for example, breaking the passage she was to read into short sections facilitated her comprehension. As she recovered, the amount of written information that she could process accurately increased, although at the time of discharge, 14 months after the injury, she still had not started to read for pleasure again. She complained, at this time, that she did not understand the story.

Writing

Like her reading, her written language improved quickly, although sensory problems in her right hand and her need to use her left non-dominant hand interfered with activities involving handwriting skills. Jane suffered fatigue easily while writing so a typewriter or computer often was used. It was the spelling of the small abstract words such as "the," "as," and so forth, that gave her the greatest difficulty. She would omit them or interchange them indiscriminately (e.g., use "was" for "the" without seeing that it was incorrect).

A letter received from Jane some 2 years after her injury had no spelling mistakes and her syntax was correct. A note added by her mother said that Jane had written most of the letter herself without help.

Behavior

When admitted to a school for handicapped children Jane was unhappy with her class placement. She wanted to return to her former school and found it difficult to settle into the educational situation with other disabled children, many in wheelchairs. Throughout the duration of her rehabilitation Jane was anxious that all staff involved in her treatment be aware of her previous school achievements. She would constantly remind staff that she had been first in her class and that most of the activities done in therapy she used to be able to do easily. She also would keep her workbooks from her former school with her and often bring them to therapy. She was determined to succeed and return to her former school. Consequently, she worked hard at school, in therapy and at home in a very supportive family environment. However, she often was frustrated by her inability to do some activity.

Therapy

Close liaison was maintained with Jane's teacher and having a school on the same premises as the therapy departments was a distinct advantage for language treatment. Language tasks, whether they were verbal or written, mostly involved work that she would be using in class or had difficulty completing at school. School and therapy staff worked closely together; for example, when the occupational therapist planned a cooking session with Jane she would take photos of the sequence of steps and these would be used later in Jane's language session for both verbal and written tasks. Likewise, her family would send photos of special occasions or of recent outings and these would also be incorporated into language treatment sessions.

Treatment was daily and covered many areas. The main focus of therapy, however, was on Jane's word-retrieval difficulties and her problems processing varying amounts of verbal and written language. Word-retrieval strategies included: sentence completion using all parts of speech, associations and categorization tasks, questions about Jane's home and school environments, description of objects in a "Twenty Questions" format, rhyming words, and antonyms, synonyms, and homonyms. Initially, word retrieval was significantly helped by visual cues. When she played various card games with matching cards or association cards Jane could, herself, facilitate the retrieval of the word required, for example, "I want something that goes with the cage." At this stage she would be holding the picture of the cage. This would then facilitate the sentence, "I want the bird." Strategies which Jane used to retrieve words were brought to her awareness and she was encouraged to use them in all situations, for example, thinking of what letter started the word or what was the object's function such as "It flies. It is a bird."

When helping Jane with processing verbal and written information, stories from school reading programs were used, photocopied and cut into workable units starting with two sentences and increasing gradually until Jane was able to do the complete card without any modification. The computer proved a highly motivating therapy tool. Computer reading programs were used for both verbal and reading exercises because the content was easy to modify. For example, the story could be read by the clinician and Jane was asked to read silently the three answers given and choose the correct one. The game of "Hangman" on the computer helped her with spelling. Verbal reasoning was facilitated with problem-solving computer games (e.g., "Who done it" type mysteries). Fourteen months after the injury Jane was discharged. She had achieved her preinjury grade level in mathematics (still a year below her age-appropriate level) and a further grade below this level in English. Her language recovery

had not plateaued and she was referred for further language therapy.

Concluding Note

In recent contact with the family, 3 years and 3 months after the injury, her mother reported that Jane was doing extremely well in all areas. In sport she had won her age championship for the best all-round performance. She was learning the clarinet and coping well although she still had some sensory deficits in her right hand. She remained left-handed for writing because, as Jane herself commented, she could write much faster with it, but she did practice with her right hand occasionally.

In the speech and language area, her mother felt that she was still improving. Jane was placed in a normal classroom situation where she was 12 to 18 months older than most of her peers. Her report card showed that she was above average in her academic marks, particularly in mathematics, and the teacher commented that she coped far better with mathematical processes than with language. In the areas of language, mathematics, and science her teacher also reported that Jane had excellent problem-solving skills and thought of the solution to many of the problems herself. She was also able to predict the outcome of science experiments. From further comments on her school report she appears to have difficulty understanding some abstract terms such as "parallel" and in music has problems understanding rhythmic patterns. Generally, her report card showed marked improvement in all areas of language.

Jane's written narrative was cohesive although some sentence structures were incorrect and obscured the meaning (e.g., "There he was stolen up in the hills called The Fox View," meaning the horse was stolen and hidden in the hills.). Her mother reported that she was reading for pleasure again. Her main difficulty in the language area appeared to be with spelling. When tested with a new list of words at the beginning of the school week Jane only got two or three correct out of 15 but after learning them she would usually achieve 12 or 13 correct, which she then remembered. She appeared to have a problem transferring from the oral to the written form. Her mother reported that she would spell the word correctly orally but then write it incorrectly transposing letters. Jane believed that she had no problems with word finding and during the phone conversation there was no indication of any difficulty. Her mother commented that Jane was almost back to her previous personality. Her confidence had improved with her recent achievements and she had assumed a leadership role again among her peers. She was determined to do well in all areas.

Although overall Jane made a good recovery, some aphasic symptoms persisted in the higher level language areas. However, it seems probable that in time Jane may overcome many of her difficulties because she has good problem-solving skills and uses strategies to help her achieve in academic areas.

References

Backus, O., & Beasley, J. (1951). *Speech therapy with children*. Boston, MA: Houghton Mifflin.

Blank, M., Rose, S. A., & Berlin, L. J. (1978). Preschool language assessment instrument. Orlando, FL: Harcourt Brace Jovanovich.

Bloom, L., & Lahey, M. (1978). *Language development and language disorders*. New York, NY: John Wiley & Sons.

Boehm, A. E. (2000). Boehm test of basic concepts (3rd ed.). San Antonio, TX: Harcourt Assessment.

Bowers, L., Huisingh, R., & LoGiudice, C. (2005). Test of problem solving 3-elementary. East Moline, IL: LinguiSystems.

Bowers, L., Huisingh, R., LoGiudice, C., & Orman, J. (2004). *Word Test 2–Elementary*. East Moline, IL: LinguiSystems.

Carrow-Woolfolk, E. (1985). Test of auditory comprehension of language–revised. Allen, TX: DLM Teaching Resources.

Chapey, R. (1981). The assessment of language disorders in adults. In R. Chapey (Ed.), *Language intervention strategies in adult aphasia*. Baltimore, MD: Williams & Wilkins.

Chapey, R. (1986). The assessment of language disorders in adults. In R. Chapey (Ed.), *Language intervention strategies in adult aphasia* (2nd ed.). Baltimore, MD: Williams & Wilkins.

Crystal, D. (1982). *Profiling linguistic disability*. London, UK: Edward Arnold.

Crystal, D., Fletcher, P., & Garman, M. (1982). *The grammatical analysis of language disability*. London, UK: Edward Arnold.

Damico, J. S. (1985). Clinical discourse analysis. A functional language assessment technique. In C. S. Simon (Ed.), *Communication skills and classroom success: Assessment of language-learning disabled students* (pp. 125–150). San Diego, CA: College-Hill Press.

DiSimoni, F. G. (1978). Token test for children. Higham, MA: Teaching Resources.

Docking, K. M., Murdoch, B. E., & Ward, E. C. (2003). High level language and phonological awareness abilities of children following management for supratentorial tumour: Part II. *Acta Neuropsychologica, 1*, 367–381.

Dunn, L. M., & Dunn, D. M. (2007). Peabody picture vocabulary test-4th edition. Bloomington, IN: Pearson.

Dunn, L. M., & Smith, J. O. (1965). *Peabody language development kits.* Circle Pines, MN: American Guidance Service.

Edwards, S., Fletcher, P., Garman, M., Hughes, A., Letts, C., & Sinka, I. (1997). Reynell development scales–III. London, UK: Nelson.

Fisher, J. P., & Glenister, J. M. (1992). *The Hundred Picture Naming Test.* Melbourne, Australia: ACER.

Foxx, R. M. (1985). Social skills training: The current status of the field. *Australian and New Zealand Journal of Developmental Disabilities, 10,* 237–243.

Fried-Oken, M. (1987). Qualitative examination of children's naming skills through test adaptations. *Language, Speech and Hearing Services in Schools, 18,* 206–216.

Gaddes, W. H., & Crockett, D. J. (1975). The Spreen–Benton aphasia tests, normative data as a measure of normal language development. *Brain and Language, 2,* 257–280.

Guilford, A. M., & Nawojczyk, D. C. (1988). Standardization of the Boston Naming Test at the kindergarten and elementary school levels. *Language, Speech and Hearing Services in Schools, 19,* 395–400.

Hammill, D. D., Brown, V. L., Larsen, S. C., & Wiederholt, J. L. (2007). Test of adolescent language (4th ed.). Austin, TX: Pro-Ed.

Hammill, D. D., & Newcomer, P. L. (1997a). Test of language development–intermediate (3rd ed.). Austin, TX: Pro-Ed.

Hammill, D. D., & Newcomer, P. L. (1997b). Test of language development-primary (3rd ed.). Austin, TX: Pro-Ed.

Holland, A. L., Frattali, C., & Fromm, D. (1999). *Communicative Abilities in Daily Living.* Austin, TX: Pro-Ed.

Hresko, W. P., Reid, K., & Hammill, D. D. (1999). *Test of early language development* (3rd ed.). Austin, TX: Pro-Ed.

Hudson, L. J., & Murdoch, B. E. (1992). Chronic language deficits in children treated for posterior fossa tumour. *Aphasiology, 6,* 135–150.

Huisingh, R., Bowers, L., LoGiudice, C., & Orman, J. (2005). WORD test 2-Adolescent. East Moline, IL: LinguiSystems.

Irwin, E. C. (1975). Facilitating children's language development through play. *Speech Teacher, 24,* 10–12.

Jordan, F. M., & Murdoch, B. E. (1993). A prospective study of the linguistic skills of children with closed head injuries. *Aphasiology, 7,* 503–512.

Jordan, F. M., Murdoch, B. E., Buttsworth, D. L., & Hudson-Tennent, L. J. (1995). Speech and language performance of brain-injured children. *Aphasiology, 9,* 23–32.

Jorgensen, C., Barrett, M., Huisingh, R., & Zachman, L. (1981). The word test: A test of expressive vocabulary and semantics. East Moline, IL: LinguiSystems.

Kaplan, E., Goodglass, H., & Weintraub, S. (1983). The Boston naming test. Philadelphia, PA: Lea & Febiger.

Manochiopining, S., Sheard, C., & Reed, V. A. (1992). Pragmatic assessment in adult aphasia: A clinical review. *Aphasiology, 6,* 519–534.

Miller, J. F. (1981). *Assessing language production in children.* Baltimore, MD: University Park Press.

Murdoch, B. E., & Hudson-Tennent, L. J. (1994). Differential language outcomes in children following treatment for posterior fossa tumours. *Aphasiology, 8,* 507–534.

Penn, C. (1999). Pragmatic assessment and therapy for persons with brain damage: What have clinicians gleaned in two decades. *Brain and Language, 68,* 535–552.

Porch, B. E. (1974). *Porch Index of Communicative Ability in Children.* Palo Alto, CA: Consulting Psychologists Press.

Prutting, C. A., & Kirchner, D. M. (1983). Applied pragmatics. In T. M. Gallagher & C. A. Prutting (Eds.), *Pragmatic assessment and intervention issues in language.* San Diego, CA: College-Hill Press.

Prutting, C. A., & Kirchner, D. M. (1987). A clinical appraisal of the pragmatic aspects of language. *Journal of Speech and Hearing Disorders, 52,* 105–119.

Ripich, D. N., & Spinelli, F. M. (1985). *School discourse problem.* London, UK: Taylor & Francis.

Semel, W., Wiig, E. H., & Secord, W. (2003). Clinical evaluation of language fundamentals (4th ed.). San Antonio, TX: Harcourt Assessment.

Shultz, T. R. (1976). A cognitive-developmental analysis of humour. In A. J. Chapman, H. C. Foot (Eds.), *Humour and laughter: Theory, research and applications*. London, UK: John Wiley & Sons.

Simon, C. S. (1985). *Communication skills and classroom success: Therapy methodologies for language-learning disabled students*. London, UK: Taylor & Francis.

Spreen, O., & Benton, A. L. (1977). *Neurosensory Center Comprehensive Examination for Aphasia: Manual of directions* (Rev. ed.). Victoria, B.C.: University of Victoria.

Torgesen, J. K., & Bryant, B. R. (1994). *Test of Phonological Awareness*. Austin, TX: Pro-Ed.

Wallach, G. P., & Butler, K. G. (1984). *Language learning disabilities in school-age children*. Baltimore, MD: Williams & Wilkins.

Westby, C. E. (1984). Development of narrative language abilities. In G. P. Wallach & K. G. Butler (Eds.), *Language learning disabilities in school-age children*. Baltimore, MD: Williams & Wilkins.

Wiig, E. H. (1982). *Let's talk inventory for adolescents*. Columbus, OH: Charles E. Merrill.

Wiig, E. H., & Secord, W. A. (1989). *Test of Language Competence–expanded edition*. New York: Psychological Corp.

Wiig, E. H., & Secord, W. A. (1992). *Test of Word Knowledge*. San Antonio, TX: Psychological Corp.

Wiig, E. H., Secord, W. A., & Semel, E. (2006). Clinical evaluation of language fundamentals-preschool (2nd ed.). Marrickville, Australia: Harcourt Assessment.

Wiig, E. H., & Semel, E. (1974). Development of comprehension of logical grammatical sentences by grade school children. *Perceptual and Motor Skills, 38*, 171–176.

Wiig, E. H., & Semel, E. (1984). *Language assessment and intervention for the learning disabled*. Columbus, OH: Charles E. Merrill.

Wilks, V., & Monaghan, R. (1988). *The graphic conversational profile: A possible intervention tool for people with communication deficits following closed head injuries*. Paper presented at the Annual Conference of the Australian Association of Speech and Hearing, Brisbane, Australia.

Zachman, L., Barrett, M., Huisingh, R., Orman, J., & Blagden, C. (1991). Test of problem testing–adolescent. East Moline, IL: LinguiSystems.

Zachman, L., Huisingh, R., Barrett, M., Orman, J., & LoGiudice, C. (1994). Test of problem solving-elementary. East Moline, IL: LinguiSystems.

Informal Assessment of Acquired Childhood Aphasia

Name:

Etiology   Date of Onset

Items	✓	X	Comments/Observations
Yes/No Questions (1) Is your name? (2) Are you a boy/girl? (3) Do you go to . . . school (4) Are you in school now?			
Body Parts (1) Show me your nose (2) Show me your leg (3) Show me your arm (4) Show me your eyes (5) Show me your ears			
Two-Stage Commands (1) Touch your nose and your leg (2) Touch your ear and your arm (3) Close your eyes, and then open your mouth (4) Move your arm, nod your head			
Three-Stage Commands (1) Touch your nose, leg, and arm (2) Touch your eye, leg, and nose (3) Close your eyes, open your mouth, and move your arm			
Matching *Object to Object* chair, bed, bath *Object to Photo* bed, car, table			

Items	✓	X	Comments/Observations
Matching *Photo to Photo* bath, table, chair *Photo to Picture* bed, chair, bath			
Function (1) Which one do you sleep in? (2) Which one do you wash in? (3) Which one do you drive in? (4) Which one do you sit in?			
Size (1) Show me the big chair (2) Point to the small bed (3) Give me the little person (4) Which is the biggest boy?			
Semantic Relations (1) Are you older than your Dad? (2) Are you heavier than a car? (3) Is a plane faster than a motorbike? (4) Do you have lunch before breakfast? (5) Does Christmas come after Easter? (6) The ball was in the cupboard. The cupboard was in the house. Was the ball in the house? (7) Bill came behind John. Who was in front? (8) Mary stood next to June. Was June beside Mary? (9) The lion was chased by the hunter. Who was chased? (10) Daniel was hurt by Tim. Was Tim hurt?			

Items	✓	X	Comments/Observations
Concepts			
(1) Put the girl on the table			
(2) Put the man under the bed			
(3) Put the boy in the box			
(4) Who's under something?			
(5) Who's in something?			
(6) Who's on something?			
Naming			
What's this?			
bed, chair, bath, table, man, car, box, boy			
Semantic cue			
Sentence completion cue			
Phonemic cue			
Function			
What do you do with this?			
bed, chair, bath, table, car, box			
Behavior			
(1) Alert to situation			
(2) Greeting behaviors			
(3) Eye contact			
(4) Appropriate social interaction			
(5) Turn-taking			
(6) Cooperation			
(7) Attention to task			

Materials Required:

Toys—Two of everything matching: kitchen table and chair, lounge chair, bed, bath, car (large enough for a toy person to sit in), box

Photography—Two sets of photographs of the above toys

Pictures—One set of pictures (e.g., from a language test), similar but not the same, of the above toys

Observational Checklist

Language Behaviors	Number	Examples/Comment
Syntax		
In, on, under		
Plural "s"		
ing		
Possessive-s		
Articles		
Regular past-tense		
Contractible copula "be"		
Irregular past		
Regular 3rd person singular -s		
Irregular 3rd person singular -s		
Uncontractible copula "be"		
Contractible auxillary "be"		
Uncontractible auxillary "be"		
Semantics		
Existence		
Nonexistence		
Recurrence		
Rejection		
Denial		
Attribution		
Possession		
Action		
Locative action		
Locative state		
Other:		

Pragmatics	Appropriate	Inappropriate	Comment
Intelligibility			
Fluency			
Prosody			
Facial Expression			
Eye gaze			
Lexical/Specificity/ Accuracy			
Work order			
Ability to take speaker and listener roles			
Maintain topic			
Turn-taking			
Repair/Revision/ Contingency			
Pause time			
(1) Was the message received by the listener?			
General impressions (Comment)			

PART B:

Acquired Motor Speech Disorders in Childhood

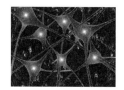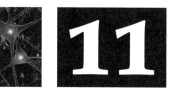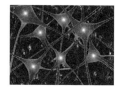

11

Acquired Dysarthria and Apraxia of Speech in Childhood

Introduction

As outlined in Chapter 1, dysarthria and apraxia of speech are both motor speech disorders involving disruption of the processes that occur within the nervous system responsible for the motor control of speech. According to Darley, Aronson, and Brown (1975), the term "dysarthria" is "a collective name for a group of related speech disorders that are due to disturbance in muscular control of the speech mechanism resulting from impairment of any of the basic motor processes involved in the execution of speech" (p. 2). According to this definition, speech disorders resulting from either somatic structural abnormalities (e.g., cleft palate, congenitally enlarged pharynx, malocclusion, etc.) or psychological disorders (e.g., psychogenic aphonia) are not classified as dys-

arthrias. Rather, the term "dysarthria" is used only to describe those speech disorders that result from damage to either the central or peripheral nervous system. The present chapter confines itself to a discussion of acquired neurogenic speech disorders occurring in children as a result of injury to the brain or peripheral nerves following head trauma, cerebrovascular accidents, neoplasms, anoxic episodes, and so forth. Discussion of speech disorders associated with congenital conditions such as cerebral palsy is not included.

Although classified as a motor speech disorder, apraxia of speech differs from dysarthria in several important ways. Whereas in dysarthria the speech disorder results from either paralysis, weakness, or incoordination of the muscles of the speech mechanism, apraxia of speech is a disorder of motor speech programming in which the individual has difficulty speaking because of a cerebral lesion that prevents him or her executing voluntarily, or on command, the complex sequence of muscle contractions involved in speaking. In the apraxic speaker, the muscles of the speech mechanism are neither weak nor paralyzed, as can be demonstrated by the child's ability to carry out movements of the face, tongue, and so forth during reflex activities such as licking the lips to retrieve a crumb. The disorder of motor speech programming is manifest in the child's speech primarily by errors in articulation and secondarily by what are thought by many researchers to be compensatory alterations of prosody (e.g., pauses, slow speech rate, equalization of stress, etc.). Although both developmental and acquired forms of apraxia of speech have been identified, the present chapter deals only with the acquired form of apraxia of speech.

Acquired Childhood Dysarthria

Systemic studies of acquired dysarthria in children are rare. Consequently, traditionally childhood dysarthria has been described and classified according to criteria pertaining to the adult dysarthric population. Despite this trend, it must be remembered that children, depending on age, either are beginning to develop or are still developing speech concurrent with damage to the nervous system. Consequently, unlike adults, motor speech disorders in children are complicated by the interaction between the acquired and developmental components of the disorder (Murdoch & Hudson-Tennant, 1994). The impact of a

congenital or acquired central nervous system lesion on the developmental continuum of speech however is, unclear, as is the contribution of developmental speech patterns to the perceived congenital or acquired dysarthria and to its resolution or progression (Murdoch & Hudson-Tennant, 1994).

Another factor that limits the application of adult findings to pediatric dysarthrias is the difference in recovery potential between the two populations. The potential of the central nervous system to recover from brain trauma sustained at a young age has often been reported as favorable relative to the recovery expected following brain damage in adults (Robinson, 1981). It also is possible that the relationship between site of lesion and the type of dysarthria determined in adults will not be readily applicable to the developing central nervous system. In fact, investigations reported to date that have attempted to associate features of pediatric dysarthria with a lesion site have not proved conclusive (e.g., Bak, van Dongen, & Arts, 1983; Stark, 1985).

The impact of a central nervous system lesion on a child who is still developing adult speech is clearly influenced by a number of variables which are unique to that population. Unfortunately as indicated above, descriptions of the nature and course of specific forms of acquired childhood dysarthria only rarely have been reported (Bak et al., 1983; Murdoch & Hudson-Tennant, 1994). Consequently, the literature on dysarthria in children has little to offer the clinician in either the diagnosis or treatment of these children. Although the difficulty of applying terminology, classification systems and theories developed for adult dysarthria to children, particularly those still developing speech, is acknowledged, until further studies of childhood dysarthria are completed, it appears such terminology, classification systems, and models are all that are currently available to help clinicians in the assessment and treatment of children with dysarthria.

Classification of Acquired Childhood Dysarthria

Childhood dysarthrias are broadly classified as being either acquired or congenital (developmental). Acquired dysarthrias result from some disease or event (e.g., traumatic brain injury, cerebrovascular accident, brain tumor, etc.) that onset during the pediatric period (0 to 15 years of age) but usually following a period of normal speech and language development. In contrast, congenital dysarthrias are associated with diseases present at birth and therefore, are also labeled "developmental dysarthrias." Examples of developmental dysarthrias include those seen with cerebral palsies and with Möbius syndrome.

A variety of different systems have been used to classify the dysarthrias. The more commonly used systems applied to childhood dysarthria include those based on etiology, site of lesion, and pathophysiology. Dwokin and Hartman (1988) presented a dysarthria classification system based on etiology that defined eight different categories of dysarthria including vascular, infectious, traumatic/toxic, anoxic, metabolic, idiopathic, neoplastic, and degenerative/demyelinating. Although devised for classification of adult neurogenic communication disorders, the Dworkin and Hartman (1988) system is also of some use in classifying the causes of childhood dysarthria. A classification system

based on site of lesion was developed by Espir and Rose (1983) for classifying childhood dysarthrias. Their system identified five types of childhood dysarthria including: muscle; lower motor neuron; upper motor neuron; extrapyramidal; and cerebellar dysarthria. The Espir and Rose (1983) system, however, has been criticized for lack of inclusion of a mixed dysarthria classification, as motor systems may be multiply involved in children as they are in adults.

The most widely used system for the classification of dysarthrias, at least with respect to adult disorders, however, has been the neurobehavioral system devised by Darley, Aronson, and Brown (1969a, 1969b). Their system, also known as the Mayo Clinic Classification System, identifies six different types of dysarthria, including: flaccid; spastic; hypokinetic; hyperkinetic; ataxic; and mixed dysarthria. The various speech disorders identified by the Mayo Clinic classification presumably reflect underlying pathophysiology (i.e., spasticity, weakness, etc.) and correlates with the site of lesion in the nervous system. Unfortunately, no such neurobehavioral classification system exists in acquired childhood dysarthria. This is possibly due in part to the relative lack of systematic studies of acquired childhood dysarthria relative to the adult literature. Furthermore, the relatively few pediatric based studies that have been reported have focused either on characterizing the speech behavior with a noticeable lack of attention given to the precise neural basis of the dysarthria, or on the neural basis with little description of the speech characteristics of the disorder. In the absence of a pediatric based system, use of the Mayo Clinic system with childhood dysarthrias was advocated by Murdoch, Ozanne, and

Cross (1990). However, in that the system was devised primarily for adult dysarthrias, some limitations to the application of the Mayo Clinic system to childhood dysarthrias have been identified in the literature. For instance, the Mayo Clinic system identifies a category of dysarthria for disorders either rarely or not seen in children (e.g., Parkinson disease). Furthermore, some authors have suggested that the terms spastic, flaccid, and so forth, which are derived from descriptions of limb and trunk motor disturbances, may not be appropriate for disturbances of oral muscles (Abbs, Hunker, & Barlow, 1983) due to differences in physiologic and neurophysiologic control of the subsystems governing speech movements versus limb movements. van Mourik, Catsman-Berrevoets, Paquier, Yousef-Bak, and van Dongen (1997) appear to have been the first to challenge whether an adult classification system could be validly applied to children.

More recently, Morgan and Liégeois (2010) further questioned the validity of applying an adult diagnostic model to acquired dysarthria in childhood, suggesting that a child-specific diagnostic model would yield more sensitive diagnosis and management. In particular, Morgan and Liégeois (2010) proposed that empirical determination of child-based brain-behavior profiles of acquired childhood dysarthria is contingent on pooling of brain and speech outcome data across large international collaborations. Until such time that empirical speech data are available to enable derivation of a classification system specific to childhood dysarthrias, however, it would seem appropriate that the Mayo Clinic system of classification be used to define dysarthria in children in the same way as it is to define the equivalent speech disorders in adults.

Neuroanatomic and Neuropathologic Substrate of Acquired Childhood Dysarthria

The muscles of the speech mechanism are regulated by nerve impulses originating in the motor cortex that are conveyed to the muscles of the speech mechanism by way of the descending motor pathways. Overall, the control of muscular activity can be considered as if the nervous system involved a series of levels of functional activity in which the higher levels dominate the lower levels.

The lowest level of motor control is provided by the neurons that connect the central nervous system to the skeletal muscle fibers. These neurons, referred to as lower motor neurons, have their cell bodies located in either nuclei in the brainstem (in which case their axons run in the cranial nerves having a motor function) or the anterior horns of gray matter of the spinal cord (in which case their axons run in the various spinal nerves). The lower motor neurons form the only route by which nerve impulses can travel from the central nervous system to cause contraction of the skeletal muscle fibers and, for this reason, are also known as the final common pathway.

The motor areas of the cerebral cortex responsible for the initiation of voluntary muscle activity constitute the highest level of motor control. These areas are responsible for the initiation of voluntary muscle activity and can dominate the lower motor neurons arising from the brainstem and spinal cord, either via the direct descending motor pathways (also called the pyramidal system) or the indirect descending motor pathways (formerly called the extrapyramidal system). [Note: The term "pyramidal system" takes its name from the fact that the majority of the direct connections between the motor areas of the cerebral cortex and the lower motor neurons pass through the pyramids of the medulla oblongata. However, in that some of the direct pathways, namely the corticobulbar and corticomesencephalic tracts (see below) do not pass through the pyramids, the use of the term "extrapyramidal system" to describe the indirect motor pathways has recently been discouraged.] The indirect pathways are so called because they are multisynaptic pathways and involve a multiplicity of connections with various subcortical structures, but particularly with the basal ganglia. The neurons that comprise the direct (pyramidal) and indirect (extrapyramidal) descending motor pathways are collectively referred to as upper motor neurons.

The type of dysarthria manifest as a result of disruption to these descending motor pathways is dependent on the site of the lesion(s) within the central and/or peripheral nervous systems. Lesions causing dysarthria may occur in the motor areas of the cerebral cortex, the cerebellum, basal ganglia system, brainstem or peripheral nervous system. In addition dysarthria can also result from diseases of the neuromuscular junction (e.g., myasthenia gravis) or from diseases of the muscles themselves (e.g., Duchenne muscular dystrophy). The neuropathological substrate and etiologies of the different acquired childhood dysarthrias classified according to the Mayo Clinic classification system are listed in Table 11–1.

Acquired Childhood Dysarthria in Relation to Site of Lesion

On the basis of acoustic-perceptual judgments of speech and neuroanatomical data, Darley et al. (1969a, 1969b) identified six different types of dysarthria in adults including: flaccid, spastic, hypokinetic, hyperkinetic, ataxic, and mixed (e.g., spastic-ataxic dysarthria).

Flaccid Dysarthria (Lower Motor Neuron Dysarthria). Lower motor neurons form the ultimate pathway through which nerve impulses are conveyed from the central nervous system to the skeletal muscles, including the muscles of the speech mechanism. The cell bodies of the lower motor neurons are located in either the anterior horns of the spinal cord or in the motor nuclei of the cranial nerves in the brainstem. From this location, the axons of the lower motor neurons pass via the various spinal and motor cranial nerves of the peripheral nervous system to the voluntary muscles. Lesions of the motor cranial nerves and spinal nerves represent lower motor neuron lesions and interrupt the conduction of nerve impulses from the central nervous system to the muscles. As a consequence, voluntary control of the affected muscles is lost. At the same time, because the nerve impulses necessary for the maintenance of muscle tone are also lost, the muscles involved become flaccid (hypotonic).

In addition to loss of muscle tone, lower motor neuron lesions are characterized by muscle weakness, a loss or reduction of muscle reflexes, atrophy of the muscle involved and fasciculations (spontaneous twitches of individual muscle bundles—fascicles). All or some of these characteristics may be exhibited in the muscles of the speech mechanism in a patient with flaccid dysarthria. In particular, however, the degree of muscle atrophy may show some variability depending on the nature of the underlying neurologic disorder and fasciculations are not manifest in all of the diseases that can cause damage to lower motor neurons.

Table 11–1. Neuropathologic Substrate, Clinical Features, and Etiologies of the Acquired Dysarthrias in Childhood

Type of Dysarthria	Neuropathologic Substrate	Clinical Features	Etiologies
1. FLACCID	Damage to the lower motor neurons supplying speech muscles, their nuclei, neuromuscular junctions, and the muscles they innervate. In particular, damage to cranial nerves V, VII, X, and XII.	MUSCLES: hypotonic, weak, absent or decreased reflexes, atrophy, and fasciculations. SPEECH: nasal emission, hypernasality, monopitch, imprecise consonants, audible respiration, breathiness.	Severe CHI, viral infection (e.g., poliomyelitis), tumors, CVA, or degenerative disorders.
2. SPASTIC	Damage to the upper motor neuron supplying bulbar cranial nerve nuclei. Lesions—cerebral cortex, internal capsule, cerebral peduncles, or brainstem. Bilateral corticobulbar lesions are usually required to cause permanent or severe spastic dysarthria.	MUSCLES: spastic paralysis or paresis, little or no atrophy, weakness, hyperactive muscle stretch reflexes and pathologic reflexes present. SPEECH: imprecise consonants, reduced rate, low pitch, harsh voice, strained-strangled phonation.	Bilateral lesions resulting from: severe CHI, bilateral CVA, multiple sclerosis, motor neuron disease, tumors, congenital disorders, or encephalitis.
3. HYPERKINETIC	Damage to the basal ganglia system (basal ganglia, red nucleus, thalamus, subthalamic nuclei, and substantia nigra.	MUSCLES: abnormal or involuntary muscle contractions (quick or slow), that disturb the rhythm and rate of normal movements. SPEECH: Quick—harsh voice, imprecise consonants, and prolonged intervals. Slow—harsh and strained-strangled voice, monopitch, monoloudness.	Myoclonic jerks—epilepsy, and infectious or toxic disorders of the CNS. Tics—idiopathic Chorea—Huntington disease and Sydenham chorea. Athetosis—disordered development of the brain and birth injury. Dyskinesia—Tardive dyskinesia Dystonia—CHI, toxicity, and encephalitis.

Type of Dysarthria	Neuropathologic Substrate	Clinical Features	Etiologies
4. HYPOKINETIC	Damage to the basal ganglia system. In particular disruption in the dopaminergic pathway of the substantia nigra.	MUSCLES: tremor, rigidity, akinesia, loss of normal postural fixing reflexes. SPEECH: difficulty initiating speech, festination, imprecise consonants, disturbed prosody, reduced loudness, and inappropriate silences.	Hypokinetic dyskinesia, drug-induced parkinsonism, postencephalitic parkinsonism, post-traumatic parkinsonism (caused by CHI).
5. ATAXIC	Damage to the cerebellum and/or its connections.	MUSCLES: Incoordination. Muscles are slow, inaccurate, and irregular. SPEECH: Breakdown in articulatory and prosodic aspects of speech.	Posterior fossa tumors, infections, degenerative disorders, toxic, metabolic and endocrine disorders, and severe CHI.
6. MIXED	Damage to more than one level of the neuromuscular system.	Muscular and speech characteristics are dependent on area of the neuromuscular system that is damaged.	Wilson disease, tumors, inflammatory disease, degenerative disease, CVA, and severe, diffuse CHI.

CVA = Cerebrovascular Accident; CHI = Closed-Head Injury.

Damage to either the lower motor neurons (including those that innervate the respiratory musculature and/or those that run in the cranial nerves to innervate the speech musculature) and/or the muscles of the speech mechanism results in speech changes collectively referred to as flaccid dysarthria, although the term peripheral dysarthria has been used by some authors (Edwards, 1984). The actual name, flaccid dysarthria, is of course derived from the major symptom of lower motor neuron damage, flaccid paralysis. The speech characteristics of each patient with flaccid dysarthria, however, varies depending on which particular nerves are affected and the relative degree of weakness resulting from the damage. In addition to lesions in the lower motor neurons themselves, flaccid dysarthria can also result from either impaired nerve impulse transmission across the neuromuscular junction (such as occurs in myasthenia gravis) or disorders which involve the muscles of the speech mechanism themselves (e.g., muscular dystrophy). The actual lower motor neurons which, if damaged, may be associated with flaccid dysarthria are listed in Table 11–2.

With the exception of the muscles of respiration, the muscles of the speech mechanism are innervated by the motor cranial nerves which arise from the bulbar region (pons and medulla oblongata) of the brainstem. These nerves include cranial nerves V, VII, IX, X, XI, and XII.

Table 11–2. Lower Motor Neurons Associated with Flaccid Dysarthria

Speech Process	Muscle	Site of Cell Body	Nerves Through Which Axons Pass
Respiration	Diaphragm	3rd to 5th cervical segments of spinal cord	Phrenic nerves
	Intercostal and abdominal	1st to 12th thoracic and 1st lumbar segments of the spinal cord	Intercostal nerves. 6th thoracic to 1st lumber spinal nerves
Phonation	Laryngeal muscles	Nucleus ambiguus in medulla oblongata	Vagus nerves (X)
Articulation	Pterygoid, masseter, temporalis, etc.	Motor nucleus of trigeminal in pons	Trigeminal nerves (V)
	Facial expression, e.g., orbicularis oris	Facial nucleus in pons	Facial nerves (VII)
	Tongue muscles	Hypoglossal nucleus in medulla oblongata	Hypoglossal nerves (XII)
Resonation	Levator veli palatini	Nucleus ambiguus in medulla oblongata	Vagus nerves (X)
	Tensor veli palatini	Motor nucleus of trigeminal in pons	Trigeminal nerves (V)

Trigeminal Nerve (V). The trigeminal nerves emerge from the lateral sides of the pons and are the largest of the cranial nerves (Figure 11–1). Each trigeminal nerve is composed of three branches, the ophthalmic branch, the maxillary branch and the mandibular branch. Of the three branches, the ophthalmic and maxillary are both purely sensory, whereas the mandibular is mixed sensory and motor. A large ganglion, the Gasserian ganglion, which is homologous to the dorsal root ganglion of the spinal nerve, is located at the point where the trigeminal nerves divide into three branches.

The ophthalmic branch exits the skull through the superior orbital fissure and provides sensation from the cornea, ciliary body, iris, lacrimal gland, conjunctiva, nasal mucous membrane, and the skin of the eyelid, eyebrow, forehead, and nose. The maxillary branch leaves the skull through the foramen rotundum and supplies sensory fibers to the skin of the cheek, lower eyelid, side of the nose and upper jaw, teeth of the upper jaw, and mucous membrane of the mouth and maxillary sinus.

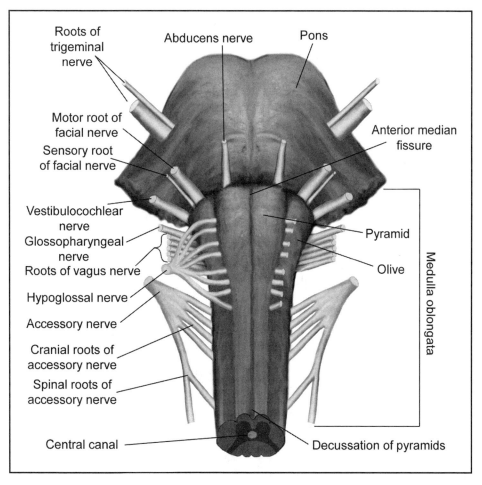

FIGURE 11–1. Anterior view of the pons and medulla oblongata showing the origins of cranial nerves V to XII. [From Murdoch, 2010]

The mandibular branch unites with the motor root immediately after it has exited from the cranial cavity via the foramen ovale. The motor root arises from the motor nucleus of the trigeminal in the pons. Because the trigeminal nerve is mainly sensory, the motor root is much smaller than the sensory portion. Sensory fibers in the mandibular branch provide sensation from the skin of the lower jaw and the temporal region. In the mouth they supply the lower teeth and gums and the mucous membrane covering the anterior two-thirds of the tongue. The motor fibers of the mandibular branch innervate the muscles of mastication which include the temporalis, masseter and medial and lateral pterygoid muscles. In addition, the motor fibers also supply the mylohyoid, anterior belly of the digastric, the tensor veil palatini, and the tensor tympani of the middle ear.

The functioning of the motor portion of the trigeminal nerve can be tested clinically by observing the movements of the mandible. Normally, when the mouth is opened widely, the mandible is depressed in the midline. In unilateral trigeminal lesions, however, the mandible deviates towards the paralyzed side due to the unopposed contraction of the pterygoid muscles on the active side (i.e., the side opposite to the lesion) when the mouth is opened. As a further test of trigeminal function, the masseter and temporalis muscles should be palpated while patients clench their teeth. In patients with unilateral lesions, it is noted that the muscles of mastication on the same side as the lesion will either fail to contract or contract only weakly. Where bilateral trigeminal lesions are present, the muscles of mastication on both sides will undergo flaccid paralysis.

Facial Nerve (VII). Each facial nerve emerges from the lateral aspect of the brainstem at the lower border of the pons, in the ponto-medullary sulcus, in the form of two distinct bundles of fibers of unequal size (see Figure 11–1). The larger more medial bundle arises from the facial nucleus of the pons and carries motor fibers to the muscles of facial expression. The smaller, more lateral bundle, carries autonomic fibers and is known as the nervus intermedius. The two roots run together for a short distance in the posterior cranial fossa to enter the internal auditory meatus in the petrous temporal bone along with the VIIIth nerve (auditory nerve). Within the temporal bone the facial nerve passes through the facial canal and eventually emerges from the skull at the stylomastoid foramen. From here the motor fibers are distributed to the muscles of facial expression including the occipitofrontalis, orbicularis oris, and buccinators. Other muscles supplied by the facial nerve include the stylohyoid and the posterior belly of the digastric. Within the facial canal, a small number of motor fibers are given off to supply the stapedius muscle in the middle ear.

The autonomic fibers pass into two fine branches of the facial nerve which emerge independently from the temporal bone. One of these is the chorda tympani, which exits the skull via the petro-tympanic fissure to join the lingual nerve, a branch of the mandibular division of the trigeminal nerve. The lingual nerve delivers the fibers of chorda tympani to the submandibular ganglion. Here they synapse with postganglionic neurons which pass to the submandibular and sublingual salivary glands. The chorda tympani also conveys taste sensation from the anterior two-thirds of the tongue. The second small branch which carries autonomic fibers supplies the lacrimal gland in the orbit and is known as the greater petrosal nerve.

The motor portion of the facial nerve is tested by observing the patient's face, both at rest and during the performance of a variety of facial expressions such as pursing the lips, smiling, corrugating the forehead, blowing out the cheeks, showing the teeth, and closing the eyes against resistance. Normally, all facial movements should be equal bilaterally. Unilateral facial nerve lesions cause weakness or paralysis of the half of the face on the same side as the lesion. At rest, the face of patients with unilateral flaccid paralysis of the muscles of facial expression appears to be asymmetric. The mouth on the affected side droops below that on the unaffected side and saliva may constantly drool from the corner. In addition, due to loss of muscle tone in the orbicularis oris muscle, the lower eyelid may droop causing the palpebral fissure on the affected side to be somewhat wider than on the normal side. When the patient smiles, the mouth is retracted on the active side but not on the affected side. Likewise, when asked to frown, the frontalis muscle on the contralateral side will corrugate the forehead, however, on the side ipsilateral to the lesion, no corrugation will occur.

In bilateral facial nerve paralysis, as might occur in Möbius syndrome, saliva may drool from both corners of the mouth. The seal produced by compression of the lips may be so weak that the patient cannot puff out their cheeks and the lips may be slightly parted at rest.

Glossopharyngeal Nerve (IX). Each glossopharyngeal nerve arises from the medulla oblongata as a series of rootlets at the upper end of the postolivary sulcus. The IXth nerve leaves the cranial cavity via the jugular foramen along with the vagus and the accessory nerves.

The glossopharyngeal nerve contains both sensory and motor as well as autonomic fibers. The motor fibers arise from the nucleus ambiguus and innervate the stylopharyngeus muscle. The sensory fibers provide sensation from the pharynx, the posterior one-third of the tongue, the fauces, tonsils, and soft palate. They also carry the sense of taste from the posterior one-third of the tongue.

The autonomic fibers within the IXth nerve pass to the otic ganglion where they synapse with postganglionic neurons which in turn regulate secretion from the parotid salivary gland.

Vagus Nerve (X). Each vagus nerve arises from the lateral surface of the medulla oblongata by numerous rootlets which lie immediately inferior to those which give rise to the glossopharyngeal nerve. It then leaves the cranial cavity via the jugular foramen.

The vagus nerve contains sensory, motor and autonomic fibers and is the only cranial nerve to venture beyond the confines of the head and neck, supplying structures within the thorax and the upper parts of the abdominal cavity.

After emerging from the jugular foramen, the vagus receives additional motor fibers from the cranial portion of the accessory nerve. The motor fibers of the vagus arise from the nucleus ambiguus and in combination with those from the accessory nerve, supply the muscles of the pharynx, larynx, and the levator veli palatini, and musculus uvulae of the soft palate. The first branch of the vagus nerve important for speech is the pharyngeal nerve which supplies the levator muscles of the soft palate. As the vagus descends in the neck it gives off a second branch, the superior laryngeal nerve, which supplies the cricothyroid muscle (the chief tensor muscle of the vocal folds). At a lower level in the neck, a third branch is given off, the recurrent laryngeal nerve, which supplies all of the intrinsic muscles of the larynx except for the cricothyroid and is, therefore, responsible for regulating adduction of the vocal folds for phonation and abduction of the vocal folds for unvoiced phonemes and inspiration.

Prior to entering the larynx, the left recurrent laryngeal nerve descends into the thorax, loops under the aortic arch and then ascends along the lateral aspects of the trachea to enter the larynx from below and behind the left cricothyroid joint. The right recurrent laryngeal nerve enters the larynx at the equivalent point on the right side but descends in the neck only as far as the right subclavian artery before commencing its ascent to the larynx. Looping of the left recurrent laryngeal nerve under the aortic arch makes it vulnerable to compression by intrathoracic masses (e.g., lung tumors) and aortic arch aneurysms.

The autonomic component of the vagus supplies organs in the thorax and abdomen including the heart, lungs, major airways and blood vessels and the upper part of the gastro-intestinal system.

Functioning of the vagus nerve can be easily checked clinically by noting: (1) the quality of the patient's voice; (2) their ability to swallow; and (3) the position and movements of the soft palate at rest and during phonation. Unilateral vagus nerve lesions cause paralysis of the ipsilateral vocal fold leading to dysphonia. The paralyzed vocal fold can be neither abducted nor adducted. By asking patients to open their mouth and say /ah/, movements of the soft palate can be observed. Normally, the uvula and soft palate rise in the midline during phonation. However, unilateral lesions of the vagus nerve cause the palate to deviate to the contralateral side (the side opposite to the lesion) during phonation. In addition, the distance between the soft palate and the posterior pharyngeal wall is less on the paralyzed side and the arch of the palate at rest will droop on the side of the lesion.

In bilateral lesions of the vagus nerves, both sides of the soft palate and vocal folds may be paralyzed. Both sides of the soft palate rest at a lower level than normal, although their symmetry at rest may appear normal to inexperienced clinicians. However, despite the apparent symmetry, there is less space under the arches of the soft palate and the curvature is flatter. The extent of movement on phonation is reduced and in severe cases, the palate may not rise at all. When observed by either direct or indirect laryngoscopy, abduction and adduction of both vocal folds is severely impaired.

Accessory Nerve (XI). There are two parts to each accessory nerve, a cranial portion that arises from the nucleus ambiguus in the medulla oblongata and a spinal portion that arises from the first five segments of the cervical region of the spinal cord (see Figure 11–1). The cranial accessory emerges from the lateral part of the medulla oblongata in the form of four to five rootlets immediately below those that form the vagus nerve. Prior to leaving the cranial cavity via the jugular foramen, the cranial accessory is joined by the spinal accessory to form the accessory nerve. The spinal accessory fibers arise from the anterior horns of the first five cervical segments of the spinal cord. These fibers emerge from the lateral parts of the spinal cord and unite to form a single nerve trunk which ascends alongside the spinal cord and enters the skull through the foramen magnum to join the cranial accessory.

After exiting through the skull, the cranial accessory leaves the spinal accessory and joins the vagus nerve and is distributed by that nerve to provide motor supply to the muscles of the pharynx, larynx, musculus uvulae, and levator veli palatini muscles. The spinal accessory on the other hand, provides the motor supply to the trapezius muscle and the upper portion of the sternocleidomastoid muscle.

Disorders of the cranial accessory are recognized clinically as disorders of the vagus nerve while disorders of the spinal accessory are evident in atrophy and paralysis of the trapezius and sternocleidomastoid muscles.

Hypoglossal Nerve (XII). Each hypoglossal nerve arises from motor cells in the hypoglossal nucleus and emerge from the medulla oblongata as a series of rootlets in the groove that separates the pyramid and olive. The nerves leave the cranial cavity via the hypoglossal canal which lies in the margin of the foramen magnum.

The hypoglossal nerves provide the motor supply to the muscles of the tongue. Tongue muscles can be divided into two groups, the intrinsic muscles, which lie entirely within the substance of the tongue and are responsible for changes in its shape, and the extrinsic muscles. The latter muscles are attached at one end to structures outside the tongue and are responsible for moving the tongue within the mouth. The hypo-

glossal nerves innervate all of the tongue muscles with exception of the palatoglossus. Other muscles in the region of the neck also supplied by the hypoglossal nerves include the sternohyoid, sternothyroid, inferior belly of the omohyoid, and the geniohyoid muscles.

Functioning of the hypoglossal nerves can be tested by observing the tongue at rest and during movement. Unilateral hypoglossal nerve damage is associated with atrophy and fasciculations in the ipsilateral side of the tongue. When observed in the mouth the tongue on the side of the lesion may appear smaller and the surface corrugated, indicative of atrophy. Fasciculation of the tongue in some cases may be the earliest sign of lower motor neuron disease. When the patients are asked to protrude their tongue, it will deviate to the paralyzed side. Another test for weakness of the tongue is to have patients press their tongue against their cheek while the examiner presses against the bulging cheek with the hand.

In bilateral hypoglossal involvement, both sides of the tongue may be atrophied and show fasciculations. Although protrusion occurs in the midline, the degree of protrusion may be severely limited by weakness and in the more severe cases the patient may not be able to extend the tongue far beyond the lower teeth. Elevation of the tip and body to contact the alveolar ridge or hard palate may be difficult or impossible.

Neurologic Disorders Associated with Lower Motor Neuron Lesions in Children. The lower motor neurons that innervate the muscles involved in speech production can be damaged by a variety of neurologic diseases, including viral infections (e.g., poliomyelitis), tumors, cerebrovascular accidents (e.g., embolization resulting from congenital heart disease), degenerative disorders and traumatic head injury. The general name applied to flaccid paralysis of the muscles supplied by nerves arising from the bulbar regions of the brainstem (which, with the exception of the respiratory muscles, include the muscles of the speech mechanism) is bulbar palsy. Bulbar palsy can be caused by pathologic conditions that affect either the cell body of the lower motor neurons in the cranial nerve nuclei or the axon of the lower motor neuron as it courses through the peripheral nerve. In particular, damage to cranial nerves V (trigeminal), VII (facial), X (vagus), and XII (hypoglossal) in their peripheral course can lead to flaccid dysarthria.

Trigeminal Nerve Disorders. The trigeminal nerves supply the muscles of mastication (temporalis, masseter, pterygoids) which in turn regulate the movement of the mandible. In children with unilateral trigeminal lesions, the mandible deviates toward the paralyzed side when a child is asked to open his or her mouth widely. This deviation is brought about by the unopposed contraction of the pterygoid muscles on the active side (i.e., the side opposite to the lesion). In addition, the child will show a loss or reduction of muscle tone and atrophy in the muscles of mastication on the side of the lesion. Only minor alterations in speech occur, however, as a result of unilateral trigeminal lesions, in that movements of the mandible are impaired to only a small extent. A much more devastating effect on speech occurs following bilateral trigeminal lesions, the muscles responsible for the elevation of the mandible being too weak in many cases to approximate the man-

dible and maxilla. This inability, in turn, may prevent the tongue and lips from making the necessary contacts with oral structures for the production of labial and lingual consonants and vowels. Unilateral trigeminal lesions in children may result from traumatic head injury and brainstem tumors involving the pons. Bilateral flaccid paralysis of the masticatory muscles, on the other hand, may be seen in bulbar poliomyelitis.

Facial Nerve Disorders. The muscles of facial expression (e.g., orbicularis oris, buccinators, etc.) are supplied by the facial nerves. Unilateral facial nerve lesions cause flaccid paralysis of the muscles of facial expression on the same side as the lesion. Consequently, children with such lesions present with drooping of the mouth on the affected side and saliva may constantly dribble from the corner. In addition, as a result of loss of muscle tone in the orbicularis oculi muscle, the lower eyelid may also droop. During smiling the mouth is retracted on the active side but not on the child's affected side. Likewise, during frowning, the frontalis muscle on the side contralateral to the lesion will corrugate the forehead; however, on the side ipsilateral to the lesion no corrugation will occur. In cases of bilateral facial nerve paralysis, saliva may drool from both corners of the mouth and the lips may be slightly parted at rest.

Both unilateral and bilateral facial nerve lesions affect speech production. Children with facial nerve lesions are unable to seal their lips tightly and during speech air escapes between their lips during the buildup of intraoral pressure. Consequently, unilateral facial nerve lesions cause distortion of bilabial and labiodental consonants. Speech impairments associated with bilateral facial nerve lesions range from distortion to complete obliteration of bilabial and labiodental consonants.

A number of different acquired disorders can cause malfunctioning of the facial nerves in children. In some cases the facial palsy may have an idiopathic origin, such as in Bell palsy. Bell palsy usually causes unilateral facial paralysis. Prognostically, in the region of 80% of Bell palsy cases recover in a few days or weeks. Unilateral facial paralysis can also result from closed-head injuries, damage to one or other facial nerve during the course of a forceps delivery, compression of the facial nerve by tumor (e.g., acoustic neuroma) and damage to the facial nucleus by brainstem tumors (e.g., glioma).

Bilateral facial paralysis may occur in idiopathic polyneuritis (Guillain-Barré syndrome). In addition, sarcoidosis, bulbar poliomyelitis and some forms of basal meningitis may also cause facial diplegia as can some congenital disorders such as congenital hypoplasia of the nuclei of the VIIth and VIth cranial nerves (Möbius syndrome).

Vagus Nerve Disorders. Among other structures, the vagus nerves supply the muscles of the larynx and the levator muscles of the soft palate. Lesions of the vagus nerves, therefore, can affect either the phonatory or resonatory aspects of speech production or both, depending upon the location of the lesion along the nerve pathway. Lesions that involve the nucleus ambiguus in the medulla (as occurs in lateral medullary syndrome following occlusion of the posterior inferior cerebellar artery) or the vagus nerve near to the brainstem (e.g., in the region of the

jugular foramen) cause paralysis of all the skeletal muscles supplied via the vagus. Children with this type of lesion present with a flaccid dysphonia characterized by moderate breathiness, harshness, and reduced volume. Other voice problems that also may be present include diplophonia, short phrases, and inhalatory stridor. These voice abnormalities result from paralysis of the vocal fold on the side of the lesion which tends to lie in a slightly abducted position. In addition to the voice problem, these children also present with hypernasality due to paralysis of the soft palate on the affected side.

Lesions of the vagus which involve the nerve at a point distal to the exit of the pharyngeal nerve (which supplies the levator of the soft palate) but proximal to the exit of the superior laryngeal nerve, have the same effect on phonation as brainstem lesions. These lesions, however, do not cause hypernasality since the functioning of the levator veli palatini is not compromised. In those cases where the recurrent laryngeal nerve is involved, dysphonia in the absence of hypernasality is also present. In these latter cases, however, the cricothyroid muscles (the principal tensor muscles of the vocal folds) are not affected and the vocal folds are paralyzed closer to the midline (the paramedian position). Consequently, although the voice is likely to be harsh and reduced in loudness, there is likely a lesser degree of the breathiness than is seen in those children with brainstem lesions involving the nucleus ambiguus. The recurrent laryngeal nerve can be injured during surgery to the neck (e.g., thyroidectomy) or occasionally during chest surgery, especially on the left side where the nerve loops around the aortic arch. Bilateral damage to the recurrent laryngeal nerves is rare.

Hypoglossal Nerve Disorders. With the exception of the palatoglossus, all the extrinsic and all the intrinsic muscles of the tongue are controlled by the hypoglossal nerves. Unilateral hypoglossal nerve damage therefore, as might occur in either brainstem conditions such as medial medullary syndrome or peripheral nerve lesions such as submaxillary tumors that compress one or other hypoglossal nerves, is associated with flaccid paralysis, atrophy, and fasciculations in the ipsilateral side of the tongue. On protrusion, the tongue deviates to the affected side.

In bilateral hypoglossal involvement, both sides of the tongue may be atrophied and show fasciculations. Although in this case protrusion occurs in the midline, the degree of protrusion may be severely limited. In addition, elevation of the tip and body to contact the alveolar ridge or hard palate may be difficult or impossible.

Although both phonation and resonation remain normal, lesions of the hypoglossal nerves therefore cause disturbances in articulation by interfering with normal tongue movement. The articulatory imprecision occurs especially during production of linguodental and linguopalatal consonants. In the case of unilateral lesions the articulatory imprecision may be temporary in that most patients learn to compensate for unilateral tongue weakness within a few days. More serious articulatory impairments, however, are associated with bilateral hypoglossal nerve lesions. As indicated above, tongue movement in such cases may be severely restricted and speech sounds such as high front vowels and consonants that require ele-vation of the tongue tip to contact the upper alveolar ridge or hard palate (e.g., /t/, /d/, /l/, etc.) may be grossly distorted.

Hypoglossal nerve lesions are rare in children and more commonly result from damage to the hypoglossal nucleus in the brainstem than from damage to the peripheral nerve itself. Some isolated cases of damage to the hypoglossal nerve are seen as the result of the child falling with something (usually a pencil) in their mouth.

Multiple Cranial Nerve Disorders. In addition to individual damage to each of the bulbar cranial nerves, flaccid dysarthria can also result from simultaneous damage to a number of cranial nerves. For example, lesions in the region of the jugular foramen (the exit point of the IXth, Xth, and XIth nerves) can cause the concurrent dysfunctioning of the pharynx, soft palate, and larynx. The nerves passing through the jugular foramen can be affected by disorders such as tumors with the jugular foramen (i.e., glomus jugulare tumors), metastases involving the base of the skull and sarcoidosis.

Spastic Dysarthria (Upper Motor Neuron Dysarthria). The term "spastic dysarthria" was first used by Darley et al. (1969a, 1969b) to describe the speech disturbance seen in association with damage to the upper motor neurons that convey nerve impulses from the motor areas of the cerebral cortex to the lower motor neurons originating from the bulbar cranial nerve nuclei. The lesions associated with spastic dysarthria can involve either the cortical motor areas from which the descending motor pathways originate (primarily the precentral gyrus and premotor cortex) or the descending tracts themselves as they pass through the internal capsule, cerebral peduncles or the brainstem. The speech characteristics of spastic dysarthria are presumed to reflect the effects of hypertonicity (spasticity) and weakness of the bulbar musculature in a way that slows movement and reduces its range and force (Murdoch, Thompson, & Theodoros, 1997). The reference to "spastic" in the term "spastic dysarthria" is therefore a reflection of the clinical signs of upper motor neuron damage which include: spastic paralysis or paresis of the involved muscles; hyperreflexia (e.g., hyperactive jaw-jerk); little or no muscle atrophy (except for the possibility of some atrophy associated with disuse); and the presence of pathologic reflexes (e.g., sucking reflex). One of the basic features of upper motor neuron lesions is that reflex arcs remain anatomically intact, whereas in lower motor neuron lesions the reflex arc is disrupted and reflexes become absent or diminished. Table 11–3 compares the major signs associated with upper versus lower motor neuron lesions.

Neuroanatomy of the Upper Motor Neuron System. The two major components comprise the upper motor neu-

ron system, including a direct and an indirect component. The direct component, also known as the pyramidal system, is comprised of neurons that project their axons from their cell bodies located in the cortical motor areas directly to the level of the lower motor neurons without synapsing along the way. In contrast, the indirect component (previously referred to as the extrapyramidal system) involves multisynaptic pathways that originate from the motor cortex but then pass to the level of the lower motor neurons via multisynaptic connections that involve structures such as the basal ganglia, various brainstem nuclei, the reticular formation, cerebellum, and thalamus. For instance, many of the extrapyramidal fibers descend from the motor cortex in the internal capsule and cerebral peduncles to the pons and then are relayed to the cerebellum from which projections then pass to either the brainstem or back of the cerebral cortex via the thalamus. Many other extrapyramidal fibers descend from the motor cortex via the internal capsule to the basal ganglia where they are relayed by a variety of pathways to the excitatory and inhibitory centers of the brainstem. Overall, the extrapyramidal system is said to comprise all of

Table 11–3. Clinical Signs of Upper and Lower Motor Neuron Lesions

Upper Motor Neuron Lesions	Lower Motor Neuron Lesions
• Hypertonus (spasticity)	• Hypotonus (flaccidity)
• Mild atrophy of disuse	• Atrophy of individual muscles
• Hyperactive muscle stretch reflexes (e.g. jaw-jerk)	• Muscle stretch reflexes decreased or absent
• Positive sucking reflex	• Negative sucking reflex
• Positive Babinski sign	• Negative Babinski sign

those tracts, besides the pyramidal system, that transmit motor signals from the cortical motor areas to the lower motor neurons. The final pathways for transmission of extrapyramidal signals to the lower motor neurons include the vestibulospinal tracts, the tectospinal tracts, the rubospinal tracts, and the reticulospinal tracts (Figure 11–2).

The extrapyramidal system appears to be primarily responsible for postural arrangements and the orientation of movement in space, whereas the pyramidal system is chiefly responsible for controlling the far more discrete and skilled voluntary aspects of a movement.

Because in most locations (e.g., internal capsule) the two systems lie in close anatomical proximity, lesions that affect one component usually will also involve the other component. The term "upper motor neuron lesion" usually is not applied to disorders affecting only the extrapyramidal system (e.g., in basal ganglia lesions). Such disorders are termed "extrapyramidal syndromes" and are discussed further below.

The Pyramidal System. Based on their projections to either the spinal cord, midbrain or bulbar region of the brainstem, three major fiber groups are

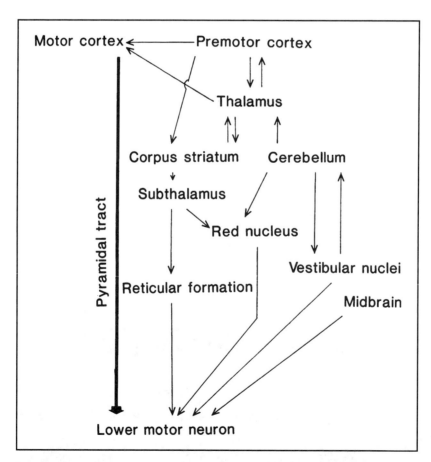

FIGURE 11–2. Schematic diagram of the direct (pyramidal) and indirect (extrapyramidal) motor pathways. [From Murdoch, 2010]

recognized as comprising the pyramidal system. These groups include: the corticospinal tracts (pyramidal tracts proper), the cortico mesencephalic tracts and the corticobulbar tracts.

The corticospinal tracts descend from the cerebral cortex to various levels of the spinal cord where they synapse with lower motor neurons. Although the greatest proportion of fibers arise from the motor cortex (primarily the precentral gyrus), the corticospinal tracts originate from both the motor and sensory areas of the cerebral cortex. The corticospinal tract in each cerebral hemisphere enters the subcortical white matter from the cortex in a fan-shaped distribution of fibers called corona radiata (radiating crown). The common central mass of white matter in each cerebral hemisphere which contains commissural, association, and projection fibers and into which the pyramidal fibers pass, has an oval appearance in horizontal sections of the brain and, therefore, is called the centrum semiovale. From the corona radiata the fibers of the corticospinal tracts converge into the posterior limb of the internal capsule and then pass via the cerebral peduncles of the midbrain to the pons. As the fibers of the corticospinal tracts are closely grouped together as they pass through the internal capsule, even small lesions in this area can have a devasting effect on the motor control of the limbs on one half of the body. After traversing the pons, the fibers group together to form the pyramids of the medulla oblongata. It is from the pyramids that the term "pyramidal tracts" is derived. Near to the junction of the medulla oblongata and the spinal cord, the majority (85 to 90%) of the fibers in each pyramid cross to the opposite side, interlacing as they do so and forming the decussation of the pyramids. It is the crossing that provides the contralateral motor control of the limbs, the motor cortex controlling movement of the right limbs and vice versa. The fibers that cross then descend in the lateral funiculus of the spinal cord as the lateral corticospinal tracts. Of those fibers that remain uncrossed, most descend in the ventral funiculus as the anterior corticospinal tracts. Most of these latter fibers descussate to the opposite side further down the spinal cord.

The corticomesencephalic tracts are comprised of fibers which descend from the cerebral cortex to the nuclei of cranial nerves III, IV, and VI which provided the motor supply to the extrinsic muscles of the eye. These fibers arise from the fontal eye field which is that part of the cerebral cortex of the frontal lobe that lies immediately anterior to the premotor cortex.

The fibers of the corticobulbar tracts start out in company with those of the corticospinal tracts but take a divergent route at the level of the midbrain. They terminate by synapsing with lower motor neurons in the nuclei of cranial nerves V, VII, IX, X, and XII. For this reason, they form the most important component of the pyramidal system in relation to the occurrence of spastic dysarthria. Although the majority of corticobulbar fibers cross to the contralateral side, uncrossed (ipsilateral) connections also exist. In fact, most of the motor nuclei of the cranial nerves in the brainstem receive bilateral upper motor neuron connections. Consequently, although to a varying degree the predominance of upper motor neuron innervation to the cranial nerve nuclei comes from the contralateral hemisphere, in most instances there is also considerable ipsilateral upper motor neuron innervation.

One important exception to the above upper motor neuron innervation of the cranial nerve nuclei is that part of the facial nucleus that gives rise to the lower motor neurons that supply the lower half of the face. It appears to receive only a contralateral upper motor neuron connection (Sears & Franklin, 1980; Snell, 1980). (Figure 11–3).

Clinically, the presence of a bilateral innervation to most cranial nerve nuclei has important implications for the type of speech disorder that follows unilateral upper motor neuron lesions. Although a mild and usually transient impairment in articulation may occur subsequent to unilateral corticobulbar lesions, in general bilateral corticobulbar lesions are required to produce a permanent dysarthria.

Unilateral upper motor neuron lesions located in either the motor cortex or internal capsule, and so forth cause a spastic paralysis or weakness in the contra-lateral lower half of the face but not the upper part of the face which may be associated with a mild, transient dysarthria due to weakness of orbicularis oris. There is no weakness of the forehead, muscles of mastication, soft palate (i.e., no hypernasality), pharynx (i.e., no swallowing problems), or larynx (i.e., no dysphonia). A unilateral motor neuron lesion however, may, pro-

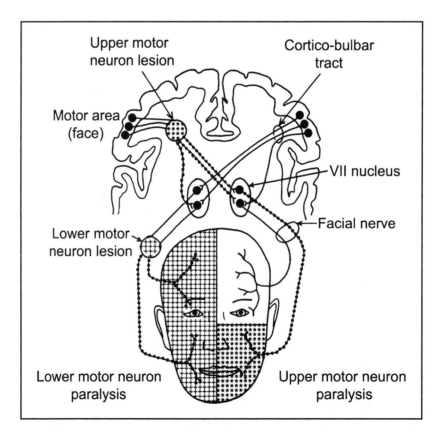

FIGURE 11–3. The effects of unilateral disruption to the upper and lower motor neuron supply to the muscles of facial expression. [From Murdoch, 2010]

duce a mild unilateral weakness of the tongue on the side opposite the lesion. In the case of such a unilateral lesion it appears, therefore, that the ipsilateral upper neuron is adequate to maintain near formal function of most bulbar muscles, except those in the tongue. Although most authors agree that the hypoglossal nucleus receives bilateral upper motor neuron innervation, for some reason, the ipsilateral connection appears to be less effective than in the case of other cranial nerve nuclei. Snell (1980) suggested that the part of the hypoglossus nucleus that supplies the genioglossus muscle (the only muscle that can protrude the tongue) receives upper motor neuron innervation from only the contralateral cerebral hemisphere.

Clinical Features of Spastic Dysarthria.

To date, systematic studies of spastic dysarthria in children are lacking. Consequently, in order to predict the potential effects of disruption to the upper motor neurons on speech in childhood, it is necessary to turn to reports of the clinical features of spastic dysarthria based on examination of adult cases.

Darley et al. (1975) identified four major symptoms of muscular dysfunction subsequent to disruption of the upper motor neuron supply to the speech musculature in adults that reflect in the speech output: spasticity, weakness, limited range of movement, and slowness of movement. Consequently, these physiologic features are characteristically identified as the underlying basis of the majority of the deviant speech behaviors observed in individuals with spastic dysarthria, a condition characterized by slow, dragging, labored speech that is produced with some effort. The most prominent perceptible speech devi-

ations reported to be associated with spastic dysarthria include: imprecise consonants, monopitch, reduced stress, harsh voice quality, monoloudness, low pitch, slow rate, hypernasality, strained-strangled voice quality, short phrases, distorted vowels, pitch breaks, continuous breathy voice, and excess and equal stress (Darley et al., 1969b). The deviant speech characteristics cluster primarily into the areas of articulatory/resonatory incompetence, phonatory stenosis, and prosodic insufficiency.

Neurologic Disorders Associated with Upper Motor Neuron Lesions in Children.

Persistent spastic dysarthria is caused by bilateral disruptor of the upper motor neuron supply to the bulbar cranial nerve nuclei. Lesions of upper motor neurons that can cause dysarthria may be located in the cerebral cortex, the internal capsule, the cerebral peduncles or the brainstem. Clinical signs of upper motor neuron lesions include: spastic paralysis or paresis of the involved muscles, little or no muscle atrophy, hyperactive muscle stretch reflexes (e.g., hyperactive jaw-jerk) and the presence of pathologic reflexes (e.g., positive Babinski sign, positive rooting reflex, etc.).

In the majority of the cranial nerve nuclei receive a bilateral upper motor neuron innervation, in general bilateral corticobulbar lesions are required to produce a permanent and severe spastic dysarthria. Usually, only a transient impairment in articulation occurs subsequent to unilateral corticobulbar lesions. Such lesions cause a spastic paralysis or weakness in the contralateral lower half of the face, but not the upper part of the face, which may be associated with a mild, transient dysarthria due to weakness of the orbicularis oris. There is, however, no weakness of the forehead, muscles of mastication, soft palate (therefore no hypernasality), pharynx (therefore no swallowing problems), or larynx (therefore no dysphonia). In addition to the lower facial weakness, however, unilateral upper motor neuron lesions may produce a mild weakness of the tongue on the side opposite the lesion.

The general name given to spastic paralysis of the bulbar musculature as a result of bilateral upper motor neuron lesions is pseudobulbar palsy (supranuclear palsy). Pseudobulbar palsy, which takes its name from its clinical resemblance to bulbar palsy, may be associated with a variety of neurologic disorders that bilaterally affect the upper motor neurons anywhere from their cell bodies, located in the motor cortex, through to their synapses with the appropriate lower motor neurons. Bilateral cerebrovascular accidents, multiple sclerosis, motor neuron disease, extensive neoplasms, congenital disorders, encephalitis, and severe brain trauma are all possible causes of this syndrome. All aspects of speech production, including phonation, resonation, articulation, and respiration are affected in pseudobulbar palsy, but to varying degrees. Overall, pseudobulbar palsy is characterized by features such as bilateral facial paralysis, dysphagia, hypophonia, bilateral hemiparesis, incontinence, and bradykinesia.

Hypoxic ischemic encephalopathy is the most common cause of spastic dysarthria in childhood. In most cases this is associated with intrapartum asphyxia, although severe anoxic brain damage at any stage can cause the same disorder. Brainstem ischemia with infarction resulting from embolization in association with congenital heart disease can also cause pseudobulbar palsy in children (as it can bulbar palsy).

Spastic dysarthria may also be seen in children who have suffered head injuries with elevated intracranial pressure and a midbrain or upper brainstem shearing injury (as a result of a deceleration/acceleration type of injury). Although a common cause of pseudobulbar palsy in adolescents and young adults, disseminated sclerosis is not a common cause of spastic dysarthria in prepubertal children. Degenerative disorders, such as metachromatic leukodystrophy can also cause childhood pseudobulbar palsy.

Dysarthria Associated with Extrapyramidal Syndromes. The term "extrapyramidal system" was first used by Wilson (1912) to refer to those parts of the central nervous system concerned with motor function but which are not a part of the pyramidal system. The extrapyramidal system, as described above, consists of a complex series of multisynaptic pathways which indirectly connect the motor areas of the cerebral cortex to the level of the lower motor neurons. The major components of the extrapyramidal system include the basal ganglia (Figure 11–4) within the cerebral hemispheres plus the various brainstem nuclei that contribute to motor functioning. These latter nuclei include the paired substantia nigra, the red nuclei, and the subthalamic nuclei.

Diseases that selectively affect the extrapyramidal system without involving the pyramidal pathways are referred to as "extrapyramidal syndromes" and include a number of clinically defined disease states of diverse etiology and often obscure pathogenesis. Extrapyramidal syndromes share a number of related symptoms and the major pathologic changes noted in these disorders are located within the various extrapyramidal nuclei. Movement disorders are the

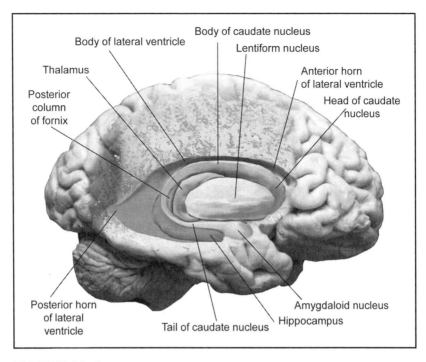

FIGURE 11–4. Lateral view of the right cerebral hemisphere dissected to show the position of the different basal ganglia. [From Murdoch, 2010]

primary features of the extrapyramidal syndromes and, where the muscles of the speech mechanism are involved, disorders of speech may occur. The clinical signs and symptoms that characterize extrapyramidal syndromes and help tie these various disorders together fall into the following four groups: (1) hypokinesia (akinesia)—slowness and poverty of spontaneous movement; (2) hyperkinesia—abnormal involuntary movements; (3) rigidity of the muscles; and (4) loss of normal postural reactions.

Overall, the extrapyramidal system appears to control muscle tone for the maintenance of posture and for supporting movements (i.e., those muscle actions which provide a firm base of support against which skilled voluntary acts can take place).

As in the case of movement disorders of basal ganglia origin affecting limb and trunk muscles, dysarthrias associated with lesions in the basal ganglia take the form of hypo- and hyperkinetic movement disorders. In general, hypokinetic disorders (e.g., Parkinson disease) are associated with increased basal ganglia output, whereas hyperkinetic movement disorders (e.g., Huntington disease) are associated with decreased output. Hypokinetic disorders are characterized by significant impairments in movement initiation (akinesia) and reduction in the velocity of voluntary movements (bradykinesia) and are usually accompanied by muscular rigidity and tremor at rest. By contrast, hyperkinetic disorders are characterized by excessive motor activity in the form of involuntary movements (dyskinesia) with varying degrees of hypotonia. With regard to their effect on the speech production mechanism, these disorders manifest as hypokinetic dysarthria (classically associated with Parkinson disease) and hyperkinetic dysarthria (seen in association with a range of hyperkinetic conditions such as Huntington disease, dystonia, etc.).

Hypokinetic Dysarthria in Childhood. The term "hypokinetic dysarthria" was first used by Darley et al. (1969a, 1969b) to describe the resultant complex pattern of perceptual speech characteristics associated with Parkinson's disease. Parkinsonism occurs most commonly in persons in their 50s and 60s. However, a syndrome which, like idiopathic Parkinson disease in adults, is associated with either a reduced level of dopamine in the substantia nigra or blockage of the dopamine receptors in the basal ganglia, also occurs in childhood. This syndrome is referred to as hypokinetic dyskinesia. In addition, a number of other conditions also predispose to the occurrence of Parkinson disease in childhood. Drug-induced parkinsonism, for instance, can occur at all ages and subacute meningitis, such as that seen in association with measles may also present with a Parkinsonian-like picture. Furthermore, in past years, postencephalitic parkinsonism secondary to epidemic encephalitis was common in children.

Overall, the speech characteristics associated with hypokinetic dysarthria follow largely from the generalized pattern of hypokinetic movement disorders, which includes marked reductions in the amplitude of voluntary movement (akinesia), initiation difficulties, slowness of movement (bradykinesia), muscular rigidity, tremor at rest, and postural reflex impairments. Although impairments in all aspects of speech production (i.e., respiration, phonation, resonance, articulation, and prosody) involving the various subsystems of the speech production mechanism have been identified in adults with hypokinetic dysarthria, these individuals are most likely to exhibit disturbances of prosody, phonation, and articulation. According to Darley et al. (1975) features of the speech disorder seen in adult Parkinson patients include: difficulty in initiating speech, once speech is started the speech becomes faster (festinant speech), reduced loudness, variable speech rate between subjects, some patients speaking at a slower than normal rate and others speaking at a slightly faster than normal rate, and disturbed prosody (e.g., monopitch, reduced stress, monoloudness).

Hyperkinetic Dysarthria in Childhood. A variety of extrapyramidal disorders may cause hyperkinetic dysarthria. Each of these disorders is characterized by the presence of abnormal involuntary muscle contractions of the limbs, trunk, neck, face, and so forth which disturb the rhythm and rate of normal, motor activities, including those involved in speech production. The major extrapyramidal disorders that cause hyperkinetic dysarthria include myoclonic jerks, tics, chorea, athetosis, dyskinesia, and dystonia. The abnormal involuntary movements involved vary considerably in their form and locus across the different diseases of the basal ganglia. Consequently, there is considerable heterogeneity in the deviant speech dimensions that manifest as the speech disorders collectively termed "hyperkinetic dysarthria." Any or all of the major subcomponents of the speech production apparatus may be involved, with disturbances in prosody also being present. In that the various different types of hyperkinetic dysarthria are each associated with one of the hyperkinetic movement disorders, clinically the hyperkinetic dysarthrias are usually described in the context of the underlying movement disorders causing the speech disturbance.

According to the nature of the abnormal involuntary movements, hyperkinetic disorders are divided into quick hyperkinesias (e.g., myoclonic jerks, tics, and chorea) and slow hyperkinesias (e.g., athetosis, dyskinesia, and dystonia). In quick hyperkinesias, the abnormal involuntary movements are rapid and either unsustained or sustained only very briefly and occur at random in terms of the body part affected. In contrast, the abnormal involuntary movements seen in slow hyperkinesias built up to a peak slowly and are sustained for at least one second or longer. Muscle tone waxes and wanes producing a variety of distorted postures.

Myoclonic Jerks. These are abrupt, sudden, unsustained muscle contractions that occur irregularly. The muscles of the limbs as well as those of the speech mechanism can be affected. The muscles of the face, soft palate, larynx, diaphragm, and so forth may be either involved individually or in combination (e.g., palatopharyngolaryngeal myoclonus). Myoclonic jerks may be seen in children in associated with diffuse metabolic infections or toxic disorders of the central nervous system such as diffuse encephalitis and toxic encephalopathies. In addition, they also are associated with convulsive disorders (epilepsy).

Tics. Tics are recurrent, but brief, unsustained compulsive movements that involve a relatively small part of the body. One distinctive childhood disease characterized by the progressive development of tics involving the face, neck, upper limbs, and eventually the entire body is Gilles de la Tourette's syndrome. In this condition, which usually has an onset between 2 and 15 years of age, uncontrolled vocalizations (e.g., grunting, coughing, barking, hissing, and snorting) occur often as a result of involuntary contractions of the muscles of the speech mechanism. In addition stuttering-like repetitions, unintelligible sounds, and echolalia are also present in some cases. The cause of the condition is unknown, although it has been suggested that the pathophysiologic basis of the disease is increased dopamine activity.

Chorea. Slower than myoclonic jerks, choreic contractions involve a single, unsustained, isolated muscle action that produces a short, rapid, uncoordinated jerk of part of the body, such as the trunk, limb, face, tongue, and so forth. These contractions are random in their distribution and their timing is irregular and unpredictable. When superimposed on the normal movements of the speech mechanism during speech production, choreiform movements can cause momentary disturbances to the course of contextual speech. In fact, all aspects of speech can be disrupted in patients with chorea and the hyperkinetic dysarthria of chorea is characterized by a highly variable pattern of interference with articulation, phonation, resonation, and respiration.

There are two major diseases in which choreic movements are present: Sydenham chorea and Huntington disease. The onset of Sydenham chorea usually occurs between 5 and 10 years of age, females being affected more than males. In many instances, Sydenham's chorea appears to be associated with either streptococcal infections (strep-throat) or rheumatic heart disease. Huntington's disease is an inherited disorder which, although it can manifest in childhood, usually has its onset in adult life.

Athetosis. Athetoid movements are characterized by a continuous, arrhythmic, slow, writhing-type of muscle movement. These movements are always the same in the same patient and cease only during sleep. Although athetoid movements primarily involve the limbs, the muscles of the speech mechanism, including the muscles of the face, tongue, etc. may also be affected, causing facial grimacing, protrusion and writhing of the tongue and difficulty in speaking and swallowing. Athetoid movements disrupt these functions by interfering with the normal contraction of the muscles involved. In most cases athetosis forms part of a complex of neurologic signs, including those of cerebral palsy, that result from disordered development of the brain, birth injury, or other etiologic factors. The condition is usually associated with pathologic changes in the corpus striatum and cerebral cortex.

Dyskinesia (lingual-facial-buccal dyskinesia). Miller and Keane (1978) defined dyskinesia as "impairment of the power of voluntary movements." Although, according to this definition, all involuntary movements could be described as dyskinetic, only two dyskinetic disorders are described under this heading: tardive dyskinesia and levodopa-induced dyskinesia. Tardive dyskinesia is a well recognized side effect of long-term neuroleptic treatment (treatment with a pharmacologic agent having an antipsychotic action), whereas levodopa-induced dyskinesia results from the use of levadopa in the treatment of Parkin-

son disease. In that the muscles of the tongue, face and oral cavity are often most affected, these two disorders are also termed lingual-facial-buccal dyskinesias. In both conditions, the basic pattern of abnormal involuntary movement is one of repetitive, slow writhing, twisting, flexing, and extending movements, often with a mixture of tremor.

Dystonia. Dystonia tends to involve large parts of the body. The abnormal involuntary movements are slow and sustained for prolonged periods of time and may produce grotesque posturing and bizarre writhing movements. Although these involuntary movements mostly involve the trunk, neck, and proximal parts of the limbs, the muscles of the speech mechanism can also be affected. A variety of conditions lead to dystonia, including encephalitis, head trauma, vascular diseases, and drug toxicity (especially the more potent tranquillizers).

Ataxic Dysarthria (Cerebellar Dysarthria). The cerebellum is responsible for the coordination of muscular activity throughout the body. Although it does not itself initiate any muscle contractions, the cerebellum monitors those areas of the brain that do in order to coordinate the action of muscle groups and time their contractions so that movements involving the skeletal muscles are performed smoothly and accurately. Damage to the cerebellum or its connections leads to a condition called ataxia in which movements become uncoordinated. Although even simple movements are affected by cerebellar damage, the movements most disrupted by cerebellar disorders are the more complex, multicomponent sequential movements, such as those involved in speech production. Following damage to the cerebellum, complex movements tend to be broken down or decomposed into their individual sequential components each of which may be executed with errors of force, amplitude, and timing leading to uncoordinated movements. If the ataxia affects the muscles of the speech mechanism, the production of speech may become abnormal leading to a cluster of deviant speech dimensions collectively referred to as ataxic dysarthria.

Neuroanatomy of the Cerebellum. Located posterior to the brainstem, the cerebellum occupies most of the poste-

rior cranial fossa and is separated from the occipital and temporal lobes of the cerebrum by the tentorium cerebelli.

The cerebellum is composed of two large cerebellar hemispheres that are connected by a midportion called the vermis (wormlike) (Figure 11–5). The cerebellar surface or cerebellar cortex consists of complexly folded ridges of gray matter while the central core of the cerebellum consists of white matter in which are located several nuclear gray masses called the deep (cerebellar) nuclei.

A series of deep and distinct fissures divide the cerebellum into a number of lobes. Although different authors have classified the cerebellar lobes in

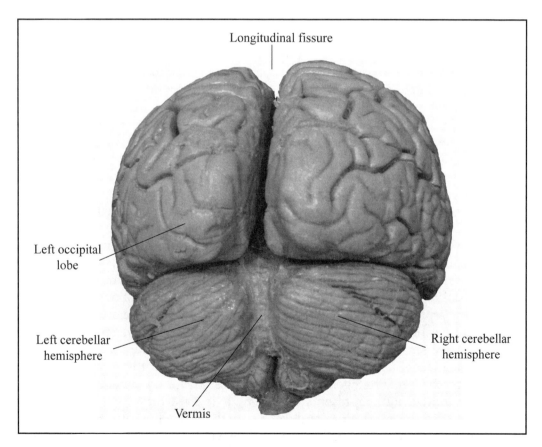

FIGURE 11–5. Posterior view of the brain showing the two cerebellar hemispheres located below the occipital lobes. [From Murdoch, 2010]

different ways, most neurologists recognize three different cerebellar lobes. These include: the anterior lobe; the posterior lobe; and the flocculonodular lobe (includes the paired flocculi and the nodulus). The anterior lobe, which can be seen from a superior view of the cerebellum, is that portion of the cerebellum that lies anterior to the primary fissure. It roughly corresponds to that part of the cerebellum called the paleocerebellum. The anterior lobe has a significant role in the regulation of muscle tone and receives its primary input from proprioceptors and exteroceptors in the head and body, including some from the vestibular system.

The largest portion of the cerebellum is the posterior lobe, also referred to as the neocerebellum. It is located between the other two lobes and is phylogenetically the newest portion of the cerebellum, being best developed in those animals such as primates that have a well-developed cerebral cortex. It functions in close association with the cerebral cortex and is most concerned with the regulation of voluntary movements. In particular, it plays an essential role in the coordination of phasic movements and is the most important part of the cerebellum for the coordination of speech movements. The flocculonodular lobe is composed of the nodulus and the paired flocculi and occupies the inferior-rostral region of the cerebellum. The nodulus represents the rostral portion of the inferior vermis whereas the flocculi are two small irregular-shaped appendages attached to the inferior region of the cerebellum. Phylogenetically, the flocculonodular lobe represents the oldest portion of the cerebellum and is also known as the archicerebellum. It functions in close association with the

vestibular system and is therefore important in maintaining equilibrium and keeping the individual oriented in space.

The cerebellum is made up of both gray and white matter. As in the cerebral hemispheres, most of the gray matter is found covering the surface of the cerebellum as cortex. The cerebellar cortex is highly folded into thin transverse folds or folia. As a consequence of this extensive folding, in the region of 85% of the cerebellar cortex is concealed and its surface area is much larger than might be expected (about three-quarters of that of the cerebrum). Unlike the cerebral cortex, the cerebellar cortex is uniform throughout its structure. The central core of the cerebellum is made up of white matter in which are embedded four gray masses on either side of the midline. These gray masses are referred to as the cerebellar or deep nuclei. The largest and most medially placed of these nuclei is the dentate nucleus. Medial to the dentate nucleus are two smaller nuclei, the globose and emboliform nuclei (taken together called the interpositus), and most medial of all the deep nuclei is the fastigial nucleus. The cerebellum is attached to the brainstem on either side by three structures called the cerebellar peduncles. These peduncles are composed of bundles of nerve fibers that convey impulses either to or from the cerebellum. In order to coordinate muscular contractions, the cerebellum is linked to a large number of other parts of the nervous system by an extensive system of afferent and efferent fibers. Damage to these pathways can cause cerebellar dysfunction and possibly ataxic dysarthria the same as damage to the cerebellum itself. Overall, the extensive afferent and efferent connections of the cerebellum form a feedback loop by which the cerebellum can both monitor and modify motor activities taking place in various parts of the body to produce a smooth, coordinated motor action. Through its afferent supply, the cerebellum receives input from a number of different regions of the nervous system regarding motor activities either already in progress or about to occur. Furthermore, by means of its efferent connections, the cerebellum is able to modify motor actions initiated elsewhere in the central nervous system.

Clinical Signs of Damage to the Cerebellum. Clinically the signs of damage to the cerebellum include ataxia, dysmetria, decomposition of movement, dysdiadochokinesia, hypotonia, asthenia, tremor, rebound phenomena, disturbance of posture and gait, nystagmus, and dysarthria. Clinically, signs usually appear on the same side of the body as the cerebellar lesion. Different symptoms result from cerebellar damage depending on the part of the cerebellum involved. Broadly, cerebellar disorders can be divided into those that affect the vestibulocerebellum (flocculonodular lobe) and those affecting the main mass of the cerebellum (the corpus cerebelli, which includes both the anterior and posterior lobes). Obviously, in many disorders both the corpus cerebelli and the flocculonodular lobe are involved.

Isolated damage to the flocculonodular lobe is most commonly associated with the presence of a tumor, usually a medulloblastoma, and is associated with a disturbance in equilibrium called archicerebellar syndrome. Patients are unsteady and have a tendency to fall either backward, forward or to one side when standing on a narrow base with their eyes open. Some patients, in fact,

are unable to maintain an upright position. Their gait is staggering and they tend to walk on a wide base. Other signs may also be present if the tumor later invades other parts of the cerebellum.

Damage to the corpus cerebelli or its connections is associated with a group of symptoms commonly collectively called neocerebellar syndrome, although the paleocerebellum is usually involved. Destruction of small portions of the corpus cerebelli causes no detectable abnormality in motor function. It appears that the remaining areas of the cerebellum can compensate for the damaged part. More severe and enduring dysfunction of the cerebellum, however, occurs if either the deep nuclei or superior cerebellar peduncle are involved. When the lesion involves the cerebellum unilaterally, as is usually the case, the motor disturbance occurs on the same side as the lesion.

Complex movements, such as required for speech production or the movement of an entire limb to a new position, depend on the proper sequencing of composite simple movements (composition). Furthermore, they also are dependent on the contraction of synergistic muscles to provide postural fixation of certain joints to allow for the precise movement of other joints (synergia: cooperative action of muscles). Cerebellar dysfunction causes errors in both of these parameters leading to slowing, dysmetria, dyssynergia, and decomposition of movement. In the case of alternating movements, dysdiadochokinesia also results. The resulting uncoordinated, clumsy and disorganized muscular activity is termed ataxia. Ataxia is the principal sign of cerebellar dysfunction.

The presence of dysmetria is exhibited by the patient's inability to stop a movement at the desired point. For example, when reaching for an object, the patient's hand may either overshoot the intended point or stop short of the intended point. Dyssynergia is reflected in the separation of a series of voluntary movements that normally flow smoothly and in sequence into a succession of mechanical or puppetlike movements (decomposition of movement). It also may be manifest as movement abnormalities such as delayed starting and stopping of movements. Dysdiadochokinesia refers to an inability to perform rapid alternating movements, such as rapidly moving the tongue from one side of the mouth to the other and back several times. To be performed rapidly such movements require considerable coordination by the cerebellum and therefore are severely disturbed in patients with cerebellar disorders.

A decrease in the muscle (hypotonia) is also usually evident in cerebellar disorders (as can be ascertained by palpation of the muscles) and muscles affected by cerebellar lesions tend to be weaker and tire more easily than normal muscles (asthenia). The reduction in muscle tone may result from reduced muscle spindle sensitivity possibly because of an inadequate alpha motor neuron discharge as a result of the cerebellar damage. Tremor is another feature of cerebellar disease. It usually takes the form of an intention tremor and is seen during movement but is absent at rest. Disturbances of posture and gait may be very pronounced, the patient possibly being unable to maintain an upright posture and walking in a staggering fashion with a broad base of support.

The presence of rebound phenomenon can be demonstrated by asking patients to flex their elbow against resistance offered by the observer when their hand is only a small distance from their face and then suddenly releasing the forearm. Normally, the movement of the forearm in the direction of flexion (i.e., towards the face) is quickly arrested by contraction of the extensor muscle (triceps). Cerebellar damage, however, delays this contraction with the result that patients may strike themselves in the face. Nystagmus may also be present, especially if the lesion encroaches upon the vermis.

Finally, as a result of dyssynergy and decomposition of the movement of the muscles of the speech mechanism during speech production, ataxic dysarthria may be present in association with some cerebellar lesions.

Clinical Features of Ataxic Dysarthria. The most predominant features of ataxic dysarthria include a breakdown in the articulatory and prosodic aspects of speech. According to Brown, Darley, and Aronson (1970), the 10 deviant speech dimensions most characteristic of ataxic dysarthria can be divided into three clusters: articulatory inaccuracy, characterized by imprecision of consonant production, irregular articulatory breakdowns, and distorted vowels; prosodic excess, characterized by excess and equal stress, prolonged phonemes, prolonged intervals, and slow rate; and phonatory-prosodic insufficiency, characterized by harshness, monopitch, and monoloudness. The dysprosody, resulting in slow, monotonous, and improperly measured speech has been termed "scanning speech" by some authors.

Diseases of the Cerebellum Associated with Ataxic Dysarthria. The cerebellum can be affected by a variety of different pathologic conditions (Table 11–4), all of which may be associated with the occurrence of ataxic dysarthria.

Table 11–4. Diseases of the Cerebellum Associated with Ataxic Dysarthria

Diseases	Example	General Features
Congenital anomalies	Cerebellar agenesis	Partial to almost total nondevelopment of the cerebellum. May in some cases not be associated with any clinical evidence of cerebellar dysfunction. In other cases, however, a gait disturbance may be evident in addition to limb ataxia (especially involving the lower limbs) and dysarthria.
Chromosomal disorders	Trisomy	Diffuse hypotrophy (underdevelopment) of the cerebellum may be present which may be associated with either no clinical symptoms of cerebellar dysfunction through to marked limb ataxia.
Trauma	Penetrating head wounds (e.g., bullet wounds)	May be associated with either mild slowly developing cerebellar dysfunction or rapid, severe cerebellar dysfunction.
Vascular disease	Occlusion of anterior-inferior cerebellar artery	Hypotonia and ipsilateral limb ataxia.
	Occlusion of posterior-inferior cerebellar artery	Dysarthria, nystagmus, ipsilateral limb ataxia, and disordered gait and station
	Occlusion of superior cerebellar artery	Disordered gait and station. Ipsilateral hypotonia, ipsilateral limb ataxia, and intention tremor. Occasionally dysarthria.
Infections	Cerebellar abscess	Most frequently caused by purulent bacteria but can also occur with fungi. Cerebellar abscesses most frequently arise by direct extension from adjacent infected areas such as the mastoid process or from otologic disease.
Tumors	Medulloblastomas, astrocytomas, and ependymomas	Primary tumors of the cerebellum occur more frequently in children than adults. Medulloblastomas occur most commonly in the midline of the cerebellum in children and usually have a rapid course with a poor prognosis. Astrocytomas are more benign than medulloblastomas and generally occur in children of an older age group than medulloblastomas. Ependymomas are relatively slow growing and again are more common in children than adults.

continues

345

Table 11–4. *continued*

Diseases	Example	General Features
Toxic metabolic and endocrine disorders	Exogenous toxins, e.g., industrial solvents, carbon tetrachloride, heavy metals, etc.	Signs of cerebellar involvement usually associated with symptoms of diffuse involvement of the central nervous system following these intoxications rather than appearing in isolation to other neurologic deficits.
	Enzyme deficiencies, e.g., pyruvate dehydrogenase deficiency	Ataxia most marked in the lower limbs.
	Hypothyroidism	Cretins show poor development of the cerebellum. Ataxia present in 20 to 30% of myxoedema cases.
Hereditary ataxias	Friedreich ataxia	The most commonly encountered spinal form of hereditary ataxia. Pathologic degeneration primarily involves the spinal cord with degeneration of neurons occurring in the spinocerebellar tracts. Some degeneration of neurons in the dentate nucleus and brachium conjunctivum also may occur. The first clinical sign of the disease is usually clumsiness of gait. Later, limb ataxia (especially involving the lower extremities) also occurs. A large percentage of cases also exhibit dysarthria and nystagmus and cognitive deficits may also be present
Demyelinating disorders	Multiple sclerosis	Usually associated with demyelination in a number of regions of the central nervous system including the cerebellum. Consequently, the dysarthria, if present, usually takes the form of a mixed dysarthria rather than purely an ataxic dysarthria. Paroxysmal ataxic dysarthria may occur as an early sign of multiple sclerosis.

More specifically, major causes of acquired ataxia in childhood include: posterior fossa tumors (e.g., medulloblastomas, cerebellar astrocytomas, etc.), traumatic head injury, infections (cerebellar abscess), hereditary ataxias (e.g., Friedreich ataxia), degenerative disorders (e.g., metachromatic leukodystrophy), and toxic (e.g., heavy metal poisoning), metabolic and endocrine disorders.

Mixed Dysarthria. Some disorders of the nervous system affect more than one level of the neuromuscular system. Consequently, in addition to the more "pure" forms of dysarthria outlined above, clinicians may also be confronted by patients who exhibit "mixed dysarthrias." These may be caused by a variety of conditions including cerebrovascular accidents, head trauma, brain tumors, inflammatory diseases, and degenerative conditions. For example a mixed ataxic-hypokinetic-spastic dysarthria may be seen in children with Wilson disease. Wilson disease, or hepatolenticular degeneration, is a rare inborn metabolic disorder caused by the body's inability to process dietary copper. As a result, copper accumulates in the tissues of the body, especially in the brain, liver, and cornea of the eye. The most severely affected parts of the brain are the basal ganglia, although lesser degrees of copper deposition may also occur in the cerebellum, brainstem, and other parts of the cerebrum. The condition is inherited as an autosomal recessive disorder. The most common clinical signs and symptoms of the disease include Parkinsonian and hyperkinetic neurologic behaviors. A mixed ataxic-hypokinetic-spastic dysarthria is a prominent feature of Wilson disease although the combination of dysarthria types and the level of severity varies widely among individuals with the disease.

Acquired Childhood Dysarthria of Different Etiologies

The major etiologies of acquired childhood dysarthria include traumatic brain injury, intracerebral tumors, cerebrovascular accidents, and infectious disorders. In addition, genetic disorders are also sometimes the cause of childhood dysarthria, including Duchenne muscular dystrophy, Friedreich ataxia, and Huntington disease.

Acquired Childhood Dysarthria Following Traumatic Brain Injury. Persistent dysarthria is a commonly reported sequelae of severe TBI in children. Despite this, few studies have investigated the incidence and nature of dysarthria following TBI acquired in childhood. The majority of studies that do exist tend to report only the presence or frequency of dysarthria but do not go on to provide an analysis of the speech disorder. The small number of the studies that have attempted to further define the nature of dysarthria subsequent to TBI in children have been case studies (Cahill, Murdoch, & Theodoros, 2000; Murdoch & Horton, 1998; Murdoch, Pitt, Theodoros, & Ward, 1999) or have examined only one aspect of the speech production mechanism (Stierwalt, Robin, Solomon, Weiss, & Max 1996). Murdoch and colleagues (1999), in a study of the effects of real-time continuous visual biofeedback in the treatment of speech breathing disorders, examined the motor speech function of one child with severe dysarthria subsequent to TBI using perceptual and instrumental measures, and observed impairments in all of the speech subsystems. Similarly, Murdoch and Horton (1998) identified a range of impairments across the speech production mechanism, using both perceptual and instrumental assessments, in single case studies of children with dysarthria subsequent to TBI. In the most comprehensive series of studies completed to date, Cahill, Murdoch, and Theodoros (2002, 2003, 2005) examined 24 children who had acquired a TBI, using both perceptual and instrumental measures, and found that each child presented with a differing profile of speech subsystem deficits, ranging from no dysarthria through to moderate-severe dysarthria.

These findings are not unexpected given that the diffuse, non-specific nature of TBI can lead to damage in many areas of the central nervous system, resulting in impairment in one or more of the motor speech subsystems (for a description of the biomechanics and neuropathophysiology of traumatic brain injury see Chapter 3). More specifically, the perceptual and instrumental analysis of speech function in the group of children with TBI examined by Cahill and colleagues identified substantial impairments in prosody, velopharyngeal and articulatory function, as well as reduced lung capacity and impaired respiratory-phonatory control for speech but little impairment in laryngeal function. A more complete description of dysarthria associated with childhood traumatic brain injury is presented in Chapter 12.

Acquired Childhood Dysarthria Associated with Brain Tumors. Dysarthria has been reported to occur subsequent to the diagnosis and treatment of posterior fossa tumors, with the presentation of the speech impairment ranging from transient mutism, to mild dysarthria, through to a persistent developmental speech disorder. The literature, to date, predominantly documents the presence of transient cerebellar mutism subsequent to surgery for a posterior fossa tumor and that resolution to normal speech involves a period of dysarthria. There is some evidence, however, that in some individuals treated for posterior fossa tumors speech does not return to premorbid levels, implying the presence of a persistent dysarthria. The majority of reports, however, are not only based on small numbers of children, but are also restricted to descriptions of the speech impairment based on perceptual speech analyses. A number of studies have labeled the speech disorder evident as cerebellar or ataxic dysarthria utilizing the Mayo Clinic classification. Unfortunately, in many of these studies the actual clinical features of the speech disorder were not elaborated, using the overall term of ataxic dysarthria only as a descriptor.

In a recent published series of studies based on perceptual, acoustic, and physiologic assessments, Cornwell, Murdoch, and Ward (2003, 2005) and Cornwell, Murdoch, Ward, and Kellie (2004) determined that, although not all children treated for posterior fossa tumors exhibit a persistent dysarthria, in those cases where it does occur the nature of the deviant perceptual features usually reflects those associated with dysarthria in adults with cerebellar or lower motor neuron damage, dependent on tumor location within the posterior cranial fossa. In particular, where the tumor is primarily cerebellar in location the child usually exhibits a predominance of phonatory, articulatory, and prosodic disturbances. Examination of the individual components of the speech musculature revealed that there was impairment to lip, tongue, and laryngeal function both at rest and during performance of nonspeech and speech tasks, along with more minor deficits in palatal and respiratory function. A more comprehensive description of the dysarthria associated with posterior fossa tumors in children is presented in Chapter 13. A detailed description of the various types of posterior fossa tumors can be found in Chapter 4.

Acquired Childhood Dysarthria Following Cerebrovascular Accident. Although cerebrovascular disorders constitute a much smaller proportion of neurologic diseases of childhood than of adulthood, they are a significant cause of morbidity and mortality in the childhood population. Although dysarthria associated with cerebrovascular accidents is therefore less common than in adults, cerebrovascular disorders are an acknowledged cause of dysarthria in children being observed in both occlusive and hemorrhagic conditions (Horton, Murdoch, Theodoros, & Thompson, 1997).

The majority of the diseases of blood vessels that affect adults at some time may also affect children. The causes of vascular diseases of the brain in children, however, differ from those in adults. Although some vascular diseases of the brain, such as embolism arising from subacute or acute bacterial endocardial vascular disease, occur at all ages, others such as cerebrovascular disorders associated with congenital heart disease, are peculiar to childhood. At the other extreme, degenerative disorders of the vascular system such as atherosclerosis affect primarily middle-aged and elderly people and are rare in childhood.

Vascular anomalies are the most common cause of primary central nervous system hemorrhage in infants and children. The most important of these are angiomas. Rather than being vascular neoplasms, angiomas represent developmental malformations and can be classified as arteriovenous, venous, cavernous, or capillary. In addition to vascular abnormalities, cerebral hemorrhage in children can occur secondary to hematologic diseases such as leukemia, sickle cell disease, hemophilia, and thrombocytopenic purpura as well as traumatic head injury.

Arterial occlusion in childhood is most frequently the consequence of congenital dysplasia of the vessels, cerebral arteritis, trauma, or thromboembolic disease, the latter condition usually occurring in infants or children with congenital heart disease. Occlusive vascular disease in children has been observed in cases of sickle cell disease and moyamoya disease and as an outcome of complications of certain hereditary metabolic diseases such as homocystinuria and Fabry disease.

Despite being a recognized sequelae of cerebrovascular disorders, very few detailed descriptions of dysarthria resulting from cerebrovascular disorders in children have been reported (for a comprehensive description of the cerebrovascular disorders affecting children see Chapter 2). Horton et al. (1997) have provided the only detailed description of a child with dysarthria associated with basilar artery stroke based on a comprehensive assessment using both perceptual and physiologic techniques. The physiologic assessments indicated the most severe motor speech deficits to be in the respiratory and velopharyngeal subsystems with significant deficits also being apparent in the articulatory subsystem, collectively resulting in severely reduced intelligibility. Bak et al. (1983) described the perceptual features of the speech disorder exhibited by a child with a brainstem infarct following occlusion of the basilar artery. Specifically, the dysarthria in their case was characterized by imprecise consonants, distorted vowels, hypernasality, and a breathy voice.

Acquired Childhood Dysarthria Associated with Infectious Disorders.

Infectious disorders of the central nervous system are a recognized cause of dysarthria in both children and adults. These infectious disorders include those caused by bacterial, spirochetal, viral, and other less common microorganisms. In particular, major infectious disorders that have been documented in the literature as causing dysarthria in children include: meningitis, encephalitis, bulbar polioencephalitis (bulbar form of poliomyelitis), Reye syndrome, Sydenham chorea, and cerebellar abscesses.

Acquired Apraxia of Speech

Acquired apraxia of speech is a motor speech programming disorder characterized primarily by errors in articulation and secondarily by alterations in prosody. Although most of what we know about this disorder comes from studies on adult subjects, it has been speculated that acquired verbal apraxia can also occur in children with brain injuries. Unfortunately only scant information regarding the nature and occurrence of this disorder in childhood is available in the literature, with the presence of apraxia of speech occasionally being noted by authors as one of the speech-language disorders to occur amongst other following brain injury, but with few details being provided. As in adults, it appears that acquired apraxia of speech usually occurs in combination with an acquired aphasia and/or dysarthria. One possible reason for the lack of attention paid to acquired apraxia of speech in the literature is that the condition appears to resolve quickly.

This is true whether the apraxia is oral or verbal in nature. The only two articles which make reference to acquired apraxia of speech in children either documents its recovery or notes its presence in the early stages postonset. Aram, Rose, Rekate, and Whitaker (1983) described the oral apraxia in a 7-year-old right-handed girl with acquired capsular/striatal aphasia. On day four after onset, the child was totally mute and unable to produce nonspeech oral movements on command but could produce them on imitation. Two days later these nonspeech movements were initiated on command as was phonation. Within another two days a full range of tongue movements was possible and vowel sounds could be imitated. At this time two word phrases were spontaneously produced. Some weakness of the right facial muscles was present but no dysarthria was noticeable. No further mention of speech disturbances was made, although aphasic symptoms were still present.

Three out of the 15 cases of children with acquired aphasia described by Cooper and Flowers (1987) presented with apraxia of speech one month after onset. One case was head-injured whereas two of the three cases had suffered hematomas. All three cases were communicating orally at the time the apraxia was noted. Therefore, an apraxia of speech can be assumed. No information on the apraxia symptoms or their recovery was given. Therefore, in the absence of detailed descriptions of apraxia of speech symptoms in children one must again turn to the adult literature.

Features of apraxia of speech seen in adults include:

1. Visible and audible groping to achieve correct individual articulatory postures and sequence of postures to produce sounds and words.
2. Highly variable articulatory errors (e.g., /v/ may at different times be produced /v/, /z/, /p/, /f/, /r/, /b/, /h/, and /w/).
3. Based on perceptual analysis with the naked ear, articulatory errors appear to involve substitutions rather than distortions of individual phonemes as occurs in dysarthria.
4. A greater number of articulatory errors occur during repetition than during conversational speech.
5. The number of articulatory errors increases as the complexity of the articulatory exercise increases— few errors are made on single consonants whereas more errors occur on consonant clusters.
6. In addition to articulatory disturbances, as these patients speak, they slow down their rate of speech, space their words and syllables more evenly and stress them more equally.
7. Speech output is nonfluent because of pausing and hesitating while the individual gropes for articulatory placement and makes repeated efforts to produce words correctly.

Differentiation of Apraxia of Speech from Acquired Dysarthria

Although apraxia of speech and dysarthria are both motor speech disorders, each represents a breakdown at a different level of speech production. Individuals with apraxia, on neurologic examination, show no significant evidence of slowness, weakness, incoordination, paralysis, or alteration of tone of the muscles of the speech production mechanisms that can account for the associated speech disturbance. Individuals with dysarthria, on the other hand, dependent on the type of dysarthria present, may exhibit either hyper- or hypotonus of the speech muscles, a restricted range of movement, and so forth. Whereas individuals with dysarthria often show variable disturbances in all of the basic motor processes that underlie speech production including respiration, phonation, resonation, articulation, and prosody, in apraxia of speech the continuing impairment is specifically articulatory, with prosodic alterations occurring as compensatory phenomena. Furthermore, the nature of the articulatory disturbance differs between the two conditions. In dysarthria, the errors of articulation are characteristically errors of simplification (e.g., distortions or omissions), whereas in apraxia of speech, the articulatory errors largely take the form of complications of speech (e.g., substitution of one phoneme for another, addition of phonemes, repetitions of phonemes, etc.).

Case Examples

Case 1: Dysarthria

Rebecca was a 13-year-old, right-handed female who sustained a severe closed-head injury (Glasgow Coma Score = 5) when hit by a motor vehicle. A computed tomographic (CT) scan performed shortly after admission to hospital revealed a large soft tissue hematoma over the temporal and parietal regions of her left and right cerebral hemispheres with a further small lesion localized to the left lenticular nucleus. Rebecca was mute for 4 months postinjury. Although from that time speech did begin to return, Rebecca remained moderately dysarthric until referred to the Centre for Neurogenic Communication Disorders Research at 10 months postinjury. A perceptual analysis of Rebecca's speech conducted at that time revealed the presence of deficits in all five aspects of the speech production process (prosody, respiration, articulation, resonance, and phonation). A comprehensive instrumental assessment using a range of physiologic instruments capable of assessing the functioning of the various components of the speech production apparatus confirmed the presence of impairments at all five levels. In particular, the major features contributing to Rebecca's dysarthria included severely reduced tongue function and moderately reduced lip, velopharyngeal and laryngeal function, and a mild-moderately reduced respiratory function. Her speech was moderately unintelligible with decreased rate of speech, reduced variability of pitch and imprecision of consonants. The single greatest contributor to Rebecca's unintelligibility appeared to be the dysfunction in the articulatory system, especially the impaired tongue function. Following an intensive three-month period of traditional therapy supplemented with biofeedback therapy (using electropalatographic feedback) aimed at improving Rebecca's tongue and lip function, her speech had improved to a level where intelligibility was rated as being only mildly impaired. Subsequently, Rebecca was able to return to school with renewed confidence in her spoken output and to pursue a more active and natural social life.

Case 2: Acquired Apraxia of Speech

Lauren, at 8 years, 4 months of age suffered a cerebrovascular accident involving the left middle cerebral artery shortly after an operation to repair a faulty heart valve. Unfortunately for Lauren, the operation had triggered an embolus which had traveled up the left internal carotid artery to lodge in her left middle cerebral artery. Prior to her neurologic episode Lauren had been developing normally and was enjoying third grade at school. Initially, Lauren presented with a severe right hemiparesis that affected her upper and lower limbs. Her right arm was more severely affected than her right leg, her right hand having no functional grasp and release. Lauren was unable to walk without assistance and her visual-perceptual abilities were affected. She also had a severe oral and verbal apraxia with a suspected expressive aphasic component. Her right upper motor neuron weakness was associated with drooling from the right side of her mouth. Lauren's range of tongue movement appeared adequate for eating and speech. When required to imitate oral movements, gross attempts and groping movements were noted. She was unable to repeat single sounds and her spontaneous speech output consisted of a single vowel and an attempt to say "no." Tests indicated that Lauren's auditory comprehension skills were intact and she responded appropriately to conversation and was able to follow 4-stage commands. Lauren used facial expression, gross gestures, and vowel sounds for expressive communication. She was provided with a communication board to aid her communication. Nine months after her stroke, Lauren's speech was intelligible in all situations and her oral and verbal apraxia had resolved to being mild. Her rigid lower facial muscle weakness had also resolved. She was unable to volitionally elevate her tongue tip but when eating a cookie she cleaned her top lip without effort. Imitations of single sounds revealed only an inability to make voiced and voiceless /the/ and mild distortions of /l/ and /r/. Repetition of phoneme sequences and syllable sequences were still marked by delayed responses and slow rate of repetition with some visible searching behaviors, but these problems did not appear to hamper her functional communication. A mild prosodic impairment, mainly a reduced rate of speech, was present when her syntactic construction was complex or when a polysyllabic word she used was new to her vocabulary. There was little detectable muscle weakness. Mild word-related problems remained. Lauren was able to return to school eight weeks poststroke. Her teacher reported that she was coping with the work in grade 3 and was just below the average in a class of 30 students.

References

Abbs, J. H., Hunker, J. C., & Barlow, S. M. (1983). Differential speech motor subsystem impairments with suprabulbar lesions: Neurophysiological framework and supporting data. In W. R. Berry (Ed.), *Clinical dysarthria* (pp. 21–56). San Diego, CA: College-Hill Press.

Aram, D. M., Rose, D. F., Rekate, H. L., & Whitaker, H. A. (1983). Acquired capsular/striatal aphasia in childhood. *Archives of Neurology, 40,* 614–617.

Bak, E., van Dongen, H. R., & Arts, W. F. M. (1983). The analysis of acquired dysarthria in childhood. *Developmental Medicine and Child Neurology, 25,* 81–94.

Brown, J. R., Darley, F. L., & Aronson, A. E. (1970). Ataxic dysarthria. *International Journal of Neurology, 7,* 302–318.

Cahill, L. M., Murdoch, B. E., & Theodoros, D. G. (2000). Variability in speech outcome following severe childhood traumatic brain injury: A report of three cases. *Journal of Medical Speech-Language Pathology, 8,* 347–352.

Cahill, L. M., Murdoch, B. E., & Theodoros, D. G. (2002). Perceptual analysis of speech following traumatic brain injury in childhood. *Brain Injury, 16,* 415–446.

Cahill, L. M., Murdoch, B. E., & Theodoros, D. G. (2003). Perceptual and instrumental analysis of laryngeal function following traumatic brain injury in childhood. *Journal of Head Trauma Rehabilitation, 18,* 268–283.

Cahill, L. M., Murdoch, B. E., & Theodoros, D. G. (2005). Articulatory function following traumatic brain injury in childhood: A perceptual and instrumental analysis. *Brain Injury, 19,* 41–58.

Cooper, J. A., & Flowers, C. R. (1987). Children with a history of acquired aphasia: Residual language and academic impairments. *Journal of Speech and Hearing Disorders, 52,* 251–262.

Cornwell, P. L., Murdoch, B. E., & Ward, E. C. (2003). Perceptual evaluation of motor speech following treatment for childhood cerebellar tumour. *Clinical Linguistics and Phonetics, 17,* 597–615.

Cornwell, P. L., Murdoch, B. E., & Ward, E. C. (2005). Differential motor speech outcomes in children treated for mid-line cerebellar tumour. *Brain Injury, 19,* 119–134.

Cornwell, P. L., Murdoch, B. E., Ward, E. C., & Kellie, S. (2004). Acoustic investigation of vocal quality following treatment for childhood cerebellar tumour. *Folia Phoniatrica et Logopaedica, 56,* 93–107.

Darley, F. L., Aronson, A. E., & Brown, J. R. (1969a). Differential diagnostic patterns of dysarthria. *Journal of Speech and Hearing Research, 12,* 246–269.

Darley, F. L., Aronson, A. E., & Brown, J. R. (1969b). Clusters of deviant speech dimensions in the dysarthrias. *Journal of Speech and Hearing Research, 12,* 462–496.

Darley, F. L., Aronson, A. E., & Brown, J. R. (1975). *Motor speech disorders.* Philadelphia, PA: W. B. Saunders.

Dworkin, J. P., & Hartman, D. E. (1988). *Cases in neurogenic communicative disorders.* Boston, MA: Little, Brown.

Edwards, M. (1984). *Disorders of articulation: Aspects of dysarthria and verbal dyspraxia.* Vienna, Austria: Springer-Verlag.

Espir, M. L. E., & Rose, F. C. (1983). *The basic neurology of speech.* Philadelphia, PA: F. A. Davis.

Horton, S. K., Murdoch, B. E., Theodoros, D. G., & Thompson E. C. (1997). Motor speech impairment in a case of childhood basilar artery stroke: Treatment directions derived from physiological and perceptual assessment. *Pediatric Rehabilitation, 1,* 163–177.

Miller, B. F., & Keane, C. B. (1978). *Encyclopedia and dictionary of medicine, nursing, and allied health.* Philadelphia, PA: W. B. Saunders.

Morgan, A. T., & Liégeois, F. (2010). Rethinking diagnostic classification of the dysarthrias: A developmental perspective. *Folia Phoniatrica et Logopaedica, 62,* 120–126.

Murdoch, B. E. (2010). *Acquired speech and language disorders: A neuroanatomical and functional neurological approach* (2nd ed.). Oxford, UK: Wiley-Blackwell.

Murdoch, B. E., & Horton, S. K. (1998). Acquired and developmental dysarthria in childhood. In B. E. Murdoch (Ed.), *Dysarthria: A physiological approach to assessment and treatment* (pp. 373–427). Cheltenham, UK: Stanley Thornes.

Murdoch, B. E., & Hudson-Tennent, L. J. (1994). Speech disorders in children treated for posterior fossa tumours: Ataxic and developmental features. *European Journal of Disorders of Communication, 29,* 379–397.

Murdoch, B. E., Ozanne, A. E., & Cross, J. A. (1990). Acquired childhood speech disorders: Dysarthria and dyspraxia. In B. E. Murdoch (Ed.), *Acquired neurological speech/language disorders in childhood* (pp. 308–341). London, UK: Taylor & Francis.

Murdoch, B. E., Pitt, G., Theodoros, D. G., & Ward, E. C. (1999). Real-time visual biofeedback in the treatment of speech breathing disorders following childhood traumatic brain injury: A report of one case. *Pediatric Rehabilitation, 3,* 5–20.

Murdoch, B. E., Thompson, E. C. & Theodoros, D. G. (1997). Spastic dysarthria. In M. R. McNeil (Ed.), *Clinical management of sensorimotor speech disorders* (pp. 287–310). New York, NY: Thieme.

Robinson, R. (1981). Equal recovery in child and adult brain. *Developmental Medicine and Child Neurology, 23,* 379–383.

Sears, E. S., & Franklin, G. M. (1980). Diseases of the cranial nerves. In R. N. Rosenberg (Ed.), *Neurology* (Vol. 5, pp. 471–493). New York, NY: Grune & Stratton.

Snell, R. S. (1980). *Clinical neuroanatomy for medical students.* Boston, MA: Little, Brown.

Stark, R. E. (1985). Dysarthria in children. In J. K. Darby (Ed.), *Speech and language evaluation in neurology: Childhood disorders* (pp. 185–217). Orlando, FL: Grune & Stratton.

Stierwalt, J. A. G., Robin, D. A., Solomon, N. P., Weiss, A. L., & Max, J. E. (1996). Tongue strength and endurance: Relation to speaking ability of children and adolescents following traumatic brain injury. In D. A. Robin, K. M. Yorkston, & D. R. Beukelman (Eds.), *Disorders of motor speech: Assessment, treatment and clinical characteristics* (pp. 241–256). Baltimore, MD: Paul H. Brooks.

van Mourik, M., Catsman-Berrevoets, C. E., Paquier, P. F., Yousef-Bak, E., & van Dongen, H. R. (1997). Acquired childhood dysarthria: Review of its clinical presentation. *Pediatric Neurology, 17,* 299–307.

Wilson, S. K. A. (1912). Progressive lenticular degeneration: Familial nervous disease associated with cirrhosis of the liver. *Brain, 34,* 295.

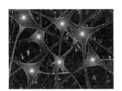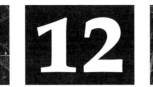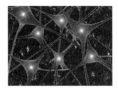

Dysarthria Subsequent to Traumatic Brain Injury in Childhood

Introduction

Dysarthria, a motor speech disorder resulting from neuromuscular impairments, is a commonly reported sequelae of traumatic brain injury (TBI) in children (Bak, van Dongen, & Arts, 1983; Cahill, Murdoch, & Theodoros, 2002; Costeff, Groswasser, & Goldstein, 1990). Rate, strength, and coordination of the muscles subserving speech may be impaired to different degrees, affecting articulation, prosody, resonance, respiration, and phonation (Darley, Aronson, & Brown, 1975). The reported incidence of dysarthria in children with TBI varies. Stierwalt, Robin, Solomon, Weiss, and Max (1996) reported that 30% (7 of 23) of their children with TBI had dysarthria whereas Cahill et al. (2002) noted that two-thirds (16 of 24) of their cases were classified as dysarthric. Based on a long-term follow-up study of children who had suffered severe TBI, Ylvisaker (1986) observed that 10% of children

and 8% of adolescents in his study were unintelligible. One feature of the dysarthria following TBI often reported is the persistent nature of the condition (Costeff, Groswasser, Landman, & Brenner, 1985; Rusk, Block, & Lowmann, 1969; Thomsen, 1984). Costeff et al. (1985) found that 14 out of 36 children with severe TBI presented with dysarthria 2 years postinjury, whereas only one child remained aphasic. Hécaen (1976) reported that, second to writing disorders, articulation disorders were the most prevalent and persistent communication deficit in a group of 15 children with severe closed-head injuries. Boyer and Edwards (1991) studied 220 children and adolescents with severe TBI who were admitted consecutively to a rehabilitation program. They reported that dysarthria was present in 33% of cases, whereas 25% were nonspeaking 1 to 3 years postinjury.

Partly as a consequence of the persistent nature of the condition, dysarthria can seriously compromise the child's quality of life, including withdrawal from family, social and academic activities. Furthermore, long-term vocational outcomes and social reintegration can also be negatively influenced by the presence of a persistent communication deficit (Brooks, McKinlay, Symington, Beattie, & Campsie, 1987; Malkmus, 1989), with some authors even suggesting that communicative abilities may play the pivotal role in determining the quality of life post-TBI (Najenson, Sazbon, Fiselzon, Becker, & Schechter, 1978).

Despite its frequent occurrence in the pediatric population, its persistent nature and potential negative impact on the quality of life of affected children, until recently there has been a relative paucity of research into the clinical features and neuropathophysiologic basis of dysarthria in children with TBI. Previously, it has been assumed that the physiologic impairment underlying dysarthria in children is the same as in adults and consequently the adult classification of dysarthria correlating with the pathophysiology of the motor systems has usually been applied to describe childhood dysarthria. More recently, it has been suggested that acquired dysarthria occurring in children requires its own classification (Morgan & Liégeois, 2010; van Mourik, Catsman-Berrevoets, Paquier, Yousef-Bak, & van Dongen, 1997) given that there are a number of reasons why the physiologic manifestation of dysarthria in children with TBI may differ from that in adults with TBI. These include: children may still be developing speech; there may be differences in recovery potential for children and adults; and there may be different mechanisms of neurologic damage in children and adults. The recognition of these potential differences between chil-

dren and adults has in recent years provided the impetus for further research into the nature of the physiologic functioning of the motor speech impairment in children with TBI. The most comprehensive series of physiologically based studies of children with TBI reported to date are those conducted by Cahill et al. (2002) and Cahill, Murdoch, and Theodoros (2002, 2003, 2005). The findings of these studies are and discussed later in this chapter.

This chapter aims to provide a contemporary overview of the major clinical characteristics of dysarthria in children with TBI in terms of its perceptual, acoustic, and physiologic features.

Traumatic Brain Injury in Childhood

Epidemiology

TBI is the leading cause of death and permanent disability in children and adolescents (Guyer & Ellers, 1990) and is one of the most frequent neurologic conditions resulting in hospitalization of children under 19 years of age (Field, 1976). Overall the incidence of TBI in children has been reported to be approximately 200 per 100,000 (Kraus, 1995) or 1 in every 550 school-aged children under 15 years of age (Kraus, Fife, Cox, Ramstein, & Conroy, 1986). In the United States, more than 200,000 children are hospitalized as a result of TBI each year, with approximately 15,000 of these children experiencing a severe TBI (Di Scala, Osberg, Gans, Chin, & Grant, 1991). A recent Swedish study reported that, after exclusion of concussion and other mild injuries, a mean incidence rate for TBI in children and adolescents of 12 per 100,000, with 6 in every 100,000 cases being left with permanent functional impairment indicating that serious brain injury is a significant cause of permanent neurological disability in the pediatric age group (Emanuelson & von Wendt, 1997).

It is well documented that the incidence of TBI varies across different age groups with the peak incidence of TBI reported to occur between the ages of 15 and 24 years (Kraus, Rock, & Hemyari, 1990; Mira, Tucker, & Tyler, 1992). With regard to children and adolescents, Sterling (1994) reported that 17.8% of injuries occur between the ages of 5 and 7 years, 35.6% between 8 and 11 years, 34.4% between 12 and 15 years, and 12% between 16 and 18 years. Likewise, the cause of injury also varies across the different age groups. The most common causes of TBI in infants, toddlers, and preschoolers are abuse and falls whereas the predominant cause of TBI in children aged 5 to 14 years appears to be motor vehicle accidents involving pedestrians or bicycles, and sporting injuries. High-speed motor vehicle accidents are reported to be the major cause of severe TBI in high school students and late adolescents (Annegers, 1983; Di Scala et al., 1991; Goldstein & Levin, 1987; Kraus et al., 1986).

As in the case of adult TBI, male children have a higher incidence of TBI than female children with ratios between 2 to 1 and 3 to 1 being reported (Goldstein & Levin, 1987; Rimel & Jane, 1983). Reasons for this gender difference include: males are more likely to be involved in motor vehicle accidents and to sustain sporting-related injuries; males are more involved in risk-taking behaviors and more aggressive sporting activities (Klauber, Barrett-Connor, Hofsetter, & Micik, 1986).

Prognostic Factors

Depending on the type of injury, the specific area of the brain affected and the severity of injury, the specific nature of impairment following TBI varies for each child (Bigler, Clark, & Farmer, 1996). Furthermore, factors such as age, developmental level, academic achievement, and behavioral adjustment interact with the brain injury itself to determine the child's presentation and long-term outcome (Rivara et al., 1994). Importantly, factors influencing the outcome of TBI in children vary from those that affect adults. Although the prognosis for recovery shown by children who have suffered mild TBI has been reported to be excellent (Bijur, Haslum, & Goldring, 1990) the prognosis for recovery from severe TBI (defined by a postresuscitation Glasgow Coma Score of 8 or less) is less certain, but reported to be far better for children than adults (Craft, Shaw, & Cartlidge, 1972). This difference may result from three factors. First, it may be due to the greater plasticity of the child's brain. TBI in childhood has been documented to recover more rapidly than that endured in adulthood as a consequence of distinctive neuroplasticity mechanisms (Levin, Benton, & Grossman, 1982). Second, it may be due to the different nature of the impacts causing head injury in children versus adults. Third, it may be related to differences in the basic mechanisms of brain damage following TBI in adults and children which in turn are related to differences in the physical characteristics of children's heads and adult heads.

As indicated above, most childhood accidents result from falls (this is particularly the case for infants and toddlers) or low-speed (30 to 60 km/h) pedestrian or bicycle accidents that involve a motor vehicle. Consequently many pediatric head injuries are associated with a lesser degree of rotational acceleration and, therefore, presumably with a lesser amount of brain damage (Levin et al., 1982). Adults, on the other hand, as well as persons in their late teens, are more likely to sustain TBI as a result of high-speed motor vehicle accidents, which by their nature yield greater diffuse brain injury. Some authors have noted the presence of persistent neurological deficits only in children injured in road traffic accidents (Jamison & Kaye, 1974). Likewise Moyes (1980) reported road traffic accidents to be the most common cause of long-term morbidity following head injury in childhood.

The reported greater capacity of young children to survive severe TBI, as compared with adults, has also been attributed to anatomic and physical features of head injury that differ between the two populations (Levin, Ewing-Cobbs, & Benton, 1984) thereby contributing to different patterns of brain injury following head trauma in each group. First, an infant's brain weight at birth is 15% of body weight, progressing through to only 3% in adults. By the end of the second year of life, brain weight is 75% of adult brain weight and reaches 90% of adult brain weight by the end of the sixth year (Jellinger, 1983). Second, the presence of unfused sutures and open fontanelles makes the skull of an infant and young child pliable. Some authors have suggested that, because of its elasticity and greater degree of deformation, the skull of an infant absorbs the energy of the physical impact and thereby protects the brain better than the skull of an adult (Craft et al, 1972; Menkes & Till, 1995). Other authors, however, believe that the greater pliability of the heads of infants

makes them more susceptible to external forces than older children and adults. According to Menkes and Till (1995), although the deformation of the head absorbs much of the energy of the impact, thereby reducing the effects of acceleration/deceleration, it adds to the risk of tearing blood vessels.

At the time of impact, as a result of external forces, the brain moves within the skull, making contact with its rigid walls, with the greatest degree of contact occurring between the soft temporal and frontal lobes and the bony prominences of the skull. A third anatomic difference in the skulls of children versus adults that may aid a better prognosis in the former group is that the floors of the middle cranial fossa and the orbital roofs continue to be relatively smooth and offer little resistance to the shifting brain. Overall, it would appear that the pathophysiologic mechanisms underlying childhood TBI may be disparate to those which take hold in the adult brain, particularly when considered within the context of developmental hierarchies, type of injury, and neuroplasticity capabilities (Levin et al., 1982). Consequently, it is possible that functioning of the major components of the speech apparatus will be affected differently in children and adults following TBI. Furthermore, it cannot be assumed that children will recover from TBI or respond to rehabilitative measures in the same manner as adults.

Dysarthria in Childhood Traumatic Brain Injury

As outlined in Chapter 11, acquired childhood dysarthria traditionally has been described and classified using criteria pertaining to the adult dysarthric population. However, children with TBI may still be developing speech, and therefore the resultant motor speech disorder may well be an interaction of developmental and acquired components of this disorder (Murdoch & Hudson-Tennant, 1994). In particular, communication disorders such as dysarthria have not been comprehensively studied in childhood TBI. Until recently, there has been little information regarding the nature of dysarthria in children subsequent to TBI available in the literature. In the absence of a model of motor speech disorders for children most investigators have used the adult model of dysarthria, which correlates the type of dysarthria with the pathophysiology of the motor subsystems. This model is not totally satisfactory, particularly for younger children, whose speech and language skills are still developing. Therefore, there is an obvious need to investigate the specific nature of the speech disturbance following TBI as it relates to the pediatric population.

The few studies that have attempted to further define the nature of dysarthria subsequent to TBI in children have largely been case studies (Cahill et al., 2000; Murdoch & Horton, 1998; Murdoch, Pitt, Theodoros, & Ward, 1999). Murdoch et al. (1999) examined the effects of real-time continuous visual biofeedback as a treatment for speech breathing disorders in a child with severe dysarthria following TBI. Based on a series of perceptual and physiologic measures they reported the presence of a level of impairment in all of the subcomponents of the speech production mechanism including respiration, phonation, resonation, and articulation. Similarly, Murdoch and Horton (1998) identified a range of impairments across

the speech production mechanism, using both perceptual and instrumental assessments, in single case studies of children with dysarthria subsequent to TBI. The most comprehensive series of studies of dysarthria subsequent to childhood TBI reported to date was completed by Cahill et al. (2002, 2003, 2005). Based on the findings of both perceptual and physiologic assessments, these latter researchers found that each child presented with a differing profile of speech subsystem deficits, ranging from no dysarthria to moderate-severe dysarthria. The heterogeneity of the speech impairments identified in this series of studies is not unexpected, given that the diffuse, nonspecific nature of TBI can lead to damage in many areas of the central nervous system (see Chapter 3 for a more complete description of the biomechanics of TBI). More specifically, the perceptual and instrumental analysis of speech function in the group of children with TBI examined by Cahill et al. (2002, 2003, 2005) identified substantial impairments in prosody, velopharyngeal and articulatory function, as well as reduced lung capacity and impaired respiratory-phonatory control for speech but little impairment in laryngeal function. These findings are described more fully below.

Functioning of the Speech Production Mechanism Following Childhood Traumatic Brain Injury

Cahill and colleagues (2002, 2003, 2005) assessed the perceptual and physiologic features of speech functioning in a group of 22 individuals who sustained a TBI during childhood. All four functional components of the speech mechanism (respiratory, laryngeal, velopharyngeal, and articulatory function) were assessed using a variety of perceptual and instrumental procedures (for a comprehensive description of perceptual, acoustic, and physiologic assessment of dysarthria see Chapter 14). Of the 22 subjects assessed, 10 were classified as dysarthric, on the basis of a perceptual analysis, and 12 were nondysarthric. Fourteen (64%) of the total sample of TBI subjects were male (M = 13.52 years; SD = 3.16; range = 8 to 18 years), and eight were female (M = 11.35 years; SD = 3.26; range = 5 to 15 years). The mean age of the total sample of TBI subjects was 12.73 years (SD = 3.29), with ages ranging from 5 to 18 years. All subjects were at least 6 months postinjury. The biographical and clinical details of the 22 children with TBI assessed by Cahill and colleagues are presented in Table 12–1.

Perceptual Speech Features in Childhood Traumatic Brain Injury

The battery of perceptual assessments used by Cahill et al. (2002, 2003, 2005) to assess the speech abilities of their 22 children with TBI included:

■ Assessment of Intelligibility of Dysarthric Speech (Yorkston & Beukelman, 1981)
■ Frenchay Dysarthria Assessment (Enderby, 1983)
■ Fisher-Logemann Test of Articulation Competence (Fisher & Logemann, 1971)
■ Speech sample analysis (SSA)

The Assessment of Intelligibility of Dysarthric Speech (ASSIDS; Yorkston & Beukelman, 1981) provides an index of the severity of dysarthric speech by quantifying both single-word and sentence intelligibility as well as the speaking rate (words per minute), the rate of intelligible speech (i.e., the number of intelligible words per minute [IWPM]), and the communication efficiency ratio (CER) of dysarthric speakers. The test is designed for use with the adult population, but can be modified (by having the child repeat the words and sentences rather than read them) for children with reading difficulties or for those children who had not yet reached a reading level appropriate for administration of the test. The Frenchay Dysarthria Assessment (FDA; Enderby, 1983) provides a standardized assessment of speech neuromuscular activity, presented in a composite profile form and is easily administered to children. The Fisher-Logemann Test of Articulation Competence (Fisher & Logemann, 1971) provides an articulation profile and may be analyzed further to establish the presence of phonological processes, especially the presence of any developmental errors. Finally, a sample of the child's reading is analyzed perceptually (SSA). The children are asked to read aloud the standardized passage "The Grandfather Passage" (Darley et al., 1975) or, if the child cannot read, a picture description task is used. This sample is then rated by two experienced speech language pathologists on a series of 33 different dimensions of speech, encompassing prosody, respiration, phonation, resonance, and articulation (Fitz-Gerald, Murdoch, & Chenery, 1987). Full details of these assessments are presented in Chapter 14.

The perceptual analysis of the speech of the 22 TBI subjects, when compared to an age- and gender-matched control group, revealed a significant disturbance in various aspects of prosody, resonance, phonation, and articulation.

Table 12–1. Biographical and Clinical Details of the TBI Subjects Assessed by Cahill et al. (2002, 2003, 2005)

Subject	Age at Assess. (years)	Sex	Months Postinjury	Nature of Accident	GCS	Site of Lesion(s) Confirmed by CT/MRI	Severity of Dysarthria
1	15.17	M	7	HBT	4	Depressed skull; diffuse cerebral edema	Mild
2	11.17	M	6	MV/B	3	Right parietal skull #	Absent
3	9.17	M	10	MV/B	8	Mild cerebral swelling	Absent
4	8.25	M	25	MV/B	8	Left upper hematoma, narrowing of ventricular system; linear fracture left frontal lobe	Absent
5	8.57	F	14	BA	4	Skull #; left frontal contusion; edema	Absent
6	15.00	F	31	MV/P	3	# right petrous temporal bone & left maxilla; small bleed in right basal ganglia	Absent
7	16.08	M	19	MV/B	9	Subdural hemorrhage temporoparietal region; edema left cerebral hemisphere	Absent
8	14.67	M	29	MV/P	3	# through occipital & basal regions with severe diffuse cerebral edema	Absent
9	14.33	M	21	MV/P	8	Left frontal petechial hemorrhage with diffuse cerebral edema swelling, left > right	Absent
10	11.00	F	36	MV/P	12	Deep white matter changes consistent with diffuse axonal injury	Absent
11	5.42	F	8	MVA	12	# right parietal bone; hematoma right temporoparietal area	Absent
12	12.08	F	40	Fall	3	Depressed compound # left parietooccipital region; edema	Absent
13	15.17	M	72	MV/B	3	Diffuse axonal injury	Mild-moderate

continues

Table 12–1. *continued*

Subject	Age at Assess. (years)	Sex	Months Postinjury	Nature of Accident	GCS	Site of Lesion(s) Confirmed by CT/MRI	Severity of Dysarthria
14	15.42	F	24	MV/P	3	Cerebral edema; subarachnoid & intraventricular hemorrhage	Mild
15	10.75	M	42	Fall	7	Diffuse axonal injury; right cerebral edema & hematoma	Absent
16	18.25	M	10	MV/B	3	Right temporoparietal, cerebral edema	Moderate-severe
17	9.83	M	18	MBA	5	Posterior interhemispheric hematoma extending over left tentorium; profuse edema; dilation of temporal horns	Moderate
18	16.00	M	78	MV/B	4	Edema and effacement of sulci & compression of ventricles; hematoma in left parietal lobe lateral to thalamus	Severe
19	17.17	M	40	MV/B	4	Intracranial petechial hemorrhages and contusion right basal ganglia	Moderate
20	11.08	F	13	MV/B	3	Brainstem/pontine hemorrhage; prominent lateral ventricles secondary to diffuse axonal injury	Moderate
21	13.25	M	6	MV/B	7	Brainstem hemorrhages; diffuse bilateral cerebral contusions and axonal injury	Moderate
22	12.25	F	78	MV/P	3	Pneumoencephaly, contrecoupe lesions parietal lobes; depressed right parietal #; pituitary fossa #; obliteration of basal cisterns, third and fourth ventricle effacement; hemorrhage into right thalamus	Moderate

GCS = Glasgow Coma Score; HBT = hit by train; MV/B = motor vehicle/bicycle accident; BA = bicycle accident; MV/P = motor vehicle/pedestrian accident; MVA = motor vehicle accident; MBA = motorbike accident; # = fracture.

In addition, assessment on the ASSIDS revealed that the group with TBI demonstrated a significant reduction in the rate of speech, intelligible words per minute, and communication efficiency, when compared to the control group, with the dysarthric subjects with TBI also demonstrating a reduced sentence intelligibility. The group with TBI also exhibited significant impairment in reflex, lip, palate, laryngeal, and tongue function, when the results of the FDA were compared to the control group. The SSA revealed that the children with TBI displayed significant impairment on 5 of the 33 speech dimensions, compared to the matched control group. Specifically, the group with TBI as a whole demonstrated: a lack of pitch variation, a decreased general rate of speech, hypernasality, glottal fry, and imprecision of consonants.

When the 10 dysarthric children with TBI were compared to the control group, 9 of the 33 dimensions were noted to be significantly impaired. Three of these deviant speech dimensions related to prosody (lack of variation in pitch, decreased general rate of speech, and excess stress on usually unstressed parts of speech) and two related to articulation (imprecision of consonants, and increased length of phonemes). In addition, the dysarthric children with TBI were noted to have significantly impaired breath support for speech, significant degrees of hypernasality and glottal fry, and a significant reduction in speech intelligibility, when compared to the control group. The frequency of occurrence of each deviant speech dimension exhibited by the group with TBI as a whole was also determined to provide a descriptive measure of the perceptual speech sample analysis. The most frequently occurring deviant speech dimen-

sion was that of imprecision of consonants, with 59% of all children with TBI being rated with some degree of consonant imprecision, ranging from a mild to a severe degree. The speech dimensions of hypernasality, inappropriate pitch level, lack of variation in pitch, and glottal fry were present in 54% of the subjects. Excess stress for the context was the next most frequently occurring deviant speech dimension, being present in 41% of all children with TBI. Impaired breath support for speech, a shortened phrase length, increased length of phonemes, and hoarseness were present in 36% of all subjects. Other frequently occurring deviant speech dimensions included maintenance of rate, prolonged intervals, and decreased overall intelligibility (27%). Maintenance of loudness, hyponasality, and imprecision of vowels were noted to be present in 22% of subjects. The speech dimensions of mixed nasality, harshness, strain-strangled phonation, intermittent breathiness, wetness, pitch breaks, excessive fluctuation of rate and pitch, excessive loudness variation, short rushes of speech, forced inspiration/ expiration, and audible inspiration were noted in only one of two children.

Based on the results of the ASSIDS, the group with TBI as a whole was found to exhibit significant reductions in rate of speech (WPM), intelligible words per minute (IWPM), and communication efficiency (CER), compared to the control children. Although the sentence intelligibility score was lower for the group with TBI, it was not significantly different from that of the control group. However, when the dysarthric children with TBI were compared to the control group, significant reductions were noted in sentence intelligibility as well as in WPM, CER, IWPM, and an increase was noted in unintelligible words per minute (UWPM).

It also was noted that the nondysarthric children with TBI demonstrated significantly reduced WPM, CER, and IWPM, when compared to the control group. Therefore, although not perceived to be dysarthric, certain elements of speech intelligibility, such as rate of speech, as measured on the ASSIDS, were found to be impaired in the nondysarthric group, compared to their control counterparts.

Evaluation on the FDA indicated that, when compared to the control group, the performance of the children with TBI was significantly impaired on 19 of the 25 subsystem components. The group with TBI demonstrated impairments in all subsystems of the speech mechanism, except for jaw and respiratory function. Furthermore, the 10 dysarthric speakers were found to demonstrate significantly impaired function on all measures of lip, tongue, and laryngeal function, with impairment also noted in respiration during speech and palatal function. Interestingly, the nondysarthric children with TBI also demonstrated significantly impaired function in many areas of lip, tongue, and laryngeal function, when compared to the control group. Therefore, some degree of subclinical impairment in speech neuromuscular activity was evident in the speech of these speakers, even though they had been rated perceptually as nondysarthric.

Physiologic Functioning of the Speech Mechanism Following Childhood Traumatic Brain Injury

Physiologic assessment of speech function conducted by Cahill and Colleagues (2002, 2003, 2005) identified varying degrees of impairment across all speech subsystems in the children with TBI compared to their control group. Velopharyngeal function was found to be the most impaired subsystem with significantly increased nasality present in all the group with TBI's nonnasal utterances. Articulatory function in the children with TBI was also found to be significantly impaired, with lip function being more impaired than tongue function. Spirometric assessment of respiratory function identified significantly reduced mean predicted values for VC and FEV_1 in the children with TBI which were associated with reduced syllables per breath and syllables per minute. Kinematic assessment revealed relatively normal respiratory values with the exception of a reduced lung volume initiation (LVI) and abdominal volume initiation (ABVI), when expressed as a percentage of VC, during conversation. Assessment of laryngeal function on aerodynamic and electroglottographic measures identified no areas of significant impairment in the children with TBI, with the exception of a reduced ad/abduction rate. A summary of the deviant physiologic speech features of the children with TBI can be found in Table 12–2.

Respiratory Function. Respiratory function was assessed using both spirometric and kinematic techniques. The group with TBI was found to have a significant reduction in the mean predicted values for both VC (74%) and FEV_1 (69%), when compared to their control group (VC = 91%; FEV_1 = 83%). The 10 dysarthric children with TBI were found to have a significantly reduced VC (68%), but not FEV_1 (70%).

Kinematic evaluation revealed essentially normal respiratory function in the children with TBI, with the exception of a reduced lung volume initiation (LVI) when expressed as a percentage of VC, during conversational speech. This could largely be accounted for by a

Table 12–2. Summary of the Deviant Physiologic Speech Features Identified in the Childhood TBI Group

Speech Subsytem		Deviant Physiologic Speech Features
Respiratory		↓ vital capacity
		↓ FEV$_1$
		↓ LVI in conversation
		↓ ABVI in conversation
		↓ syllables per breath
		↓ syllables per minute
Velopharyngeal		↑ nasality NN sounds
		↑ nasality NN words
		↑ nasality NN sentences
		↑ nasality NN utterances
Laryngeal		↓ ad/abduction rate
Articulatory	Lip	↓ maximum lip pressure
		↓ sustained maximum lip pressure
		↓ lip pressure in repetitive tasks
	Tongue	↓ rate in fast tongue repetition task

↓ = decreased; ↑ = increased; LVI = lung volume initiation; ABVI = abdominal volume initiation; FEV$_1$ = forced expiratory volume in one second; NN = nonnasal.

decrease in abdominal volume initiation (ABVI) in conversation. Even though the respiratory kinematics of the group with TBI were relatively normal, significant impairments in breath control and speaking rate were noted, with significant reductions in syllables per breath (M = 6.52) and syllables per minute (M = 114.98), when compared to the control group (M = 10.51 syllables per breath; M = 174.31 syllables per minute). The dysarthric speakers with TBI also demonstrated a significantly reduced number of syllables per breath (M = 4.55) and syllables per minute (M = 84.55), supporting the perceptual findings of significantly impaired breath support for speech on both the FDA and SSA.

Laryngeal Function. Laryngeal function was assessed by Cahill et al. (2003) using both electroglottographic (laryngograph) and aerodynamic (Aerophone II) measures (see Chapter 14). No significant differences were detected between the group with TBI and the control group on the various electroglottographic measures. As well as this, no significant differences were found between the dysarthric speakers in the TBI group, the nondysarthric speakers, and a control group. The results of the aerodynamic assessment indicated that the ad/abduction rate was significantly reduced in the group with TBI as a whole and the 10 dysarthric children with TBI , when compared to a control group. The lack of statistically significant differences on most physiologic measures of laryngeal function between these groups is interesting, given that the presence of glottal fry was detected by these authors in 54% of their children with TBI, and 36% were reported as being hoarse. Similarly, all measures of laryngeal function measured on the FDA were reported to be significantly impaired. Several factors have contributed to these conflicting results. The wide age range of the children with TBI meant that children with prepubertal and pubertal stages of laryngeal development were included in the group with TBI, and the effect of endocrinological changes on the vocal qualities of both male and female adolescents is well documented (Hollien & Malcik, 1967; Michel, Hollien, & Moore, 1966). Another reason may be that the FDA and the physiologic assessments are assessing quite different measures of laryngeal function. Other factors suggested by Cahill et al. (2003) that may have influenced the results include the relatively low number of dysarthric speakers with TBI, and the intersubject variability present in the electroglottographic and aerodynamic data. Therefore it may be more appropriate that analysis of laryngeal function involves the identification of subgroupings of participants with similar ages and/or similar vocal function to allow for these confounding influences.

Velopharyngeal Function. Results of accelerometric assessment conducted by Cahill et al. (2002, 2003, 2005) indicated that the group with TBI as a whole exhibited a significant degree of increased nasality on all non-nasal utterances, when compared to a control group. Similarly, assessment on the Nasometer revealed that the group with TBI and the dys-

arthric subjects with TBI demonstrated significantly higher nasalance levels than the control subjects. These results support the results of the perceptual assessment conducted by these researchers, which identified hypernasality as the second most frequently occurring deviant speech dimension in the children with TBI, with 54% perceived to have some degree of hypernasality in their speech.

Articulatory Function. Instrumental assessment of lip function by Cahill et al. (2005) revealed significant impairment in the group with TBI as a whole, and in the dysarthric and nondysarthric children with TBI, when compared to a control group, in the areas of maximum lip pressure, sustained maximum lip pressure, repetition of maximum lip pressure, and a reduced pressure in the fast lip repetition task. These results supported the perceptual findings of Cahill et al. (2002) of consonant imprecision and impaired lip function on the FDA. The presence of significantly impaired lip function in the nondysarthric children with TBI indicated that, although speech was perceived to be normal in this group, there were in fact subclinical impairments present in lip function. This fact was supported by the presence of significantly impaired function on the FDA in the areas of lips at rest and alternating lip movements in the nondysarthric children with TBI, when compared to the control group.

Physiological assessment of tongue function completed by Cahill (2005) identified a significantly reduced rate of tongue movement in the fast tongue repetition task in the group with TBI, when compared to the control group. This finding supported their perceptual finding of a reduced general rate of speech in the children with TBI. However, it is surprising that other elements of impaired tongue function were not identified on the instrumental assessment, given that significant impairment was noted in all areas of tongue function on the FDA. The most obvious reason for this discrepancy is that the FDA evaluates quite different measures of tongue function than the instrumental assessment of tongue function. The tongue pressure transduction system utilized by Cahill et al. (2005) assesses static measures of tongue strength, endurance, fine force control, and rate of repetitive movements, whereas the FDA rates range and coordination of tongue movements. Stierwalt and colleagues (1996), in their study of children and adolescents with TBI, also found that their group with TBI did not differ from controls in terms of maximal tongue strength. They did, however, identify significant correlations between the nonspeech measures of tongue performance and the perceptual judgments of overall speech defectiveness and articulatory imprecision in their children with TBI. This discrepancy in results highlights the need for more dynamic assessment of tongue function during speech, using procedures such as electropalatography and electromagnetic articulography.

Case Examples

Case 1: James

James, an 18-year-old male sustained a severe TBI (Glasgow Coma Score = 3) at the age of 9 years 11 months when knocked from his bicycle by a motor vehicle. A CT scan taken on the day of admission to hospital indicated a skull fracture in the right frontoparietal region, some blood in the third ventricle and ethmoid sinuses, and mild cerebral edema on the right side of the brain with compression of the right anterior horn of the lateral ventricle. James was mute for a period of six months postinjury and remained moderately dysarthric at the time of referral to the Centre for Neurogenic Communication Disorders Research at The University of Queensland 8 years 1 month postinjury.

A battery of perceptual and physiologic tests conducted at that time revealed that James displayed varying degrees of dysfunction at all levels of the speech production apparatus (respiratory, laryngeal, velopharyngeal, and articulatory subsystems). He was rated as having a moderate flaccid dysarthria. Table 12–3 presents a summary of the results of his perceptual and physiologic assessments.

Respiratory Function

Spirometric assessment of James's respiratory function revealed that both the vital capacity (VC = 45%) and forced expiratory volume (FEV$_1$ = 47%), when compared to their predicted values, were markedly reduced. Kinematic assessment indicated increased lung volume initiation ($\uparrow$ 3.24 SD), lung volume termination ($\uparrow$ 1.75 SD) and lung volume excursion ($\uparrow$ 2.67 SD) during reading, when compared to a control group. This pattern of speech breathing indicated that James was using the higher end of lung volume during this task, which was inconsistent with a normal pattern.

Laryngeal Function

Perceptual assessment of James's laryngeal subsystem on the FDA indicated

Table 12–3. Case 1: Results of Perceptual and Physiologic Assessments

Case 1: 18-year-old male assessed 8.5 years post-MVA (hit from bike). GCS = 3.
CT scan data indicated damage in the right parietal region and mild cerebral edema.
He was rated as having a moderate flaccid dysarthria.

Speech Subsystem	Perceptual Assessment	Physiologic Assessment
Respiratory	FDA—Very mild impairment at rest	↓ vital capacity
	SSA—Mod. ↓ breath support for speech	↓ forced expiratory volume
	—Mild intermittent breathiness	
Laryngeal	FDA—Mod./severe impairment	↓ peak air pressure
	SSA—Mild ↓ in pitch variation	↓ phonatory resistance
	—Mild ↓ in loudness level	↓ adduction/abduction rate
	—Mild intermittent breathiness	
Velopharyngeal	FDA—Mod. ↓ in palatal function	Moderate ↑ nasality in nonnasal utterances
	SSA—Severe hypernasality	
Articulatory		
Lip	FDA—Mod./severe impairment	↓ maximum lip strength
	SSA—Mod. consonant imprecision	↓ rate of repetitive lip movements
		↓ lip endurance
Tongue	FDA—Mod./severe impairment	↓ maximum tongue strength
	SSA—Mod. consonant imprecision	↓ rate of repetitive movements
	—Mod. ↓ in general rate	↓ tongue endurance
		↓ fine force control
Intelligibility	ASSIDS—Sentence intelligibility 45% of normal	
	—↓ rate of speech	
	SSA—Moderate ↓ in speech intelligibility	
	—Moderate ↓ in general rate of speech	

FDA = Frenchay Dysarthria Assessment; SSA = speech sample analysis; ASSIDS = Assessment of Intelligibility of Dysarthric Speech; ↑↓ = greater than 1 standard deviation above or below a control group mean. (Laryngeal values are compared to a single matched-control subject.)

moderate-to-severe impairment of laryngeal characteristics. Electroglottographic measures (fundamental frequency, closing time, and duty cycle) were found to be comparable to a matched control subject. However, aerodynamic measures (Aerophone II) of laryngeal function revealed decreased phonatory resistance and adduction/abduction rate, when compared to a control subject matched for age and sex. These factors are consistent with hypofunctioning of the laryngeal valving mechanism, and with the diagnosis of flaccid dysarthria.

The discrepancies in the perceptual and physiologic assessment results highlight the need to identify the underlying physiological impairment and not rely solely on the perceptual analysis of speech, especially when planning therapy. Theodoros and Murdoch (1994) stated that an understanding of the physiologic nature of the laryngeal subsystem is very important, since this component of the speech mechanism not only provides the acoustic medium through which speech is delivered, but also contributes to the suprasegmental and articulatory features of speech.

Velopharyngeal Function

Accelerometric assessment of James's speech indicated an increased degree of nasality in the production of nonnasal utterances ($\uparrow$ 2.07 SD), which confirmed the perceptual rating of moderate hypernasality. An inadequate velopharyngeal mechanism can place increased burdens on the respiratory system, which, in turn, may lead to shortened phrases and phonatory abnormalities involving pitch and loudness as well as articulatory disturbance (Johns & Salyer, 1978).

Articulatory Function

The perceptual analysis of James's speech sample (SSA) identified moderate impairment of articulation and prosody in the form of imprecision of consonants, decreased overall speech intelligibility, and a slowed rate of speech. Results of the FDA, in which moderate-to-severe impairment of the lips and tongue were observed, and a reduced sentence intelligibility score (45%) on the ASSIDS, support the perceptual finding of articulatory imprecision.

Lip and tongue pressure transducer analyses demonstrated impaired labial and lingual function, when compared to a control group. Significant impairments were noted in the areas of lip strength ($\downarrow$ 1.82 SD) and sustained maximal lip pressure ($\downarrow$ 1.83 SD) and in the repetitive movement tasks, where both the rate ($\downarrow$ 1.38 SD) and pressure ($\downarrow$ 1.76 SD) were reduced, when compared to a control group. Tongue function was also significantly impaired, most noticeably in the areas of tongue strength ($\downarrow$ 3.04 SD), endurance ($\downarrow$ 2.38 SD), repetition of maximum tongue pressure ($\downarrow$ 2.91 SD), and rate in the fast repetition task ($\downarrow$ 2.91 SD). On the basis of these assessments, it was noted that tongue function appeared to be more severely affected than lip function. This finding may account for the perception of articulatory imprecision, as well as a reduction in the general rate of speech and in the perception of prolonged intervals during speech production.

Summary and Implication for Treatment

James presented with a moderate flaccid dysarthria characterized by a decreased rate of speech, moderate hypernasality, moderate imprecision of consonants, and moderately decreased speech intelligibility. Physiological assessment revealed impairments across all speech subsystems. Based on both the perceptual and instrumental assessments, treatment would concentrate on the following areas:

1. Articulatory function:

    Increase tongue strength and endurance

    Increase lip strength and endurance

    Increase rate and maintenance of pressure on repetitive lip and tongue tasks

2. Velopharyngeal function:

    Decrease nasality in speech/increase oral resonance

3. Laryngeal function:

    Increase phonatory effort to improve vocal fold adduction

4. Respiratory function:

    Increase vital capacity to improve breath support for speech

James would benefit from a multisystem approach to therapy, working on respiratory, laryngeal, and velopharyngeal function to facilitate adequate breath and voice to support articulation. As the velopharyngeal system plays an important role in the maintenance of intraoral pressure for the production of plosive and fricative sounds, therapy should also be focused on increasing velopharyngeal valving. Treatment aimed at increasing laryngeal valving could also incorporate exercises aimed at increasing respiratory support, vocal fold adduction, and volume, pitch, and loudness variation. Both traditional and biofeedback techniques could be used to remediate lip and tongue deficits.

Case 2: Leonard

Leonard sustained a severe TBI (Glasgow Coma Score = 3) at age 10 years 7 months when the bicycle he was riding was struck by a motor vehicle. A CT scan taken shortly after admission to hospital revealed a skull fracture in the right parietal region. He was assessed at the Centre for Neurogenic Communication Disorders Research, The University of Queensland, 7 months postinjury at age 11 years 2 months. A battery of perceptual and physiologic tests of Leonard's speech performed at the time revealed minimal deficits and he was not deemed to demonstrate any perceptible dysarthria. Table 12–4 presents a summary of Leonard's perceptual and physiologic assessments.

Respiratory Function

Perceptual assessment of Leonard's speech (FDA, SSA) identified no areas of impairment in respiratory function. Spirometric assessment, however, identified reduced vital capacity (VC = 67%) and forced expiratory volumes (FEV_1 = 45%), when compared with their predicted values. Kinematic assessment indicated that LVI and LVT during reading were reduced when compared to a control group, and that Leonard produced a reduced number of syllables per breath during reading, which supports the notion that respiratory support for speech was not totally adequate.

Table 12–4. Case 2: Results of Perceptual and Physiologic Assessments

Case 2: 11-year-old male assessed 7 months post-MVA (hit from bike). GCS = 3. CT scan data indicated a right parietal fracture. He was rated as nondysarthric.

Speech Subsystem	Perceptual Assessment	Physiologic Assessment
Respiratory	FDA—No impairment noted	↓ vital capacity
	SSA—No features noted	↓ forced expiratory volume
		↓ syllables/breath
Laryngeal	FDA—No impairment noted	↑ phonatory flow rate
	SSA—No features noted	↓ phonatory resistance
		↓ adduction/abduction rate
Velopharyngeal	FDA—Mild hyponasality noted	↑ nasality in nonnasal sounds & sentences
	SSA—Mild hyponasality noted	
Articulatory		
Lip	FDA—Very mild ↓ in coordination	↓ lip pressure in fast repetition tasks
	SSA—No features noted	
Tongue	FDA—Very mild ↓ in coordination	↓ maximum tongue strength
	SSA—No features noted	↓ tongue pressure in fast repetition tasks
Intelligibility	ASSIDS—Mild decrease in rate of speech	
	SSA—No features noted	

FDA = Frenchay Dysarthria Assessment; SSA = speech sample analysis; ASSIDS = Assessment of Intelligibility of Dysarthric Speech; ↑↓ = greater than 1 standard deviation above or below a control group mean. (Laryngeal values are compared to a single matched-control subject.)

Laryngeal Function

Aerodynamic assessment (Aerophone II) identified an increased phonatory flow rate, decreased phonatory resistance, and a decreased adduction/abduction rate, when compared to a matched control subject, consistent with mild hypofunctioning of the laryngeal valve. However, all measures taken from the electroglot-tographic assessment were found to be comparable to the control subject matched for age and sex. Perceptual analysis of Leonard's speech found no evidence of laryngeal dysfunction.

Velopharyngeal Function

Perceptual assessment of Leonard's speech identified mild hyponasality, which was in direct contrast to the findings of the accelerometric assessment, which identified moderately increased nasality in non-nasal utterances ($\uparrow$ 2.86 SD).

Articulatory Function

Perceptual assessment on the FDA identified mild incoordination of the lips and tongue. No deviant features relating to articulatory function were noted on the SSA. Physiological assessment of lip and tongue function, using pressure transduction systems, identified mild subclinical deficits in articulatory function, especially apparent in tasks requiring rapid repetitive movements of the tongue. These results support the perceptual finding of mild incoordination of lip and tongue movements noted on the FDA.

Summary and Implications for Treatment

Perceptually Leonard presented as non-dysarthric, with only a mild degree of hyponasality noted in his speech. However, mild subclinical deficits in some speech subsystems were noted on instrumental assessment. The nature and degree of these deficits, however, would not be sufficient to recommend any intervention. The absence of dysarthria in this child is interesting, given that he sustained an injury of similar type and severity to Case 1. This disparity highlights the differential nature of speech outcome that can occur following TBI in childhood.

Case 3: Rodney

Rodney presented at the Centre for Neurogenic Communication Disorders Research, The University of Queensland, for assessment at the age of 15 years. He had sustained a severe TBI (Glasgow Coma Score = 3) 6 years earlier when his bicycle was hit by a motor vehicle. A CT scan taken on the day of admission to hospital revealed diffuse axonal injury. Rodney was reportedly mute for several weeks post-injury.

Perceptual and physiologic assessment of Rodney's speech revealed mild-to-moderate impairment in articulatory, laryngeal, and velopharyngeal function, but essentially normal respiratory function. His speech was characterized by prosodic disturbances such as reduced pitch variation, decreased general rate of speech, and excess stress for context, resulting in an overall rating of mild-to-moderate ataxic dysarthria. Table 12–5 presents a summary of the results of his perceptual and physiologic assessments.

Respiratory Function

Spirometric assessment of respiratory function revealed that Rodney's vital capacity and forced expiratory volumes were within normal limits. Kinematic assessment indicated essentially normal respiration patterns when compared to a control group, with the exception of a reduced LVI during reading. These results confirm the perceptual rating on the FDA and SSA of normal respiratory function. The exception to this was the finding of a reduced number of syllables per breath. However, it is possible that the reduced syllables per breath were a result of Rodney's slowed rate of speech rather than impaired respiratory function per se.

Laryngeal Function

Although perceptual analysis on the FDA indentified moderate impairment in pitch, volume, and vocal quality, the

Table 12–5. Case 3: Results of Perceptual and Physiologic Assessments

Case 3: 15-year-old male assessed 6 years post-MVA (hit from bike). GCS = 3. CT scan revealed evidence of diffuse axonal injury. He was rated as having a mild-to-moderate ataxic dysarthria.

Speech Subsystem	Perceptual Assessment	Physiologic Assessment
Respiratory	FDA—No impairment noted SSA—No features noted	↓ syllables/breath
Laryngeal	FDA—Mod. Impairment noted SSA—Mild ↓ in pitch variation	↓ peak air pressure ↓ phonatory resistance ↑ closing time
Velopharyngeal	FDA—Mild impairment noted SSA—Mild hypernasality noted	Mod. ↑ nasality in nonnasal utterances
Articulatory		
Lip	FDA—Mild impairment in lip function SSA—No features noted	↓ maximum lip strength ↓ pressure in fast repetition tasks ↓ fine force control of lips
Tongue	FDA—Mild/mod. ↓ in tongue function SSA—Mild ↓ in general rate of speech	↑ maximum tongue pressure ↓ rate in fast repetition task
Intelligibility	ASSIDS—↓ sentence intelligibility —↓ rate of speech SSA—Intelligibility rated as within normal range	
Prosody	SSA—Mild decrease in general rate of speech —Mild decrease in pitch variation —Moderate excess of stress for context	

FDA = Frenchay Dysarthria Assessment; SSA = speech sample analysis; ASSIDS = Assessment of Intelligibility of Dysarthric Speech; ↑↓ = greater than 1 standard deviation above or below a control group mean. (Laryngeal values are compared to a single matched-control subject.)

373

only feature rated as deviant on the SSA was mildly impaired variation of pitch. Aerodynamic assessment (Aerophone II) of laryngeal function identified decreased peak air pressure and decreased phonatory resistance, while electroglottographic assessment (Laryngograph) revealed an increased closing time, when compared to a matched control subject. In general, these features are consistent with hypofunctioning of the laryngeal valve.

Velopharyngeal Function

Instrumental assessment of Rodney's velopharyngeal function, when compared to a control group, revealed a moderate-to-severe degree of hypernasality on production of nonnasal utterances ($\uparrow$ 3.64 SD). This finding conflicts with the perceptual rating on both the FDA and SSA, which indicated only mildly increased nasality. This inconsistency highlights the need to confirm perceptual judgments with physiologic information before commencing therapy. A finding of only mildly increased nasality may not warrant specific intervention, and the deficit may remain untreated. Hypernasality typically results from paralysis, paresis, or incoordination of the muscles involved in velopharyngeal closure (Johns & Salyer, 1978). However, it has also been suggested by Hoodin and Gilbert (1989) that a decreased rate of speech may affect velopharyngeal closure. In their study of subjects with Parkinson disease, Hoodin and Gilbert (1989) found that these subjects demonstrated a break in the velopharyngeal seal at slower speaking rates. Therefore, it is conceivable that the increased nasality identified instrumentally in Rodney's speech could be due to poor functioning of the velopharyngeal valve, or possibly could be a side effect of his reduced rate of speech.

Articulatory Function

Perceptual assessment of articulatory function using the FDA identified mild impairment in lip function and mild-to-moderate impairment in tongue function. A mild decrease in the general rate of speech was identified perceptually on the SSA, and a decreased number of words per minute (77 WPM, $\downarrow$ 3.13 SD) was identified on the ASSIDS. Physiologic assessment of tongue function identified an increased maximum tongue pressure ($\uparrow$ 1.35 SD), but a reduction in the rate of rapid repetitive tongue movements ($\downarrow$ 1.29 SD), when compared to the control group. This finding of reduced rate of tongue movements would contribute directly to the perceptual finding of a reduction in the general rate of speech.

Instrumental assessment of lip function revealed decreased maximum lip strength ($\downarrow$ 1.30 SD) and decreased pressure in repetition of maximum lip pressure, when compared to a control group. It is surprising that, despite these impairments in lip function, Rodney was perceived as having normal consonant precision. It has been suggested (Robin, Goel, Somodi, & Luschei, 1992) that there is a "critical level" of strength reduction (i.e., the degree of strength reduction that is sufficient to affect speech production). Although there was a considerable reduction in lip strength, the weakness appears not to be within the critical range that affects the accuracy of consonant production.

Prosodic Aspects of Speech

The most salient aspect of Rodney's speech was a decreased general rate of speech, with reduced pitch variation and excess stress for context. With the absence of impairments in the area of breath support for speech, Rodney's decreased rate of speech would most likely be explained by the reduced rate of tongue movements identified in repetitive tasks. The decreased pitch variation may be related to the presence of hypofunctioning of the laryngeal valve, which results in reduced laryngeal tone and a subsequent reduction in pitch range (because of the impaired ability of vocal folds to increase tone). It also is likely that Rodney's slowed rate of speech contributes to the perception of decreased pitch variation and excess stress for context.

Summary and Implications for Treatment

Rodney presented perceptually with a mild-to-moderate ataxic dysarthria, characterized by a slowed rate of speech, decreased pitch variation, excess stress for context, and mild-to-moderate hypernasality. Instrumental assessment of the speech mechanism identified mild-to-moderate impairment in all subsystems except respiration, when compared to the control group. Based on these findings, the following treatment regimen would be suggested to address the underlying pathophysiology of the dysarthric speech pattern exhibited by this subject.

1. Prosody:

    Increase speech rate

2. Velopharyngeal function:

    Decrease nasality in speech/ increase oral resonance

3. Articulatory function:

    Increase rate and maintenance of pressure of repetitive lip and tongue tasks

4. Laryngeal function:

    Increase phonatory effort to improve vocal fold adduction

As velopharyngeal functioning appears to be the most severely impaired aspect of speech production, based on instrumental assessment, treatment should initially commence in this area. However, therapy aimed at increasing articulatory function, especially rapid repetitive movements of the tongue, would be beneficial in increasing Rodney's rate of speech, and hence improve prosody. Treatment aimed at increasing laryngeal valving may also benefit Rodney by increasing air pressure essential for the production of bilabial sounds.

Case Examples: Summary

The differential nature of speech outcome following TBI in childhood was highlighted by these three cases. Despite the similar age at injury, and the comparable type and severity of injury, each case presented with a different profile of speech subsystem impairment. The diffuse, nonspecific nature of TBI means that damage may occur to many areas of the central nervous system, resulting in impairment in one or more of the motor speech subsystems. Using a combination of perceptual and instrumental investigations allows for a more accurate determination of the underlying pathophysiology of the speech disorder, and hence, enables more effective planning for therapy programs.

References

Annegers, J. F. (1983). The epidemiology of head trauma in children. In K. Shapiro (Ed.), *Pediatric head trauma* (pp. 1–10). Mount Kisco, NY: Futura.

Bak, E., van Dongen, H. R., & Arts, W. F. M. (1983). The analysis of acquired dysarthria in childhood. *Developmental Medicine and Child Neurology, 25,* 81–94.

Bigler, E. D., Clark, E., & Farmer, J. (1996). Traumatic brain injury: 1990s update—Introduction to the special series. *Journal of Learning Disabilities, 29*(5), 512–513.

Bijur, P. E., Haslum, M., & Golding, J. (1990). Cognitive and behavioural sequelae of mild head injury in children. *Paediatrics, 86,* 337–344.

Boyer, M. G., & Edwards, P. (1991). Outcome 1 to 3 years after severe traumatic brain injury in children and adolescents. *Injury: British Journal of Accident Surgery, 22*(4), 315–320.

Brooks, N., McKinlay, W., Symington, C., Beattie, A., & Campsie, L. (1987). Return to work within the first seven years of severe head injury. *Brain Injury, 1,* 5–19.

Cahill, L. M., Murdoch, B. E., & Theodoros, D. G. (2000). Variability in speech outcome following severe childhood traumatic brain injury: A report of three cases. *Journal of Medical Speech-Language Pathology, 8,* 347–352.

Cahill, L. M., Murdoch, B. E., & Theodoros, D. G. (2002). Perceptual analysis of speech following traumatic brain injury in childhood. *Brain Injury, 16,* 415–446.

Cahill, L. M., Murdoch, B. E., & Theodoros, D. G. (2003). Perceptual and instrumental analysis of laryngeal function following traumatic brain injury in childhood. *Journal of Head Trauma Rehabilitation, 18,* 268–283.

Cahill, L. M., Murdoch, B. E., & Theodoros, D. G. (2005). Articulatory function following traumatic brain injury in childhood: A perceptual and instrumental analysis. *Brain Injury, 19,* 41–58.

Costeff, H., Groswasser, Z., & Goldstein, R. (1990). Long-term follow-up review of 31 children with severe closed head trauma. *Journal of Neurosurgery, 73,* 684–687.

Costeff, H., Groswasser, Z., Landman, Y., & Brenner, T. (1985). Survivors of severe traumatic brain injury in childhood. Late residual disability. *Scandinavian Journal of Rehabilitation Medicine, Supplement 12,* 10–15.

Craft, A. W., Shaw, D. A., & Cartlidge, N. E. F. (1972). Head injuries in children. *British Medical Journal, 4,* 200–203.

Darley, F. L., Aronson, A. E., & Brown, J. R. (1975). *Motor speech disorders.* Philadelphia, PA: W. B. Saunders.

Di Scala, C., Osberg, J. S., Gans, B. M., Chin, L. J., & Grant, C. C. (1991). Children with traumatic brain injury: Morbidity and postacute treatment. *Archives of Physical Medicine and Rehabilitation, 72*(9), 662–666.

Emanuelson, I., & von Wendt, L. (1997). Epidemiology of traumatic brain injury in children and adolescents in southwestern Sweden. *Acta Paedratrica, 86,* 730–735.

Enderby, P. M. (1983). Frenchay dysarthria assessment. San Diego, CA: College-Hill Press.

Field, J. H. (1976). *Epidemiology of head injury in England and Wales: With particular application to rehabilitation.* Leicester, UK: Willsons.

Fisher, H. B., & Logemann, J. A. (1971). *The Fisher-Logemann test of articulation competence.* Boston, MA: Houghton Mifflin.

FitzGerald, F. J., Murdoch, B. E., & Chenery, H. J. (1987). Multiple sclerosis: Associated speech and language disorders. *Australian Journal of Human Communication Disorders, 15,* 15–33.

Goldstein, F. C., & Levin, H. S. (1987). Epidemiology of pediatric closed head injury: Incidence, clinical characteristics, and risk factors. *Journal of Learning Disabilities, 20,* 518–524.

Guyer, B., & Ellers, B. (1990). Childhood injuries in the United States. *American Journal of Diseases of Children, 144,* 649–652.

Hécaen, H. (1976). Acquired aphasia in children and the ontogenesis of hemispheric functional specialization. *Brain and Language, 3,* 114–134.

Hollien, H., & Malcik, E. (1967). Evaluation of cross-sectional studies of adolescent voice changes in males. *Speech Monographs, 34,* 80–84.

Hoodin, R. B., & Gilbert, H. R. (1989). Nasal airflows in Parkinsonian speakers. *Journal of Communication Disorders, 22,* 169–180.

Jamison, D. L., & Kaye, H. H. (1974). Accidental head injury in children. *Archives of Disease of Childhood, 49,* 376–381.

Jellinger, K. (1983). The neuropathology of pediatric head injuries. In K. Shapiro (Ed.), *Pediatric head trauma* (pp. 143–194). Mount Kisco, NY: Futura.

Johns, D. F., & Salyer, K. E. (1978). Surgical and prosthetic management of neurogenic speech disorders. In D. Johns (Ed.), *Clinical management of neurogenic communication disorders* (pp. 311–331). Boston, MA: Little, Brown.

Klauber, M. R., Barrett-Connor, E., Hofsetter, C. R., & Micik, S. H. (1986). A population-based study of non-fatal childhood injuries. *Preventive Medicine, 15,* 139–149.

Kraus, J. F. (1995). Epidemiological features of brain injury in children: Occurrence, children at risk, causes and manner of injury, severity, and outcomes. In S. H. Broman & M. E. Michel (Eds.), *Traumatic head injury in children* (pp. 22–39). New York, NY: Oxford University Press.

Kraus, J. F., Fife, D., Cox, P., Ramstein, K., & Conroy, C. (1986). Incidence, severity, and causes of pediatric brain injury. *American Journal of Diseases in Children, 140,* 687–693.

Kraus, J. F., Rock, A., & Hemyari, P. (1990). Brain injuries among infants, children, adolescents, and young adults. *American Journal of Diseases in Children, 144,* 684–691.

Levin. H. S., Benton, A. L., & Grossman, R. G. (1982). *Neurobehavioral consequences of closed head injury.* New York, NY: Oxford University Press.

Levin, H. S., Ewing-Cobbs, L., & Benton, A. L. (1984). Age and recovery from brain damage: A review of clinical studies. In S. W. Scheff (Ed.), *Aging and recovery of function in the central nervous system* (pp. 169–205). New York, NY: Plenum.

Malkmus, D. D. (1989). Community re-entry: Cognitive-communication intervention within a social skill context. *Topics in Language Disorders, 9,* 50–66.

Menkes, J. H., & Till, K. (1995). Postnatal trauma and injuries by physical agents. In J. H. Menkes (Ed.), *Textbook of child neurology* (pp. 557–597). Baltimore, MD: Williams & Wilkins.

Michel, J. F., Hollien, H., & Moore, P. (1966). Speaking fundamental frequency characteristics of 15, 16 and 17-year-old girls. *Language and Speech, 9,* 46–51.

Mira, M. P., Tucker, B. F., & Tyler, J. S. (1992). *Traumatic brain injury in children and adolescents: A sourcebook for teachers and other school personnel.* Austin, TX: Pro-Ed.

Morgan, A. T., & Liégeois, F. (2010). Rethinking diagnostic classification of the dysarthrias: A developmental perspective. *Folia Phoniatrica et Logopaedica, 62,* 120–126.

Moyes, C. D. (1980). Epidemiology of serious head injuries in childhood. *Child, Care, Health and Development, 6,* 1–9.

Murdoch, B. E., & Horton, S. K. (1998). Acquired and developmental dysarthria in childhood. In B. E. Murdoch (Ed.), *Dysarthria: A physiological approach to assessment and treatment* (pp. 373–427). Cheltenham, UK: Stanley Thornes.

Murdoch, B. E., & Hudson-Tennent, L. J. (1994). Speech disorders in children treated for posterior fossa tumours: Ataxic and developmental features. *European Journal of Disorders of Communication, 29,* 379–397.

Murdoch, B. E., Pitt, G., Theodoros, D. G., & Ward, E. C. (1999). Real-time visual biofeedback in the treatment of speech breathing disorders following childhood traumatic brain injury: A report of one case. *Pediatric Rehabilitation, 3,* 5–20.

Najenson, T., Sazbon, L., Fiselzon, J., Becker, E., & Schechter, I. (1978). Recovery of communication functions after prolonged traumatic coma. *Scandinavian Journal of Rehabilitative Medicine, 10,* 15–21.

Rimel, R. W., & Jane, J. A. (1983). Characteristics of the head-injured patient. In M. R. Rosenthal, M. R. Bond, J. D. Miller, & E. R. Griffith (Eds.), *Rehabilitation of the head injured adult* (pp. 9–12). Philadelphia, PA: Davis.

Rivara, J. B., Jaffe, K. M., Polissar, N. L., Fay, N. L., Martin, G. C., Shurtleff, H. A., & Liao, S. (1994). Family functioning and children's academic performance and behavior problems in the year following traumatic brain injury. *Archives of Physical Medicine and Rehabilitation, 75,* 269–279.

Robin, D. A., Goel, A., Somodi, C. B., & Luschei, E. S. (1992). Tongue strength and endurance: Relation to highly skilled movements. *Journal of Speech and Hearing Research, 35,* 1239–1245.

Rusk, H., Block, J., & Lowmann, E. (1969). Rehabilitation of the brain-injured patient: A report of 157 cases with long-term follow-up of 118. In E. Walker, W. Caveness, & M. Critchley (Eds.), *The late effects of head injury* (pp. 327–332). Springfield, IL: Charles C. Thomas.

Sterling, L. (1994). *Students with acquired brain injuries in primary and secondary schools.* Canberra, Australia: Government Printing Service.

Stierwalt, J. A. G., Robin, D. A., Solomon, N. P., Weiss, A. L., & Max, J. E. (1996). Tongue strength and endurance: Relation to speaking ability of children and adolescents following traumatic brain injury. In D. A. Robin, K. M Yorkston, & D. R Beukelman (Eds.), *Disorders of motor speech: Assessment, treatment and clinical characteristics* (pp. 241–256). Baltimore, MD: Paul H. Brookes.

Theodoros, D. G., & Murdoch, B. E. (1994). Laryngeal dysfunction in dysarthric speakers following severe closed head injury. *Brain Injury, 8,* 667–684.

Theodoros, D. G., Murdoch, B. E., & Chenery, H. J. (1994). Perceptual speech characteristics of dysarthric speakers following severe closed head injury. *Brain Injury, 8,* 101–124.

Thomsen, I. V. (1984). Late outcome of severe blunt head injury: A ten to fifteen-year second follow-up. *Journal of Neurology, Neurosurgery and Psychiatry, 38,* 713–718.

van Mourik, M., Catsman-Berrevoets, C. E., Paquier, P. F., Yosef-Bak, E., & van Dongen, H. R. (1997). Acquired childhood dysarthria: Review of its clinical presentation. *Pediatric Neurology, 17,* 299–307.

Ylvisaker, M. (1986). Language and communication disorders following pediatric head injury. *Journal of Head Trauma Rehabilitation, 1,* 48–56.

Yorkston, K. M., & Beukelman, D. R. (1981). Assessment of intelligibility of dysarthric speech. Austin, TX: Pro-Ed.

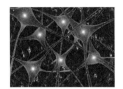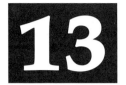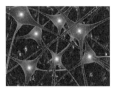

13

Dysarthria Following Treatment for Childhood Brain Tumors

Introduction

Brain tumors are a recognized cause of acquired speech disorder in childhood (Ammirati, Mirzai, & Samii, 1989; Brown, 1985; Cornwell, Murdoch, & Ward, 2005; Cornwell, Murdoch, Ward, & Kellie, 2003a; Hudson, 1990; Hudson, Murdoch, & Ozanne, 1989; Murdoch & Hudson-Tennent, 1994; Rekate, Grubb, Aram, Hahn, & Ratcheson, 1985; Volcan, Cole, & Johnston, 1986). The nature and distribution of brain tumors differ, however, in children compared to adults. Tumors located in the posterior cranial fossa (i.e., infratentorial tumors involving the cerebellum, fourth ventricle, and/or brainstem) account for up to 70% of all pediatric intracranial neoplasms (Farwell, Dohrmann, & Flannery, 1977; Gjerris, 1978; Kadota, Allen, Hartman, & Spruce, 1989; Russell & Rubinstein, 1989). Although infratentorial tumors are more common than supratentorial tumors in children, infratentorial tumors

account for only 25 to 30% of intracranial space-occupying lesions in adults (Menkes & Till, 1995). In children under age 1, as in adults, supratentorial tumors are the most common brain tumors (Menkes & Till, 1995). Due to the greater prevalence of posterior fossa tumors in children in general, however, the majority of reported literature relating to pediatric intracranial neoplasms has focused on tumors involving the cerebellum, fourth ventricle, and/or brainstem.

Neurologic symptoms produced by brain tumors include both general and local symptoms. General symptoms result from increased intracranial pressure that results directly from progressive enlargement of the tumor within the limited space of the cranial cavity. Local symptoms result from the effects of the tumor on contiguous areas of the brain. In that a tumor located in the posterior cranial fossa will inevitably involve the cerebellum, ataxic features may be anticipated in any associated speech disorder. Indeed, a number of authors have reported the occurrence of "cerebellar dysarthria" subsequent to surgical excision of a posterior fossa tumor in childhood (Brown, 1985; Hudson, Murdoch, & Ozanne 1989; Murdoch & Hudson-Tennent, 1994). Other symptoms associated with posterior fossa tumors include bifrontal headache, nausea and vomiting, gait disturbance, depressed cerebral function (manifested as apathy and irritability), neck stiffness and neck pain, dizziness, papilledema squint and nystagmus, alteration of muscle tone, tendon reflex changes, dorsiflexor plantar response, tilting the head from the side of the tumor, visual impairment and paresis of the limbs, and language disturbances (Delong & Adams, 1975; Gol, 1963; Hudson et al., 1989; Kadota et al., 1989; Tew, Feibel, & Sawaya, 1984). Although rare, facial weakness and deafness also have been reported (Delong & Adams, 1975). Treatment for posterior fossa tumors is by way of surgical excision of the tumor. Children with malignant tumors may also undergo a course of radiotherapy and, in the case of highly malignant tumors, a course of chemotherapy as well. Those children with low-grade tumors (e.g., low grade astrocytomas) may be spared both radiotherapy and chemotherapy, a factor which has been suggested as a reason for their lower incidence of neuropsychological sequelae, including speech and language disorders (Huber, Bradley, Spiegler, & Dennis, 2007; Hudson, Buttsworth, & Murdoch, 1990).

The most common posterior fossa tumors are medulloblastomas, astrocytomas, and ependymomas. The basic features of these types of tumors are outlined below, however, for a more comprehensive description of the various posterior fossa tumors see Chapter 4.

Based on a sample of 151 children with posterior fossa tumors, Menkes and Till (1995) reported that 34.4% had medulloblastomas, 21.9% had astrocytomas, and 10.6% had ependymomas. Brainstem neoplasms were present in 26.5% of the 151 cases.

Medulloblastomas are highly malignant brain tumors derived from primitive neurons, the neuroblasts. In particular, the majority of these tumors are thought to arise from embryonal cell rests in the posterior medullary velum of the cerebellum. Although these tumors originate from the cerebellum, they subsequently invade the subarachnoid spaces, fourth ventricle, and spinal canal. As the tumor grows it tends to extend backward and may occlude the foramen magnum and infiltrate the meninges. Most medulloblastomas are situated in the midline of the cerebellum (i.e., the vermis). Characteristically, on CT scans, medulloblastomas appear as relatively well-defined, noncalcified, noncystic, slightly dense inferior vermian masses. Children have been diagnosed with medulloblastomas between 4 months and 16 years of age with there being a slightly higher (1.3:1) incidence in male children. The primary concern for patients with medulloblastomas is the risk of tumor recurrence in the posterior cranial fossa and/or the development of supratentorial, spinal cord or systemic metastases. Where they occur, recurrences usually arise in the first 2 to 3 years following treatment with an average survival time for patients with recurrence of only 19 months. The prognosis for patients with recurrent medulloblastomas is therefore poor. Currently, the overall 5-year disease-free survival rate for medulloblastomas is approximately 50% for patients treated with surgery and craniospinal irradiation (Menkes & Till, 1995).

As the name implies, astrocytomas are derived from the astrocytic neuroglial cells. Although they can occur above or below the tentorium cerebelli, as pointed out earlier, infratentorial astrocytomas are more common in children. These tumors, when located in the posterior cranial fossa, can arise from either the vermis or lateral lobes of the cerebellum and tend to be well circumscribed and often cystic, containing one or more sacs of clear yellow or brown fluid. Geissinger and Bucy (1971) reported the average age at diagnosis of cerebellar astrocytoma to be 8 years and 9 months. However, children presenting with this type of tumor at clinics for treatment of associated dysarthria could be expected to vary in age from infancy through to adolescence. Males and females appear to be affected equally. Cerebellar astrocytomas are usually low grade with regard to malignancy and, therefore, associated with a favorable prognosis postsurgical removal. Although some more malignant forms of astrocytoma exist, tumor recurrence although reported is rare. In general, therefore, recovery from astrocytomas is favorable, particularly when the tumor does not involve the brainstem.

The third most frequently encountered type of tumor found in the posterior cranial fossa is the ependymoma. These tumors are derived from the ependymal cells lining the ventricles of the brain. Although they can arise from any part of the ventricular system, the roof and the floor of the fourth ventricle are the most common origins for ependymomas in children. From there the tumor grows to occlude the cavity of the fourth ventricle, protrudes into the cisterna magna or may extend through the foramen magnum to overlap the cervical segments of the spinal cord.

Ependymomas are slow growing and predominantly benign tumors. Due to their origins in the roof or floor of the fourth ventricle, however, complete surgical resection is not possible so that recurrence of the tumors in the primary site is common. Development of metastases in other sites, however, is unusual. Tumor recurrence rates as high as 90% have been reported (Menkes & Till, 1995) with a 5-year progression-free survival rate of approximately 40% (Naidich & Zimmerman, 1984). Overall, the prognosis for a child with an ependymoma is poor in terms of ultimate cure.

In addition to the more common posterior fossa tumors outlined above, acquired childhood dysarthria can also be associated with a variety of brainstem tumors. The initial presentation of brainstem tumors in children vary from case to case. All, however, show a uniformly fatal progression. The tumors themselves may vary from benign astrocytomas through to highly malignant glioblastomas. The majority are in general malignant and arise from the pons. Manifestations of brainstem tumors in children appear at 2 to 12 years of age with peak incidence at 6 years. Neurological signs may include cranial nerve palsies (including associated speech disturbances if cranial nerves supplying the speech production mechanism are involved), pyramidal tract signs and cerebellar signs. Vomiting and disturbances of gait are the most common presenting complaints. Cranial nerves most commonly affected are nerves VII and VI, with the facial weakness being of the lower motor neuron type and associated with a degree of flaccid dysarthria. Other cranial nerves may also be affected with increasing numbers involved over time. Progression of symptoms is relentless with patients becoming unable to speak (anarthric) or swallow and the extremities becoming paralyzed. Eventually damage to the reticular formation, cardiac, and respiratory centers leads to cardiac and respiratory problems, coma, and death. Average survival time post initial hospital admission is 15 months (Panitch & Berg, 1970).

Due to the prevalence of posterior fossa tumors in childhood, a large proportion of the literature relating to speech disorders associated with pediatric intracranial neoplasms has been focused on tumors involving the cerebellum, fourth ventricle, and/or brainstem. Dysarthria has been reported to occur subsequent to the diagnosis and treatment of posterior fossa tumors, with the presentation of this disorder ranging from transient mutism, to mild dysarthria, through to a persistent developmental speech disorder. The literature, has to date, predominantly documented the existence of a condition referred to as transient cerebellar mutism subsequent to surgery for a posterior fossa tumor and that resolution to normal speech involves a period of dysarthria (Aguiar, Plese, Cinquini, & Marino, 1995; Balasubramaniam, Subramaniam, & Balasubramaniam, 1993; Catsman-Berrevoets et al. 1999; Frim & Ogilvy, 1995; Jansen et al., 1998; Pollack, Polinko, Albright, Towbin, & Fitz, 1995; Rekate et al., 1985).

In recent times a number of studies have indicated that in some cases speech does not return to its premorbid level, implying a persistent speech disorder (Murdoch, Horton, Theodoros, & Thompson, 1996; Murdoch & Hudson-Tennent, 1994; van Dongen, Catsman-Berrevoets & van Mourik, 1994; van Mourik, Catsman-Berrevoets, Paquier, Yousef-Bak & van Dongen, 1997; van Mourik, Catsman-Berrevoets, van Dongen,

& Neville, 1997; van Mourik, Catsman-Berrevoets, Yousef-Bak, Paquier, & van Dongen, 1998). These same studies have attempted to describe the speech features that characterize the speech disorder in children treated for posterior fossa tumors. Many of these descriptions are based not only on small numbers of children but are also restricted to perceptual speech analyses (Murdoch & Hudson-Tennent, 1994; van Dongen et al., 1994; van Mourik, Catsman-Berrevoets, Paquier, et al., 1997; van Mourik, Catsman-Berrevoets, van Dongen, et al., 1997; van Mourik et al., 1998). Although the speech disorder exhibited by children who have undergone treatment for posterior fossa tumors has often been labeled "ataxic dysarthria" in accordance with the Mayo Clinic Classification System (Darley, Aronson, & Brown, 1975), in the majority of studies the specific features of the speech disorder are not described in detail. The most comprehensive series of studies based on perceptual, acoustic, and physiologic assessments, reported to date are those conducted by Cornwell et al. (2003a, 2005) and Cornwell, Murdoch, Ward, and Kellie (2004). The findings of these latter studies are described more fully below.

Posterior Fossa Syndrome and Mutism

Posterior fossa syndrome is a well recognized clinical entity that represents a complication of surgery to remove posterior fossa tumors in children. Transient cerebellar mutism is a central feature of this syndrome in the majority of cases; however, the syndrome also covers a wider spectrum of postoperative, often transient neurobehavioral deficits that may include irritability and mood lability, poor oral intake and impaired eye opening, decreased spontaneous initiation of movements, and a lack of control of bowel and bladder. In addition, concomitant postoperative language disturbances have also been reported such as word-finding difficulties (Aarsen, van Dongen, Paquier, van Mourik, & Catsman-Berrevoets, 2004), agrammatism (Riva & Giorgi, 2000), adynamic language characterized by a lack of verbal initiative (Ozimek et al., 2004), comprehension deficits (Cornwell, Murdoch, Ward, & Morgan, 2003b), reading (Scott et al., 2001), and writing problems (Aarsen et al., 2004). During the recovery phase, mutism is frequently followed by dysarthria. Consequently, the condition has also been termed the syndrome of (cerebellar) mutism and subsequent dysarthria (MSD). The clinical features cited as typifying MSD include: (1) mutism occurs most frequently after resection of a cerebellar mass lesion; (2) there generally is a delayed onset of speech loss after a brief interval of 1 to 2 days of normal speech postsurgery; (3) mutism is transient and generally lasts from 1 day to 6 months; and (4) mutism is followed by a period of dysarthric speech which usually recovers favorably in 1 to 6 months but may persist in some cases (Aguiar et al., 1995; Ammirati et al., 1989; De Smet et al., 2007; Koh, Turkel, & Baram, 1997; Rekate et al., 1985).

The causes and anatomic basis of MSD remain controversial and not all cerebellar lesions lead to dysarthria. A complex interaction of cerebellar lesion, brainstem affection, and hydrocephalus appears likely (Gordon, 1996; van Dongen et al., 1994). Many authors have noted that involvement of the midline region of the cerebellum, in particular surgical incision of the cerebellar vermis,

increases the risk that the client will develop MSD (Al-Jarallah, Cook, Gascon, Kanaan, & Sigueira, 1994; Jansen et al., 1998; Rekate et al., 1985). In a study by Catsman-Berrevoets et al. (1999), the researchers attempted to determine the risk factors for development of MSD. They noted that if the tumor was located in the midline of the cerebellum that MSD was 8.2 times more likely to develop than when the tumor was located in the lateral parts of the cerebellar hemispheres. Based on examination of a 6-year-old boy who underwent resection of the midline cerebellar tumor, Kusano et al. (2006) concluded that his resultant cerebellar mutism was caused by bilateral damage to the dentate nuclei. A number of other authors have also implicated the dentate nucleus in the occurrence of postoperative mutism (Ozimek et al., 2004; Pollack et al., 1995). Pollack et al. (1995) postulated that cerebellar mutism is related to transient impairment of the afferent and/or efferent pathways of the dentate nuclei that are involved in the initiation of complex volitional movement. Other hypothesized pathophysiologic mechanisms that might underlie MSD include: postoperative spasm of the blood vessels that supply the cerebellum and brainstem leading to ischemia and subsequent edema (Ferrante, Mastronardi, Acqui, & Fortuna, 1990; Nagatani, Waga, & Nakagawa, 1991; Turgut, 1998) possibly accounting for the delayed appearance of mutism after a period of apparently normal speech in the immediate postoperative phase; transient dysregulation of neurotransmitter release originating from the tumor removal and the alleviation of long-lasting compression of the brainstem by the tumor (Caner, Altinörs, Benli, Calisaneller, & Albayrak, 1999); crossed cerebellocerebral diaschisis reflecting the metabolic impact of a cerebellar lesion on a distant but anatomically and functionally connected supratentorial region (Mariën, Engelborghs, Fabbro, & De Deyn, 2001; Sagiuchi et al., 2001).

Examination of individuals with infarction of the superior and posterior inferior cerebellar artery has lead a number of researchers to the conclusion that the critical region of the cerebellum for the development of dysarthria is the paravermal area of the superior cerebellum (Ackermann, Hertrich, & Hehr, 1995; Amarenco, Chevrie-Muller, Roullet, & Bousser, 1991) which corresponds to paravermal lobules VI and VII (Manto, 2002). Although some authors have proposed that only left-sided lesions of the cerebellum produce dysarthria (e.g., Amarenco et al., 1991) evidence is available to support the notion that lesions of the superior cerebellum on either side produce dysarthria (Ackermann et al., 1995). The latter suggestion has been supported by the findings of a fMRI study that demonstrated that silent repetitions of syllables by healthy individuals were associated with activation of the superior cerebellum bilaterally.

Although the pathogenesis of MSD is not known with certainty, two explanations for the postoperative development of mutism have been proposed: (1) the anarthria hypothesis; and (2) the language disorder hypothesis. According to the anarthria hypothesis postoperative cerebellar mutism is considered to be a severe form of dysarthria (anarthria) (Ackermann & Ziegler, 1994), with the affected individual being unable to articulate any sounds at all (Turgut, 1998). Support for this hypothesis is drawn from observations of the recovery process in children with cerebellar mutism. Recovery of speech following

the period of mutism initially sees the child with a severe dysarthria which gradually improves to either a mild dysarthria or in some rare cases towards premorbid speech abilities (Aguiar et al., 1995; Al-Jarallah et al., 1994; Jansen et al., 1998; Rekate et al., 1985; Riva & Giorgi, 2000; van Dongen et al., 1994). Alternatively, cerebellar mutism is regarded by some researchers as a language disorder (Riva, 1998) on the basis that some children exhibit a language impairment similar to agrammatism but not dysarthria in the postmutistic phase (Riva & Giorgi, 2000).

Incidence of Speech Deficits Subsequent to Posterior Fossa Tumor

The incidence of MSD is estimated between 8% and 31% of children undergoing surgical resection of a posterior fossa tumor (Catsman-Berrevoets et al., 1999; Dailey, McKhann, & Berger, 1995; Pollack et al., 1995; van Mourik et al., 1998). Pollack et al. (1995) compiled data on 142 children who underwent surgery for a posterior fossa tumor and reported that 8.5% of cases developed a postoperative mutism and subsequent dysarthria. Furthermore, when the tumor was located in the region of the cerebellar vermis (92 cases), postoperative mutism and subsequent dysarthria occurred at an incidence of 13%.

A study by Catsman-Berrevoets et al. (1999) found a slightly higher incidence of cerebellar mutism and subsequent dysarthria in a group of 42 children treated for a posterior fossa tumor. In their study the overall incidence of speech deficits following surgery was 29%. These researchers then subdivided their subject group into tumor type and found that 53% of children treated for a medulloblastoma developed mutism and subsequent dysarthria, whereas for ependymomas it was 33% and astrocytomas, 11%. They also concluded that the risk of developing a speech deficit subsequent to treatment for a posterior fossa tumor was increased eight-fold if the tumor was located within the cerebellar midline, including the cerebellar vermis.

The studies completed by Pollack et al. (1995) and Catsman-Berrevoets et al. (1999) did not report on cases where treatment had included radiotherapy and/or chemotherapy. The focus of these investigations was primarily on the period of time immediately postsurgery. Murdoch and Hudson-Tennent (1994) reported on a group of nineteen subjects who had all undergone surgical resection of the tumor, with thirteen of the subjects having also completed a course of radiotherapy, and one subject had received both radiotherapy and chemotherapy. In this group of 19 subjects, eleven (58%) were found to have a speech disorder and, of the 11 children who presented with speech disorders posttreatment, 10 had experienced central nervous system prophylaxis (radiotherapy and/or chemotherapy). There is limited information on the effects of radiotherapy and chemotherapy on speech production, but the disparity between incidence rates of speech disorders found by Murdoch and Hudson-Tennent (1994) and the previous two studies could possibly be attributed to treatment protocols. The findings of Richter et al. (2005) provide further support for this suggestion. These latter authors investigated the incidence of dysarthric symptoms in ten children after cerebellar surgery. They concluded that speech impairments are rare after cerebellar surgery with neither a perceptual analysis of spontaneous speech nor an acoustic analysis showing persistent speech impairments in the majority of children included in their study. It is noteworthy, however, that Richter et al. (2005) exclude children with signs of posterior fossa syndrome with temporary mutism and none of their cases had undergone either radiotherapy and/or chemotherapy. As both radiotherapy and chemotherapy are known to have detrimental effects on brain structure and function (for a full description of the effects of radiotherapy and chemotherapy on central nervous system structure and function see Chapter 4). The absence of these therapies in the cases examined by Richter et al. (2005) may well have contributed to the observed low incidence of dysarthria in their study. Furthermore, the exclusion of children with mutism postsurgery is also likely to have mitigated against the occurrence of dysarthria leading to the low incidence of speech impairment reported by Richter et al. (2005). Although some children have been reported to develop dysarthria secondary to treatment for posterior fossa tumors without entering a mute phase (Murdoch & Hudson-Tennent, 1994) it would appear that in the majority of cases dysarthria when it occurs follows a period of postsurgical mutism.

Reports in the literature are also contradictory regarding the quality of motor speech production post-mutism. Although some authors propose that mutism always progresses into dysarthria (Paquier, van Mourik, van Dongen, Catsman-Berrevoets, & Brison, 2003; van Dongen et al, 1994), others have documented cases of formerly mutistic children without dysarthria (Ozimek et al., 2004; Riva & Giorgi,

2000). Furthermore, the authors of some literature reviews consider a number of children to be dysarthric once speech returns (Turgut, 1998), whereas the same children are considered to be nondysarthric by the authors of other reviews (e.g., Ersahin, Mutluer, Cagli, & Duman, 1996). In an attempt to clarify this situation, De Smet et al. (2007) critically reviewed data on 283 children with MSD to chart the recovery of motor speech production after the mute period. Subsequent to application of stringent exclusion criteria, they determined that 98.8% of the children exhibited dysarthric speech. Further, De Smet et al. (2007) noted that recovery of motor speech function after the mute period was much less favorable than often reported.

Clinical Features of Dysarthria Associated with Posterior Fossa Tumors

Acquired dysarthria is acknowledged within the literature as an acute sequelae of surgical intervention for the treatment of posterior fossa tumors in children (Balasubramaniam et al., 1993; Catsman-Berrevoets et al., 1999; Jansen et al., 1998; Pollack et al., 1995; Rekate et al., 1985). Although, as indicated earlier, the predominant focus of research has been on the development of dysarthria during the acute phase postsurgery that in many cases resolves to normal or "near-normal" speech, speech production does not return to premorbid levels in all cases. Persistent dysarthria therefore, does develop in some cases of children treated for posterior fossa tumor (Cornwell et al., 2003a; De Smet et al., 2007; Murdoch & Hudson-Tennent, 1994; van

Dongen et al., 1994). In a study of 21 children treated for childhood cerebellar tumor, Cornwell et al. (2003a) found that for the majority of cases the dysarthria is mild in severity. However, for some children more severe specific impairments to speech production have been observed.

Perceptual Speech Characteristics of Dysarthria Associated with Posterior Fossa Tumors

Studies to date that have attempted to describe the speech disorder that arises subsequent to treatment for posterior fossa tumors have relied predominantly on perceptual analyses of speech. Given the neuroanatomical location of posterior fossa tumors and their usual involvement of the cerebellum, it could be expected that the perceptual features of the speech disorder associated with resection of posterior fossa tumors would resemble the deviant speech characteristics of ataxic dysarthria seen in adults. The characteristic features specified by Darley, Aronson, and Brown (1969a, 1969b) as most representative of cerebellar dysarthria include: imprecise consonants, irregular articulatory breakdowns, vowel distortions, equal and excess stress (scanning speech), prolonged phonemes, prolonged intervals, slow rate of speech, harsh voice, monopitch and monoloudness. Therefore it would be expected that deviant speech characteristics exhibited by children treated for posterior fossa tumors would cluster in the areas of articulation, prosody and phonation, and speech dimensions characterizing the dysarthria would be impaired stress patterns and imprecision of consonant production. Although a number of authors have labeled the speech disorder demonstrated by their cohort of children treated for posterior fossa tumor as ataxic dysarthria (Al-Jarallah et al., 1994; Kai, Kuratsu, Suginohara, Marubayashi, & Ushio, 1997; Rekate et al., 1985; Wang, Kent, Duffy, Thomas, & Fredericks, 2006), many of these studies did not elaborate on the clinical features of the speech disorder observed in their participants, instead only using the overall term as a descriptor.

Wang et al. (2006) reported the case of an 11-year-old boy who developed severe cerebellar ataxia following resection of a fourth ventricle medulloblastoma. Based on an acoustic analysis they noted that his dysarthria was highly similar to classic descriptions of ataxic dysarthria in adults, being notable for its scanning pattern, which co-occurred with a number of other abnormalities, including explosive consonants, dysphonia, and irregular articulatory breakdowns. In contrast, other authors have noted that prominent characteristics of ataxic dysarthria, such as irregular articulatory breakdown and scanning speech are not necessarily the hallmark of dysarthria following treatment for posterior fossa tumors (Cornwell et al., 2003a; De Smet et al., 2007; van Mourik et al., 1998).

Based on a perceptual analysis of 11 children treated for cerebellar tumors, Cornwell et al. (2003a) did find a preponderance of deviant speech dimensions related to prosody, and to a lesser extent articulatory and phonatory aspects of speech. However, the distinctive excess and equal stress pattern was missing. This finding is consistent with that of van Mourik et al. (1998) who reported slow speech rate to be a prominent and distinctive characteristic of the

dysarthria in children treated for posterior fossa tumors but not scanning speech and irregular articulatory breakdown. According to Ackermann, Vogel, Petersen, and Poremba (1992), the pattern of excess and equal stress may be associated with more severe types of cerebellar dysarthria and consequently may be absent in the speech of children with mild dysarthria subsequent to surgical treatment of posterior fossa tumors. They noted that a reduced rate of speech was more likely to typify milder forms of ataxic dysarthria consistent with the findings of van Mourik et al. (1998).

Overall, the deviant perceptual speech features most commonly associated with dysarthria in children treated for posterior fossa tumors include: a slow rate of speech; imprecision of consonants; distorted vowels, and a reduced overall speech intelligibility (Catsman-Berrevoets, van Dongen, & Zwetsloot, 1992; Cornwell et al., 2003a; Murdoch & Hudson-Tennent, 1994; van Dongen et al., 1994; van Mourik et al., 1998). Catsman-Berrevoets et al. (1992) reported on three cases of children who had undergone surgery for posterior fossa tumors, then subsequently developed mutism which resolved to a dysarthria. Common to all three of these cases was the presence of an articulatory disturbance, which improved to a level where difficulties were generally noted only on polysyllabic words or those that contained consonant clusters. In two of the cases slow rate of speech was observed as a characteristic feature of their speech, with respiratory support for speech also compromised. It was suggested by the authors that a reduced rate of speech could be considered a compensatory strategy used by these children due to decreased respiratory control. A mild nasality disturbance was noted in one case, whereas in another a hoarse voice quality was observed during the recovery phase.

A study by van Dongen et al. (1994) examined the speech of 15 children who underwent surgery for resection of a posterior fossa tumor. The participants were divided into three groups, eight children with no specific speech deficits, two with mild speech deficits, but not mutism, and five children who developed mutism and a subsequent dysarthria postsurgery. Common speech features noted in the children who developed dysarthria subsequent to a period of mutism included audible respiration, nasal vocal quality, articulation disturbances, slow rate of speech, difficulty with volume control, and poor vocal quality, with descriptions including harsh, hoarse or strained-strangled vocal quality. In four of the five cases reported, the children's dysarthria was observed to have resolved to mild articulatory deficits or reduced rate of speech when last followed up. Long-term follow-up of the fifth child was not possible due to medical complications that resulted in the child dying.

The perceptual features of the dysarthria evident in children diagnosed with cerebellar and brainstem tumors was reported by van Mourik et al. (1998). They rated 12 children, with six children in each of the tumor groups on 36 of the 38 speech features of Darley et al. (1969a) using audio- or video-taped speech samples that consisted of both spontaneous speech and repetition tasks. The three most prominent speech features noted in children with a cerebellar tumor were slow rate of speech, imprecise consonants, and distorted vowels. The features that occurred most com-

monly included high pitch, monopitch, and a harsh vocal quality. Speech characteristics most evident in children treated for brainstem tumors were imprecise consonants, distorted vowels, and hypernasality.

The 1994 study by Murdoch and Hudson-Tennent attempted to determine the nature of the speech disorder evident after treatment for posterior fossa tumors using perceptual assessment procedures in line with the physiological approach. The test battery included, The Frenchay Dysarthria Assessment (Enderby, 1983), The Fisher–Logemann Test of Articulation Competence (Fisher & Logemann, 1971), and an analysis of a connected speech sample using a rating scale described by FitzGerald, Murdoch, and Chenery (1987), with eleven children assessed on this battery. The results of these assessments concluded that when compared with a control group matched for sex and age, the cerebellar tumor group exhibited decreased overall intelligibility, reduced precision of consonant production, and variation in their general use of stress. Information obtained from the Frenchay Dysarthria Assessment demonstrated that the children had reduced abilities within the respiratory and laryngeal systems, as well as reduced lip and tongue function. These difficulties were observed both at rest, and during rapid speech and nonspeech movements. They concluded that these results pointed to the involvement of abnormal muscle tone and impaired coordination. Finally, they also noted that 9 of the 11 children included in the study demonstrated developmental speech errors including, phonological processes, articulatory substitutions, and/or vowel distortions.

The most salient features of the dysarthria observed in children treated for cerebellar tumors by Cornwell et al. (2003a) were the mild nature of the speech disorder and clustering of speech deficits in the prosodic, phonatory, and articulatory aspects of speech production. Overall, the deviant speech dimensions reported to contribute to the perception of dysarthria in the 11 cases examined by these researchers included: imprecision of consonants, hoarseness; decreased pitch variation; and a reduction in overall speech intelligibility for both sentences and connected speech. Cornwell et al. (2003a) noted that the finding of a mild persistent speech disorder was consistent with previously reported cases of children with cerebellar tumor, where it has been documented that despite at times quite severe disturbances to speech in the acute postoperative period, recovery of speech occurs and results in a mild degree of impairment or near-normal speech (Rekate et al., 1985; van Mourik et al., 1998). Although the majority of children treated for cerebellar tumor included in their study exhibited a mild speech disorder, Cornwell et al. (2003a) cautioned that the overall presentation of some children revealed more severe specific impairments. A perceptual speech sample analysis revealed that the degree of impairment for the dimensions of precision of consonant production, ability to vary pitch and audible inspirations were rated at a moderate level for a number of the children treated for cerebellar tumor with moderate and moderate-severe deficits in tongue function also being identified by Cornwell et al. (2003a) on the Frenchay Dysarthria Assessment. Cornwell et al. (2003a) concluded that, although the predominant group pattern suggests that the long-term dysarthria in children treated for cerebellar tumor is mild, this generaliza-

tion should be tempered by the knowledge that more severe impairments may develop in some cases.

Acoustic and Physiologic Features of Dysarthria Associated with Posterior Fossa Tumor

Research into the speech disorder following treatment for posterior fossa tumor has primarily focused on description of perceptual speech characteristics. The benefits of supplementing perceptual judgments with acoustic and/or physiologic assessment tools, however, has been widely documented (Duffy & Kent, 2001; Kent, 2000; Theodoros, Murdoch, & Chenery, 1994). To date relatively few studies have been reported that have utilized either acoustic and/or physiological procedures in combination with perceptual assessments to further define the nature of the dysarthria associated with treatment of posterior fossa tumors. Those that have been reported are best considered according to the specific subsystem of the speech production mechanism addressed.

Respiratory Function in Children Treated for Posterior Fossa Tumor

Respiratory dysfunction has been documented to occur as a result of cerebellar damage incurred during adulthood (Murdoch, Chenery, Stokes, & Hardcastle, 1991) suggesting that the same deficits may be exhibited by children treated for cerebellar tumors. Contrary to this suggestion, the deviant speech characteristics commonly associated with impaired respiratory support (decreased breath support for speech, abnormal inspirations, and forced inspirations/

expirations) have not been observed as key perceptual features in the speech of adults (Brown, Darley, & Aronson, 1970; Chenery, Ingham, & Murdoch, 1990) or children (Murdoch & Hudson-Tennent, 1994; van Mourik et al., 1998) with cerebellar damage. In part, this could be explained by the knowledge that the respiratory capacity required for speech is well below that of the total lung capacity (Yorkston, Beukelman, Strand, & Bell, 1999) and therefore some disruption to function may not be of significant magnitude to be perceived as an area of deficit in speech production (Hixon, Putnam, & Sharp, 1983). Furthermore, the respiratory system has a multifactorial role in speech production (Hixon, 1973) and so deficits in respiratory function may be expressed as, or contribute to other deviant speech features more commonly related to phonation, articulation or prosody. Alternatively, the perceptual analysis may not be sufficiently sensitive to detect the presence of subtle impairments in respiratory function. Consequently, more objective instrumental based assessment of children treated for cerebellar tumors may be necessary to detect impaired respiratory function at a physiologic level. To date only two studies have utilized physiological instrumentation to investigate speech breathing in children treated for posterior fossa tumors (Murdoch, Horton, Theodoros, & Thompson, 1996; Murdoch & Hudson-Tennent, 1993). Murdoch and Hudson-Tennent (1993) investigated respiratory function in five children treated for posterior fossa tumors using spirometric and kinematic techniques. They reported that general respiratory function (Vital Capacity [VC] and Forced Expiratory Volume in 1 second [FEV$_1$]) in the group was within normal limits. Kinematic measures of chest wall movements, however, were in agreement with the adult investigation and revealed an increased incidence of abdominal paradoxing, as well as increased numbers of slope changes during speech tasks when compared to a control group. As in the case of adults with cerebellar lesions (Murdoch et al., 1991) these kinematic abnormalities were attributed to difficulties in the temporal coordination of the components of the chest wall (Murdoch & Hudson-Tennent, 1993).

The single case reported by Murdoch et al. (1996) was an 8-year-old girl diagnosed with a large cerebellar astrocytoma two years previously. The treatment she received was surgical only, with no radiotherapy or chemotherapy considered necessary. Although a perceptual assessment indicated no disturbance in respiratory function, instrumental assessment using both spirometric and kinematic methodology revealed below-normal lung volumes and capacities, and that the child was an abdominal breather. It therefore is evident that children treated for posterior fossa tumors may exhibit subtle deficits in respiratory function which, although not clearly manifest at the perceptual level, may contribute to the overall speech deficit at the level of phonation, articulation, or prosody.

Laryngeal Function in Children Treated for Posterior Fossa Tumor

It has been suggested that the role of the cerebellum in phonation is instrumental in the control of pitch and loudness, and less important for initiation of voice production (Larson, Sutton, & Lindeman, 1978). This theory has received some support from the perceptual studies completed to date. Perceptually, a number of deviant voice qualities have been identified as associated with damage to the cerebellum including harshness, strain-strangled phonation (Chenery et al., 1990; Darley et al., 1975; Yorkston, Beukelman, & Bell, 1991); hoarseness (Yorkston et al., 1991); monopitch, decreased pitch level, excessive loudness, vocal tremor (Aronson, 1990; Chenery et al., 1990; Darley et al., 1975; Yorkston, 1991); and pitch breaks (Chenery et al., 1990; Darley et al., 1975).

Minimal attention has been given to the specific nature of laryngeal dysfunction in children with, and treated for posterior fossa tumors in the research literature. Studies to date, primarily have focused on describing the perceptual speech features noted in the speech of these children (Catsman-Berrevoets et al., 1992; Murdoch & Hudson-Tennent, 1994; van Dongen et al., 1994; van Mourik et al., 1998). In general, the deviant perceptual speech characteristics linked to disturbance phonation in the pediatric population following cerebellar lesions include deficits in pitch level, control of pitch and loudness, and vocal quality (Murdoch & Hudson-Tennent, 1994; van Mourik et al., 1998).

Disturbance in phonatory function was not identified by van Mourik and colleagues (1998) as a dimension of the acute dysarthria seen in six children treated surgically for cerebellar tumor. Examination of the individual deviant speech features documented for each child, however, revealed that five of the children exhibited at least one dimension that could result from a deficit at the laryngeal level. In most cases the deviant dimensions were linked to difficulty in controlling pitch and volume, not unexpected due to the proposed role of the cerebellum in just these functions. Two children also exhibited defi-

cits in vocal quality, predominantly harshness and hoarseness, suggesting individual variation within the deviant vocal characteristics in this population. The work of van Mourik et al. (1998) highlights the importance of considering each child individually. Furthermore, case reports of children treated for posterior fossa tumor, published by van Dongen et al. (1994) and Catsman-Berrevoets et al. (1992), noted that the children's speech can exhibit laryngeal dysfunction manifesting as reduced volume or difficulty controlling volume, hoarse vocal quality, and monopitch. Catsman-Berrevoets et al. (1992) also noted that one child had difficulty in coordinating respiration and phonation for speech. These deviant perceptual voice characteristics were noted to be evident during the acute phase but resolved in all cases.

Dysphonia, as a continuing feature of the dysarthria seen in children treated for posterior fossa tumor was documented by Murdoch and Hudson-Tennent (1994). Murdoch and Hudson-Tennent (1994), in a study of 11 children treated for posterior fossa tumor, found six of the 11 participants had speech marked by disturbances in pitch, vocal quality, and volume control, with abnormally high pitch levels the most commonly observed. The authors did not suggest that phonatory disturbance was a key feature of the speech disorder seen in children treated for posterior fossa tumor, but a component that should be considered in any management plan.

Cornwell et al. (2004) documented the acoustic parameters of voice using the Multidimensional Voice Program (MDVP, Kay Elemetrics) of a group of 9 children treated for cerebellar tumor. The findings of their acoustic evaluation of phonatory quality identified 7 of their

9 participants with impaired phonation. More specifically the MDVP revealed differences between the children treated for cerebellar tumor and control children across a number of parameters, particularly in measurements of amplitude perturbation. A prevailing characteristic of the results obtained by Cornwell et al. (2004) was that the children treated for cerebellar tumor produced voice samples within the appropriate fundamental frequency range compared to controls. However, they experienced more difficulty controlling the laryngeal mechanism, as suggested by significantly increased values for frequency perturbation and amplitude perturbation measurements compared to the control children as well as an increased number of voice breaks. A similar profile of acoustic characteristics has been documented to be representative of vocal dysfunction in adults with cerebellar damage (Colton & Casper, 1996). Cornwell et al. (2004) concluded that their findings confirmed voice dysfunction as a component of the long-term dysarthria exhibited by children treated for cerebellar tumor. The severity of the vocal disturbance generally was mild, and the deviant features of roughness, instability and breathiness characterized the vocal quality. Overall, the findings indicate that the difficulty for children treated for cerebellar tumor arises in controlling the laryngeal mechanism for smooth vibratory cycles during voice production rather than in the initiation of appropriate fundamental frequency.

Velopharyngeal Function in Children Treated for Posterior Fossa Tumor

Critically important to the evaluation of the oral mechanism in children treated for cerebellar tumor is the determination of velopharyngeal function, because impairment at this level exaggerates the impairment of other components of the speech mechanism (Yorkston et al., 1999). Velopharyngeal dysfunction impacts not only on the resonance of speech but can also contribute to decreased overall speech intelligibility, poor articulation, and phonatory quality (Moller, 1991). An inability to generate sufficient intra-oral air pressure due to poor velopharyngeal closure can impact on the production of oral stop, fricative and affricate consonants, and distort vowel quality (Moller, 1991: Yorkston et al., 1999; Zemlin, 1998). The adequacy of velopharyngeal closure is dependent on three factors, the structural status of the soft palate, its mobility (Moller, 1991; Yorkston et al., 1999), and coordination of the valving action of the soft palate with other aspects of speech production (Yorkston et al., 1999; Zemlin, 1998).

Studies evaluating the speech of children treated for cerebellar and posterior fossa tumors have failed to indicate disturbed nasality, as a perceptual correlate of velopharyngeal dysfunction, as a key deviant speech feature (Murdoch & Hudson-Tennent, 1994; van Mourik et al., 1998). Closer examination, however, of the individual results reported by Murdoch and Hudson-Tennent (1994) for 11 participants with posterior fossa tumor, revealed eight (72.7%) children exhibited disturbed nasality as a deviant speech characteristic. Six children were documented to have speech marked by increased nasality, while the other two were perceived to have decreased levels of nasality. Mild hypernasality was also detected in two of the six children treated for cerebellar tumor in a study by van Mourik and colleagues (1998). To date there have been no reported specific instrumental evaluations of velopharyngeal function in children treated for posterior fossa tumors.

Articulatory Function in Children Treated for Posterior Fossa Tumor

Articulatory dysfunction, along with a disturbance in the prosody of speech, is one of the most commonly affected aspects of speech production in dysarthria due to cerebellar damage in adults, and therefore it could be hypothesized that articulatory deficits may be present in the speech of children with cerebellar damage due to cerebellar tumor. There is a paucity of literature investigating articulatory deficits in children with cerebellar lesions, but three small group studies of the perceptual speech characteristics in children treated for cerebellar and posterior fossa tumors have documented articulatory impairment as key features (Cornwell et al., 2003a; Murdoch & Hudson-Tennent, 1994; van Mourik et al., 1998). Specifically, imprecision of consonants was common to the speech outcomes for all three studies (Cornwell et al., 2003a; Murdoch & Hudson-Tennant, 1994; van Mourik et al., 1998), whereas distorted vowels (van Mourik et al., 1998) and reduced rate of speech (Murdoch & Hudson-Tennant, 1994) were also considered indicative of impairment to the articulatory mechanism. There also are a number of reported case studies that list imprecision of consonants, distorted vowels, and slow rate of speech as deviant speech features in children treated for cerebellar tumors (Al-Jarallah et al., 1994; Humphreys, 1989; Rekate et al., 1985; van Dongen et al., 1994).

Physiologic analysis of lip and tongue function has been documented for a single case study of a child treated for a cerebellar tumor with a mild dysarthria (Murdoch & Horton, 1998). The results of the investigation of lip function revealed that the child had reduced lip pressures on both maximum effort speech tasks and lip pressures produced during bilabial consonant production; however, this did not relate to a perceivable distortion of bilabial consonants during connected speech. Tongue pressure and tongue endurance levels were reported to be within normal limits for this participant, but the child produced a significantly reduced number of repetitions which the authors indicated was a compensatory strategy to preserve pressure and accuracy of tongue movement. Murdoch and Horton (1998) stated that this finding was supported by the perceptual speech profile for their participants, where overall speech intelligibility was maintained by a reduction in speech rate.

Murdoch et al. (1996) also used instrumental techniques to investigate articulatory function in an 8-year-old girl surgically treated for a large cerebellar astrocytoma. Evidence of articulatory dysfunction was noted using strain-gauge and pressure transducers. More specifically, the results indicated that maximum lip pressures were reduced on both speech and nonspeech tasks, however, this was not considered sufficient to lead to a notable distortion of bilabial consonants. Unlike lip function, Murdoch et al. (1996) reported that tongue pressures and endurance measures for this child were not reduced, although repetitive tongue movements were slow. Furthermore, the authors suggested that the number of repetitions of the tongue movements were reduced by the child in an attempt to preserve strength and accuracy of her tongue movements.

The perceptual and acoustic characteristics of consonant production in three children with dysarthria associated with treatment for cerebellar tumor were investigated by Cornwell et al. (2004). Temporal acoustic analysis of the alveolar stop consonant /t/ provided objective evidence of a disturbance in the timing of articulatory movements in children with dysarthria subsequent to treatment for cerebellar tumor. Although all three cases reported by Cornwell et al. (2004) exhibited consonant durations that differed to those of healthy controls, variability among the participants was noted. Two children (cases A and C) exhibited increased consonant durations, whereas one child (Case B) demonstrated reduced consonant durations. Cornwell et al. (2004) noted that increased consonant duration implies slowing of the articulatory gesture for /t/, which is in keeping with earlier physiologic studies of adults with dysarthria due to cerebellar damage, and documented slowness of movements resulting in articulatory deficits (Kent & Netsell, 1975; Netsell & Kent, 1976). Although unexpected, Cornwell et al. (2004) proposed that the reduced consonant durations recorded for Case B may have been related to observed reductions in stop gap durations for this case. Cornwell et al. (2004) proposed that a possible explanation for this finding could be incomplete articulatory contact for the stop consonant, which could result in a reduced stop gap duration and has been previously documented to occur inconsistently in adults with cerebellar dysarthria (Hirose, Kiritani, Ushijima, & Sawashima, 1978). Overall the findings

of Cornwell et al. (2004) suggest that deficits in timing articulatory movements may contribute to the perception of consonant imprecision in children treated for cerebellar tumor.

Case Examples

Case 1: Randolph (Cerebellar Tumor)

Randolph was a 12-year-old male who had completed treatment for a cerebellar tumor 18 months prior to referral to the Centre for Neurogenic Communication Disorders Research at The University of Queensland. His speech was characterized by a mild dysarthria predominantly related to phonatory and articulatory impairments.

The assessment of respiratory function and speech breathing revealed deficits in aspects of general respiratory function, paradoxical movements of the chest wall during maximal effort tasks and decreased lung volume excursion during a reading task. Randolph's FEV_1 was significantly below that of the control group, as well as both VC and FEV_1 measured at below 80% which has been reported as the lower level of normal respiratory capacity. Incoordination of the rib cage and abdomen during speech production, in conjunction with reduced vital capacity, has previously been linked to the perception of decreased respiratory support for speech, which was not perceived in the present case. It should be acknowledged that, whereas respiratory support for speech was deemed to be adequate, the impact that impairment in one motor speech subsystem can have on other aspects of speech production should not be discounted. In particular, voice production (phonation) is dependent on the respiratory forces generated from the respiratory mechanism for voice production and phonatory disturbances have previously been linked to respiratory abnormalities.

Randolph was noted to have a disturbed vocal quality described as a harsh quality. Electroglottographic (EGG) and aerodynamic measures of laryngeal function failed to identify a physiologic reason for this perceived vocal quality. The tasks associated with the EGG and aerodynamic assessments were vowel prolongation and syllable repetition and this differs from the connected speech samples on which the perceptual judgments of phonatory impairment were made. It should be suggested that consideration must be given to the role that a reduction in the lung volumes during connected speech could have on Randolph's vocal quality, something not evaluated by the EGG and aerodynamic procedures.

Physiologic assessment of velopharyngeal function revealed an absence of any impairment consistent with the perceptual assessment of Randolph's speech. Randolph was reported to demonstrate mild imprecision of consonant production in the absence of decreased speech intelligibility and impairments in jaw, lip and/or tongue function on the Frenchay Dysarthria Assessment. The physiologic investigation of lip and tongue function revealed that any articulatory impairment was not due to a decrement in maximum lip or tongue pressures; however, fine control of the articulators was noted to be impaired. Fine force control tasks for both the lip and tongue revealed an inability to maintain force and position stability for both lip and tongue movements, which previously has been linked to the articulatory

deficits seen in adults with cerebellar damage. A tendency toward difficulty in coordinating lip and tongue movements was possibly evident in the fast-rate repetition tasks for lip and tongue, although the results did not reach the significance level. These findings suggest that the underlying pathophysiology to the deviant perceptual speech feature of imprecision of consonants may be a difficulty in coordinating the fine movements (timing, force, range, and accuracy) of the lips and tongue required for speech production as a result of cerebellar damage.

Case 2: Alex (Cerebellar Tumor)

Alex was a 12-year-old male treated for a cerebellar tumor 2 years prior to the assessment. His speech had been judged to exhibit a mild degree of dysarthria, with deviant perceptual speech features related to respiratory, phonatory, and resonatory function, as well as disturbance to the prosody of his speech. The Frenchay Dysarthria Assessment revealed impairments in motor speech function, specifically in the areas of laryngeal and articulatory (lip and tongue) function.

Overall, the physiological investigation of motor speech function for Alex identified some degree of impairment within the respiratory mechanism as well as isolated articulatory deficits, but found no dysfunction within the laryngeal or velopharyngeal mechanism. Specifically, spirometric assessment, using predicted values, indicated intact general respiratory function, whereas the kinematic evaluation revealed incoordination of the rib-cage and abdomen during maximal effort tasks as measured through the incidence of paradoxic movements. Lung volume excursion was decreased in a sustained phonation task that was influenced by the increased value obtained for lung volume termination (LVT). Increased values for LVT were also obtained during the conversational speech sample, although this did not negatively impact lung volume excursions on this task. The observed deviant perceptual speech feature of reduced breath support for speech did not appear to be supported by the physiologic findings. Despite the identification of paradoxical movements of the abdomen during maximal effort tasks, this did not correlate with reduced respiratory excursions during connected speech.

The instrumental assessments of laryngeal and velopharyngeal function did not detect any evidence of impairment; this is in contrast to the perceptual profile created for this child which identified phonatory and resonatory impairments. Possible explanations for the disparity in the laryngeal findings of the two modes of assessment could arise from the difficulties associated with identifying perceptual voice characteristics, particularly in the presence of other deviant perceptual speech features (respiratory and articulatory) or methodological problems. Consequently, it is not possible to conclusively exclude laryngeal impairment which leads to the need to consider further assessment (acoustic or fiberoptic endoscopic) to investigate the laryngeal mechanism in this child.

The Frenchay Dysarthria Assessment results indicated that Alex's lip and tongue function were mildly impaired; however, the physiologic investigations failed to identify significant deficits in these areas. Alex was able to produce maximum pressures within the range of control group both on maximum effort tasks and during repetition tasks. He did experience some fatigue effects during performance of a sustained submaximal lip task. The only deficit observed on the instrumental assessment of tongue function was an inability to maintain tongue position stability at low pressures. The deficits in fine force control coordination may be indicative of cerebellar dysfunction.

References

Aarsen, F. K., van Dongen, H. R., Paquier, P. F., van Mourik, M., & Catsman-Berrevoets, C. E. (2004). Long-term sequelae in children after cerebellar astrocytoma surgery. *Neurology, 62,* 1311–1316.

Ackermann H., Hertrich, I., & Hehr, T. (1995). Oral diadochokinesis in neurological dysarthrias. *Folia Phoniatrica et Logopaedica, 47,* 15–23.

Ackermann, H., Vogel, M., Petersen, D., & Poremba, M. (1992). Speech deficits in ischaemic cerebellar lesions. *Journal of Neurology, 239,* 223–227.

Ackermann, H., & Ziegler, W. (1994). Mutismus bei zentralmotorischen Störungen. *Fortschritte der Neurologie und Psychiatrie, 9,* 337–344.

Aguiar, P. H., Plese, J. P. P., Cinquini, O., Marino, R. (1995). Transient mutism following posterior fossa approach to cerebellar tumors in children: A critical review of the literature. *Child's Nervous System, 11,* 306–310.

Al-Jarallah, A., Cook, J. D., Gascon, G., Kanaan, I., & Sigueira, E. (1994). Transient mutism following posterior fossa surgery in children. *Journal of Surgical Oncology, 55,* 126–131.

Amarenco, P., Chevrie-Muller, C., Roullet, E., & Bousser, M. G. (1991). Paravermal infarct and isolated cerebellar dysarthria. *Annals of Neurology, 30,* 211–213.

Ammirati, M., Mirzai, S., & Samii, M. (1989). Transient mutism following removal of a cerebellar tumour: A case report and review of the literature. *Child's Nervous System, 5,* 12–14.

Aronson, A. E. (1990). *Clinical voice disorders: An interdisciplinary approach.* New York, NY: Thieme.

Balasubramaniam, C., Subramaniam, V., & Balasubramaniam, V. (1993). Mutism following posterior fossa surgery for medulloblastoma. *Neurology India, 41,* 173–175.

Brown, J. K. (1985). Dysarthria in children: Neurologic perspective. In J. K. Darby (Ed.), *Speech and language evaluation in neurology: Childhood disorders* (pp. 75–93). New York, NY: Grune & Stratton.

Brown, J. R., Darley, F. L., & Aronson, A. E. (1970). Ataxic dysarthria. *International Journal of Neurology, 7,* 302–318.

Caner, H., Altinörs, N., Benli, S., Calisaneller, T., & Albayrak, A. (1999). Akinetic mutism after fourth ventricle choroid plexus papilloma: Treatment with a dopamine agonist. *Surgical Neurology, 51,* 181–184.

Catsman-Berrevoets, C. E., van Dongen, H. R., Mulder, P. G. H., Geuze, D. P., Paquier, P. F., & Lequin, M. H. (1999). Tumour type and size are high risk factors for the syndrome of "cerebellar" mutism and subsequent dysarthria. *Journal of Neurology, Neurosurgery and Psychiatry, 67,* 755–757.

Catsman-Berrevoets, C. E., van Dongen, H. R., & Zwetsloot, C. P. (1992). Transient loss of speech followed by dysarthria after removal of posterior fossa tumour. *Developmental Medicine and Child Neurology, 34,* 1102–1117.

Chenery, H. J., Ingram, J., & Murdoch, B. E. (1990). Perceptual analysis of the speech in ataxic dysarthria. *Australian Journal of Human Communication Disorders, 18,* 19–28.

Colton, R., & Casper, J. K. (1996). *Understanding voice problems: A physiological perspective for diagnosis and treatment.* Baltimore, MD: Williams & Wilkins.

Cornwell, P. L., Murdoch, B. E., & Ward, E. C. (2005). Differential motor speech out-comes in children treated for mid-line cerebellar tumour. *Brain Injury, 19,* 119–134.

Cornwell, P. L., Murdoch, B. E., Ward, E. C., & Kellie, S. (2003a). Perceptual evaluation of motor speech following treatment for childhood cerebellar tumour. *Clinical Linguistics and Phonetics, 17,* 597–615.

Cornwell, P. L., Murdoch, B. E., Ward, E. C., & Kellie, S. (2004). Acoustic investigation of vocal quality following treatment for childhood cerebellar tumour. *Folia Phoniatrica et Logopaedica, 56,* 93–107.

Cornwell, P. L, Murdoch, B. E., Ward, E. C., & Morgan, A. T. (2003b). Dysarthria and dysphagia as long-term sequelae in a child treated for posterior fossa tumour. *Pediatric Rehabilitation, 6,* 67–75.

Dailey, A. T., McKhann, G. M., & Berger, M. S. (1995). The pathophysiology of oral pharyngeal apraxia and mutism following posterior fossa tumor resection in children. *Journal of Neurosurgery, 83,* 467–475.

Darley, F. L., Aronson, A. E., & Brown, J. R. (1969a). Differential diagnostic patterns of dysarthria. *Journal of Speech and Hearing Research, 12,* 246–269.

Darley, F. L., Aronson, A. E., & Brown, J. R. (1969b). Clusters of deviant speech dimensions in the dysarthrias. *Journal of Speech and Hearing Research, 12,* 462–496.

Darley, F. L., Aronson, A. E., & Brown, J. R. (1975). *Motor speech disorders.* Philadelphia, PA: W. B. Saunders.

Delong, G. R., & Adams, R. D. (1975). Clinical aspects of tumours of the posterior fossa in childhood. In P. J. Vinken & G. W. Bruyn (Eds.), *Handbook of clinical neurology: tumours of the brain and skull* (Vol. 18, Part III, pp. 387–411). Amsterdam, the Netherlands: North Holland.

De Smet, H. J., Baillieux, H., Catsman-Berrevoets, C., De Deyn P., Mariën, P., & Paquier, P. F. (2007). Post-operative motor speech production in children with syndrome "cerebellar" mutism and subsequent dysarthria: A review of the literature. *European Journal of Paediatric Neurology, 11,* 193–207.

Duffy, J. R., & Kent, R. D. (2001). Darley's contributions to the understanding, differential diagnosis and scientific study of dysarthrias. *Aphasiology, 15,* 275–289.

Enderby, P. M. (1983). Frenchay dysarthria assessment. San Diego, CA: College-Hill Press.

Ersahin, Y., Mutluer, S., Cagli, S., & Duman, Y. (1996). Cerebellar mutism: Report of seven cases and review of the literature. *Neurosurgery, 38,* 60–66.

Farwell, J. R., Dohrmann, G.J., & Flannery, J. T. (1977). Central nervous system tumors in children. *Cancer, 40,* 3123–3132.

Ferrante, L., Mastronardi, L., Acqui, M., & Fortuna, A. (1990). Mutism after posterior fossa surgery in children. *Journal of Neurosurgery, 72,* 959–963.

Fisher, H. B., & Logemann, J. A. (1971). The Fisher–Logemann test of articulation competence. Boston, MA: Houghton Mifflin.

FitzGerald, F. J., Murdoch, B. E., & Chenery, H. J. (1987). Multiple sclerosis: Associated speech and language disorders. *Australian Journal of Human Communication Disorders, 9,* 15–33.

Frim, D. M., & Ogilvy, C. S. (1995). Mutism and cerebellar dysarthria after brain stem surgery: Case report. *Neurosurgery, 36,* 854–857.

Geissinger, J. D., & Bucy, P. C. (1971). Astrocytomas of the cerebellum in children. *Archives of Neurology, 24,* 125–135.

Gjerris, F. (1978). Clinical aspects and long-term prognosis of infratentorial intracranial tumours in infancy and childhood. *Acta Neurologica Scandinavica, 57,* 31–52.

Gol, A. (1963). Cerebellar astrocytomas in children. *American Journal of Diseases in Children, 106,* 21–24.

Gordon, N. (1996). Speech, language and the cerebellum. *European Journal of Disorders of Communication, 31,* 359–367.

Hirose, H., Kiritani, S., Ushijima, T., & Sawashima, M. (1978). Analysis of abnormal articulatory dynamics in two dysarthric patients. *Journal of Speech and Hearing Disorders, 4,* 96–105.

Hixon, T. J. (1973). Respiratory function in speech. In F. Minifie, T. J. Hixon, & F. Williams (Eds.), *Normal aspects of speech, hearing and language* (pp. 75–125). Englewood Cliffs, NJ: Prentice-Hall.

Hixon, T. J., Putnam, A., & Sharp, J. T. (1983). Speech production with flaccid paralysis of the rib-cage, diaphragm and abdomen. *Journal of Speech Hearing Disorders, 48,* 315–327.

Huber, J. F., Bradley, K., Spiegler, B., & Dennis, M. (2007). Long-term neuromotor speech deficits in survivors of childhood posterior fossa tumors: Effects of tumor type, radiation, age at diagnosis and survival years. *Journal of Child Neurology, 22,* 848–854.

Hudson, L. J. (1990). Speech and language disorders in childhood brain tumours. In B. E. Murdoch (Ed.), *Acquired neurological speech/language disorders in childhood* (pp. 245–268). London, UK: Taylor & Francis.

Hudson, L. J., Buttsworth, D. L., & Murdoch, B. E. (1990). Effect of CNS prophylaxis on speech and language function in children. In B. E. Murdoch (Ed.), *Acquired neurological speech/language disorders in childhood* (pp. 269–307). London, UK: Taylor & Francis.

Hudson, L. J., Murdoch, B. E., & Ozanne, A. E. (1989). Posterior fossa tumours in childhood: Associated speech and language disorders post-surgery. *Aphasiology, 3,* 1–18.

Humphreys, R. P. (1989). Mutism after posterior fossa tumor surgery. In A. E. Marlin (Ed.), *Concepts in pediatric neurosurgery* (pp. 57–64). Basel, Switzerland: Karger.

Jansen, G., Messing-Junger, A. M., Engelbrecht, V., Gobel, U., Bock, W. J., & Lenard, H. G. (1998). Cerebellar mutism syndrome. *Klinische Padiatrie, 210,* 243–247.

Kadota, R. P., Allen, J. B., Hartman, G. A., & Spruce, W. E. (1989). Brain tumors in children. *Journal of Pediatrics, 114,* 511–519.

Kai, Y., Kuratsu, J., Suginohara, K., Marubayashi, T., & Ushio, Y. (1997). Cerebellar mutism after posterior fossa surgery: Two case reports. *Neurological Medicine Chirugica, 37,* 929–933.

Kent, R. D. (2000). Research on speech motor control and its disorders: A review and prospective. *Journal of Communication Disorders, 33,* 391–428.

Kent, R. D., & Netsell, R. (1975). A case study of an ataxic dysarthric: Cineradiographic and spectrographic observations. *Journal of Speech and Hearing Disorders, 40,* 115–134.

Koh, S., Turkel, S. B., & Baram, T. Z. (1997). Cerebellar mutism in children: Report of six cases and potential mechanisms. *Pediatric Neurology, 16,* 218–219.

Kusano, Y., Tanaka, Y., Takasuna, H., Wada, N., Tada, T., & Kakizawa, Y., . . . Hongo, K. (2006). Transient cerebellar mutism caused by bilateral damage to the dentate nuclei. *Journal of Neurosurgery, 104,* 329–331.

Larson, C. R., Sutton, D., & Lindeman, R. C. (1978). Cerebellar regulation of phonation in rhesus monkey (Macaca mulatto). *Experimental Brain Research, 63,* 596–606.

Manto, M. U. (2002). Clinical signs of cerebellar disorders. In M. U. Manto (Ed.), *The cerebellum and its disorders* (pp. 97–120). New York, NY: Cambridge University Press.

Mariën, P., Engelborghs, S., Fabbro, F., & De Deyn P. P. (2001). The lateralized linguistic cerebellum: A review and a new hypothesis. *Brain and Language, 79,* 580–600.

Menkes, J. H., & Till, K. (1995). Postnatal trauma and injuries by physical agents. In J. H. Menkes (Ed.), *Textbook of child neurology* (pp. 557–597). Baltimore, MD: Williams & Wilkins.

Moller, K. T. (1991). An approach to evaluation of velopharyngeal adequacy for speech. *Clinics in Communication Disorders, 1,* 61–75.

Murdoch, B. E., Chenery, H. J., Stokes, P. D., & Hardcastle, W. J. (1991). Respiratory kinematics in speakers with cerebellar disease. *Journal of Speech and Hearing Research, 34,* 768–780.

Murdoch, B. E., & Horton, S. K. (1998). Acquired and developmental dysarthria in childhood. In B. E. Murdoch (Ed.), *Dysarthria: A physiological approach to assessment and treatment* (pp. 373–427). Cheltenham, UK: Stanley Thornes.

Murdoch, B. E., Horton, S. K., Theodoros, D. G., & Thompson, E. C. (1996). Determination of treatment priorities in acquired childhood dysarthria: A role for physiological instrumentation. In J. Ponsford, P. Snow, & V. Anderson (Eds.), *International perspectives in traumatic brain injury* (pp. 267–271). Brisbane, Australia: Australian Academic Press.

Murdoch, B. E., & Hudson-Tennent, L. J. (1993). Speech breathing anomalies in children with dysarthria following treatment for posterior fossa tumours. *Journal of Medical Speech-Language Pathology, 1*(2), 107–119.

Murdoch, B. E., & Hudson-Tennent, L. J. (1994). Speech disorders in children treated for posterior fossa tumours: Ataxic and developmental features. *European Journal of Disorders of Communication, 29,* 379–397.

Nagatani, K., Waga, S., & Nakagawa, Y. (1991). Mutism after removal of a vermian medulloblastoma: Cerebellar mutism. *Surgical Neurology, 36,* 307–309.

Naidich, T. P., & Zimmerman, R. A. (1984). Primary brain tumors in children. *Seminars in Roentgenology, 19,* 100–114.

Netsell, R., & Kent, R. (1976). Paroxysmal ataxic dysarthria. *Journal of Speech and Hearing Disorders, 41,* 93–109.

Ozimek, A., Richter, S., Hein-Kropp, C., Schoch, B., Gorissen, B., Kaiser, O., . . . Timmann, D. (2004). Cerebellar mutism: Report of four cases. *Journal of Neurology, 251,* 963–972.

Panitch, H. S., & Berg, B. D. (1970). Brain stem tumours of childhood and adolescence. *American Journal of Disorders of Childhood, 119,* 465–472.

Paquier, P. F., van Mourik, M., van Dongen, H., Catsman-Berrevoets, C., & Brison, A. (2003). Syndrome de mutisme cérébelleux et dysarthrie subséquente: Étude de trois enfants et revue de la littérature. *Revue Neurologique (Paris), 159,* 1017–1027.

Pollack, I. F., Polinko, P., Albright, A. L., Towbin, R., & Fitz, C. (1995). Mutism and pseudobulbar symptoms after resection of posterior fossa tumors in children: Incidence and pathophysiology. *Neurosurgery, 37,* 885–893.

Rekate, H. L., Grubb, R. L., Aram, D. M., Hahn, J. F., & Ratcheson, R. A. (1985). Muteness of cerebellar origin. *Archives of Neurology, 42,* 697–698.

Richter, S., Schoch, B., Ozimek, A., Gorissen, B., Hein-Kropp, C., Kaiser, O., . . . Timmann, D. (2005). Incidence of dysarthria in children with cerebellar tumors: A prospective study. *Brain and Language, 92,* 153–167.

Riva, D. (1998). The cerebellar contribution to language and sequential functions: Evidence from a child with cerebellitis. *Cortex, 34,* 279–287.

Riva, D., & Giorgi, C. (2000). The cerebellum contributes to higher functions during development. Evidence from a series of children surgically treated for posterior fossa tumours. *Brain, 123,* 1051–1061.

Russell, D. S., & Rubinstein, L. J. (1989). *Pathology of tumours of the nervous system.* London, UK: Williams & Wilkins.

Sagiuchi, T., Ishii, K., Aok, Y., Utsuki, S., Tanaka, R., Fujii, K., . . . Hayakawa, K. (2001). Bilateral crossed cerebello-cerebral diaschisis and mutism after surgery for cerebellar medulloblastoma. *Annals of Nuclear Medicine, 15,* 157–160.

Scott, R. B., Stoodley, C. J., Anslow, P., Paul, C., Stein, J. F., Sugden, E., . . . Mitchell, C.. (2001). Lateralized cognitive deficits in children following cerebellar lesions. *Developmental Medicine and Child Neurology, 43,* 685–691.

Tew, J. M., Feibel, J. H., & Sawaya, R. (1984). Brain tumors: Clinical aspects. *Seminars in Roentgenology, 19,* 115–128.

Theodoros, D. G., Murdoch, B. E., & Chenery, H. J. (1994). Perceptual speech characteristics of dysarthric speakers following severe closed head injury. *Brain Injury, 8,* 101–124.

Turgut, M. (1998). Transient "cerebellar" mutism. *Child's Nervous System, 14,* 161–166.

van Dongen, H. R., Catsman-Berrevoets, C. E., & van Mourik, M. (1994). The syndrome of 'cerebellar' mutism and subsequent dysarthria. *Neurology, 44,* 2040–2046.

van Mourik, M., Catsman-Berrevoets, C. E., Paquier, P. F., Yousef-Bak, E., & van Dongen, H. R. (1997). Acquired childhood dysarthria: Review of its clinical presentation. *Pediatric Neurology, 17,* 299–307.

van Mourik, M., Catsman-Berrevoets, C. E., van Dongen, H. R., & Neville, B. G. R. (1997). Complex orofacial movements and the disappearance of cerebellar mutism: Report of five cases. *Developmental Medicine and Child Neurology, 39,* 686–690.

van Mourik, M., Catsman-Berrevoets, C. E., Yousef-Bak, E., Paquier, P. F., & van Dongen, H. R. (1998). Dysarthria in children with cerebellar or brainstem tumors. *Pediatric Neurology, 18,* 411–414.

Volcan, I., Cole, G. P., & Johnston, K. (1986). A case of muteness of cerebellar origin. *Archives of Neurology, 43,* 313–314.

Wang, Y. T., Kent, R. D., Duffy, J. R., Thomas, J. E., & Fredericks, G. V. (2006). Dysarthria following cerebellar mutism secondary to resection of a fourth ventricle medulloblastoma: A case study. *Journal of Medical Speech-Language Pathology, 14,* 109–127.

Yorkston, K. M., Beukelman, D. R., & Bell, K. R. (1991). *Clinical management of dysarthric speakers.* Austin, TX: Pro-Ed.

Yorkston, K. M., Beukelman, D. R., Strand, E. A., & Bell, K. R. (1999). *Management of motor speech disorders in children and adults.* Austin, TX: Pro-Ed.

Zemlin, W. R. (1998). *Speech and hearing science: Anatomy and physiology.* Boston, MA: Allyn and Bacon.

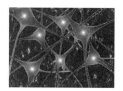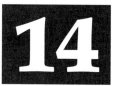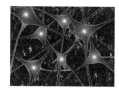

14

Assessment and Treatment of Acquired Motor Speech Disorders in Childhood

Introduction

Specific descriptions of the nature, course, and prognosis of pediatric motor speech disorders are few in number. Consequently, reports in the literature have little to offer the clinician in either the diagnosis or treatment of acquired motor speech disorders in children. Most of the assessment and treatment strategies for dysarthria and acquired apraxia of speech have therefore been developed by researchers working with the adult population (Darley, Aronson, & Brown, 1975; Nemec & Cohen, 1984; Netsell & Cleeland, 1973; Theodoros, Murdoch, & Chenery, 1994). These strategies have been adapted for use with children. However, there is some concern about the validity of such practices as the characteristics of children with motor speech disorders may be different from those in adults (Catsman-Berrevoets, van Dongen, & Zwetsloot, 1992). As

pointed out in Chapter 11, the criteria for classifying acquired dysarthria in adults may not apply to children. Depending on the time of onset of the dysarthria the child's speech and language development may not be complete, forcing a developmental perspective onto that of an acquired disorder. Murdoch and Hudson-Tennent (1994) acknowledge this difficulty and urge that a child's phonological development prior to the onset of dysarthria be taken into consideration. Any developmental components in the speech disorder need to be identified as such. Differential diagnosis of acquired motor speech problems, articulation difficulties, and phonological delays is important if appropriate treatment goals are to be formulated (Murdoch, Ozanne, & Cross, 1990). As with adults a subsystems approach to the analysis and management of the acquired motor speech disorders of childhood has long been accepted (Love, 1992).

Assessment of Acquired Motor Speech Disorders in Childhood

Careful and detailed assessment of acquired neurologic speech disorders in children is essential to aid clinicians in their formulation of a diagnosis and for determination of specific treatment priorities. The assessment should involve the gathering of relevant information, the observation of the child's abilities in a variety of settings and the systematic testing, combined with an objective evaluation scale, of the speech mechanism during nonspeech and speech activities with attention being paid to the involuntary and voluntary control of the speech mechanism. The information should include a description of the child's phonological system before the lesion and a neurologic report on the site of the brain lesion and the nature of the neurologic impairment.

Several assessment tools designed for the adult client (e.g., Frenchay Dysarthria Assessment (FDA) [Enderby, 1983], Working With Dysarthrics [Robertson & Thomson, 1986], and the Apraxia Battery for Adults [Dabul, 1979]) may be used successfully with children although some modification may be necessary. These modifications may include the simplification of instructions, the use of play situations when asking the child to sustain a sound (e.g., "Let's see how long you can sound the siren on your fire engine.") or the substitution of a child-oriented articulation test and a selection of multisyllabic words of increasing complexity all of which would be in the child's receptive vocabulary. In some cases tests used to assess acquired childhood motor speech disorders rep-

resent adaptations of assessments devised for testing developmental speech disorders. For example, the Nuffield Centre Dyspraxia Programme (Nuffield Hearing and Speech Centre, 1985) designed primarily for the child with developmental dyspraxia is also a useful assessment and treatment tool with children with acquired motor speech disorders.

The tools mentioned above represent a systematic approach to the assessment of the child's speech mechanism but no assessment would be complete without an analysis of the child's functional speech and nonspeech activities. Judgments need to be made on how well the child is understood at home, in school, with peers, and in the community. If the child's message breaks down, why does it fail? An analysis of a speech sample should follow a similar systematic approach to that detailed in the assessment profiles (e.g., Respiration: How does the child's respiratory cycle affect his speech? Is his or her breath control poor? Prosody: Does the child phrase incorrectly so that the meaning of the utterance is lost? Is his or her rate of speech too slow?). Also, included in these observational sessions would be a judgment of the child's eating skills.

Darley et al. (1975) suggested five parameters requiring assessment when diagnosing motor speech disorders:

Respiration: the volume and control of the exhaled air.

Phonation: the quality, harshness, duration, pitch, steadiness, and loudness of the voice.

Resonance: the hypernasality or hyponasality of speech. The testing for nasal emission of the airstream during speech.

Articulation: the precision of isolated sounds, sound combinations, single words, and phrases.

Prosody: the rate, intonation, stress, and other suprasegmental features of oral communication and overall intelligibility.

Robertson and Thomson (1986) in devising their assessment tool included the five areas mentioned by Darley et al. (1975) but also added the following:

Facial musculature: the function of jaws, lips, tongue, and palate during speech.

Diadochokinesis: the rate and precision of repetitive movements using speech sounds and oral movements.

Reflexes: the presence of drooling during eating or speech, the cough reflex, chewing, and swallowing of liquids and solids.

Intelligibility: the overall integration and coordination of all motor speech processes.

A range of assessment techniques are available to the clinician to assist in formulation of a diagnosis and determination of specific treatment priorities. A comprehensive assessment of children affected by neurologic impairments should include the following components: A detailed case history; an oromotor examination; determination of the key features of the speech disorder and identification of their neural substrates based on an integrated perceptual, acoustic, and physiologic assessment of their

speech disorder. Assessment procedures are similar for acquired dysarthria and apraxia of speech as these two motor speech disorders, together with aphasia, often coexist.

Case History

Prior to undertaking any formal tests it is informative and necessary for the clinician to first collect a case history from the client. A detailed case history can inform the clinician of the salient features of the disorder from the perspective of the client. It is not unusual that a skilled clinician can arrive at a tentative diagnosis based on information gained from the case history alone. Essential background information to be collected as part of the case history should include the following client details: age, education level, academic abilities, and prior history of speech-language impairments (including developmental conditions experienced earlier in childhood); onset and course of the disorder (how long has the client had the condition? Is it progressive or stable? etc.); associated deficits (e.g., drooling, swallowing impairments, hemiplegia, etc.); emotional disturbances; prior treatment and management regimens; client's awareness and understanding of the disorder; and consequences of the disorder for the client (e.g., disruption to school, family life, social activities, etc.). Details of any available neurologic and neuroimaging reports should also be documented.

Oromotor Examination

An oromotor examination primarily involves visual and tactual observation of the speech production mechanism during performance of a range of non-speech activities and provides important information about the size, strength, symmetry, range, tone, steadiness, speech, and accuracy of movements of the face, jaw, tongue, and velum (soft palate). Each of these four components of the speech production system is observed in the following conditions: at rest; during sustained postures (e.g., retraction of the lips, protrusion of the tongue, etc.); and during movement (e.g., alternate pursing and retraction of the lips). While each structure is at rest the clinician should observe whether or not the structure is symmetric or deviated to one side (e.g., at rest does the face, tongue, jaw, and velum appear symmetric). Further, while at rest the presence of any involuntary movements (e.g., twitching of the tongue muscle) and muscle wastage (atrophy) need to be noted as both of these features may be indicative of the presence of a neurologic impairment such as a lower motor neuron lesion. The strength of the tongue and jaw can be tested by having the client move these structures against a force applied by the clinician (e.g., the client can be asked to press their tongue against the cheek to oppose a force imposed externally on the cheek by the hand of the clinician). The presence and absence of both normal and pathologic reflexes also can be good indicators of the presence of disease in either the peripheral or central nervous systems. For example, the absence of a normal reflex such as the gag reflex or jaw jerk can indicate the presence of pathology. Likewise, the presence of primitive or pathologic reflexes (i.e., reflexes absent in non-neurologically impaired individuals) such as the sucking reflex is also indicative of neurologic impairment.

Determination of the Principal Features of the Speech Disorder

Techniques available for determining the principal features of the neurological speech disorder exhibited by a client and their neuropathologic substrates can be broadly divided into three major categories: perceptual techniques—these assessments are based on the clinicians impression of the auditory-perceptual attributes of the client's speech; acoustic techniques—assessments in this category are based on the study of the generation, transmission, and modification of sound waves emitted from the vocal tract; and physiologic techniques—these methods are based on instrumental assessment of the functioning of the various subsystems of the speech production mechanism in terms of their movements, muscular contractions, and so forth. In addition to these techniques, as indicated above it is also important to assess the child's functional or pragmatic speech abilities.

Perceptual Assessment

Perceptual analysis of neurological speech disorders has been the "gold standard" and preferred method by which clinicians have made differential diagnoses and defined treatment programs for their clients for many years. In fact, many clinicians still rely almost exclusively on auditory-perceptual judgments of speech intelligibility, articulatory accuracy, or subjective ratings of various speech dimensions on which to base their diagnosis of dysarthria and apraxia of speech and plan their intervention. Various perceptual assessment regimes have been used with children with motor speech disorders. Examples from the literature of the perceptual assessments used and the types of child cases tested are shown in Table 14–1.

Table 14–1. Examples of Perceptual Assessments Used to Assess Children with Dysarthria

Authors	Perceptual Assessments Included in the Investigations	Subject Details
Finley, Niman, Standley, and Wansley (1977)	Oromotor examination including breath support (breaths/min & panting), phonatory control (sustained sounds /a/, /e/) and syllable production tasks	Four children (2 males, 2 females) ages between 6 to 10 y with spastic cerebral palsy
Love, Hagerman, and Taimi (1980)	Perceptual rating of speech proficiency; Irwin integrated articulation test for cerebral palsied children: feeding skills; examination of retention of reflexes	Sixty subjects aged between 3 to 22 y with spastic, athetoid, and mixed spastic/athetoid cerebral palsy
Vogel and von Cramon (1982)	Phoniatric examination, phonetic testing, articulation testing, phonatory skills, respiration, spontaneous speech tasks. All tasks were evaluated by 2 phoneticians for phonatory features	Two female subjects (aged 12 and 15 y) who had suffered a CHI
Bak, van Dongen, and Arts (1983)	Neurologic exam of the speech musculature; audiotaped samples of repeated words, phrases, spontaneous speech and singing. All speech samples rated perceptually using the Darley et al. (1969a, 1969b, 1975) three-point rating scales	One 6 y/o male following brainstem infarct caused by basilar artery occlusion
De Feo and Schaefer (1983)	Oromotor evaluation, observation of nonspeech tasks, Fisher-Logemann Test of Articulation Competence; connected speech analyzed for pitch, prosody, rate, nasality, and intelligibility; evaluation of respiratory behavior	Three-year-old male with bilateral facial paralysis
Hardcastle, Morgan-Barry, and Clark (1987)	Impressionistic auditory appraisals of speech, Edinburgh Articulation Test	Four articulation disordered children, two of whom were diagnosed as dysarthric aged between 7 to 9 y/o

continues

405

Table 14–1. *continued*

Authors	Perceptual Assessments Included in the Investigations	Subject Details
van Dongen, Arts, and Yousef-Bak (1987)	Neurologic examination of the speech musculature; tape recording of word and sentence repetition and spontaneous speech. Speech tasks perceptually rated using the Darley et al. (1969a, 1969b, 1975) three-point rating scales	Eight subjects consisting of: 15 y/o female with bilateral 7th nerve palsy, 12 y/o male with bilateral 7th, 9th, and 10th nerve palsies, 11 y/o male with bilateral facial and bulbar weakness, 6 y/o male with basilar artery occlusion, 13 y/o female with bilateral facial and lingual weakness, 14 y/o female with acute encephalopathy, 10 y/o male with bilateral cerebral contusion
Hudson, Murdoch, and Ozanne (1989)	The Fisher–Logemann Test of Articulation Competence analyzed both for articulatory competence and presence of phonological processes; The Frenchay Dysarthria Assessment; connected speech sample perceptually analyzed for the 10 predominant features of ataxic dysarthria (Darley et al., 1969a,1969b)	Five subjects including 6 y/o male with medulloblastoma, 8 y/o male with posterior fossa tumor, 8 y/o posterior fossa ependymoma, 11 y/o solid cerebellar astrocytoma, 15 y/o male ependymoma, 16 y/o male recurrent posterior fossa astrocytoma and extradural hematoma
Jordan and Murdoch (1990)	The Frenchay Dysarthria Assessment; Articulation subtest of the Neurosensory Center Comprehensive Examination of Aphasia	7 y/o female following CHI
Jordan (1990)	The Frenchay Dysarthria Assessment; Articulation subtest of the Neurosensory Center Comprehensive Examination of Aphasia	9 y/o female following CHI
Milloy and Morgan-Barry (1990)	Edinburgh Articulation Test; Phonological Assessment of Child Speech (PACS); Informal observation	Two subjects: 9 y/o female with mild spastic quadriplegia, 8 y/o male with cyclomegalovirus infection in utero

Authors	Perceptual Assessments Included in the Investigations	Subject Details
Murdoch, Ozanne, and Cross (1990)	Frenchay Dysarthria Assessment; spontaneous speech samples	13 y/o male following cerebral anoxia
Robin and Eliason (1991)	Assessment of the structure and movement of the speech mechanism; Templin-Darley Test of Articulation (1969a,b); informal ratings of intelligibility and nasality during conversational speech; diadochokinetic rates for syllables, prosodic evaluation of sentences using particular intonation and stress patterns judged on a forced-choice paradigm	Seven children aged between 5 to 16 y/o with von Recklinghausen's disease
Workinger and Kent (1991)	Recorded sample of sustained vowels, sentence repetitions, counting and spontaneous speech. Speech rated perceptually on 22 dimensions from Seif et al. (1981)	Eighteen children aged between 7 to 14 y/o
Catsman-Berrevoets, van Dongen, and Zwetsloot (1992)	Videotape recordings of speech perceptually analyzed using Darley et al. (1969a,b, 1975) three point rating scales; neurologic examination of the speech musculature	Three subjects: 6 y/o male medulloblastoma, 8 y/o female medulloblastoma and posterior fossa epidural hematoma, 8 y/o male medulloblastoma
Wit, Maassen, Gabreëls, and Thoonen (1993)	Phoneme discrimination test; imitation of short sentences; imitation of pitch changes and duration changes while sustained /a/; oromotor tasks, observation of speech organs; recorded sample of spontaneous speech	7 males, 4 females aged 6 to 11 y with spastic dysarthria due to cerebral palsy
Murdoch and Hudson-Tennent (1994)	Frenchay Dysarthria Assessment, Fisher–Logemann Test of Articulation Competence; connected speech sample from either reading passage or a picture description task. Speech samples rated using the 32 perceptual dimensions described by Darley et al. (1969a, 1969b,1975) and modified by FitzGerald, Murdoch, and Chenery (1987)	Nineteen children aged 4 to 16 y with posterior fossa tumors

continues

Table 14–1. *continued*

Authors	Perceptual Assessments Included in the Investigations	Subject Details
Wit, Maassen, Gabreëls, Thoonen, and de Swart (1994)	Recorded sample of spontaneous speech and imitated sentences rated for intelligibility, and severity of dysarthria	12 y/o male with spastic dysarthria following CHI, 13 y/o female with spastic dysarthria following CHI, 7 children aged between 10 to 16y with spastic dysarthria due to cerebral palsy
Stierwalt, Robin, Solomon, Weiss, Max, and Luschei (1994)	Repetition of 10 sentences from the Carrow Elicited Language Inventory (CELI) and a cartoon description task. Perceptual ratings on a 7-point scale of articulatory precision and overall speech defectiveness	Twenty-three children who had sustained a traumatic brain injury
Cahill, Murdoch, and Theodoros (2002)	Frenchay Dysarthria Assessment, Fisher–Logemann Test of Articulation Competence, Assessment of Intelligibility of Dysarthric Speech; connected speech sample from a reading passage rated using 32 dimensions outlined by FitzGerald, Murdoch, and Chenery (1987)	Twenty-four children who sustained a traumatic brain injury
Cornwell, Murdoch, Ward, and Kellie (2003)	Frenchay Dysarthria Assessment, Verbal Motor Production Assessment for Children, Children's Speech Intelligibility Measure, Assessment of Intelligibility of Dysarthric Speech, Fisher–Logemann Test of Articulation Competence; connected speech sample from a reading passage rated using 32 dimensions outlined by FitzGerald, Murdoch, and Chenery (1987)	Twenty-one children treated for a cerebellar tumor

The use of auditory perceptual assessments to characterize the different types of dysarthria and to identify the spectrum of deviant speech characteristics associated with each was pioneered by Darley, Aronson, and Brown (1969a, 1969b, 1975). It was from findings of their auditory-perceptual studies of dysarthria that the system of classification of dysarthria most frequently used in clinical settings was developed. Darley et al. (1969a, 1969b) assessed speech samples taken from 212 dysarthric speakers with a variety of neurologic conditions on 38 speech dimensions which fell into seven categories: pitch, loudness, voice quality (including both laryngeal and resonatory dysfunction), respiration, prosody, articulation, and two summary dimensions relating to intelligibility and bizarreness. A key component of their research was the application of the "equal-appearing intervals scale of severity" which utilized a seven-part scale of severity.

Rating scales have also been used by a number of other researchers to determine the deviant speech characteristics of various neurologic speech disorders. For example, a modification of Darley's original seven-point rating scale developed by FitzGerald, Murdoch, and Chenery (1987) has been used to investigate speech disorders in patients with multiple sclerosis, Parkinson disease, pseudobulbar palsy, stroke, and ataxic dysarthria among others. Another example of how symptoms of dysarthria are assessed and measured on a rating scale is the FDA (Enderby, 1983). The FDA is the only published diagnostic test of dysarthria and utilizes a nine-point rating scale presented vertically as a bar graph (Figure 14–1). As in the Darley et al. (1975) seven-point rating scale, a rating of 1 corresponds to more severe disruption with 9 representing normal

function. The 28 dimensions rated in the FDA are grouped under the headings of reflex, respiration, lips, jaw, palate, laryngeal, tongue, and intelligibility.

In addition to rating scales, other perceptual assessments used to investigate neurologic speech disorders include the application of intelligibility measures, phonetic transcription studies and articulation inventories. According to Duffy (2005), "intelligibility is the degree to which a listener understands the acoustic signal produced by a speaker" (p. 96). Quantifiable intelligibility measures are clinically important because they can monitor change during treatment and document functional level or adequacy of communication. Although most comprehensive perceptual assessments such as those developed by Darley et al. (1975) and FitzGerald et al. (1987) mentioned above, provide a single measure of overall intelligibility, this measure represents a global rating of the overall impact of the speech on the listener and considers how much effort is involved by the listener in understanding the speech sample. Thus, these global measures are based on the entire sample of speech, usually spoken paragraph such as the "Grandfather Passage" (Darley et al., 1975). A more valid method of estimating dysarthric speech intelligibility is to obtain a number of more detailed and comprehensive measures of intelligibility. The Assessment of Intelligibility of Dysarthric Speech (ASSIDS) (Yorkston & Beukelman, 1981) provides an index of severity of dysarthric speech by quantifying both single–word and sentence intelligibility as well as the speaking rate of individuals. It requires the client to read or imitate 50 randomly selected words and 22 randomly selected sentences that range in length from 5 to 15 words. A number of

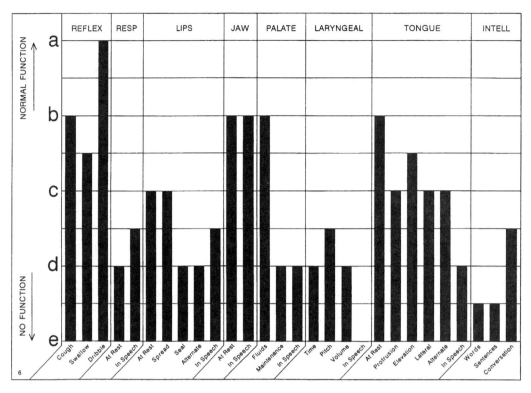

FIGURE 14–1. Example of Frenchay Dysarthria Assessment Profile of a dysarthric speaker.

dimensions are calculated in the ASSIDS, including: a percentage intelligibility for single words; a percentage intelligibility for sentences; a total speaking rate; a rate of intelligible speech expressed as intelligible words per minute; and a communication efficiency ratio.

Where necessary, such as for research purposes, more detailed perceptual analyses of neurological speech disorders can involve the use of phonetic transcription of selected speech stimuli (e.g., production of a series of single-syllable real and nonsense words) to provide detailed information about the pattern of articulatory deficits. In addition, articulatory inventories can be used to characterize the articulation abilities of individuals with dysarthria and apraxia of speech. For example, an articulation test such as the Fisher–Logemann Test

of Articulation Competence (Fisher & Logemann, 1971) can be used to provide an articulation profile and may be analyzed further to establish the presence of developmental features such as phonological processes.

The major advantages of perceptual assessment are those that have lead to its preferred use as a tool for characterizing and diagnosing dysarthric speech. Perceptual assessments are readily available and require only limited financial outlay. In addition all students of speech-language pathology are taught how to test for and identify perceptual symptoms. Finally, perceptual assessments are useful for monitoring the effects of treatment on speech intelligibility and the adequacy of communication.

Clinicians need to be aware, however, that there are a number of inherent inadequacies with perceptual assessment that may limit their use in determining treatment priorities. First, accurate, reliable perceptual judgments are often difficult to achieve as they can be influenced by a number of factors including the skill and experience of the clinician and the sensitivity of the assessment. In particular, raters must have extensive structured experience in listening prior to performing perceptual ratings.

Second, perceptual assessments are difficult to standardize both in relation to the patient being rated and the environment in which the speech samples are recorded. Patient variability over time and across different settings prevents maintenance of adequate intra- and inter-rater reliability. Furthermore, the symptoms may be present in certain conditions and not others. This variability is also found in the patients themselves such that characteristics of the person being rated (e.g., their age, premorbid medical history, and social history) may influence speech as well as the neurologic problem itself.

A third factor that limits reliance on perceptual assessments is that certain speech symptoms may influence the perception of others. This confound has been well reported in relation to the perception of resonatory disorders, articulatory deficits, and prosodic disturbances.

Probably the major concern of perceptual assessments, particularly as they relate to treatment planning, is that they have restricted power for determining which subsystems of the speech motor system are affected. In other words, perceptual assessments are unable to accurately identify the pathophysiologic basis of the speech disorder manifest in various types of dysarthria. It is possible that a number of different physiologic deficits can form the basis of perceptually

identified features, and that different patterns of interaction within a patient's overall symptom complex can result in a similar perceptual deviation (e.g., distorted consonants can result from reduced respiratory support for speech, from inadequate velopharyngeal functioning or from weak tongue musculature). When crucial decisions are required in relation to optimum therapeutic planning, an overreliance on only perceptual assessment may lead to a number of questionable therapy directions.

Acoustic Assessment

Acoustic analyses can be used in conjunction with perceptual assessments to provide a more complete understanding of the nature of the disturbance in dysarthric speech. In particular, acoustic assessment can highlight aspects of the speech signal that may be contributing to the perception of deviant speech production and can provide confirmatory support for perceptual judgments. For example, they may confirm the perception that speech is slow and demonstrate that the reduced rate of speech may be the result of increased interword durations and prolonged vowel and consonant production. As a further example, an acoustic analysis might be used to confirm the perception of imprecise consonant production and to show that such imprecision is the result of spirantization of consonants and reduction of consonant clusters. In addition to altered speech rate and consonant imprecision, other perceived deviant speech dimensions that can be confirmed by way of acoustic analysis include, among others, breathy voice, voice tremor, and reduced variability of pitch and loudness. Acoustic analysis is also useful for providing objective documentation of the effects of treatment and disease progression on speech production.

Acoustic measurements can be taken primarily from two different types of acoustic displays: oscillographic displays and spectrographic displays. An oscillographic display is a two-dimensional waveform display of amplitude (on the *y*-axis) as a function of time (*x*-axis). Oscillographic displays are easy to generate and can provide information on a variety of acoustic parameters such as segment duration (e.g., vowel duration, word duration, etc.), amplitude, fundamental frequency, and the presence of some acoustic cues of articulatory adequacy such as voice onset time, spirantization, and voiced-voiceless distinctions. Measurements from oscillographic displays can be made either manually or, alternatively, by using computer controlled acoustic analysis software. Some of the commonly used computerized systems and dedicated devices for acoustic speech analysis include: C Speech; CSL (Computerized Speech Lab); CSRE (Canadian Speech Research Environment); ILS-PC (Interactive Laboratory System); and MSL (Micro Speech Lab).

In contrast to the two-dimensional oscillographic display, a spectrographic display is actually a three-dimensional display, of both frequency and amplitude as a function of time, where time is on the x-axis and frequency is displayed on the y-axis. There are two different types of spectrographic displays: wideband displays (also called broadband displays) and narrowband displays. Wideband spectrographic displays are used to determine accurate temporal measurements whereas narrowband spectrograms are useful for making measurements of fundamental frequency and the prosodic aspects of speech.

Although there is no "standard" set of parameters included in all acoustic analyses, there are, however, a number of different acoustic measures which can provide important information about the acoustic features of dysarthric speech. These parameters can be loosely arranged into groups of measures including: fundamental frequency measures, amplitude measures, perturbation measures, noise-related measures, formant measures, temporal measures, measures of articulatory capability, and evaluations of manner of voicing.

Physiologic Assessment

Although perceptual evaluations contribute valuable information to the process of diagnosing and interpreting neurologic speech disorders, instrumental observation and measurement of speech and its physiologic correlates offer significant advantages over unaided perceptual judgments. By including the use of instrumental procedures in the process of diagnosing speech disorders, clinicians are able to extend their senses and objectify their perceptual observations. In particular, instrumentation has given the clinician the ability to determine the contributions of malfunctions in the various components of the speech production mechanism to the production of disordered speech. Indeed, modern instrumentation enables the clinician to assess and obtain information about the integrity and functional status of the muscle groups at each stage of the speech production process from respiration through to articulation. It is not surprising, therefore, that clinicians are beginning to appreciate the considerable advantages of instrumental analysis which provides quantitative, objective data on a wide range of different speech parameters far beyond the scope of an auditory-based impressionistic judgment. Instrumental assessment can enhance the abilities of the clinician in all stages of clinical management, including:

■ increasing the precision of diagnosis through more valid specification of abnormal functions that require modification.
■ the provision of positive identification and documentation of therapeutic efficacy.
■ the expansion of options of therapy modalities, including the use of instrumentation in a biofeedback modality.

To be of value in determining treatment priorities, instrumental assessment should be comprehensive, covering as many components of the speech production mechanism as possible. A wide variety of different types of physiologic instrumentation have been described in the literature for use in the assessment of the functioning of the various components of the speech production apparatus. Examples of physiologic instruments used to assess children with acquired dysarthria are presented in Table 14–2. Each of these instruments has been designed to provide information on a specific aspect of speech production including muscular activity, structural movements, airflows, and air pressures generated in various parts of the speech mechanism. The features of the most commonly used physiologic instruments used to assess the functioning of the respiratory system, larynx, velopharynx (soft palate), and articulators (e.g., lips, tongue, etc.) are briefly outlined below.

Instrumental Assessment of Speech Breathing. The respiratory system provides the basic energy source for all speech and voice production, regulating such important parameters as speech and voice intensity (loudness), pitch, linguistic stress, and the division of speech into units (e.g., phrases). Physiologic instruments used in the assessment of speech breathing can be divided into two major types: those that directly measure various lung volumes, capacities and airflows (e.g., spirometers) and those that indirectly measure respiratory function by monitoring movements of the chest wall, the so-called kinematic assessments (e.g., mercury strain gauges, magnetometers, respiratory inductance plethysmographs, and strain-gauge belt pneumographs).

Spirometers are specifically designed for the evaluation of respiratory volumes. The basic principle of a spirometer is to measure and record the volumes of air blown into either a tube or a fitted face mask, which is attached to the machine (Figure 14–2). By using this type of assessment, the investigator can obtain a number of valuable respiratory/airflow measures, including vital capacity, forced expiratory volume, functional residual capacity, inspiratory capacity, expiratory and inspiratory reserve volumes, as well as volume/flow relationships and tidal volume and respiration rate.

Kinematic devices allow the clinician to infer the airflow volume changes during respiration from rib cage and abdominal displacements. In that they do not require the need for restrictive mouth pieces and nose clips that can interrupt natural speech production and respiratory patterns, the kinematic method allows for more accurate measurements of the breath support during speech production. The rib cage and diaphragm-abdomen displace volume as they move and, resultingly, their combined volume displacements equal that of the lungs. In essence, therefore, the kinematic analysis involves the simultaneous but independent recording of changes in the circumference of the rib cage and abdomen.

Table 14–2. Examples of Physiologic Assessment of Children with Dysarthria

Authors	Physiologic Instrumentation	Parameters Investigated	Subjects Investigated
Hardcastle, Morgan-Barry, and Clark (1987)	Electropalatography	Details of tongue contacts with the hard palate during the repetition of target word lists	Four articulation disordered children, aged between 7 and 9 y/o, 2 of whom were diagnosed as dysarthric
Robin and Eliason (1991)	Visipitch (Kay Elemetrics)	Fundamental frequency, range of fundamental frequency, vocal tremor	Seven children aged between 5 to 16 y/o with von Recklinghausen's disease
Murdoch and Hudson-Tennent (1993)	Kinematic analysis of speech breathing using a strain-gauge belt pneumograph system	Chest wall movements during relaxed breathing, deep breathing, sustained vowel, syllable repetition and reading tasks	Five children aged between 7 to 16 y/o following treatment for posterior fossa tumor
	Spirometric assessment using Mijnhardt Vicatest-P1 Spirometer	Vital capacities and forced expiratory volumes	
Wit, Maassen, Gabreëls, and Thoonen (1993)	Acoustic analysis using the "Speech Lab" computer software program (Reetz, 1989)	Maximum performance tasks: maximum duration of sound prolongation, fundamental frequency range, maximum repetition rate of syllables, and temporal variability of syllable production	Seven males and 4 females aged between 6 to 11 y/o with spastic dysarthria due to cerebral palsy
Wit, Maassen, Gabreëls, Thoonen, and de Swart (1994)	Acoustic analyses using the "Speech Lab" computer software program (Reetz, 1989) and the "Accuracy" computer program	Maximum performance tasks: maximum duration of sound prolongation, fundamental frequency range, maximum repetition rate of syllables, and temporal variability of syllable production	Twelve y/o male with spastic dysarthria following closed-head injury (CHI), 13 y/o female with spastic dysarthria following CHI, 7 children aged between 10 to 16 y/o with spastic dysarthria due to cerebral palsy

Authors	Physiologic Instrumentation	Parameters Investigated	Subjects Investigated
Stierwalt, Robin, Solomon, Weiss, Max, and Luschei (1994)	Iowa Oral Performance Instrument (IOPI) (Robin, Somodi, and Luschei, 1991)	Maximum tongue strength and endurance measures	Twenty three children who had sustained a traumatic brain injury
Cahill, Murdoch, and Theodoros (2005)	Tongue and lip pressure transducers	Maximum tongue and lip strength and endurance measures	Twenty-four children who had sustained a traumatic brain injury
Cornwell, Murdoch, and Ward (2005)	Spirometer and Respitrace system	Lung volumes and capacities plus respiratory kinematics	Six children treated for midline cerebellar tumor
	Aerophone II and electroglottography	Laryngeal airflows, subglottal pressure, fundamental frequency, duty cycle	
	Nasometer	Nasalance scores	
	Tongue and lip pressure transducers	Maximum tongue and lip strength and endurance measures	

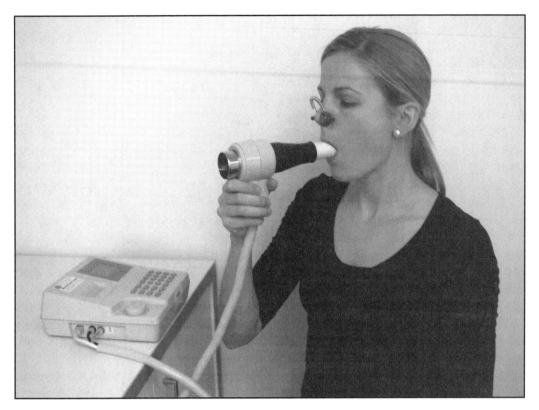

FIGURE 14–2. Respiratory spirometer.

Investigations of speech breathing using kinematic assessments have predominately used four main types of kinematic instrumentation. These include magnetometers (e.g., Solomon & Hixon, 1993); strain-gauge belt pneumograph systems (e.g., Manifold & Murdoch, 1993); mercury strain gauges (e.g., Cavallo & Baken, 1985); and respiratory inductance plethysmography (available commercially as the "Respitrace" system) (e.g., Sperry & Klich, 1992). Of these techniques, the Respitrace system is most commonly available in clinical settings. This latter system senses movements of the chest wall via the changes in electrical inductance of a zigzag of wire attached to elastic bands positioned around the rib cage and abdominal regions (Figure 14–3). Oscillators positioned in the center of the chest wall anteriorly produce a frequency-modulated signal that passes through the wires of the chest bands, the frequency of which is related to the circumference of the chest wall. Changes in the size of the chest wall circumference alter the shape and, therefore, conductance of the zigzag wires of the straps, and resultingly change the signal.

One other important indicator of respiratory function for speech production is the ability of the subject to generate subglottal air pressure during speech. Subglottal air pressure is estimated using an Aerophone II (Kay Elemetrics) air-flow measurement system (Figure 14–4). The Aerophone II consists of hand-held transducer module together with a powerful data acquisition and processing

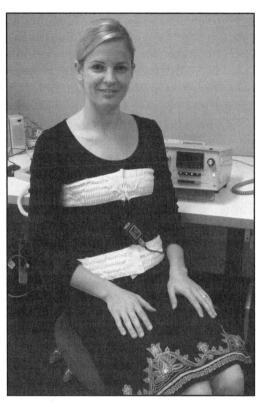

FIGURE 14–3. Respitrace system for kinematic assessment of speech breathing.

software program. The transducer module consists of miniaturized transducers capable of recording airflow, air pressure, and acoustic signals during speech. A face mask through which a thin flexible tube of silicon rubber is inserted to record intraoral pressure is attached to the hand-held transducer module. To estimate subglottal pressure the subject is asked to repeat /ipipipi/ into the face mask, with the rubber tube located in the oral cavity, for several seconds. The point of maximum intraoral pressure during the pronunciation of the voiceless stop /p/ is calculated automatically over six repetitions and used as the estimate of subglottal air pressure.

Instrumental Assessment of Laryngeal Function. Physiologic evaluation of laryngeal function is carried out using both direct and indirect techniques. Endoscopy using a rigid endoscope or nasendoscopy using a flexible fiberscope both allow for direct observation of

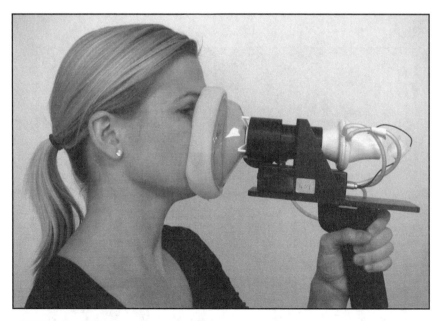

FIGURE 14–4. Aerophone II airflow measurement system.

vocal fold movement. Both systems are telescopic-type devices that illuminate the laryngeal area and allow visual inspection of the laryngeal region. The rigid endoscope is inserted through the mouth into the region of the oropharynx, allowing direct observation of the vocal folds during phonation of sustained vowels. In comparison, the flexible fiberscope is inserted through the nasal cavity and then passed down through the pharyngeal area until the tip of the scope is positioned at approximately the level of the epiglottis to allow an unobstructed view of the vocal folds. As the oral cavity is not obstructed using the nasendoscopic technique, visual record of laryngeal function can be obtained during normal speech production. Both the endoscope and nasoendoscope are connected to a video monitoring and recording system, which allows the visual image of the vocal folds to be recorded for later viewing and analysis. Videostroboscopy combines the use of a strobe light source in conjunction with the videoendoscopic procedures outlined above. Using the stroboscopic technique, the movements of the vocal folds during speech production can be "slowed" or "stopped" through the optical illusion of stroboscopy making identification of vocal fold dysfunction much more easy.

The indirect methods of evaluating physiological functioning of the larynx include electroglottography (electrolaryngography) and aerodynamic examination. Electroglottography is an electrical impedance method of estimating vocal fold contact during phonation that is designed to allow investigation of laryngeal microfunction (cycle-by-cycle periodicity and contact). The electroglottographic assessment is conducted using a Fourcin laryngograph interfaced with a Waveform Display System (Kay Elemetrics Model 6091) (Figure 14–5). The system records the degree of vocal fold contact and the vocal fold vibratory patterns during phonation, these features being displayed in the form of an Lx waveform. The Waveform Display System allows for acquisition and real-time viewing of the Lx waveform on the

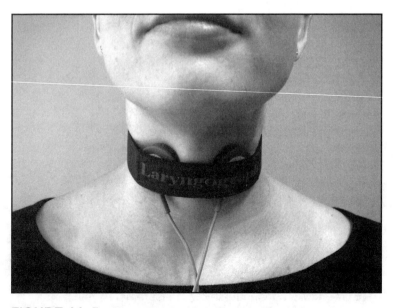

FIGURE 14–5. Client fitted with a Fourcin laryngograph.

computer monitor as well as storage and analysis of segments of the waveform. Although some caution must be used in interpreting electroglottographic results, a number of authors have acknowledged that this procedure provides a useful estimate of vocal fold contact during the glottal cycle and gives some insight into the regulation, maintenance, and quality of phonation.

Aerodynamic measures allow examination of the macrofunctions of the larynx such as laryngeal airflow, glottal pressures and glottal resistance. Estimates of these parameters are obtained by way of an Aerophone II Airflow Measurement System (see Instrumental Assessment of Speech Breathing above).

Instrumental Assessment of Velopharyngeal Function (Soft Palate). Two contemporary instruments for assessing velopharyngeal function include an accelerometric procedure and the Nasometer. The accelerometric procedure involves the use of two miniature accelerometers to detect nasal and throat vibrations during speech. One miniature accelerometer is attached to the upper side of the nose over the lateral nasal cartilage just in front of the nasal bone, while the other is attached to the side of the neck over the lamina of the thyroid cartilage. The output signals from each accelerometer are amplified by a DC amplifier and the amplified signals are then relayed to a computerized physiologic data acquisition system. The system yields an index of oral/nasal coupling during production of a range of nasal and nonnasal sounds, words, and sentences.

Another instrument available for assessment of nasality is the Nasometer (Kay Elemetrics) (Figure 14–6). The Nasometer is a computer-assisted instrument that provides a measure of nasality derived from the ratio of acoustic energy output from the nasal and oral cavities during speech. Acoustic energy is detected by two directional microphones (one placed in front of the nares and the other in front of the mouth) separated by a sound separator plate. The instrument yields a "nasalance" score made up of a ratio of nasal to oral plus nasal acoustic energy calculated as a percentage.

Instrumental Assessment of Articulatory Function. The term "articulators" is used to represent collectively the muscle groups of the lips, tongue, and jaw. Although these structures are often grouped together due to their common influence over speech production at the articulatory stage, each one functions independently and contributes differently to speech production. Consequently, a variety of instrumental techniques have been developed to examine the degree of compression force exerted by each articulator during speech and nonspeech tasks, as well as to investigate force control properties, rate of individual articulatory movements, endurance capabilities of the individual articulators, and the movement patterns during speech production of each separate aspect of the articulatory system.

Of the various types of instrumentation used to assess the articulators, strain gauge transducers, used to record articulator movement and force generating capacities, have been the most frequently used. Because of their high levels of sensitivity, strain gauge transducers are especially suited to detecting the subtle changes in movement that occur in speech production. In addition, they are relatively inexpensive, noninvasive, provide an immediate voltage analogue of movement, and can be adapted to assess lip, tongue, and jaw function during both speech and nonspeech tasks. An example of a strain

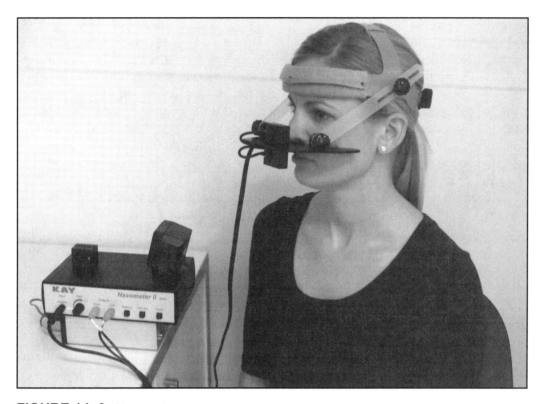

FIGURE 14–6. Nasometer.

gauge system for estimating lip strength is shown in Figure 14–7.

In addition to strain gauge transducers, pressure or force transducers can also provide valuable information regarding the functioning of the articulatory system. For example, a miniaturized pressure transducer is frequently used to assess lip function. Because of its small size the transducer is capable of being placed between the lips to generate interlabial pressure measurements during speech production without interfering with normal articulatory movements. The transducer is interfaced with a dedicated software package designed to allow for investigations of combine upper and lower lip pressures, pressure control for maximum and submaximum pressure levels, endurance, and speech pressures during production of bilabial sounds.

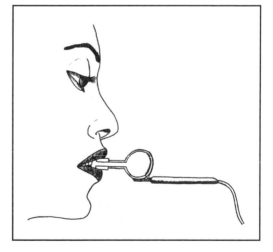

FIGURE 14–7. Example of strain gauge system for measuring lip strength.

An equivalent commercially available instrument for estimating tongue strength and endurance is the Iowa Oral Performance Instrument (IOPI), which consists of an air-filled rubber bulb attached to a pressure transducer (Figure 14–8). For testing, the bulb is placed in the mouth and the subject is instructed to squeeze the bulb against the roof of the mouth with the tongue. When the bulb is squeezed by the tongue, the amount of pressure is displayed on a digital readout.

Electromyography (EMG) is another technique that has commonly been used (primarily by researchers rather than clinicians) to examine articulator function. Using this technique, the momentary changes in electrical activity that occur when a muscle is contracting are recorded by using various types of electrodes (e.g., surface, needle or hook-wire) placed either overlying (surface electrodes) or within (e.g., hook-wire electrodes and needle electrodes) the

muscle. The data obtained from EMG assessment has proven useful for investigating the neurophysiologic bases of various disorders, such as identifying the presence of increased muscle tone (hypertonicity) or abnormal variations in the activation or inhibition of muscle activity. In addition, EMG has been used to record muscle activity simultaneously with the speech movement patterns of these same muscles, in order to examine the motor control of the articulators.

Electropalatography is another technique for examining tongue function, which provides the clinician with information on the location and timing of tongue contacts with the palate during speech. In this technique, the client wears an acrylic palate with an array of contact sensors implanted on the surface (Figures 14–9A and 14–9B).

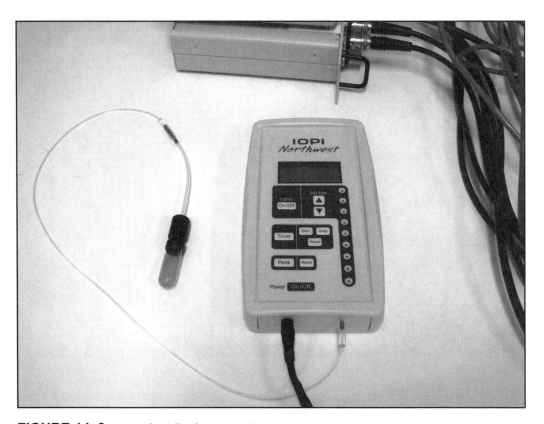

FIGURE 14–8. Iowa Oral Performance Instrument.

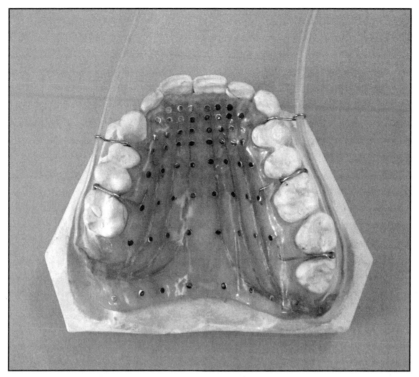

A

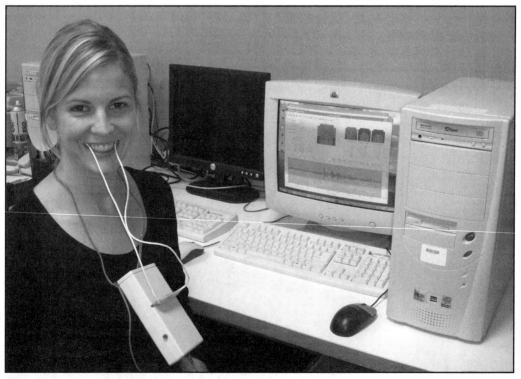

B

FIGURE 14–9. **A.** Acrylic electropalatography palate with embedded touch sensors. **B.** Client fitted with an electropalatography palate.

When contact occurs between the tongue and any of the electrodes, a signal is conducted via lead-out wires to an external processing unit, which then displays the patterns of contact on a computer screen (Figure 14–10).

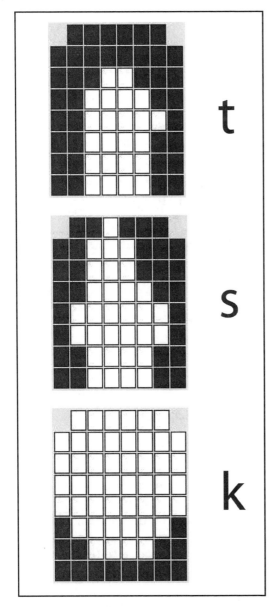

FIGURE 14–10. Electropalatographic contact pattern representing tongue contact with the palate. Adapted from McLeod, S., & Singh, S. (2008). *Speech Sounds*. San Diego, CA: Plural Publishing.

In recent years the development and introduction of a technique called electromagnetic articulography (EMA) has provided a safe, noninvasive assessment tool with which the dynamic aspects of articulatory dysfunction in various neurologic speech disorders may be investigated. Importantly, the EMA technique does not require the use of ionizing radiation. Rather the EMA system tracks articulatory movements during speech using weak alternating electromagnetic fields. Transmitter coils, housed in a plastic cube and positioned around the head, generate alternating magnetic fields at different frequencies, which in turn induce alternating signals in small receiver coils temporarily glued to the tongue, upper and lower lip, and jaw (Figure 14–11). The position of the receiver coils in relation to the transmitter coils is sampled over time and plotted on a computer, providing a visual representation of articulator movements in real time. From these data, quantitative kinematic parameters can be derived including the velocity, acceleration, distance, and duration of movements of the lips, tongue, and jaw during speech production. The most recently introduced EMA system, the AG500 is capable of tracking articulatory movements in three dimensions.

Evaluating the movements of the tongue is more difficult than assessing lip or jaw movement primarily because of the fact that the tongue functions within the confines of the mouth. In addition to the EMA technique described above, imaging techniques such as cineradiography and ultrasound have proved useful for examining the complex patterns of tongue movement during speech. Cineradiography is a high-speed x-ray motion picture technique which records the lateral view of the mouth, nose, and

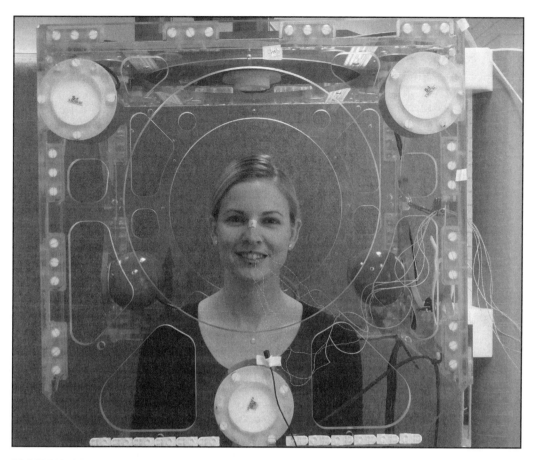

FIGURE 14–11. AG500 Electromagnetic articulograph.

pharynx. Using this technique, it is possible to view the articulatory structures during speech in order to identify gross deviations of articulatory movement such as reduced mobility of the tongue or soft palate. Unfortunately, due to its reliance on potentially harmful x-rays, cineradiography has fallen out of favor and has little potential for use as a routine clinical tool, especially for child cases. In contrast, ultrasonography involves the transmission of high-frequency sound waves through the body's tissues. Consequently, ultrasound is considered harmless and noninvasive, allowing tongue movement to be investigated for longer periods without harm or discomfort to the client. Unlike other imaging techniques, ultrasound reveals not only the surface displacement but also changes in soft tissue organization within the tongue in both the sagittal and coronal planes and can be used to record lingual movements during production of vowels and most consonants.

Limitations with ultrasound include an inability to assess tongue tip movements and to view the movements of other structures (e.g., jaw, lips, etc.) besides the tongue using this technique. In addition, specialist training and some experience in viewing ultrasound scans is required in order to interpret the information provided by these scans accurately. Furthermore, the need to place the ultrasound source below the lower jaw directly under the floor of the mouth may restrict natural jaw movement during speech. Despite these limitations, however, ultrasound has the potential to be a useful clinical tool for client evaluation.

Summary: Physiologic Assessment. In summary, although instrumentation has opened a whole new range of assessment techniques, physiologic data should be integrated with data from other appraisal procedures (i.e., combined information from perceptual, physiologic, and acoustic information) to ensure that an accurate diagnosis is made and that the subsequent remediation techniques are appropriate. In particular, the limitations of each of the instrumental procedures need to be kept in mind when making clinical decisions based on their findings. It also must be remembered that, despite the wide variety of objective instrumental measures available for documenting the physiology of speech production, to date, the clinical application of these techniques has been limited. Increasing the use of instrumentation in the clinical setting, for the purposes of both assessment and treatment, will require the implementation of training programs for the clinicians as well as an increase in clinical research projects designed to demonstrate the clinical utility of instrumental techniques and to validate the role of instrumentation in the management of neurological speech disorders.

Assessment of Pragmatic Speech Skills

The most important pragmatic skills to assess in a child with a motor speech disorder are the paralinguistic features and the nonverbal behaviors that the child uses in a communicative act. Is the child able to convey his or her attitudes or emotions by changes in intonation, pitch, stress, or emphasis? Can he or she alter the meaning of an utterance by using suprasegmental devices to signal the change rather than by altering the form? Are the child's facial expressions appropriate to the situations or is his or her face "masklike" so that the listener is unable to read the nonverbal cues? Is pause time too great leaving the dialogue partner wondering whether the listener is ignoring them, does not know the answer or is thinking? With some children, even though the formal assessment reveals near-normal motor speech skills, effective communication is hampered by their problems with some paralinguistic and nonverbal behaviors.

For example, Julia, a 12-year-old girl, who had been injured in a motor vehicle accident, was shown to have made a good recovery when a dysarthric assessment was administered 12 months after the injury. However, pragmatic problems were evident in conversation. Her volume was soft, articulation imprecise, although she had demonstrated good intelligibility with single words and sentences in the formal testing situation, and her face lacked mobility so that it was hard to tell what she might be thinking.

Assessment of Acquired Apraxia of Speech in Childhood

Although, as indicated above, the assessment for apraxia of speech may follow similar parameters to acquired dysarthria, to enable differential diagnosis of acquired apraxia of speech particular attention needs to be paid to the following:

■ an observable difference between involuntary and voluntary movement.

- the ability of the child to sequence sounds (e.g., /p/, /t/, and /p/, /t/, /k/).
- his or her ability to repeat the sequence of sounds several times.
- his or her ability to repeat minimal pairs using manner and place contrasts (e.g., bow, toe and pea, bee).
- his or her ability to articulate words of increasing complexity (e.g., butter, topcoat, crocodile, kangaroo).

Apraxia may be present when:

- involuntary movement of the articulators appears superior to volitional movement.
- inconsistent errors are demonstrated during repetitive oral movements and speech production of phonemes, words, and phrases.
- deterioration in performance is observed as the word length increases.
- automatic speech is more intelligible than propositional speech.
- searching behaviors, similar to those observed in adults with acquired apraxia, are present in the child's speech.
- the child's facial expression seems to suggest that he or she is puzzled about how to use his or her muscles of articulation to make the required sound.
- some alteration in prosody is observed (e.g., rate of speech).

Inconsistent errors are frequently heard in children who are still developing their phonological system so differential diagnosis between normal phonological processes (e.g., assimilation, final consonant deletion, etc.) and the inconsistent errors (e.g., phonemic anticipatory errors, transpositions, voicing errors, omissions) heard in the speech of an apraxic child is important when assessing children with acquired motor speech disorders. A knowledge of the child's speech development before his or her brain lesion is necessary to make this clinical judgment.

Treatment of Acquired Motor Speech Disorders in Childhood

As with assessment, current treatment methods for dysarthria in children, particularly for those with acquired dysarthria largely are modifications of adult methods. The potential problems of this approach have been pointed out earlier; however, the adult treatment methods do provide a starting point from which to proceed in planning and implementing treatment. The present chapter focuses primarily on the strategies currently being used for the treatment of acquired dysarthria in adults, with special reference to their potential use with children with acquired motor speech disorders. A range of treatment options exist in the management of dysarthria and apraxia of speech. However, the overall goal in treatment programs for individuals with neurogenic speech disorders is to improve intelligibility by enhancing physiological support for speech and by teaching compensatory speech behaviors. Occasionally, the speech-language pathologist may also be required to work in collaboration with medical professionals and specialists in order to explore surgical or prosthetic approaches to management.

Regardless of the best applicable treatment technique, the following five principles are considered practical strategies that promote greater success in the treatment of neurogenic motor speech disorders in both adult and child populations (Darley et al., 1975; Murdoch et al., 1990).

1. Compensatory strategies—Assisting the patient to utilize their remaining strengths and potential is an important strategy. Children in particular often have more of a tendency to compensate due to their ongoing development, as speech patterns prior to an acquired disturbance such as brain injury tend to be less well established than in adults.
2. Purposeful activity—As the individual becomes aware of how their articulators work and interact, they are able to more effectively learn a range of strategies designed to increase the intelligibility of their speech. What was once an automatic response now needs to be learned as a purposeful behavior.
3. Early treatment—It is essential to begin rehabilitation early. The sooner the patient becomes aware of how their speech system works, the greater the chance that effective self-monitoring skills are established.
4. Monitoring—Self-monitoring of behaviors and behavioral change is a key strategy in effectively treating neurogenic speech deficits in adults and children and generalizing. Children may find this skill more difficult to learn, but may be taught as a set strategy with steps that can be followed in contextual situations.
5. Motivation—This ingredient will ensure much higher success and better outcomes in treating the individual's speech deficit and in the reduction of unintelligibility. Children need to understand the importance of the therapy techniques they are learning and wish to put them into practice if therapy is to succeed.

A pragmatic approach, where the child can learn the consequences of both poor and intelligible communication, may reinforce the child's desire to communicate effectively. Many children make an excellent recovery with only mild difficulties with their muscles of articulation, yet subtle problems remain causing their speech to sound imprecise and monotonous. If the child does not have the motivation to monitor his or her speech, then intelligibility may remain a problem in many situations.

Treatment in the Acute Stage

During the acute stages of acquired dysarthria, when a child's symptoms are usually at their most severe, treatment strategies generally are focused on feeding and graded oral and facial stimulation (Murdoch et al., 1990). Treatment of communication skills may begin when a child is neurologically and cognitively stable.

Mutism is frequently reported in the first stages of recovery after brain trauma, (Catsman-Berrevoets et al., 1992; Jordan & Murdoch, 1990; Murdoch & Hudson-Tennent, 1994). During this phase of recovery, it is most important to establish a form of communication aside from verbal output until speech becomes more functional. This may include signals or gesture, or more formal signing to be introduced as one of the earliest treatment goals. All gestures and attempts at communication by the patient should be encouraged. Symbol systems such as Compic, the Picture Exchange Communication System (PECS), or self-made photograph communication boards may be an appropriate method of communication, particularly if physical abilities are also restricted and limit the use of sign. The communication system selected, however, should rely on the patient's cognitive level, receptive language skills, perceptual and motor abilities, and their level of desire to interact and communicate.

In some cases, the use of an augmentative communication system may facilitate the return of verbal communication. Some patients however, may have more severe motor involvement or apraxia of phonation, in which recovery may either occur spontaneously or require specific treatment. Many of these individuals, particularly children, may vocalize spontaneously in emotional situations (laughing, etc.), in play settings, or in other active therapy sessions. The speech-language clinician may therefore find it beneficial to be present and participate in team therapy sessions in order to shape and build on these vocalizations. Patients with severe involvement and poorer prognosis for recovery may require a more advanced communication device such as a voice output device or a computer-based system with context-based control options.

After this initial period of mutism the child often presents with severe dysarthria (Catsman-Berrevoets et al., 1992; Murdoch & Hudson-Tennent, 1994). At this time treatment strategies need to address the need for improving functional communication and overall intelligibility. Various treatment techniques have been designed to remediate the different functional components of the speech mechanism (i.e., diaphragm, abdomen, rib cage, larynx, velopharynx, tongue, lips, and jaw) (see below). For patients with speech impairments, at several different levels of the speech production apparatus, as identified through perceptual and physiologic assessment,

the treatment framework to be employed must be established and the treatment goals prioritized within it.

Two treatment frameworks that may be considered are:

(a) Hierarchical where each impairment is treated in order of priority.
(b) Simultaneous where specific speech impairments that are interdependent are treated together.

In many cases it is recommended that the clients should receive a treatment program based on a combination of these methods. Underlying subsystem impairments should be prioritized and treated individually and where appropriate less system specific impairments can be treated simultaneously. The bases of prioritization for the establishment of the treatment hierarchy are as follows:

(a) Severity
(b) Impact on intelligibility
(c) The effect of impairments in a subsystem on other parts of the speech mechanism.

Once the treatment hierarchy has been established the therapeutic approach needs to be determined to aid in selection of specific treatment techniques. There are a number of approaches available to the speech-language pathologist for treating severe dysarthria in children. These include:

■ Behavioral approach—The focus of this approach is to teach patients new skills or compensatory techniques that utilize traditional techniques that involve the presentation of stimulus and patient response. Due to the portability, flexibility, and low-cost nature of this approach, it is often the technique most widely used in clinical situations.

■ Biofeedback/instrumental approach —The use of biofeedback or instrumentation is based on the principle that effective motor speech learning is dependent on the patient receiving immediate and specific feedback regarding their performance across each component of the speech production mechanism. Therefore, instruments are used to determine the exact level of functioning of the tongue, lip, and jaw, and to ascertain the presence and nature of facial weakness, respiratory dysfunction, velopharyngeal incompetence, and prosodic impairment. The information is then presented in a way that facilitates the patient's control of the variable, in turn, providing a large range of possible treatment strategies.

■ Surgical and prosthetic approaches —As an alternative to traditional or biofeedback therapy techniques, surgical procedures or prosthetic involvement may be used in the management of severe cases of dysarthria. Techniques such as amplification devices, palatal lifts, or bite blocks may be used to assist the patient to compensate for reduced or impaired functioning of a specific aspect of the speech mechanism, where other approaches are not feasible. Surgical procedures such as Teflon injections, laser surgery, and pharyngeal flap surgery are often utilized in patients who have severe impairments that are unresponsive to other therapeutic approaches.

■ Pragmatic approach—Rather than focusing on improving the actual physiologic aspects of the speech mechanism, this approach aims to assist the patient in providing strategies that maximize communication within the context of daily life situations. Such methods may include altering the communicative environment (e.g., avoiding communication in dark or noisy situations, reducing distance between communicative partner, etc.), modifying utterance/sentence length, teaching repair strategies, and attention and topic orientation.

In many cases, a combined traditional and physiologic approach seems to be indicated. With regard to application of these approaches to children of the physiologic approaches documented in the literature (Netsell & Rosenbek, 1986), visual biofeedback would seem to be the most relevant. It provides real-time information regarding the effectiveness of the patient's attempt at a task, an excellent reward system to motivate the subject, and is often simple enough for children to understand and perform on their own (Michi, Yamashita, Imai, Suzuki, & Yoshida, 1993; Netsell & Daniel, 1979).

Traditional techniques also could be used including oromotor exercises with and without resistance, contrastive stress drills, relaxation, and improved posture for respiration (Crary, 1993; Netsell & Rosenbek, 1986; Newman, Creaghead, & Secord, 1985; Rosenbek & LaPointe, 1985).

One approach which seems to have specific relevance to the remediation of the dysarthria of childhood is the PROMPT System (Prompts for Restructuring Oral Muscular Phonetic Targets) devised by Hayden (1995). The system is based on neurologic, anatomic, and motor theory principles. Using the PROMPT System the phonemic system is translated directly to the neuromuscular movements required for articulatory sequences. The PROMPT System, uses a tactile basis for guiding the articulatory mechanism and has developed multidimensional prompts that may signal various phonemic components such as place, manner, muscle groups, and tension of muscle groups, closure, timing, and coarticulators influences during transitive movement, stress, and prosodic changes (Hayden & Square, 1994). Hayden has used the system with both children and adults in group and individual settings. She has targeted individuals with disorders including those of phonology, developmental delay, dysarthria, apraxia, and others. This system coupled with her Motor Speech Treatment Hierarchy (Hayden & Square, 1994) provide a useful additional approach to the assessment and intervention for children with motor speech disorders complementing those mentioned previously.

The most important consideration throughout the whole process of designing the treatment hierarchy, establishing the therapeutic approach and selecting therapy techniques is the need to provide the child with an effective functional communication system. It therefore is important to integrate the speech treatment with the treatment of other communication skills such as language and to use augmentative and alternative communication strategies if necessary.

Treatment of Acquired Dysarthria in Childhood

Specific Treatment Methods

Inherent within the main approaches to the management of dysarthria are treatment techniques that have been specifi-

cally designed to target the neurologically impaired respiratory, laryngeal, velopharyngeal, and articulatory subsystems of the speech production mechanism. In addition, a variety of techniques have been developed to address the abnormal prosodic features of dysarthric speech.

Treatment of Speech Breathing Disorders. Impaired respiratory function may be the result of a number of different factors, including: a limited or reduced respiratory supply; inadequate inspiratory control, which can limit the client's ability to produce the pattern of fast inhalations used during speech breathing; inadequate expiratory control, which can lead to the inability to sustain sufficient subglottal pressures for phonation; and the presence of incoordination of the muscles involved in respiration. Considering that one or more of these features may be present in any one client, comprehensive assessment of the respiratory system prior to intervention is crucial to ensure that the most appropriate treatment strategies are applied in each case. The remediation of respiratory deficits in individuals with dysarthria usually involves a combination of strategies to improve physiologic support and guide compensatory behaviors that will enable optimal available respiratory support for speech. A primary and commonly used behavioral strategy for this physiologic component of the speech mechanism consists of training the client to maintain adequate posture for respiration. Instrumental techniques range from simple homemade devices to complex instrumentation to provide biofeedback of respiratory function, and are extremely useful for promoting controlled exhalation. For example, using a straw to blow bubbles in a glass of water, or using a U-shaped manometer where a client blows into one end of plastic tubing to maintain a consistent water level. In those clients with more severe respiratory impairment, prosthetic approaches such as short periods of supporting the abdominal muscle with an elastic bandage have been trialed and appear to provide the client more control over expiratory breath.

Treatment of Phonatory Disorders. Techniques addressing disturbances to laryngeal function and phonation in individuals with dysarthria will vary depending on the underlying neuromuscular issue and the actual motor speech disorder. Treatment of this collection of phonation disorders in dysarthria often incorporates mostly behavioral and instrumental techniques with possible use of prosthetic compensatory devices. Surgical intervention may be required in such cases to maximize the effectiveness of the other treatment approaches. However, it is important to identify the underlying pathophysiology and the impact of other speech subsystems on phonatory disturbances that exist prior to treatment planning.

Excessive vocal fold adduction, or hyperadduction, produces varying degrees of low-pitched, strained-strangled, harsh vocal quality that ranges from a being unable to phonate at all to a more mild form of hyperadduction that presents as pitch breaks, mild vocal strain, and harshness. Intervention involves overall body and specific head and neck relaxation, and exercises to decrease tension in the vocal folds. These include the chewing method, the yawn-sigh approach, and gentle voice onsets.

Hypoadduction of the vocal folds involves inadequate adduction of the vocal folds for phonation and presents as increased airflow through the glottis

due to a decrease in laryngeal resistance, reduced loudness level, breathiness, hoarseness, and short phonation time. Treatment techniques to facilitate adduction of the vocal folds including pushing, pulling and lifting exercises performed together with phonation, hard glottal attack, and postural adjustment of the head such as turning the head to the affected side to decrease distance between the vocal folds. The Lee Silverman Voice Treatment (LSVT) (Ramig, Bonitati, Lemke, & Horii, 1994) program recently has been employed to increase phonatory effect by taking deeper breaths and carrying out more effortful vocal fold adduction.

Other phonation disorders that may present in dysarthric patients include phonatory instability and phonatory incoordination. Treatment for phonatory instability associated with dysarthria is essentially aimed at achieving steadiness and clarity of phonation, with techniques primarily centered on breath control exercises. Phonatory incoordination can refer to timing issues of respiration, laryngeal production, and/or articulation, as well as prosody disturbances. Delays in voice onset and offset can be affected by a failure to synchronize phonation with exhalation. The presence of phonatory incoordination will also significantly affect prosody of speech due to reduced ability to control speech parameters such as pressure, vocal fold tension, vocal quality, pitch, volume variation, and duration. Therefore, treatment strategies that are discussed below outlining treatment approaches for prosody and articulation can be applicable in treatment of phonation incoordination.

The accent method has application to treatment of dysarthric patients and associated phonatory disturbances, including hyperadduction, phonatory instability, and phonatory incoordination. Its premise is based on creating an appropriate balance between expiration and the force of the vocal fold muscles, and producing improved coordination between the voice produced at the level of the vocal folds and resonance, and improving prosody.

As disturbances of pitch, volume, variability, and duration of phonation consistently occur in dysarthric speech, biofeedback tools are an effective method of treatment in these patients. The most useful instruments are those that can consistently display vocal parameters such as the Vocalite (a voice-operated light source that gives feedback on vocal intensity), Visispeech Speech Viewer, and Visipitch (Kay Elemetrics). In treating phonation disorders in children, the Speech Viewer, for example, can also provide effective motivation. Children are able to watch a balloon blow up or deflate on the screen by manipulating their own vocal intensity, or help a monkey climb a tree to get coconuts based on pitch levels.

Prosthetic devices available in the treatment and or maintenance of phonatory/laryngeal disorders in dysarthric patients most commonly include electronic devices designed to compensate for vocal intensity, such as a vocal amplifier. Surgical techniques may be utilized for those patients for whom behavioral, instrumental, and prosthetic techniques do not produce enough improvement. Such intervention may be employed to produce a more appropriate valving mechanism, and is followed by other approaches to maximize vocal efficiency. However, the suitability of such procedures needs to be evaluated for each individual, as in some cases such intervention may be inap-

propriate based on the individual's medical condition or overall disability. Laryngeal nerve section, laser surgery, or botulism toxin injection may be carried out for hyperadduction of the vocal folds to restrict the movement of one or both of the folds. In cases of hypoadduction of the vocal folds, reinnervation of a unilateral paralyzed vocal fold, laryngoplasty, and collagen and Teflon implants may be utilized.

Treatment of Resonatory Disorders. Impaired velopharyngeal function associated with neurologic function is characterized by hypernasal resonance and nasal emission of air during speech. In severe cases, improving velopharyngeal function is often the first priority of treatment, as the impairment may contribute to respiratory impairments and articulation imprecision due to air loss through an inefficient velar valve. Determining the amount of palatal closure achieved through therapy tasks requires good self-judgment and in turn relates to effectiveness of treatment and outcomes. Therefore, it is important that the patient develops awareness of the velopharyngeal system and an ability to monitor nasality. Visual feedback can be achieved by using a mirror to detect air leakage through the nose. The patient also can obtain information from visual feedback by using a small light source and an angled mirror to see and monitor velar elevation during the production of single vowels. A variety of more formal instrumental biofeedback techniques are also employed in the treatment of resonatory disturbances. The use of pressure, icing, brushing, or vibration of the velum may also be of some benefit for patients with flaccid dysarthria. Speech drills using contrastive nasal and nonnasal sounds as well as drilling correct timing of palatal elevation in words and phrases have assisted progress in patients. The clinician should constantly evaluate the benefit for the patient and be prepared to explore alternative strategies if small or no improvements are made.

In cases where the soft palate is unresponsive to either behavioral or instrumental intervention, or when paralyzed, a prosthetic approach to treatment may be adopted and may involve the use of a palatal lift prosthesis. This device attaches to the teeth and is designed to improve resonance by partially lifting the soft palate and allowing contact with the lateral pharyngeal walls. This device may be utilized either as a temporary or permanent method.

Treatment of Articulation Disorders. For most dysarthric and apraxic clients, specific articulation training is required in order to establish and/or normalize speech movements. Treatment of articulation in both adults and children should take a functional approach, with compensatory strategies playing an important role in the dysarthric child. Articulation therapy in dysarthric clients is based on a combination of auditory, visual, and imitation learning, as well as speech drills to consolidate and generalize the target sounds.

Based on the underlying physiology for articulatory errors, individual treatment follows a sequential progression from basic sound level through to longer, more demanding, yet more normalized, speech segments. Compensation techniques may include using the blade of the tongue instead of the tongue tip for sounds such as /l/, /n/, /t/, and /d/, if tongue or lip movements remain restricted. When formulating articulation goals for treatment of children, consideration must be given to the develop-

mental acquisition of sounds. However, the general rule should be to choose a sound that the child is able to imitate and that will make the greatest difference to his or her intelligibility (such as /s/ sounds or in some instances /s/ clusters).

The physiologic technique that appears to offer the greatest potential for the treatment of acquired dysarthria in children is visual biofeedback. Visual biofeedback treatment originates from the notion of biofeedback theory, with the use of innovative technology. Biofeedback has been applied as early as the 1970s in areas of voice, fluency, and other clinical disorders in the field of speech-language pathology. However, to date, it still represents relatively new interventional approach to the treatment of motor speech disorders. Indeed, it has been highlighted that biofeedback is not a substitute for evaluation/management by a clinician. Rather, the suitability of its implementation with a client is usually referred by the clinician after careful consideration.

The procedures of biofeedback therapy are based upon the theories of cybernetics and learning models. Quintessentially, biofeedback treatment makes ambiguous internal cues about the physiologic system explicit and provides accurate information about the moment to moment changes in target responses during training through the use of instrumentation. The resulting electronic signal is converted into auditory, visual, tactile, or kinesthetic feedback to the individual who can, then, immediately and continuously be made aware to self-regulate the level of a physiologic event. Contrary to traditional therapy, the client assumes a much more active participatory role in biofeedback treatment, consistent with the "locus of control" perspective. Results of studies utilizing biofeedback techniques (e.g., Dagenais, 1995; Katz, Bharadwaj, & Carstens, 1999) have, so far, reported positive effects in the remediation of speech disorders.

The primary biofeedback approach used in treating articulatory disturbances has involved the use of electromyography (EMG) biofeedback to alter muscle tone and strength by decreasing or increasing muscle activity. The use of electropalatography (EPG) in articulation therapy is an additional device that has potential for use with dysarthric patients. As outlined previously, it consists of an artificial hard palate embedded with electrodes that is designed to fit into the individual's mouth. This instrument provides details of the location and timing of the tongue contact during speech. Such information may be provided to the patient to allow an alteration in tongue position in order to approximate the target sound. EPG has been used in recent years to provide a real-time visual information with regards to tongue-to-palate contact in individuals with speech disorders who did not previously respond well to traditional treatment techniques (e.g., Hartelius, Theodoros, & Murdoch, 2005; Morgan, Liégeois, & Occomore, 2007). These children had previously received long-term traditional therapy, but exhibited minimal progress. Although the studies on EPG treatment, so far, involved case studies, the results have been encouraging. Specifically, the children were found to exhibit spatial tongue-configuration patterns that resembled more closely those of normal speakers, with perceptual improvements noted in speech posttreatment.

With the visual information from EPG, the client would be able to monitor the articulatory posture and dynamic sequences necessary in the approach and release phases of sound and in the execution of complex sound sequences, for appropriate tongue-to-hard palate contact patterns. On the other hand, the EPG visual information could provide the clinician a more objective, detailed and accurate source of information on articulatory behavior. With this, the clinician could then specify instructions to the client during treatment phase with respect to tongue maneuvers which, otherwise, would not have been possible in traditional auditory-visual therapy.

An increasing number of studies have provided empirical evidence in support of the EPG serving as a valuable and effective visual feedback remediation tool with regards to tongue-to-palate contact patterns in children during speech. In view of the cost involved in the manufacture of the artificial palate, candidacy for EPG treatment becomes an important consideration (Dagenais, 1995). A challenge when involving children in EPG treatment lies in the durability of the artificial palate, as the child's mouth may outgrow the artificial palate during the course of treatment. Other factors such as oral sensitivity (i.e., tolerance for taking a dental impression, having an artificial palate within oral cavity during therapy), maturity-cognitive development (i.e., to be able to interact with the EPG system and understand the visual display patterns), and visual ability also have a role in determining suitability for the EPG treatment (Dagenais, 1995).

Although predominantly used as a research tool for assessing articulatory dynamics during speech, electromagnetic articulography (EMA) also offers potential as a biofeedback tool for the treatment of acquired motor speech disorders in children. Recent studies have reported the use of EMA in treatment of speech errors in adults with neurologic disorders and provided preliminary evidence that this tool potentially could be used to provide visual biofeedback of tongue movements (Katz et al., 1999; Katz, Bharadwaj, Gabbert, & Stetler, 2002).

Katz et al. (1999) was the first study reported to use the EMA in a 63-year-old adult with Broca's aphasia and apraxia of speech to treat /s/ and /sh/ with visual feedback of the tongue tip. This adult had previously received traditional speech treatment for the past eight years, but made minimal progress. EMA treatment was conducted over five sessions, within a one-month period. Findings of the study revealed /s/ accuracy improvement from 46% to 57% while /sh/ improved at least twice the initial reported accuracy (i.e., from 33% to 75%) and remained high at 81% 10 weeks posttreatment (as compared to [s] where the improvement returned to baseline with limited maintenance).

In another study, Katz et al. (2002) treated a 67-year-old male with aphasia and apraxia of speech, who had been found to exhibit relatively low accurate production of fricatives, affricates, and blends using EMA visual feedback. The results revealed clear increase in kinematic accuracy pre-post therapy on both the treated sounds /sh/ and /ch/. A more tightly controlled pattern was noticed following six treatment sessions in comparison to a highly spatial variable pattern noted prior to treatment. In addition, the physiologic findings corresponded with perceptual findings, revealing marked improvements in EMA treated sounds. Consistent with Katz et al. (1999), lasting improvement was observed for

/sh/ while accuracy for /ch/ returned to baseline level. Such findings with regards to accuracy being maintained for certain sounds but not others, at this stage, are not well understood.

Although both studies, to date, have involved single-cases, the results of the EMA visual biofeedback have been promising. In particular, improvements at the perceptual and physiologic level on treated sounds were noticeable over such a short period of treatment, in view that these individuals involved in the studies, each, had speech errors that did not resolve despite several years of traditional speech therapy. Indeed, with the sensor being affixed to the target articulator specific to the speech sound production, the EMA could potentially serve as a biofeedback tool to treat children with motor speech disorders in remediating place of articulation difficulties through observing tongue trajectory patterns on the visual display.

Both EPG and EMA visual biofeedback treatment may be regarded similar in that the treatment targets the underlying movements of speech, through visual representation of spatial information of the tongue movements. Indeed, the literature has reported that spatial information could be learned and represented through modeling. In fact, modeling of dynamic skills is also effective, and that such modeled information is able to contribute to learning of the qualitative features of the movement. Essentially, both EPG and EMA visual biofeedback approaches are motorically based approaches, consistent with the emerging literature that treatment of speech disorders could be undertaken via a motor skill learning approach.

Prosthetic approaches to the treatment of articulatory disorders are mainly limited to the use of a bite block, which may assist in stabilizing the jaw, and thereby optimizing function of the remaining articulators.

Treatment of Prosodic Disturbances. Three key prosodic features inclusive of stress patterns, rate, and intonation, play a vital role in treatment of neurogenic speech disorders across all populations. Attention to the area of prosody has many benefits that positively impact other systems (such as articulation) in enhancing intelligibility. Prosodic features contribute to highlighting the type (statement versus question, etc.) or overall tone of an utterance, as well as indicating the most important words in a sentence.

The most common behavioral technique for deficits in stress patterning in dysarthric patients involves the use of contrastive stress drills, where increases in pitch, vocal intensity and duration are utilized to create varying responses to questions. Intonation therapy may require the training of breath group patterning through reading tasks that are marked and practiced in accordance with the most appropriate breath group length. Variation of breath groups may also assist with excessively monotonous intonation. Rate control can be regulated by a number of strategies that include tapping or using a metronome, or more formalized tasks such as controlled reading tasks.

In children, activities designed for syntax therapy may assist children to phrase and group words appropriately so as to reduce the amount of words said on the one breath. In these activities, sentences are formulated using word boxes, such as, "The man/ is helping/ the lady/ across the road." Older children, however, may benefit from reading strategies similar to the adult population, where predetermined phrasing and breath groups are marked in reading passages. The use of carrier games such as the card game "Fish" ("Do you have a rabbit that is eating?"), may also benefit prosodic phrasing or breath group control, as well as articulation. Acting simple plays have also assisted carryover, where emphasis on stress, intonation, and rate can be incorporated into the activity.

Instrumental approaches to prosody therapy include the various modes of feedback that present information about parameters associated with stress, rate, and intonation. These include automatically controlled stimulus presentation and altered auditory feedback. The use of prosthetic treatment for prosodic deficits, however, is often reserved for the treatment of speech rate. Such rigid rate controlling techniques often limit the speaker to a one-syllable/word-at-a-time delivery with devices such as a pacing board. Although naturalness of speech is often forfeited, this approach is beneficial in patients with severe disturbances of rate control.

Treatment of Pragmatic Disturbances. Inclusion of the child in a group where the emphasis is on pragmatic skills may be beneficial, particularly if video recording is available. Role-playing activities that allow the child to practice the skills learned in individual sessions may be designed and these activities recorded and rated by his or her peers. The activities may involve daily living skill tasks (e.g., buying something at a shop, asking directions or giving information to someone) and the individual must remember appropriate volume, pitch, emphasis, and articulation. Nonverbal behaviors such as eye contact, physical proximity, body posture, gestures, and facial expression may also be discussed and modified if necessary. Some children who lack a variety of facial expressions may need to be encouraged to use head nodding or vocal fillers such and "um" to let the speaker know they are actively listening. The speech-language clinician and the occupational therapist may plan a joint outing to a community facility (e.g., shopping center or restaurant) where the individuals may put into practice therapy goals. This activity has proved beneficial and enjoyable with all ages but has had excellent results with adolescents who suddenly realize how important it is to achieve treatment goals if they are to become independent and accepted by the community.

Treatment of Acquired Apraxia of Speech in Childhood

There is little reported literature on the manifestation and recovery of acquired apraxia in children. It would seem that most often apraxia coexists with either acquired aphasia and/or acquired dysarthria. Acquired apraxia also seems to resolve either spontaneously or with intervention in the first year after the brain lesion.

Many of the treatment techniques which have been developed for the developmentally dyspraxic child may be useful in the child with acquired apraxia. However, the difficulties experienced by the child with the acquired disorder appear to resolve at a much greater pace than those of the developmentally dyspraxic child and this must be a consideration in therapy. Oral apraxia if present with verbal apraxia appears to resolve first and basic oral motor work is mostly unnecessary unless it serves as an introduction to verbal apraxic therapy or is combined with feeding therapy. Treatment goals for children with acquired apraxia may best be met by working on the child's articulation. Initially, visual and tactile cueing may be needed to help the child approximate the sound. The younger child benefits from some form of visual representation of the sound (e.g., the picture of a snail for "s" or if they are reading, the letter). Some children benefit from working in front of a mirror, in others this activity only seems to confuse them. These latter children have better success when watching the clinician make the sound after she or he has explained the placement of the articulators. Phonetic cuing as described by Vaughan and Clark (1979) and the cued articulation (Passy, 1985) method of helping individuals remember by using simple hand signs and how to pronounce and/or sequence the consonant sounds of English, may also serve as useful treatment procedures. However, the clinician's own knowledge of distinctive features of the phonemes will help him or her develop appropriate treatment techniques. There also are those children who require a "hands on" approach (e.g., the clinician helps the child with lip closure for "m") if they are to succeed in making the required sound.

Treatment of acquired apraxia may involve the following steps:

- Imitation of single sounds starting with those that the child finds easiest (vowels and consonants)
- Repetition of these sounds (e.g., /m/, /m/, /m.).

- Repetition of a sequence of sounds, first two and then three (e.g., /m/, /b/, /m/, /b/, and /p/, /t/, /k/).
- Combining of these sounds into consonant-vowel, vowel-consonant, consonant-vowel-consonant and consonant-vowel-consonant-vowel.
- Using the words in pragmatically appropriate situations (e.g., asking for more of something).
- Contrasting words by place, voice and manner (e.g., tar, car; poo, boo; taw, saw).
- Disyllabic words (e.g., puppy, pudding).
- Use of the child's expressive vocabulary in phrases and simple sentences (this work could be incorporated into language work if the child also has acquired aphasia).
- Selection of polysyllabic words which the child may have found difficult in the treatment session, at home or in the classroom. Team members can be alerted to listen for difficult words and record them for the speech-language clinician who can help the child with them at a later session.

Many of these activities will be used simultaneously (e.g., imitation of the single sounds which may have proved difficult for the child and the combination of established sounds in monosyllabic and disyllabic words). If the child has prosodic or pragmatic difficulties then the activities outlined in the section on dysarthria may be used.

The suggestions for assessment and treatment of acquired motor speech disorders in children outlined above are not conclusive. More research into the area of these acquired disorders is necessary if the most appropriate assessment and treatment procedures are to be developed.

Summary: Assessment and Treatment of Acquired Motor Speech Disorders

The reports in the literature have little to offer the clinician in either the diagnosis or treatment of acquired motor speech disorders in children. The available models for assessment and treatment of motor speech disorders have been developed for adults and until more research into acquired motor speech disorders in children is forthcoming, these models are all that is available to help the clinician with the assessment and treatment of the acquired disorders in childhood.

With acquired motor speech disorders in children 10 parameters: respiration, phonation, resonance, articulation, prosody, facial musculature, diadochokinesis, reflexes, intelligibility, and pragmatics, are assessed. In each applicable parameter the salient neuromuscular functions involved in motor speech disorders (strength, speed, range and accuracy of movement, steadiness of the contraction, and tone) are analyzed at rest, with voluntary and with involuntary movement. Differences between dysarthria and apraxia are mainly seen in the parameters of articulation, facial musculature with voluntary and involuntary movement and diadochokinesis.

Treatment goals for acquired motor speech disorders in children, when possible, should be functional and pragmatically appropriate. These goals may best be met by direct work on articulation. If children have prosodic difficulties then inclusion in a group where pragmatic problems are addressed seems beneficial. Finally, further research into the manifestation and recovery of children with acquired motor speech disorders will assist the clinician with the assessment and treatment of these children.

Case Examples

Case 1 (Brian): Cerebrovascular Accident (Dysarthria)

Brian was a 9-year-old male who suffered a brainstem infarct following basilar artery occlusion secondary to arteritis when he was five years of age. On admission to hospital he was drowsy with fluctuating cerebral and cerebellar signs. During this period of hospitalization he underwent initial neuroradiologic assessments (see below). Brian was readmitted to hospital two months later following decreased neurologic functioning (i.e., slurred speech, right facial palsy, marked stridor, irregular pulse and respiratory functioning, no voluntary movement of right hand or leg). Three days postreadmission Brian ceased talking with crying being his only vocalization. An angiogram performed on this day revealed the presence of occlusions in the right vertebral and basilar arteries. Mutism lasted for a period of approximately two months.

Two years, eight months after the original hospitalization Brian was further hospitalized for assessment of possible seizure activity which was verified and medication provided. Intermittent asthma and ataxia were reported in Brian's past medical history. Brian's mother reported him as having well developed speech and language skills prior to the CVA.

Neuroradiologic Examination

A CT scan performed on the day of Brian's admission indicated multiple infarcts in the cerebellum with no mass effects or calcification. An MRI performed 10 days postadmission correlated well with the CT scan but demonstrated many more changes including infarcts in the thalami and medial to the posterior horn of the left lateral ventricle in the deep white matter.

More recent scans showed lesions as persistent up until near the time of the perceptual and instrumental testing being reported below, that is, at three years eight months postadmission. There was evidence of widened CSF space in the posterior fossa and prominent sulci in the cerebellar hemispheres and vermis consistent with global cerebellar atrophy in the more recent scans.

Speech and Language Recovery

Brian received regular speech pathology support (four visits per week) from two weeks post readmission until nine weeks postreadmission when he was discharged. Therapy focused on improving oromotor skills and on providing Brian with an alternative and augmentative communication system. The following observations were made regarding Brian's progress during this time. Brian was initially fed nasogastrically due to decreased neurologic functioning and poor oromotor skills. He was then upgraded to a soft diet. Minimal improvement was seen in tongue functioning and Brian compensated for this by removing food pooled in the buccal cavities with his finger. Therefore, at the end of 7 weeks of treatment Brian still exhibited an impaired oral stage of swallowing.

At discharge, two months post major CVA Brian exhibited good concentration, cooperation, memory and problem solving skills. Orientation to time, place, and person was accurate. Receptive language skills were assessed as impaired, however, there appeared to be a mismatch between these results and Brian's functional capabilities in this area which appeared to be within normal limits.

During the acute period of muteness a photo board was used for expressive communication. This was then augmented by manual signing although poor fine motor control reduced the effectiveness of this mode of communication. Before regaining speech, Brian was spontaneously using signed utterances of up to four signs in length.

At two months post major CVA Brian was severely dysarthric having extreme muscular weakness and reduced range of movement of his oral structures. He exhibited reduced lip seal, drooling, and limited tongue movement. Brian could not produce any bilabial sounds. Following discharge, Brian received weekly speech pathology support through a regional Special Education facility while attending his local school.

A speech-language pathology review conducted two years seven months post admission indicated that Brian's general language skills were appropriate for his age, however, his response time, concentration and reading skills were reduced. Brian was using a verbal mode of communication with severe dysarthric qualities. Poor breath control affected amount and accuracy of articulatory movements, reducing intelligibility. Drooling was still evident and Brian had decreased rate of movement and coordination of tongue and lips. Palatal movement was affected with nasal air emission observed during speech production. Brian was using labiodental movement to achieve bilabial plosives.

At three years, eight months post-admission Brian was referred to the Centre for Neurogenic Communication Disorders Research at The University of Queensland for perceptual and instru-mental assessment of his speech. For contextual purposes please note that Brian could now walk, but was slow and unsteady and preferred to use a wheelchair, particularly at school.

Perceptual Analysis of Speech

The results of the perceptual assessment battery are summarized in Table 14–3 and discussed below. The perceptual measures indicated that Brian had a moderate dysarthric speech impairment. Tongue function was the most deviant dimension with severe impairment of the elevation and moderate impairment of the lateral movements of the tongue. Loudness, lip seal and palatal function during maintenance tasks were severely impaired. Hypernasality was obvious during speech to a moderate level. Perceptually, respiration appeared adequate for speech. Intelligibility was moderately impaired overall, however, because Brian spoke very slowly this allowed the listener more time to process and interpret his speech, increasing the possibility of understanding what was said.

Physiologic Analysis of Speech

The results of the physiologic assessment battery are presented in Table 14–3. Respiratory function assessment showed Brian to have an abnormal respiration pattern with virtually 100% rib cage contribution. He displayed a significant component of abdominal paradoxing indicating that during expiration his abdominal circumference actually expanded due to expiratory effort rather than decreased. This was a consistent pattern across all tasks and was indicative of the presence of flaccid paralysis of the abdominal wall.

Table 14-3. Summary of the Deviant Perceptual Speech Features and Physiologic Profiles for Cases 1 to 3

Subject	Deviant Oromotor and Speech Dimensions Identified Perceptually	Instrumental Assessment of Respiratory Function	Instrumental Assessment of Laryngeal Function	Instrumental Assessment of Velopharyngeal Function	Instrumental Assessment of Articulatory Function
9 y/o male CVA subject (Brian)	*Moderate*: hypernasality in speech, intelligibility *Severe*: tongue function, volume, lip function, rate, palatal function	↓ lung volume and capacity Abdominal paradoxing Severely reduced abdominal contribution	↑ F_0 ↓ DC and CT ↑ glottal resistance ↓ subglottal pressure	↑ nasality index on nonnasal utterances (hypernasality)	↓ tongue endurance ↓ tongue strength during maximum effort repetitions ↓ rate of tongue movements ↓ lip strength ↓ bilabial pressures during speech

continues

Table 14–3. *continued*

Subject	Deviant Oromotor and Speech Dimensions Identified Perceptually	Instrumental Assessment of Respiratory Function	Instrumental Assessment of Laryngeal Function	Instrumental Assessment of Velopharyngeal Function	Instrumental Assessment of Articulatory Function
14 y/o male CHI subject (David)	*Mild-Moderate*: reflexive behavior (swallowing), velopharyngeal function, respiration *Moderate*: loudness, vocal quality, lip function, respiration, intelligibility in sentences *Moderate-Severe*: tongue function, pitch *Severe*: consonant precision, rate, intelligibility in words, pitch variability	↓ lung volume and capacity ↓ lung volume excursion ↓ abdominal excursion during vowel and syllable production Lung volume initiation and termination values during speech breathing noted to be at abnormally high lung volumes	↓ ad/abduction rate ↑ glottal resistance ↓ subglottal pressure	↑ nasality index on nonnasal utterances (hypernasality)	↓ tongue strength ↓ tongue endurance ↓ range of lip movements during speech Assymetric lip movements during speech ↓ max strength and endurance of the lips ↓ bilabial lip pressures during speech
8 y/o female with posterior fossa tumor (Cindy)	*Mild*: alternate lip movements *Moderate*: alternate tongue movements, volume variability, reduced rate of speech	↓ lung volume and lung capacity ↓ lung volume excursion Largely an abdominal breather	WNL	WNL	↓ rate of repetition of tongue movements ↓ lip strength ↓ bilabial lip pressures during speech

WNL: within normal limits, CHI: closed-head injury, CVA: cerebrovascular accident, F_o – fundamental frequency, DC: duty cycle, CT: closing time.

The lack of abdominal contribution was consistent with Brian's low vital capacity which was only 33% of his predicted, taking into account his height, age, and sex. To compensate for the lack of abdominal contribution Brian utilized the secondary muscles of respiration e.g. the scalenus muscles and the sternocleidomastoid to raise the rib cage. Brian's very small abdominal contribution appeared to reflect the limited contribution of his diaphragm to the respiratory effort. This result directly conflicted with the perceptual finding of adequate respiration for speech and reflects on the difficulty in perceptually judging respiratory adequacy particularly in a wheelchair-bound patient with poor posture.

With regard to laryngeal function, it is felt that the indirect method used to calculate subglottal pressure was influenced by the poor lip seal of this client resulting in air leakage which may have caused a reduction of the estimated subglottal pressure. The presence of an elevated F_0, increased glottal resistance and reduced duty cycle may be indicative of some degree of laryngeal hyperfunction. Brian also demonstrated incomplete velopharyngeal closure which further exacerbated leakage of air from the oral cavity and reduced the recorded oral pressure.

Velopharyngeal function was assessed indirectly using accelerometric technique and the Nasometer. The results of both assessments revealed an increase in nasality indexes (HONC index and percent nasalance) during the production of nonnasal sounds, words, and sentences. These instrumental findings were consistent with perceptual judgments of hypernasality. The hypernasality may be attributed to velopharyngeal incompetence which as discussed earlier has many implications regarding the functioning of other subsystems within the speech mechanism.

On articulatory measure Brian was found to have good maximum tongue strength but very poor endurance and a very slow rate of repetition of tongue movements. It was considered that Brian's impaired tongue endurance may have contributed to his overall reduction in speech intelligibility.

Lip pressure analysis showed Brian to have reduced lip pressure on a maximum pressure task. His endurance for nonspeech tasks was appropriate for his age. However, on speech tasks Brian displayed decreased lip pressures for bilabial consonants. This finding may have been due to increased labial fatigue and an impaired ability to coordinate and execute a combination of articulatory movements during connected speech.

Once again, it may be observed that a combination of perceptual and physiological measures were required to provide a more complete picture of Brian's functional and system-specific speech skills. The difficulty in perceptually evaluation respiration was particularly highlighted in this case.

Implication for Treatment

Brian's major speech impairments contributing to his dysarthria included respiratory incoordination and insufficiency; reduced lip strength; and velopharyngeal dysfunction. His speech was moderately intelligible with decreased rate of production.

In this case the treatment hierarchy would be as follows:

(a) Treatment of Respiratory
 Dysfunction
 – Increase lung capacity.

- Increase abdominal contribution to speech breathing.

(b) Treatment of Articulatory Dysfunction
   - Increase lip strength to improve oral pressure for the production of stop consonants.

(c) Treatment of Velopharyngeal Dysfunction
   - Increase tongue strength and endurance.

(d) Treatment of Laryngeal Dysfunction
   - Decrease laryngeal hyperfunction.

Brian's speech breathing skills would be targeted first for treatment in accord with the recommendations of Rosenbek and LaPointe (1985) who indicated that this area often requires remediation before other areas of speech can be targeted. Hayden and Square (1994) also place the correction of breathing patterns and the achievement of adequate breath support for sequenced speech early in their motor speech treatment hierarchy.

Postural adjustment and increasing abdominal contribution to the respiratory process through pushing exercises along with increasing lung volumes through biofeedback therapy using kinematic instrumentation could form part of the treatment for respiration.

Case 2 (David): Traumatic Brain Injury (Dysarthria)

David was a 14-year-old, right-handed male who sustained a severe closed-head injury (CHI) when hit by a car. On admission to hospital he had a Glasgow

Coma Score (GCS) of 5. David was on a ventilator in the Intensive Care Unit for 4 days and required an extraventricular drain in the right hemisphere on day 2. He was discharged to an acute ward 5 days after admission.

Neuroradiologic Examination

A CT scan (Figure 14–12) performed on the day of admission indicated a large, soft tissue hematoma present over the right temporal region and left zygomatic region of David's left cerebral hemisphere. In addition, a small high attenuation area in the left lentiform nucleus and a small amount of associated edema was reported. Furthermore, small, high attenuation foci were scattered over the peripheral gray/white region anteriorly and superiorly. Ventri-

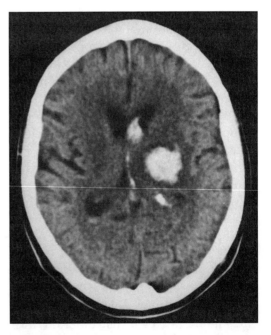

FIGURE 14–12. Case 2 (David): CT scan indicating a large, soft tissue hematoma in the right temporal region and high attenuation in the left lentiform nucleus.

cles were of normal size with no evidence of midline shift or significant mass effect noted.

Speech and Language Recovery

Speech therapy was initiated two weeks postadmission. Initial evaluation at this time indicated that David had major swallowing difficulties and oromotor impairment requiring supplementary nasogastric feeding until one month postadmission. He required intensive therapy to assist with the recovery of oromotor skills and upgrading of diet. At the time of referral to the Centre for Neurogenic Communication Disorders Research, The University of Queensland, David was able to eat a nearly normal diet with mild difficulty with chewy textures. His rate of eating and drinking, however, remained slow and he had some difficulty with saliva control.

Language recovery began with specific comprehension responses at one month post admission. Also, at the time of referral David presented with high-level comprehension difficulties. His expressive language was mild-moderately impaired with difficulties predominantly in the semantic area and with complex sentence construction.

David was mute until two and a half months post admission when he began to produce a few single word approximations. He made rapid improvements in speech from five months post admission. A speech-language pathology assessment by the hospital therapist at eight months post admission showed him to be moderately dysarthric with mildly distorted vocal quality and reduced pitch range. His resonance was hypernasal with occasional mild nasal omission on vowels. Articulation was moderately disordered with great-

est difficulty in connected speech. Lip and tongue function were impaired on the right side. Respiratory control was mildly reduced.

At eight months postadmission David was referred to the Centre for Neurogenic Communication Disorders Research, The University of Queensland for a comprehensive perceptual and physiologic analysis of his speech.

Perceptual Analysis of Speech

Table 14–3 summarizes the deviant perceptual features identified in David's speech using the perceptual assessment battery recommended by the author. Perceptual analysis of David's speech revealed a profile of speech impairments consistent with those reported by a number of researchers who have studied dysarthria following adult CHI (Sarno & Levin, 1985; Theodoros et al., 1994; Wunderli, 1962). Consistent with the findings of Theodoros et al. (1994), David exhibited deficits in all five aspects of the speech production process (prosody, respiration, articulation, resonance, and phonation). Combined, these impairments all contributed to his markedly reduced intelligibility. The overall perceptual evaluation was successful in identifying several areas of speech dysfunction. However, results from the speech sample analysis did not comply with those from the FDA in several areas notably the degree of phonatory and respiratory dysfunction. This lack of agreement may be due to the interrelated nature of these two systems, and therefore the difficulty in characterizing disordered perceptual characteristics as a result of reduced respiratory or phonatory functioning. This emphasizes the importance of instrumental investigations in identifying the physiological bases for the perceptual speech impairments.

Physiologic Analysis of Speech

Table 14–3 presents the deviant physiologic features of David's speech identified through the use and analysis of the instrumental procedures outlined earlier in the chapter. The findings of reduced lung volume and capacity and problems with two-part coordination were comparable with a group of CHI adults studied by Murdoch, Theodoros, Stokes, and Chenery (1993). David's low lung capacities may have resulted in the reduced respiratory support for speech identified in the FDA and speech sample analysis. This also may have contributed to the low subglottal pressure (SGP) discovered in the laryngeal examination. The high lung and rib cage volumes recorded during reading may have been an attempt by David to overcome the increased glottal resistance (GR) in his laryngeal valve. Thus his abnormal pattern of speech breathing may be the result of some compensatory mechanism rather than respiratory impairment.

Laryngeal function assessment using electroglottography and aerodynamic examination revealed that David exhibited some features of hyperfunctional laryngeal activity. A high incidence and wide range of laryngeal hyperfunction has been identified in the adult CHI population (Theodoros & Murdoch, 1994; von Cramon, 1981). The features of hyperfunctional laryngeal activity exhibited by David included increased GR and decreased adduction/abduction rate perhaps indicating laryngeal spasticity. The apparently conflicting result of low SGP may be a result of insufficient respiratory support or could be a result of underestimation of his actual SGP due to the instrumental method used to determine SGP. SGP is measured indirectly by the Aerophone II via an equivalent measure of the oral pressure during the production of the voiceless stop /p/. Therefore, if David had incomplete velopharyngeal closure or an inadequate bilabial seal (both of which were confirmed in later testing), leakage of air from the oral cavity may have occurred and reduced the recorded oral pressure leading to under estimation of SGP. David's GR may also be increased to compensate for the deficits in other subsystems of the speech mechanism mentioned above in an attempt to conserve expiratory airflow for speech production (LaBlance, Steckol, & Cooper, 1991).

The instrumental velopharyngeal assessment revealed that David exhibited a moderate degree of hypernasality when producing non-nasal utterances. Hypernasality has been reported as a common feature of adult CHI patients (Theodoros, Murdoch, Stokes, & Chenery, 1993). This hypernasality may be attributed to velopharyngeal incompetence (VPI). Velopharyngeal incompetence has many implications regarding the functioning of other subsystems within the speech mechanism. It is possible that David's VPI resulted in disturbances in the laryngeal and articulatory valves through wastage of airflow needed for the production of speech. As a compensatory mechanism, the laryngeal muscles may have increased the GR in an attempt to conserve airflow for speech. The high GR in turn may have resulted in the disturbances in vocal quality detected in the perceptual assessment. Wastage of air through VPI would decrease the intraoral pressure needed to produce pressure consonants. Loss of air through the nasal cavity would disrupt the airflow through the oral cavity, resulting in distorted and imprecise consonants and vowels. David's reduction in consonant and vowel precision may therefore by partly attributed to VPI.

David exhibited deficits in tongue function that were similar to those found in other studies of CHI subjects (Theodoros, Murdoch, & Stokes, 1995; Stierwalt et al., 1994). His impaired tongue endurance may have contributed to his overall reduction in speech intelligibility. A positive correlation between tongue endurance and speech intelligibility has been documented by Stierwalt et al. (1994).

The Entran Flatline pressure transducer analysis and the lip movement analysis both indicated that David's lip function was impaired. Theodoros et al. (1995) reported significant lip strength impairment in a group of adult CHI patients. The findings of decreased lip pressures during speech may have been due to increased labial fatigue and an impaired ability to coordinate and execute the combination of articulatory movements required in connected speech. David's rate of lip movement was found to be moderately reduced, consistent with the findings of Theodoros et al. (1995). This finding was suggested by Theodoros to be a compensatory mechanism to maintain higher lip pressures.

The lip movement analysis indicated that David's range of lip movement was reduced overall and furthermore showed greater reduction in the speech tasks than the nonspeech tasks. Lip symmetry analysis revealed that the right side of David's lips was weaker than the left. This asymmetry was consistent with his right arm and leg hemiparesis, thus indicating that the left cerebral hemi-

sphere was damaged as confirmed by the CT scan results. It is possible that the asymmetry of lip movement may have affected the subject's ability to maintain an adequate lip seal to build up enough intraoral pressure for successful production of bilabial consonants. This hypothesis is supported by the lip pressure analysis which revealed that David's lips sometimes did not compress together successfully when producing bilabial consonants.

Lip dysfunction may not only have affected David's articulation, but also his laryngeal function. For example, David's inadequate lip seal may have caused leakage of air from the oropharyngeal cavity, lowering the estimated value of SGP in the laryngeal valve. In addition, the high GR present in David's laryngeal muscles may have been a compensatory mechanism designed to conserve the airflow needed for the production of speech. Therefore, David's inadequate lip functioning may have contributed to the deviant vocal characteristics observed in the perceptual assessments.

In summary, it is suggested that both perceptual and instrumental assessments be administered when assessing a child with dysarthria, particularly following a CHI. In the present case the perceptual evaluation appeared to lack sensitivity and objective reliability in some of the key areas particularly laryngeal function and respiration. The instrumental assessments were able to more clearly define the physiologic nature of the dysfunctions in these subsystems and provided better direction for treatment overall. The perceptual assessments provided a functional overview of David's speech impairment and an overall indication of the severity of his dysarthria. The instrumental evaluations provided objective, reliable, and quantifiable data.

Implications for Treatment

On the basis of the findings from the perceptual and instrumental assessments the major motor speech impairments contributing to David's dysarthria included severely reduced tongue function; moderately reduced lip, velopharyngeal and laryngeal function; and a mild-moderately decreased respiratory function. His speech was moderately unintelligible with decreased rate of speech, variability in pitch, and imprecision of consonants.

Therefore the recommended treatment hierarchy would be as follows:

(a) Treatment of Articulatory Dysfunction
   - Increase tongue strength and endurance (simultaneously).
   - Increase lip strength and range of movement (simultaneously.

(b) Treatment of Laryngeal Dysfunction
   - Decrease laryngeal hyperfunction.

(c) Treatment of Velopharyngeal Dysfunction
   - Decrease nasality.

(d) Treatment of Respiratory Dysfunction
   - Increase lung vital capacity.
   - Increase abdominal contribution to speech breathing (if the mild respiratory dysfunction has not resolved through effects from the previous steps in therapy).

Furthermore, it is recommended that simultaneous treatment of rate of speech and pitch variation occur throughout the entire therapy program.

By treating David's impairments in the above order, improvement in the articulatory subsystem should effect immediate improvement in the other valves by reducing the leakage of air through the oral cavity. Furthermore, as dysfunction in the articulatory system was the greatest contributor to David's reduced intelligibility, therapy directed at that level should result in improved functional communication skills.

A combination of traditional and instrumental treatment techniques could be used with David including oromotor exercises with or without resistance and biofeedback using the tongue and lip transducers. Relaxation and tension-reducing techniques could be used to decrease laryngeal hyperfunction.

Case 3 (Cindy): Posterior Fossa Tumor (Dysarthria)

Cindy was a 6-year-old female who was admitted to hospital with a severe ataxia following a fall down the stairs.

Neuroradiologic Examination

An MRI scan taken soon after admission revealed a very large astrocytoma in the posterior fossa (Figure 14–13). There were multiple calcified areas with related soft tissue in the midline part of the mass with some extension to the right and more marked extension into the left cerebellar hemisphere. There was marked displacement of the fourth ventricle and considerable dilation of lateral and third ventricles accompanied by increased intracranial pressure.

Following stabilization of her condition over a period of six days the tumor was removed surgically. The left hemisphere of the cerebellum was completely removed along with a large portion of

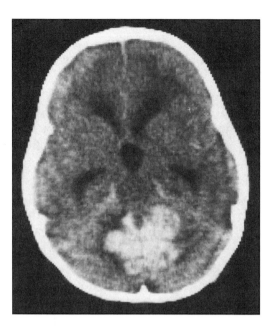

FIGURE 14–13. Case 3 (Cindy): MRI scan showing a large astrocytoma in the posterior cranial fossa.

the right cerebellar hemisphere. After surgery Cindy spent 5 days in the Intensive Care Unit. On return to the ward little improvement was noted for 4 weeks. A shunt was then inserted with immediate improvement in her condition.

Speech and Language Recovery

Daily speech-language pathology intervention was initiated soon after the initial surgery with emphasis on decreasing oral hypersensitivity, reducing gag and bite reflex and tongue thrust which were strongly influencing her ability to eat and swallow.

One month postadmission Cindy became a weekly boarder at a specialist center for children with severe multiple disabilities. Here she received daily occupational therapy, physiotherapy, and speech-language pathology sup-

port. Initially treatment concentrated on feeding skills and oromotor skills. Three months postsurgery Cindy was able to produce some babbling sounds but had difficulty initiating voice. Four months postsurgery Cindy started talking in single words. Within a fortnight she was using short sentences. Her volume and pitch were not controlled and her voice was shaky with pitch breaks. Cindy's speech was slow and deliberate and was characterized by the omission of final consonants, reduction of clusters, and difficulty with plosives and fricatives. Language comprehension appeared intact in functional situations.

Cindy then made rapid progress in all areas. She demonstrated some perseveration in conversation and had difficulty changing topics and activities. She continued in the intensive placement for another 4 months. Cindy returned home eight months postsurgery and was supported with weekly visits in her local school by a regional therapy team for several months. Speech-language pathology services were then suspended for a period of nine months. After this break Cindy received bimonthly visits from the regional speech-language pathologist to review her speech and language skills. At 30 months postsurgery Cindy began receiving weekly speech pathology intervention concentrating on developing her higher level expressive language, reasoning and narrative skills. At this time, her speech was reported to be intelligible with slow rate, and stress patterns being even and equal. When prompted Cindy was able to modulate stress for expression and emphasis during story telling.

Neuropsychological assessment carried out 23 months postsurgery indicated that Cindy's general level of cognitive functioning at that time was within the borderline range. However, her overall performance on verbal comprehension tests was significantly higher than her overall performance on visuoperceptual tests. She had some short-term memory problems and had particular difficulty with memory for visual material. Cindy's visuospatial skills were severely impaired as were visuomotor speech and visual scanning. Basic verbal fluency, higher level verbal expression and verbal comprehension were within the average range.

At 27 months postsurgery Cindy was referred to the Centre for Neurogenic Communication Disorders Research, The University of Queensland for a comprehensive perceptual and physiological analysis of her speech.

Perceptual Analysis of Speech

A summary of the deviant perceptual speech features identified by analysis of the perceptual assessment battery are presented in Table 14–3.

The perceptual assessment indicated that Cindy had a mild dysarthric speech impairment mainly characterized by the use of a slow rate of speech. Even though there was some impairment to tongue and lip movements Cindy's speech showed no reduction in intelligibility.

Physiologic Analysis of Speech

Cindy's performance on the physiologic assessment battery is presented in Table 14–3. Respiratory function as assessed through clinical spirometry showed Cindy to have lung volumes and capacity well below the predicted values for her age, sex, and height. This finding is in contrast to that reported for a group

of children with dysarthria resulting from treatment for posterior fossa tumors reported by Murdoch and Hudson-Tennent (1993). Cindy also performed differently to the group reported above in that she showed consistently high abdominal and rib cage termination values across all tasks resulting in high lung volume termination values. For syllable and reading tasks Cindy's inspiration volumes were generally lower than expected, resulting in an overall reduction in chest wall excursion leading to lower lung excursion and poorer breath support for speech. Calculation of relative volume contribution show Cindy to be a predominantly abdominal breather.

Instrumental investigation of laryngeal and velopharyngeal function indicated Cindy's skills to be within normal limits. Although Cindy had tongue pressure and endurance levels within normal limits, she produced a significantly reduced number of repetitions on a timed task. It could be hypothesized that Cindy reduced the number of repetitions in order to preserve the strength and accuracy of the movements. This would be in keeping with the perceptual observation of reduced rate of speech and maintenance of intelligibility. The Entran Flatline pressure transducer analysis indicated that Cindy's maximum lip pressure on nonspeech tasks was reduced as was her lip pressure during bilabial consonant production in speech. However, this did not appear to lead to noticeable bilabial consonant distortion as this was not noted as deviant in the perceptual assessment.

Implications for Treatment

Cindy presented with a mild dysarthria characterized by prosodic changes detected by the perceptual assessment.

Physiologic assessment revealed respiratory and articulatory system difficulties which were not detected perceptually and which may well contribute to the major area of concern that is, reduced rate of speech. It may be hypothesized that Cindy may be reducing speech rate in order to conserve expiratory output and ensure accuracy and strength of articulatory movements. Treatment would therefore concentrate on the following areas:

(a) Treatment of prosodic aspects of speech particularly rate and intonation
   – Increase speech rate.
   – Improve use of intonation patterns.

(b) Treatment of Respiratory Dysfunction
   – Increase lung volumes and capacities.
   – Decrease abdominal and rib cage termination volumes during speech.

(c) Treatment of Articulatory Dysfunction
   – Increase lip strength.
   – Increase tongue strength.

Owing to the nature of the systems requiring treatment and their interrelatedness the treatment framework would be more concurrent rather than hierarchical. It is believed in this case that the treatment of prosodic dysfunction will enhance Cindy's communication skills. Treatment techniques for prosody could include the use of breath group patterning in concert with treatment for respiratory-phonatory control to enable Cindy to produce longer breath groups. The use of reading and drama-based activities could be successful as it was mentioned above that Cindy was able to read short passages "with expression."

Case 4 (Jasmine): Cerebrovascular Accident (Apraxia)

Jasmine, at 6 years, 3 months of age, suffered an embolic cerebrovascular accident of the left middle cerebral artery during the perioperative period after the repair of anomalous pulmonary venous drainage. Before the neurological episode she had been developing normally and was in first grade at school.

Neurologic History

Initially, Jasmine presented with a dense right hemiparesis that generally was hypotonic in both upper and lower extremities. Her arm was more severely affected than her leg, her right hand having no functional grasp and release. There was no apparent primitive reflex activity or obvious motor planning problems. Her general awareness of her right hand and arm was poor. She was unable to walk without assistance and her protective reactions were sluggish. Her visual perceptual abilities were affected, particularly figure-ground, visual memory, and visual sequential memory. She also had a severe oral and verbal apraxia with a suspected expressive dysphasic component.

Eight months after the insult, Jasmine was walking with the aid of a below-knee caliper and was using her left hand for writing. Sensation was generally intact on the right side but she continued to neglect her right arm and had to be reminded to use it in bilateral activities. Visual perception was age-appropriate. Some inattention to task and poor concentration was still noted in her behavior.

Assessment of Speech

One week after the cerebrovascular accident, Jasmine was informally assessed. She presented with a right upper motor neuron weakness with associated drooling from the right side of her mouth. Her lips drooped on the right but the range of movement when she puckered was only mildly reduced. Her range of tongue movement appeared adequate for eating and speech. When she was required to imitate oral movements, gross attempts and groping movements were noted. She was unable to repeat single sounds. Her spontaneous output consisted of an undifferentiated vowel and an attempt at "no." Informal assessment indicated adequate auditory comprehension skills; she responded appropriately to conversation and was able to follow 4-stage commands. An expressive dysphasia was suspected. Jasmine used facial expression, gross gestures, and vowel sounds for expressive communication. A Blissymbol communication board was introduced.

One month after the accident, Jasmine's muscle weakness was resolving with only some occasional drooling. Informal testing revealed that the range and strength of the lip movements were mildly reduced on the right side with a mild oral apraxia persisting. She had no eating or drinking difficulties. Jasmine was able to imitate /b,m,p,n,d,t,s/ in consonant-vowel combinations. Her spontaneous verbalizations included consonant-vowel and consonant-vowel-consonant syllables as word approximations. She continued to use a Blissymbol communication board for expressive communication.

Two months after onset, Jasmine presented with moderate verbal apraxia. An informal assessment using elicited single words revealed the following errors—stopping of liquids and affricates, inconsistent stopping of fricatives, fricative simplification, cluster reduction and simplification, inconsistent deletion of unstressed syllables, and inconsistent assimilation. A spontaneous speech sample showed she also had difficulty with velar phonemes as well as the above errors. Repetition of phoneme sequences and syllable sequences was marked by substitutions, transposition errors, delayed responses, and visual and audible searching. Speech was intelligible if the listener had some contextual cues. A moderate prosodic impairment, that is, a reduced rate of speech and reduced modulation of pitch and duration was present.

Jasmine's expressive language at this time was functional and the use of the communication board was discontinued. From a language sample it was noted that her utterances were characterized by restricted syntactic constructions with many phrase structure elements (determiners, prepositions, pronouns, copula, auxiliary verbs) and morphological inflections (irregular plurals, "ing," "ed," third person singular "s") omitted. She responded to semantic and phonetic cueing. Verbal paraphasias were present in her language and made up half of all error responses. Her receptive language, using the Reynell Developmental Language Scale-Revised (Reynell, 1977), comprehension scale only, revealed a mild difficulty. On the Token Test for Children (DiSimoni, 1978), Jasmine's score on subtests II, III, IV, and V were below one and two standard deviations. On subtest I she was average. These scores confirmed observations that she was having difficulty with instructions of increasing length and complex linguistic concepts.

Eight months after the accident, Jasmine's speech was intelligible in all situations. The Nuffield Centre Dyspraxia Programme (Nuffield Hearing and Speech Centre, 1985) was administered. Jasmine could not volitionally elevate her tongue tip but when eating a biscuit she cleaned her top lip without effort. Imitations of single sounds revealed by an inability to make voiced and voiceless /the/ and mild distortions of /l/ and /r/. An analysis of a video tape recording of Jasmine before the cerebrovascular accident showed no difficulties in her phonological system. Cluster simplification, involving these same phonemes (e.g., /fl/ became /fw/ and /br/ became /bw/) as well as fricative simplification /the/ voiceless became /f/, was present. Repetition of phoneme sequences and syllable sequences were still marked by delayed responses and slow rate of repetition with some visible searching behaviors but these problems did not seem to hamper her functional communication. Repetition of contrasting consonant-vowel structures (e.g., bee, me) were accurate and slow but not effortful. A mild prosodic impairment, mainly a reduced rate of speech, was present when her syntactic construction was complex or when a polysyllabic word she used was new to her vocabulary. Word retrieval and syntactic difficulties exacerbated this problem. There was little detectable muscle weakness.

Her language abilities improved daily. In 5 months Jasmine progressed from using single words to phrases and syntactically correct simple sentences. Language testing on the TOLD-2 Primary (Newcomer & Hammill, 1988)

placed her in the below average range on most subtests except the vocabulary subtests which were in the average range. On the Peabody Picture Vocabulary Test (Dunn, 1965) she scored at the 70th percentile. Spontaneous language samples revealed that verbal paraphasias had decreased and rarely occurred in conversational speech. Word-retrieval difficulties were still apparent but only when the linguistic demands in the situation increased, for example, with narrative tasks or when she was explaining something that had happened at school and the information she was giving was new to the listener. Her utterances had increased in length and she was using "and," and "then," and "because" as conjunctions as well as "who," "what," "where," and "why" questions. Embedded clause structures were not used consistently.

Jasmine had returned to school 7 weeks postonset. Her teacher reported that she was coping with the work in Grade 1 and was just a little below average in a class of 25. She was to go into Grade 2 in the new school year.

Treatment

Jasmine's treatment was intensive, daily at first and then three times per week when she returned to school. It also was as functional as possible. Blissymbols were introduced 2 weeks postonset and she learned to use approximately 90 symbols in one and two symbol constructions. Intensive articulation therapy was carried out beginning with the imitation of single phonemes, using visual and tactile cuing. The sounds which were easiest for her to imitate were incorporated into consonant-vowel combinations and if these made words or approximations of words, for example, "more" or "ba" for "ball" they were then used in pragmatically appropriate situations. For example, the physiotherapist often played ball with Jasmine who loved this activity, and she would require Jasmine to request the game.

The Nuffield Centre Dyspraxia Programme was used successfully with Jasmine who loved the pictures representing the sounds and sound sequencing exercises. However, as soon as Jasmine was able to produce monosyllabic words as consonant-vowel or vowel-consonant they were introduced into early verbal expressive language therapy. Within 2 months of her cerebrovascular accident, most apraxic therapy goals were met in language activities, for example, playing a game of "Fish" with contrasting /sh/ and /ch/ sounds. Treatment goals required her to ask the question and to pronounce correctly the "sh" or "ch" sound. As her articulation improved no specific speech goals were formulated. Polysyllabic words that gave her trouble during language activities were noted and her mother also noted the ones with which she had problems at home. They were then worked on directly in therapy and incorporated into some language activity. Very little basic motor work was necessary as her oral apraxia resolved quickly and she had no eating or drinking difficulties. At 8 months postonset, Jasmine was still in the active recovery phase. Her right lower facial muscle weakness had resolved. Oral and verbal apraxia was mild with her expressive dysphasia being her main problem. Speech and language therapy would continue.

Summary

Jasmine made an excellent recovery of communicative abilities since she first presented with a severe oral and verbal apraxia. Initially, a Blissymbol communication board was used to give her some form of communication but this was discontinued after approximately 2 months when her verbal expression was functional. Treatment involved imitation and repetition of single phonemes, consonant-vowel, vowel-consonant, consonant-vowel-consonant combinations, minimal pairs, disyllabic, and polysyllabic words. As Jasmine's articulation improved, an expressive dysphasic component became apparent and subsequent treatment incorporated apraxic therapy and language therapy. Eight months after the cerebrovascular accident, Jasmine presented with a mild apraxia of speech that did not hamper her functional communication and a mild-to-moderate expressive dysphasia.

References

Bak, E., van Dongen, H. R., & Arts, W. F. M. (1983). The analysis of acquired dysarthria in childhood. *Development Medicine and Child Neurology, 25,* 81–94.

Cahill, L. M, Murdoch, B. E., & Theodoros, D. G. (2002). Perceptual analysis of speech following traumatic brain injury in childhood. *Brain Injury, 16,* 415–446.

Cahill, L. M., Murdoch, B. E., & Theodoros, D. G. (2005). Articulatory function following traumatic brain injury in childhood: A perceptual and instrumental analysis. *Brain Injury, 19,* 41–58.

Catsman-Berrevoets, C. E., van Dongen, H. R., & Zwetsloot, C. P. (1992). Transient loss of speech followed by dysarthria after removal of posterior fossa tumour. *Developmental Medicine and Child Neurology, 34,* 1102–1117.

Cavallo, S. A., & Baken, R. J. (1985). Prephonatory laryngeal and chest wall dynamics.

Journal of Speech and Hearing Research, 28, 79–87.

Cornwell P. L., Murdoch, B. E., & Ward, E. C. (2005). Differential motor speech outcomes in children treated for mid-line cerebellar tumour. *Brain Injury, 19,* 119–134.

Cornwell, P. L., Murdoch, B. E., Ward, E. C., & Kellie, S. (2003). Perceptual evaluation of motor speech following treatment for childhood cerebellar tumour. *Clinical Linguistics and Phonetics, 17,* 597–615.

Crary, M. A. (1993) *Developmental motor speech disorders.* San Diego, CA: Singular.

Dabul, B. (1979). *Apraxia Battery for Adults.* Tigard, OR: C.C. Publications.

Dagenais, P. A. (1995). Electropalatography in the treatment of articulation/phonological disorders. *Journal of Communication Disorders, 28,* 303–329.

Darley, F. L., Aronson, A. E., & Brown, J. R. (1969a). Differential diagnostic patterns of dysarthria. *Journal of Speech and Hearing Research, 12,* 246–269.

Darley, F. L., Aronson, A. E., & Brown, J. R. (1969b). Clusters of deviant speech dimensions in the dysarthrias. *Journal of Speech and Hearing Research, 12,* 462–496.

Darley, F. L., Aronson, A. E., & Brown, J. R. (1975). *Motor speech disorders.* Philadelphia, PA: W. B. Saunders.

De Feo, A. B., & Schaefer, C. M. (1983). Bilateral facial paralysis in a preschool child: Oral-facial and articulatory characteristics (a case study). In W. R. Berry (Ed.), *Clinical dysarthria* (pp. 165–186). Boston, MA: College-Hill Press.

DiSimoni, F. G. (1978). *The Token Test for Children.* Hingham, MA: Teaching Resources.

Duffy, J. R. (2005). *Motor speech disorders: Substrates, differential diagnosis and management* (2nd ed.). St. Louis, MO: Elsevier Mosby.

Dunn, L. M. (1965). *Peabody Picture Vocabulary Test.* Circle Pines, MN: American Guidance Service.

Enderby, P. M. (1983). *Frenchay Dysarthria Assessment.* San Diego, CA: College-Hill Press.

Finley, W. W., Niman, C. A., Standley, J., & Wansley, R. A. (1977). Electrophysiologic behavior modification of frontal EMG in cerebral-palsied children. *Biofeedback and Self-Regulation, 2*(1), 59–79.

Fisher, H. B., & Logemann, J. A. (1971). *The Fisher–Logemann Test of Articulation Competence.* Boston, MA: Houghton Mifflin.

FitzGerald, F. J., Murdoch, B. E., & Chenery, H. J. (1987). Multiple sclerosis: Associated speech and language disorders. *Australian Journal of Human Communication Disorders, 15,* 15–33.

Hardcastle, W. J., Morgan-Barry, R. A., & Clark, C. J. (1987). An instrumental phonetic study of lingual activity in articulation-disordered children. *Journal of Speech and Hearing Research, 30*(June), 171–184.

Hartelius, L., Theodoros, D. G., & Murdoch, B. E. (2005). The use of electropalatography in the treatment of disordered articulation following traumatic brain injury: A case study. *Journal of Medical Speech-Language Pathology, 13,* 189–204.

Hayden, D. A. (1995). The *P.R.O.M.P.T. System. Extended Level 1: Certification manual* (Rev. Ed.). Toronto, Ontario: The PROMPT Institute.

Hayden, D. A., & Square, P. A. (1994). Motor speech treatment hierarchy: A systems approach. *Clinics in Communication Disorders, 4*(3), 162–174.

Hudson, L. J., Murdoch, B. E., & Ozanne, A. E. (1989). Posterior fossa tumours in childhood: Associated speech and language disorders post-surgery. *Aphasiology, 3,* 1–18.

Jordan, F. M. (1990). Speech and language disorders following childhood closed head injury. In B. E. Murdoch (Ed.), *Acquired neurological speech/language disorders in childhood* (pp. 124–147). London, UK: Taylor & Francis.

Jordan, F. M., & Murdoch, B. E. (1990). Unexpected recovery of functional communication following a prolonged period of mutism post-head injury. *Brain Injury, 4,* 101–108.

Katz, W.F., Bharadwaj, S.V., & Carstens, B. (1999). Electromagnetic articulography treatment for an adult with Broca's aphasia and apraxia of speech. *Journal of*

Speech, Language and Hearing Research, 42, 1355–1366.

Katz, W. F., Bharadwaj, S. V., Gabbert, G., & Stetler, M. (2002). Visual augmental knowledge of performance: Treating place-of-articulation errors in apraxia of speech using EMA. *Brain and Language, 83,* 187–189.

LaBlance, G., Steckol, K., & Cooper, M. (1991). Non-invasive assessment of phonatory and respiratory dynamics. *Ear, Nose, and Throat Journal, 70*(10), 691–696.

Love, R. J. (1992). *Childhood motor speech disability.* New York, NY: Merrill.

Love, R. J., Hagerman, E. L., & Tiami, E. G. (1980). Speech performance, dysphagia and oral reflexes in cerebral palsy. *Journal of Speech and Hearing Research, 45,* 59–75.

Manifold, J., & Murdoch, B. E. (1993). Speech breathing in young adults: Effect of body type. *Journal of Speech and Hearing Research, 36,* 657–671.

Michi, K., Yamashita, Y., Imai, S., Suzuki, N., & Yoshida, H. (1993). Role of visual feedback treatment for defective /s/ sounds in patients with cleft palate. *Journal of Speech and Hearing Research, 36,* 277–285.

Milloy, N., & Morgan-Barry, R. (1990). Developmental neurological disorders. In P. Grunwell (Ed.), *Developmental speech disorders: Clinical issues and practical implications* (pp. 109–132). Edinburgh, UK: Churchill Livingstone.

Morgan, A. T., Liégeois, F., & Occomore, L. (2007). Electropalatography treatment for articulation impairment in children with dysarthria post-traumatic brain injury. *Brain Injury, 21,* 1183–1193.

Murdoch, B. E., & Hudson-Tennent, L. J. (1993). Speech breathing anomalies in children with dysarthria following treatment for posterior fossa tumours. *Journal of Medical Speech-Language Pathology, 1,* 107–119.

Murdoch, B. E., & Hudson-Tennent, L. J. (1994). Speech disorders in children treated for posterior fossa tumours: Ataxic and developmental features. *European Journal of Disorders of Communication, 29,* 379–397.

Murdoch, B. E., Ozanne, A. E., & Cross, J. A. (1990). Acquired childhood speech disorders: Dysarthria and dyspraxia. In B. E. Murdoch (Ed.), *Acquired neurological speech/language disorders in childhood* (pp. 308–341). London, UK: Taylor & Francis.

Murdoch, B., Theodoros, D., Stokes, P., & Chenery, H. (1993). Abnormal patterns of speech breathing in dysarthric speakers following severe closed head injury. *Brain Injury, 7*(4), 295–308.

Nemec, R. E., & Cohen, K. (1984). EMG biofeedback in the modification of hypertonia in spastic dysarthria: case report. *Archives of Physical Medicine and Rehabilitation, 65,* 103–104.

Netsell, R., & Cleeland, C. S. (1973). Modification of lip hypertonia in dysarthria using EMG feedback. *Journal of Speech and Hearing Disorders, 38,* 131–140.

Netsell, R., & Daniel, B. (1979). Dysarthria in adults: Physiologic approach in rehabilitation. *Archives of Physical Medicine and Rehabilitation, 60,* 502–508.

Netsell, R., & Rosenbek, J. (1986). Treating the dysarthrias. In R. Netsell (Ed.), *A neurobiologic view of speech production and the dysarthrias* (pp. 123–152). San Diego, CA: College-Hill Press.

Newcomer, P. L., & Hammill, D. D. (1988). *Test of Language Development-2 Primary.* Austin, TX: Pro-Ed.

Newman, P. W., Creaghead, N. A., & Secord, W. (1985). *Assessment and remediation of articulatory and phonological disorders.* Columbus, OH: Charles E. Merrill.

Nuffield Hearing and Speech Centre. (1985). *Nuffield Centre dyspraxia programme.* London, UK: Nuffield Hearing and Speech Centre.

Passy, J. (1985). *Cued articulation.* Victoria, Australia: J. Passy.

Ramig, L. O., Bonitati, C. M., Lemke, J. H., & Horii, Y. (1994). Voice treatment for patients with Parkinson's disease: Development of an approach and preliminary efficacy data. *Journal of Medical Speech-Language Pathology, 2,* 191–209.

Reetz, H. (1989). A fast expert program for pitch extraction. *Proceedings of Euro-Speech, 1,* 476–479.

Reynell, J. (1977). *Reynell Developmental Language Scales-Revised.* Oxford, UK: NFER.

Robertson, S. J., & Thomson, F. (1986). *Working with dysarthrics: A practical guide to therapy for dysarthria*. Bicester, UK: Winslow Press.

Robin, D. A., & Eliason, M. J. (1991). Speech and prosodic problems in children with neurofibromatosis. In C. A. Moore, K. M. Yorkston, & D. R. Beukelman (Eds.), *Dysarthria and apraxia of speech: Perspective on management* (pp. 137–144). Baltimore, MD: Paul H. Brookes.

Robin, D. A., Somodi, L. B., & Luschei, E. S. (1991). Measurement of strength and endurance in normal and articulation disordered subjects. In C. A. Moore, K. M. Yorkston, & D. R. Beukelman (Eds.), *Dysarthria and apraxia of speech: Perspectives on management* (pp. 173–184). Baltimore, MD: Paul H. Brookes.

Rosenbek, J. C., & LaPointe, L. L. (1985). The dysarthrias: description, diagnosis, and treatment. In D. Johns (Ed.), *Clinical management of neurogenic communication disorders* (pp. 97–152). Boston, MA: Little, Brown.

Sarno, M. T., & Levin, H. S. (1985). Speech and language disorders after closed head injury. In J. K. Darby (Ed.), *Speech and language evaluation in neurology: Adult disorders* (pp. 323–339). New York, NY: Grune & Stratton.

Solomon, N., & Hixon, T. (1993). Speech breathing in Parkinson's disease. *Journal of Speech and Hearing Research, 36,* 294–310.

Sperry, E. E., & Klich, R. J. (1992). Speech breathing in senescent and younger women during oral reading. *Journal of Speech and Hearing Research, 35,* 1246–1255.

Stierwalt, J. A. G., Robin, D. A., Solomon, N. P., Weiss, A. L., Max, J. E., & Luschei, M. (1994). *Dysarthria following traumatic brain injury: Strength, endurance and speech ability*. Paper presented at the Conference on Motor Speech. Sedona, AZ.

Theodoros, D. G., & Murdoch, B. E. (1994). Laryngeal dysfunction in dysarthric speakers following severe closed head injury. *Brain Injury, 8,* 667–684.

Theodoros, D. G., Murdoch, B. E., & Chenery, H. J. (1994). Perceptual speech characteristics of dysarthric speakers following severe closed head injury. *Brain Injury, 8,* 101–124.

Theodoros, D. G., Murdoch, B. E., & Stokes, P. D. (1995). A physiological analysis of articulatory dysfunction in dysarthric speakers following severe closed head injury. *Brain Injury, 9,* 237–254.

Theodoros, D. G., Murdoch, B. E., Stokes, P. D., & Chenery, H. J. (1993). Hypernasality in dysarthric speakers following severe closed head injury: A perceptual and instrumental analysis. *Brain Injury, 7,* 59–69.

van Dongen, H. R., Arts, W. F. M., & Yousef-Bak, E. (1987). Acquired dysarthria in childhood: An analysis of dysarthric features in relation to neurologic deficits. *Neurology, 37,* 296–299.

Vaughan, G. R., & Clark, R. M. (1979). *Speech facilitation: Extraoral and intraoral stimulation technique for improvement of articulation skills*. Springfield, IL: Charles C. Thomas.

Vogel, M., & von Cramon, D. (1982). Dysphonia after traumatic midbrain damage: A follow-up study. *Folia Phoniatrica et Logopaedica, 34,* 150–159.

von Cramon, D. (1981). Traumatic mutism and the subsequent reorganization of speech functions. *Neuropsychologia, 19,* 801–805.

Wit, J., Maassen, B., Gabreëls, F. J. M., & Thoonen, G. (1993). Maximum performance tests in children with developmental spastic dysarthria. *Journal of Speech and Hearing Research, 36,* 452–459.

Wit, J., Maassen, B., Gabreëls, F., Thoonen, G., & de Swart, B. (1994). Traumatic versus perinatally acquired dysarthria: Assessment by means of speech-like maximum performance tasks. *Developmental Medicine and Child Neurology, 36,* 221–229.

Workinger, M. S., & Kent, R. D. (1991). Perceptual analysis of the dysarthrias in children with athetoid and spastic cerebral palsy. In C. A. Moore, K. M. Yorkston, & D. R. Beukelman (Eds.), *Dysarthria and apraxia of speech: Perspectives on management* (pp. 109–206). Baltimore, MD: Paul H. Brookes.

Wunderli, J. (1962). Über Anarthrie und Dysarthria bei Parkinsonismus infantiler

Pseudobulbarparalyse und Schadel-trauma. *Schweizer Archiv für Neurologie, Neurochirurgie und Psychiatrie (Zürich), 90,* 74–103.

Yorkston, K. M., & Beukelman, D. R. (1981). *Assessment of Intelligibility of Dysarthric Speech.* Austin, TX: Pro-Ed.

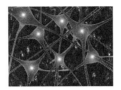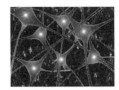

Index

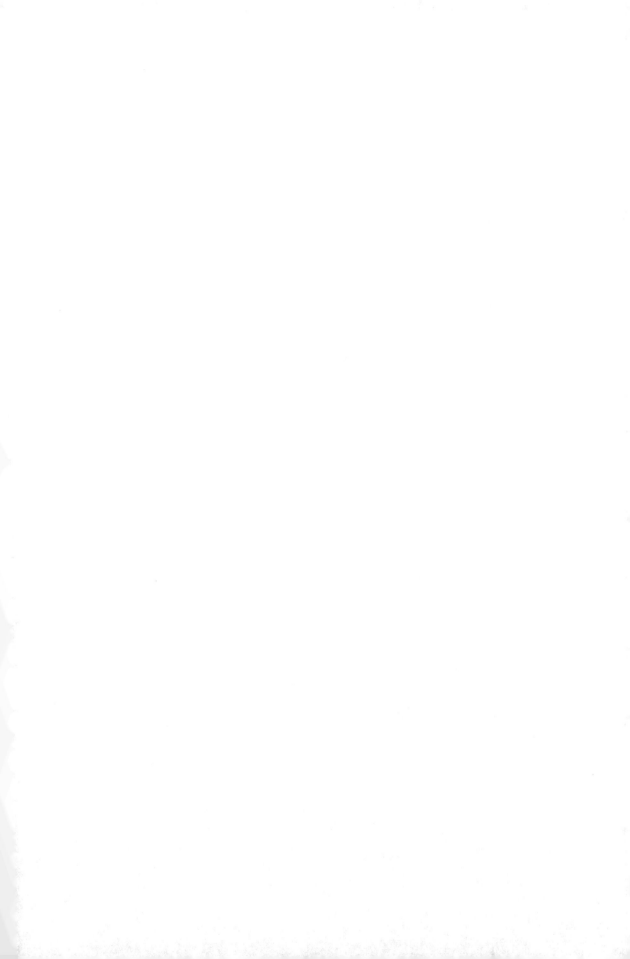